Handbook of Biomaterial Properties

Handbook of Biomaterial Properties

Edited by

Jonathan Black

Professor Emeritus of Bioengineering
Clemson University
USA

and

Garth Hastings

Professor and Director of the Biomaterials Programme
Institute of Materials Research and Engineering
National University of Singapore

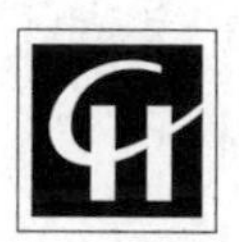

CHAPMAN & HALL
London · Weinheim · New York · Tokyo · Melbourne · Madras

Published by Chapman & Hall, an imprint of
Thomson Science, 2–6 Boundary Row, London SE1 8HN, UK

Thomson Science, 2–6 Boundary Row, London SE1 8HN, UK

Thomson Science, 115 Fifth Avenue, New York, NY 10003, USA

Thomson Science, Suite 750, 400 Market Street, Philadelphia, PA 19106, USA

Thomson Science, Pappelallee 3, 69469 Weinheim, Germany

First edition 1998

Thomson Science is a division of International Thomson Publishing

Typeset in 10/12 pt Times by Florencetype Ltd, Stoodleigh, Devon
Printed in Great Britain by T.J. International Ltd, Padstow, Cornwall

ISBN 0 412 603306

A catalogue record for this book is available from the British Library

Contents

Foreword

Progress in the development of surgical implant materials has been hindered by the lack of basic information on the nature of the tissues, organs and systems being repaired or replaced. Materials' properties of living systems, whose study has been conducted largely under the rubric of tissue mechanics, has tended to be more descriptive than quantitative. In the early days of the modern surgical implant era, this deficiency was not critical. However, as implants continue to improve and both longer service life and higher reliability are sought, the inability to predict the behavior of implanted manufactured materials has revealed the relative lack of knowledge of the materials properties of the supporting or host system, either in health or disease. Such a situation is unacceptable in more conventional engineering practice: the success of new designs for aeronautical and marine applications depends exquisitely upon a detailed, disciplined and quantitative knowledge of service environments, including the properties of materials which will be encountered and interacted with. Thus the knowledge of the myriad physical properties of ocean ice makes possible the design and development of icebreakers without the need for trial and error. In contrast, the development period for a new surgical implant, incorporating new materials, may well exceed a decade and even then only short term performance predictions can be made.

Is it possible to construct an adequate data base of materials properties of both manufactured materials and biological tissues and fluids such that *in vitro* simulations can be used to validate future implant designs before *in vivo* service? While there are no apparent intellectual barriers to attaining such a goal, it clearly lies in the distant future, given the complexity of possible interactions between manufactured materials and living systems.

However, a great body of data has accumulated concerning the materials aspects of both implantable materials and natural tissues and fluids. Unfortunately, these data are broadly distributed in many forms of publication and have been gained from experimental observations of varying degrees of accuracy and precision. This is a situation very similar to that in general engineering in the early phases of the Industrial Revolution. The response then was the publication of engineering handbooks, drawing together, first in general publications and later in specialty versions, the known and accepted data of the time. In this spirit, we offer this *Handbook of Biomaterial Properties*.

Biomaterials, as manufactured for use in implants, do not exist usefully out of context with their applications. Thus, a material satisfactory in one application can be wholly unsuccessful in another. In this spirit, the Editors have given direction to the experts responsible for each part of this *Handbook* to consider not merely the intrinsic and interactive properties of biomaterials but also their appropriate (and in some cases inappropriate) applications as well as their historical context. It is hoped that the results will prove valuable, although in different ways, to the student, the researcher, the engineer and the practicing physician who uses implants.

A handbook like this necessarily becomes incomplete immediately upon publication, since it will be seen to contain errors of both omission and commission. Such has been the case with previous engineering handbooks: the problem can only be dealt with by providing new, revised editions. The Editors would appreciate any contributions and/or criticisms which the users of this handbook may make and promise to take account of them in future revisions.

Introduction

It is a feature of any developing science and its accompanying technology that information relating to different aspects is scattered throughout the relevant, and sometimes not so relevant literature. As the subject becomes more mature, a body of information can be categorized and brought together for the use of practitioners. In providing this *Handbook of Biomaterial Properties* the Editors believe that the latter stage has been reached in several parts of the vast field of biomaterials science and engineering.

Many of the properties of the synthetic materials have been available for some time, for example those of the various metallic alloys used in clinical practice have been specified in various International, European and National Standards and can be found by searching. In the case of polymeric materials, while the information is in commercial product literature and various proprietary handbooks, it is diverse by the nature of the wide range of materials commercially available and the search for it can be time consuming. The situation is much the same for ceramic and composite materials: there the challenge is finding the appropriate properties for the specific compositions and grades in use as biomaterials.

However, when information is sought for on materials properties of human tissues, the problem is more acute as such data are even more scattered and the methods for determination are not always stated or clearly defined. For the established worker this presents a major task. For the new researcher it may make establishing a project area a needlessly time consuming activity. The biomaterials bulletin boards (on the Internet) frequently display requests for help in finding characterization methods and/or reliable properties of natural materials, and sometimes the information is actually not available. Even when it is available, the original source of it is not always generally known.

In approaching their task, the Editors have tried to bring together into one source book the information that is available. To do this they have asked for the help of many colleagues worldwide to be contributors to the *Handbook*. It has not been possible to cover all the areas the Editors had hoped. Some topics could not be covered, or the information was judged to be too fragmentary or unreliable to make it worth including. This is inevitably the sort of project that will continue to be incomplete; however, new information will be provided as more experiments are done and as methods for measurement and analysis improve. The aim has been to make this *Handbook* a ready reference which will be consulted regularly by every technician, engineer and research worker in the fields of biomaterials and medical devices.

We have tried, not always successfully, to keep the textual content to a minimum, and emphasize tabular presentation of data. However, in some cases it has been decided to include more text in order to establish the background of materials properties and use and to point to critical features in processing or production which would guide the worker looking for new applications or new materials. For example, in polymer processing, the need to dry materials thoroughly before fabrication may not be understood by those less well versed in production techniques.

It is hoped that the *Handbook* will be used and useful, not perfect but a valuable contribution to a field that we believe has matured sufficiently to merit such a publication. The *Handbook* is divided into synthetic and natural materials and the treatment is different in each part. More background was felt to be needed for the synthetic materials since processing and structural variations have a profound effect on properties and performance. Biological performance of these materials depends on a range of chemical, physical and engineering properties and the physical form can also influence *in vivo* behavior. We have not attempted to deal with issues of biological performance, or biocompatibility, but have dealt with those other features of the materials which were felt to be relevant to them as potential biomaterials. Only materials having apparent clinical applications have been included.

The biological materials have more dynamic properties since, *in vivo*, they respond to physiological stimuli and may develop modified properties accordingly. The treatment of their properties has been limited to those determined by well characterized methods for human tissues, with a few exceptions where data on other species is deemed to be applicable and reliable. These properties determined almost totally *in vitro* may not be directly predictive of the performance of the living materials *in vivo*, but are a guide to the medical device designer who wishes to determine a device design specification. Such a designer often finds it hard to realize the complexity of the task of dealing with a non-engineering system. What really are the parameters needed in order to design an effectively functioning joint endoprosthesis or a heart valve? Do tissue properties measured post explantation assist? Is individual patient lifestyle an important factor? There is immediately a degree of uncertainty in such design processes, and total reliability in performance cannot be given a prospective guarantee. However, the more we learn about the materials and systems of the human body and their interaction with synthetic biomaterials, the closer we may perhaps become to the ideal 'menotic' or forgotten implant which remains in 'menosis' – close and settled union from the Greek μενω – with the tissues in which it has been placed.

Three final comments:

Although the Editors and contributors frequently refer to synthetic and, in some cases, processed natural materials as 'biomaterials,' nothing herein should be taken as either an implied or explicit warrantee of the usefulness, safety or efficacy of any material or any grade or variation of any material in any medical device or surgical implant. Such determinations are an intrinsic part of the design, development, manufacture and clinical evaluation process for any device. Rather, the materials listed here should be considered, on the basis of their intrinsic properties and, in many cases, prior use, to be *candidates* to serve as biomaterials: possibly to become parts of successful devices to evaluate, direct, supplement, or replace the functions of living tissues.

The Editors earlier refer to absences of topics and of data for particular synthetic or natural materials. While this may be viewed, perhaps by reviewers and users alike, as a shortcoming of the *Handbook*, we view it as a virtue for two reasons:

- Where reliable data are available but were overlooked in this edition, we hope that potential contributors will come forward to volunteer their help for hoped for subsequent editions.
- Where reliable data are not available, we hope that their absence will prove both a guide and a stimulus for future investigators in biomaterials science and engineering.

The Editors, of course, welcome any comments and constructive criticism.

JB
GWH

Professor Garth W. Hastings
Institute of Materials Research & Engineering – IMRE,
Block S7, Level 3, Room 17B,
National University of Singapore,
10 Kent Ridge Crescent, Singapore 119260.
Tel: +65 771 5249
Fax: +65 872 5373

Professor Emeritus Jonathan Black
Principal: IMN Biomaterials
409 Dorothy Drive
King of Prussia, PA 19406–2004, USA
Tel/Fax: +1 610 265 6536

Contributors

COMMISSIONED BY J. BLACK:

T.O. Albrektsson
University of Gothenburg
Handicap Research, Institute for Surgical Sciences
Medicinaregatan 8
Gothenburg S-413 90, Sweden

J.M. Anderson
University Hospitals of Cleveland
Department of Pathology
Case Western Reserve University
2074 Abington Road
Cleveland, OH 44106–2622, USA

T.V. Chirila
Lions Eye Institute
2 Verdun Street, Block A, 2nd Floor
Nedlands, W. Australia 6009

Professor J.D. Currey
Department of Biology
York University
York YO1 5DD, United Kingdom

X. Deng
Laboratorie de Chirugie Exp
Agriculture Services
Room 1701 Services Building
Université Laval
Québec G1K 7P4, Canada

S.E. Gabriel
Division of Rheumatology
Mayo Clinic
200 First Street Southwest
Rochester, MN 55905, USA

V.M. Gharpuray
Department of Bioengineering
401 Rhodes Eng. Res. Ctr.
Clemson University
Clemson, SC 29634–0905, USA

R. Guidoin
Laboratorie de Chirugie Exp
Agriculture Services
Room 1701 Services Building
Université Laval
Québec G1K 7P4, Canada

S.R. Hanson
Division of Hematology/Oncology
PO Box AJ
Emory University
Atlanta, GA 30322, USA

K.E. Healy
Department of Biological Materials
Northwestern University
311 E. Chicago Ave.
Chicago, IL 60611–3008, USA

Y. Hong
Lions Eye Institute
2 Verdun Street, Block A, 2nd Floor
Nedlands, W. Australia 6009

T.M. Keaveny
Department of Mechanical Engineering
Etcheverry Hall
University of California at Berkeley
Berkeley, CA 94720, USA

R.E. Levine
Musculoskeletal Research Centre
University of Pittsburgh
1011 Liliane S. Kaufmann Building
3741 Fifth Avenue
Pittsburgh PA 15213, USA

Arthur K.T. Mak
Rehabilitation Engineering Centre
Hong Kong Polytechnic
Hunghom, Kowloon, Hong Kong

S.S. Margules
Department of Bioengineering
105D Hayden Hall
University of Pennsylvania
Philadelphia, PA 19104–6392, USA

D.F. Meaney
Department of Bioengineering
105E Hayden Hall
University of Pennsylvania
Philadelphia, PA 19104–6392, USA

K. Merritt
17704 Stoneridge Dr.
Gaithersburg, MD 20878, USA

Professor J.R. Parsons
Orthopaedics-UMDNJ
185 South Orange Avenue
University Heights
Newark, NJ 07103–2714, USA

M.G. Rock
Department of Orthopaedics
Mayo Clinic
200 First Street Southwest
Rochester, MN 55905, USA

S.M. Slack
Department of Biomedical Engineering
University of Memphis, Campus Box 526582,
Memphis, TN 38152–6502, USA

V. Turitto
Department of Biomedical Engineering
University of Memphis
Memphis, TN 38152, USA

Professor D.F. Williams
Department of Clinical Engineering
Royal Liverpool University Hospital
PO Box 147
Liverpool L69 3BX, United Kingdom

S.L.-Y. Woo
Musculoskeletal Research Center
University of Pittsburgh
1011 Liliane S. Kaufmann Building
3741 Fifth Avenue
Pittsburgh, PA 15213, USA

M. Zhang
Rehabilitation Engineering Centre
Hong Kong Polytechnic
Hungham, Kowloon, Hong Kong

COMMISSIONED BY G.W. HASTINGS:

L. Ambrosio
Department of Materials and Production Engineering
University of Naples Federico II
Institute of Composite Materials Technology CNR
Piazzale Techio, 80
80125 Naples, Italy

M.A. Barbosa
INEB-Ma
Rua do Campo
Alegre 823
4150 Porto, Portugal

V. Biehl
Lehrstuhl für Metallische Werkstoff
Universität des Saarlandes
Saarbrücken, Germany

J.C. Bokros
Medical Carbon Research Institute
8200 Cameron Road
Suite A-196
Austin TX 78754–8323, USA

J.W. and S.J. Boretos
Consultants for Biomaterials
6 Drake Court
Rockville
Maryland 20853, USA

H. Breme
Lehrstuhl für Metallische Werkstoffe
Universität des Saarlandes
Saarbrücken, Germany

G. Carotenuto
Department of Materials and Production Engineering
University of Naples Federico II
Institute of Composite Materials Technology CNR
Piazzale Technio, 80
80125 Naples, Italy

A.D. Haubold
Medical Carbon Research Institute
8200 Cameron Road
Suite A-196
Austin TX 78754–8323, USA

L. Hench
Imperial College
Department of Materials
Prince Consort Road
London SW7 2BP, United Kingdom

T. Kookubo
Division of Material Chemistry
Faculty of Engineering
Kyoto University, Sakyo-ku,
Kyoto 606–01, Japan

M. LaBerge
Associate Professor
School of Chemical and Materials Engineering
401 Rhodes Research Center
Clemson University,
Clemson, SC 29634–0905, USA

P.J. Li
Centre for Oral Biology
Karolinska Institute
Huddinge S 141–4, Sweden

R.B. More
Medical Carbon Research Institute
8200 Cameron Road
Suite A-196
Austin TX 78754–8323, USA

L. Nicolais
Department of Materials and Production Engineering
University of Naples Federico II
Institute of Composite Materials Technology CNR
Piazzale Technio, 80
80125 Naples, Italy

H. Oomamiuda
Department of Orthapaedic Surgery
Artificial Joint Section and Biomaterial Research Laboratory
Osaka-Minami National Hospital
677–2 Kido-Cho, Kawachinagano-shi,
Osaja, Japan

H. Oonishi
Department of Orthopaedic Surgery
Artificial Joint Section and Biomaterial Research Laboratory
Osaka-Minami National Hospital
677–2 Kido-Cho, Kawachinagano-shi,
Osaka, Japan

Z.G. Tang
BIOMAT Centre
National University of Singapore
Singapore 119260

S.H. Teoh
Institute of Materials Research & Engineering – IMRE
Block S7, Level 3, Room 17B
National University of Singapore
10 Kent Ridge Crescent
Singapore 119260

PART I

Cortical bone

A1

J. Currey

A1.1 COMPOSITION

A1.1.1 Overall

The main constituents are the mineral hydroxyapatite, the fibrous protein collagen, and water. There is some non-collagenous organic material.

Highly mineralized bone (petrosal bones of some non-human mammals) has little organic material (8% in the horse petrosal to 3% in the tympanic bulla) [3]. (Almost certainly human ear bones will be somewhere near or in this region, though they seem not to have been studied.)

A1.1.2 Organic

The main organic component is collagen. Most is Type I, but there are small amounts of Type III and Type VI, found in restricted locations [4]. Slowly heated collagen shrinks at a particular temperature, giving an indication of the stability of the molecules. Bone collagen in men has a shrinkage temperature of about 61.5°–63.5°C up to the age of about 60, but about 60°C over that age. Bone from women showed much greater variability [5]. About 10% of the bone organic material is non-collagenous, mainly non-collagenous protein, NCP. The main ones are listed below. They have supposed functions that change rapidly.

- Osteocalcin (OC), or bone Gla protein (BGP)
- Osteonectin (ON), or SPARC
- Osteopontin (OPN) or secreted phosphoprotein I (SPPI)
- Bone sialoprotein (BSP)

Handbook of Biomaterial Properties. Edited by J. Black and G. Hastings.
Published in 1998 by Chapman & Hall, London. ISBN 0 412 60330 6.

Table A1.1 Composition of Cortical Bone

	Water	*Organic*	*Ash*	*Source*
Mass %	12.0	28.1	59.9	[1]
Volume %	23.9	38.4	37.7	[1]
Volume %	15.5	41.8	39.9	[2]

The relative amounts of these proteins can vary greatly. Ninomiya *et al.* [6] report far more osteocalcin (31 times) in cortical bone than in trabecular bone, and far more osteonectin (29 times) in trabecular bone than in cortical bone.

A1.1.3 Mineral

The mineral has a plate-like habit, the crystals being extremely small, about 4 nm by 50 nm by 50 nm. The mineral is a variant of hydroxyapatite, itself a variant of calcium phosphate: $Ca_{10}(PO_4)_6(OH)_2$ [7]. The crystals are impure. In particular there is about 4–6% of carbonate replacing the phosphate groups, making the mineral technically a carbonate apatite, *dahllite*, and various other substitutions take place [8].

A1.1.4 Cement line

The cement line round Haversian systems (secondary osteons) contains less calcium and phosphorus, and more sulphur than nearby parts of bone. This may indicate the presence of more sulphated mucosubstances, making the cement line viscous [9].

A1.2 PHYSICAL PROPERTIES

A1.2.1 Density

Table A1.2 Density of Cortical Bone

Wet bone	1990 kg m^{-3} [1]

A1.2.2 Electromechanical behavior

Strained bone develops electrical potential differences. These used to be attributed to piezoelectric effects. However, the size of the piezoelectric effects is small compared with those produced by streaming potentials [10]. Furthermore, there were various anomalies with the potentials generated, which did not always accord with theory. The consensus now is that 'SGPs' (stress-generated potentials) are overwhelmingly caused by streaming potentials [10, 11]. Scott and Korostoff [12] determined, amongst other things, the relaxation time constants of the stress generated potentials, which varied greatly as a function of the conductivity and viscosity of the permeating fluid. As an example of their findings: a step-imposed loading moment which produced a peak strain of 4×10^{-4} induced an SGP of 1.8 mV, yielding a value of the SGP/strain ratio of 4500 mV. The SGP decayed rapidly at constant strain, reaching zero within about one second. For more detail, the complex original paper must be consulted.

A1.2.3 Other Physical Properties

Behari [10] gives a useful general review of many 'solid state' properties of bone, both human and non-human, many of which are not dealt with here. These properties include the Hall effect, photo-electric effects, electron paramagnetic resonance effects and so on.

A1.3 MECHANICAL PROPERTIES

A1.3.1 General

There is a great range for values in the literature for many reasons. Amongst these are:

(a) Different treatment of specimens

Drying bone and then re-wetting it produces some small differences [13], as does formalin fixation [14]. Testing bone dry produces results quite different from those in wet bone; dry bone is stiffer, stronger, and considerably more brittle. Very small samples produce values for stiffness and strength less than those from larger samples [15, 16]. High strain rates generally produce a higher modulus of elasticity, a higher strength [17], and a greater strain to failure than specimens tested at low strain rate.

(b) Different age and health of donors

Age may affect intrinsic properties. Osteoporotic bone may differ from 'normal' bone in ways other than the fact that it is more porous; there is evidence that the collagen is different from that in similar-aged non-osteoporotic subjects [18]. Bone from osteogenesis imperfecta patients has a higher proportion of Type III and Type V collagen compared with Type I collagen, than bone from normal subjects [19].

Bone collagen from osteopetrotic subjects is in general older than that from normal subjects, and has correspondingly different properties [5].

(c) Differences between bones, and sites in the bones

The ear bones (ossicles) and portions of the temporal bones (petrosals) are highly mineralized, and will undoubtedly be stiffer and more brittle than others (though they seem not to have been investigated in humans). Long bones differ along their length and around their circumference. The distal femur is less highly mineralized and weaker in tensile and compressive static loading, and at any level the posterior part is similarly less mineralized and weaker [20].

The values reported below should be considered paradigmatic, that is, to be valid for a well-performed test on bone obtained from a middle aged person with no disease. Other values are reported in such a way as to make it clear how some property is a function of other features of the specimen.

A1.3.2 Stiffness

(a) General

There are two ways of testing bone: mechanically by relating stresses to strains; ultrasonically, by subjecting the bone to ultrasound and measuring the velocity of the sound. From a knowledge of the density one can then obtain a stiffness matrix. If this is inverted it becomes a compliance matrix, the reciprocal of the individual terms of which are equivalent to the so-called technical moduli derived by mechanical testing [21]. Reilly and Burstein [22] give mechanical values, and Ashman *et al.* [23] give ultrasonic measurements. Reilly and Burstein [22] assumed transverse isotropy (that is, symmetry around the longitudinal axis of the bone), while Ashman *et al.* [23] assumed orthotropy (that is, that the values for stiffness could be different in the longitudinal, radial and tangential directions).

Reilly and Burstein [22] give values for Young's modulus at a number of intermediate angular orientations, but they do not form a very uniform set.

(b) Tensile modulus versus compressive modulus

Reilly *et al.* [24] tested femoral specimens specifically to determine whether the value for Young's modulus was different in tension and compression. A paired Student's 't' test showed no significant difference between the compressive and tensile moduli at the 95% confidence level. Calculations on their data show the the 95% confidence interval ranged

Table A1.3 Mechanical Properties

	Femur Tension [23]	*Femur Tension [22]*	*Femur Compression [22]*
Elastic moduli (GPa):			
E_1	12.0	12.8	11.7
E_2	13.4	12.8	11.7
E_3	20.0	17.7	18.2
Shear moduli* (GPa):			
G_{12}	4.5	–	–
G_{13}	5.6	3.3	–
G_{23}	6.2	3.3	–
Poisson's ratios:			
ν_{12}	0.38	0.53	0.63
ν_{13}	0.22	–	–
ν_{23}	0.24	–	–
ν_{21}	0.42	0.53	0.63
ν_{31}	0.37	0.41	0.38
ν_{32}	0.35	0.41	0.38

Subscript 1: radial direction relative to the long axis of the bone, 2: tangential direction, 3: longitudinal direction.
* Shear values are included under tension for convenience.

from compression modulus 1.72 GPa higher to tension modulus 0.27 GPa higher. The load–deformation traces showed no change of slope going from compression into tension and vice versa.

(c) Very small specimens

The bending modulus of very small specimens was 6.62 GPa [5].

(d) Locational variations: Metaphysis versus diaphysis

Young's modulus has been determined in three-point bending for extremely small plates (7 mm by 5 mm by (about) 0.3 mm) from the femoral metaphyseal shell and from the diaphysis of the same bones [16].

The differences between these values and those reported by Reilly and Burstein [22] are probably attributable not to the difference in testing mode, since bending and tension tests from the same bone generally give similar values for Young's modulus, but to the very small size of the specimen, and to the rather low density of the specimens.

Table A1.4 Locational Variations in Modulus

Location	*Longitudinal (GPa)*	*Transverse (GPa)*	*Source*
Metaphysis	9.6	5.5	[16]
Diaphysis	12.5	6.0	[16]

(e) Compression; effect of mineral

The compressive behavior of cubes, relating the properties to the density of the specimens gives, using ρ_a (fat-free mass divided by anatomical volume, g cm^{-3}) as the explanatory variable:

Young's modulus (GPa) = $3.3\rho_a^{2.4}$ for compact bone [25].

The higher values of ρ_a were of the order of 1.8 g cm^{-3}(=1800 kg m^{-3}); this equation [25] predicts a value of 13.5 GPa for such a specimen. Multiple regression analysis showed that the dependence of Young's modulus on density was caused by the effect of porosity on density, and that, in these specimens, the effect of mineral content was insignificant.

(f) Single secondary osteons

Ascenzi and co-workers [26–29] distinguish two types of secondary osteon: 'longitudinal' osteons, whose collagen fibres have a basically longitudinal orientation, and 'alternate' osteons, whose fibres have markedly different courses in neighboring lamellae. (This difference is a contentious issue.)

N.B.: These studies of Ascenzi and co-workers [26–29] are widely quoted, so beware of some apparent anomalies (apart from changes in nomenclature between papers). The bending modulus is remarkably low compared with the tension and compression moduli. The torsional (shear) modulus is remarkably high, compared both with the shear modulus values obtained by others (above), and with the tension and compression values. Torsional moduli are expected, on theoretical grounds, to be less than the tension and compression moduli. Furthermore, the large differences between the tension and compression moduli have not been reported elsewhere.]

(g) Strain rate effects

Calculations [30], incorporating data from non-human as well as human material, predict that Young's modulus is very modestly dependent upon strain rate:

$$E = 21402\ (\text{strain rate}\ (s^{-1}))^{0.050}\ \text{MPa}$$

Table A1.5 Moduli of Osteons

Modulus (GPa)	*Longitudinal Osteons*	*'Alternate' Osteons*	*Source*
Tension	11.7	5.5	[26]
Compression	6.3	7.4	[27]
Bending	2.3	2.6	[28]
Torsional*	22.7	16.8	[29]

* Values for an 80-year-old man excluded.

[N.B. statements about strain rate effects in bone are suspect unless it is clear that the workers have taken machine compliance into account!]

(h) Viscoelastic-damage properties

Viscoelastic time constant (the value τ (s) in the equation):

$$\epsilon(t) = \beta_1 \exp[(t_o - t)/\tau] + \beta_2,$$

where the betas are parameters, t is time (s), t_o is time at which the specimen is held at a constant stress below the creep threshold: 6.1 s [31]. For reference, its value in bovine bone: 3.6 s.

A1.3.3 Strength

(a) Overall

Table A1.6 Strength of Cortical Bone [22]

Mode	*Orientation*	*Breaking Strength (MPa)*	*Yield Stress (MPa)*	*Ultimate Strain*
Tension	Longitudinal	133	114	0.031
	Tangential	52	–	0.007
Compression	Longitudinal	205	–	–
	Tangential	130	–	–
	Shear	67	–	–

(b) Combined loading

Cezayirlioglu *et al.* [32] tested human bone under combined axial and torsional loading. The results are too complex to tabulate, but should be consulted by readers interested in complex loading phenomena.

(c) Metaphysis versus diaphysis

Same specimens as reported for modulus above (Table A1.4) [16]. 'Tensile' strength calculated from the bending moment, using a 'rupture factor' to take account of the non-uniform distribution of strain in the specimen.

Table A1.7 Locational Variations in Strength

Location	*Longitudinal (MPa)*	*Transverse (MPa)*	*Source*
Metaphysis	101	50	[16]
Diaphysis	129	47	[16]

(d) Effect of mineral

Keller [25], using the same specimens as above, provides the following relationship:

$$\text{Strength} = 43.9\rho_a^{2.0}\ (\text{MPa})$$

[N.B.: The effect of mineralization, as opposed to density, is possibly of importance here; the original paper must be consulted.]

(e) Single secondary osteons

The same nomenclature applies as for moduli of osteons (Table A1.5).

Table A1.8 Strength of Osteons

Strength (MPa)	*Longitudinal Osteons*	*'Alternate' Osteons*	*Source*
Tension	120	102	[26]
Compression	110	134	[27]
Bending	390	348	[28]
Torsional*	202	167	[29]

* Values for an 80 year old man excluded.

[N.B. The bending strengths and torsional strengths seem very high, even bearing in mind that no allowance has been made in bending for non-elastic effects.]

(f) Strain rate effects

Bone will bear a higher stress if it is loaded at a higher strain (or stress) rate. Carter and Caler [17] found an empirical relationship that failure stress (σ_f (MPa)) was a function of either stress rate ($\dot{\sigma}$) or strain rate ($\dot{\epsilon}$):

$$\sigma_f = 87\ \dot{\sigma}^{0.053}$$

$$\sigma_f = 87\ \dot{\epsilon}^{0.055}$$

N.B. These relationships imply an increase of 44% in the failure stress if the stress rate is increased one thousandfold. This relationship has been found to be roughly the same in other, non-human, mammals.

(g) Creep

Creep threshold (the stress below which no creep occurs): 73 MPa [31]. The equivalent value for bovine bone is 117 MPa [31]. Specimens in tension or compression were held at particular stresses [33]. The time (seconds) to failure is given as a function of normalized stress (stress/Young's modulus (MPa/MPa)):

Tension: Time to failure = 1.45×10^{-36} (normalized stress)$^{-15.8}$

Compression: Time to failure = 4.07×10^{-37} (normalized stress)$^{-17.8}$

(h) Fatigue

Some workers report the log of the number of cycles as a function of the applied stress levels, some report the log cycle number as a function of log stress levels, and some report log stress levels as a function of log cycle number. [The last seems wrong, since the applied stress can hardly be a function of the number of cycles the specimen is going to bear, but it is frequently used in fatigue studies. It is not possible simply to reverse the dependent and independent axes because the equations are derived from regressions with associated uncertainty.] The variation between the results for different testing modes is considerable.

Carter *et al.* [34] report on the effect of Young's modulus of elasticity and porosity in their specimens. They find that Young's modulus is positively associated with fatigue life, and porosity is negatively associated:

$$\log N_f = -2.05 \log \Delta\sigma_o \qquad \text{(S.E. 0.599)}$$

$$\log N_f = -4.82 \log \Delta\sigma_o + 0.186\,E \qquad \text{(S.E. 0.387)}$$

$$\log N_f = -2.63 \log \Delta\sigma_o - 0.061\,P \qquad \text{(S.E. 0.513)}$$

$$\log N_f = -4.73 \log \Delta\sigma_o + 0.160\,E - 0.029\,P \qquad \text{(S.E. 0.363)}$$

where N_f: number of cycles to failure; $\Delta\sigma_o$: initial stress range (these experiments were carried out under strain control, so stress range decreased as damage spread and the specimens became more compliant); E: Young's modulus (GPa); P: porosity (%). Incorporating Young's modulus into the equation has a marked effect in reducing the standard error; porosity has a much less strong effect.

[N.B. Many workers normalize their data in an effort to reduce the effect that variations in Young's modulus have in increasing the scatter of the results.]

Choi and Goldstein [15] provide alternate, somewhat higher values.

(i) Effect of remodeling

Vincentelli and Grigorov [35] examined the effect of Haversian remodelling on the tibia. The specimens they reported were almost entirely primary or Haversian, with few specimens having a scattering of secondary osteons. [Unfortunately they probably (it is not clear) allowed their specimens to dry out, so it is not sure that bone *in vivo* would show the same behavior. However, their results are similar to those found in non-human specimens.]

Table A1.9 Effect of Remodeling [35]

Property	*Primary Osteons*	*Haversian Osteons*
Tensile Strength (MPa)	162	133
Ultimate Strain	0.026	0.022
Young's modulus (GPa)	19.7	18.0

ADDITIONAL READING

Cowin, S.C. (ed.)(1989) *Bone Mechanics* Boca Raton: CRC Press.

A more rigorous, less chatty and less biologically, oriented approach than the following books by Currey and by Martin and Burr. The chapters on mechanics (2, 6 and 7), written by Cowin himself, are particularly authoritative.

Currey, J.D. (1984) *The Mechanical Adaptation of Bones* Princeton: University Press.

Out of print, new edition in preparation. Tries to deal with all aspects of mechanical properties of bone as a material and of whole bones. Not overly technical. Written from a general biological perspective, thus, does not concentrate on human material.

Martin, R.B. and Burr, D.B. (1989) *Structure, Function and Adaptation of Compact Bone* New York: Raven Press.

There are not many values of mechanical properties here, but the treatment of the biology of bone, and of fatigue of bone tissue, is excellent and the discussion of remodeling, although now somewhat out of date, is a very good introduction to this intellectually taxing topic.

Nigg, B.M. and Herzog, W. (eds)(1994) *Biomechanics of the Musculoskeletal System* John Wiley: Chichester.

Deals with many aspects of biomechanics, including locomotion, with an emphasis on human material. There is a full treatment of the measurement of many biomechanical properties.

REFERENCES

1. Gong, J.K., Arnold, J.S. and Cohn, S.H. (1964) Composition of trabecular and cortical bone. *Anat. Rec.*, **149,** 325–331.
2. Biltz, R.M. and Pellegrino, E.D. (1969) The chemical anatomy of bone I. A comparative study of bone composition in sixteen vertebrates. *J. Bone Joint Surg.*, **51A,** 456–466.

3. Lees, S. and Escoubes, M. (1987) Vapor pressure isotherms, composition and density of hyperdense bones of horse, whale and porpoise. *Con. Tiss. Res.*, **16,** 305–322.
4. Keene, D.R., Sakai, L.Y. and Burgeson, R.E. (1991) Human bone contains type III collagen, type VI collagen, and fibrillin: Type III collagen is present on specific fibers that may mediate attachment of tendons, ligaments, and periosteum to calcified bone cortex. *J. Histochem. Cytochem.*, **39,** 59–69.
5. Danielsen, C.C., Mosekilde, Li., Bollerslev, J. *et al.* (1994) Thermal stability of cortical bone collagen in relation to age in normal individuals and in individuals with osteopetrosis. *Bone*, **15,** 91–96.
6. Ninomiya, J.T., Tracy, R.P., Calore, J.D., *et al.* (1990) Heterogeneity of human bone. *J. Bone Min. Res.*, **5,** 933–938.
7. Lowenstam, H.A. and Weiner, S. (1989) *On Biomineralization*, Oxford University Press, New York.
8. McConnell, D. (1962) The crystal structure of bone. *Clin. Orthop. Rel. Res.*, **23,** 253–68.
9. Burr, D.B., Schaffler, M.B. and Frederickson, R.G. (1988) Composition of the cement line and its possible mechanical role as a local interface in human compact bone. *J. Biomech.*, **21,** 939–945.
10. Behari, J. (1991) Solid state bone behavior. *Prog. Biophys. Mol. Biol.*, **56,** 1–41.
11. Martin, R.B. and Burr, D.B. (1989) *Structure, Function, and Adaptation of Compact Bone*, Raven Press, New York.
12. Scott, G.C. and Korostoff, E. (1990) Oscillatory and step response electromechanical phenomena in human and bovine bone. *J. Biomech.*, **23**, 127–143.
13. Currey, J.D. (1988) The effects of drying and re-wetting on some mechanical properties of cortical bone. *J. Biomech.*, **21**, 439–441.
14. Sedlin, E.D. (1967) A rheological model for cortical bone. *Acta Orthop. Scand.*, (Suppl. 83), 1–78.
15. Choi, K. and Goldstein, S.A. (1992) A comparison of the fatigue behavior of human trabecular and cortical bone tissue. *J. Biomech.*, **25,** 1371–1381.
16. Lotz, J.C., Gerhart, T.N. and Hayes, W.C. (1991) Mechanical properties of metaphyseal bone in the proximal femur. *J. Biomech.*, **24,** 317–329.
17. Carter, D.R. and Caler, W.E. (1985) A cumulative damage model for bone fracture. *J. Orthop. Res.*, **3,** 84–90.
18. Bailey, A.J., Wotton, S.F., Sims, T.J. *et al.* (1993) Biochemical changes in the collagen of human osteoporotic bone matrix. *Con. Tiss. Res.*, **29,** 119–132.
19. Bateman, J.F., Chan, D., Mascara, T. *et al.* (1986) Collagen defects in lethal perinatal osteogenesis imperfecta. *Biochem. J.*, **240,** 699–708.
20. Saito, S. (1983) (Distribution of the X-ray density, compressive and tensile breaking strength in the human femoral shaft) Die Verteilung von Dichte, Druck und Festigkeit im menslichen Femurschaft. *Anat. Anzeiger Jena*, **154,** 365–376.
21. Cowin, S.C. (1989) *Bone Mechanics*, CRC Press, Boca Raton.
22. Reilly, D.T. and Burstein, A.H. (1975) The elastic and ultimate properties of compact bone tissue. *J. Biomech.*, **8,** 393–405.
23. Ashman, R.B., Cowin, S.C., Van Buskirk, W.C. *et al.* (1984) A continuous wave technique for the measurement of the elastic properties of cortical bone. *J. Biomech.*, **17,** 349–361.

24. Reilly, D.T. and Burstein, A.H. (1974) The mechanical properties of cortical bone. *J. Bone Joint Surg.*, **56A,** 1001–1022
25. Keller, T.S. (1994) Predicting the compressive mechanical behavior of bone. *J. Biomech.*, **27,** 1159–1168.
26. Ascenzi, A. and Bonucci, E. (1967) The tensile properties of single osteons. *Anat. Rec.*, **158,** 375–386.
27. Ascenzi, A. and Bonucci, E. (1968) The compressive properties of single osteons. *Anat. Rec.*, **161,** 377–391.
28. Ascenzi, A., Baschieri, P., and Benvenuti, A. (1990) The bending properties of single osteons. *J. Biomech.*, **23,** 763–771.
29. Ascenzi, A., Baschieri, P., and Benvenuti, A. (1994) The torsional properties of single selected osteons. *J. Biomech.*, **27,** 875–884.
30. Carter, D.R. and Caler, W.E. (1983) Cycle-dependent and time-dependent bone fracture with repeated loading. *J. Biomech. Eng.*, **105,** 166–170.
31. Fondrk, M., Bahniuk, E., Davy, D.T. *et al.* (1988) Some viscoplastic characteristics of bovine and human cortical bone. *J. Biomech.*, **21,** 623–630.
32. Cezayirlioglu, H., Bahniuk, E., Davy, D.T. *et al.* (1985) Anisotropic yield behavior of bone under combined axial force and torque. *J. Biomech.*, **18,** 61–69.
33. Caler, W.E. and Carter, D.R. (1989) Bone creep-fatigue damage accumulation *J. Biomech.*, **22,** 625–635.
34. Carter, D.R., Caler, W.E., Spengler, D.M. *et al.* (1981) Uniaxial fatigue of human bone. The influence of tissue physical characteristics. *J. Biomech.*, **14,** 461–70.
35. Vincentelli, R., and Grigorov, M. (1985) The effect of haversian remodeling on the tensile properties of human cortical bone. *J. Biomech.*, **18,** 201–207.

Cancellous bone

A2

T.M. Keaveny

A2.1 STRUCTURE

Trabecular bone consists primarily of lamellar bone, arranged in packets that make up an interconnected irregular array of plates and rods, called trabeculae. These trabeculae, on average, have thicknesses in the range of 100–200 microns, dependent upon both anatomic site and donor age [1]. The space between trabeculae is filled with bone marrow, and the precise architectural arrangement of the trabecular plates and rods also depends on anatomic site, making trabecular bone (at the continuum level) a highly heterogeneous material. Most mechanical properties of trabecular bone depend to a large degree on the apparent density, defined as the product of the density of the individual trabeculae (the 'tissue density') and the volume fraction of bone present in the bulk specimen. Volume fraction typically ranges from 0.60 for dense trabecular bone to 0.05 for porous trabecular bone [2,3]. The (wet) tissue density for human trabecular bone is fairly constant and is in the approximate range 1.6–2.0 g/cm^3 [4,5]. By contrast, the (wet) apparent density varies substantially and is typically in the range 0.05–1.0 g/cm^3 (Table A2.1). Compared to cortical bone, trabecular bone has a similar surface area-to-volume ratio (SVR, excluding lacunae and canaliculi), but SVR increases non-linearly with increasing volume fraction (VF) of bone [10]:

$$\mathrm{SVR} = 8.4\,(\mathrm{VF})^{0.705}$$

Handbook of Biomaterial Properties. Edited by J. Black and G. Hastings.
Published in 1998 by Chapman & Hall, London. ISBN 0 412 60330 6.

A2.2 COMPOSITION

Individual trabeculae have relatively uniform compositions that are similar to cortical bone tissue (chapter A1), but are slightly less mineralized and slightly more hydrated than cortical tissue.

The percent volume of water, inorganic, and organic components for hydrated trabeculae have been reported at 27%, 38%, and 35%, respectively [11], although the precise values depend on anatomic site, age, and health. Based on reported wet, dry, and ash apparent densities for specimens of defatted human lumbar spine trabecular bone [4], the percentage weights of the inorganic, organic, and water components for this tissue can be calculated at approximately 54%, 26%, and 20%, respectively.

A2.3 MECHANICAL PROPERTIES

A2.3.1 Modulus and strength

Trabecular bone is essentially linearly elastic until yielding at strains of approximately 1–2%. After yielding, it can sustain large deformations (up to 50% strain) while still maintaining its load-carrying capacity. Thus, trabecular bone can absorb substantial energy upon mechanical failure. Being a heterogeneous open cell porous solid, trabecular bone has anisotropic mechanical properties that depend on the porosity of the specimen as well as the architectural arrangement of the individual trabeculae. In order to specify its mechanical properties, one must therefore specify factors such as the anatomic site, loading direction with respect to the principal orientation of the trabeculae, and age and health of the donor. Young's modulus can vary 100-fold within a single epiphysis [12] and can vary on average by a factor of three depending on loading direction [13–16]. Pathologies such as osteoporosis, osteoarthritis, and bone cancer are known to affect mechanical properties [17,18]. Typically, the modulus of human trabecular bone is in the range 0.010–2 GPa depending on the above factors. Strength, which is linearly and strongly correlated with modulus [12,15], is typically in the range 0.1–30 MPa.

A2.3.2 Relationships between modulus and strength and density

The relationships between the static mechanical properties of trabecular bone and apparent density vary for the different types of trabecular bone because of the anatomic site-, age-, and disease-related variations in trabecular architecture. Both linear and power-law relationships can be used to describe the dependence of modulus and compressive strength on apparent density (Tables A2.2, A2.3), with typical coefficients of determination (r^2 values) in the range 0.5–0.9. Differences in the predictive

Table A2.1 Typical wet apparent densities, moduli, and compressive strengths for human trabecular bone

	Cadavers		*Specimens*	*Wet Apparent Density (g/cm^3)*		*Modulus (GPa)*		*Ultimate Strength (MPa)*		
Tissue Source	*Number*	*Ages*	*Number*	*Mean (SD)*	*Range*	*Mean (SD)*	*Range*	*Mean (SD)*	*Range*	*Source*
Proximal Tibia**	9	59–82	121	0.29 (0.10)	0.09–0.66	0.445 (0.257)	0.061–1.174	5.33 (2.93)	0.68–14.1	[6]
Femur†**	10	58–83	299‡	0.50 (0.16)	0.14–1.00	0.389 (0.270)	0.044–1.531	7.36 (4.00)	0.56–22.9	[7]
Lumbar Spine*	42	15–87	40	0.24 (0.07)	0.11–0.47	0.067 (0.044)	0.010–0.180	2.45 (1.52)	1.00–7.00	[8]
Lumbar Spine**	3	71–84	231	0.19 (0.08)	0.06–0.40	0.023 (0.015)	0.001–0.110	1.55 (1.11)	0.05–8.00	[9]

All mechanical data from tests with specimens oriented in the inferior–superior direction, unless noted.
* The ash densities that were originally reported have been converted to wet densities using Y = 1.86 X, based on data from Table 1 [4].
** The dry densities that were originally reported have been converted to wet densities using Y = 1.25 X, based on data from Table 1 [4].
† Proximal and distal femur pooled; proximal specimens oriented approximately along the femoral neck axis.
‡ Elastic modulus data for only 122 specimens.

power between the various linear and power laws are usually negligible since the range of apparent density exhibited by trabecular bone is less than one order of magnitude. Poisson's ratio is difficult to measure experimentally for a heterogeneous, cellular solid such as trabecular bone. Mean values of Poisson's ratio have been reported from close to zero to just less than one [23–26], with little known about the causes of this large range. The failure (yield and ultimate) strains of human trabecular bone have only a weak dependence, if any, on apparent density and modulus [8,9,19,27,28]. Mean (± SD) values of ultimate compressive strain for proximal tibial bone have been reported at approximately 2.0±0.4% [6]. Additional experiments are currently required to investigate potential effects of anisotropy, age and anatomic site on failure strains. On average, the tensile and compressive strengths appear to be equal [29], although the relationship between the tensile and compressive failure properties is not well understood. Elastic properties are the same in tension and compression. No reliable data exist for multiaxial failure behavior although it is unlikely that a von Mises-type criterion applies to this heterogeneous cellular solid.

A2.3.3. Viscoelastic properties

Trabecular bone is only slightly viscoelastic when tested *in vitro*, with both compressive strength and modulus being related to strain rate raised to a power of 0.06 [30,31]. The stiffening effect of marrow is negligible except at very high strain rates (10 strain/sec), although there is emerging evidence that the constraining effects of an intact cortical shell may allow hydraulic stiffening of whole bones *in vivo* under dynamic loads [32]. Minor stress relaxation has been shown to occur [33] and depends on the applied strain level [34], indicating that human trabecular bone is nonlinearly viscoelastic. The rate of change of the stress relaxation function (i.e. the ratio of stress to constant strain during relaxation) versus time for human femoral bone (tissue) varies from approximately 6.8 MPa/s to 18 MPa/s as a function of strain level [34]. Little else is known about its time dependent properties, including creep and fatigue. As a result, most finite element analyses are based on the assumption that the mechanical behavior of cancellous bone has no time dependence.

A2.3.4. Experimental problems

It should be noted that the *in vitro* mechanical test methods most often used to date suffer from 'end artifacts' [35–37], errors due to platen–specimen friction and machining-related damage of the specimen ends, which compromise the accuracy of most of the data. Modulus values are underestimated by at least 20% [36–38], with the error possibly depending

Table A2.2 Linear and power-law regressions between modulus (E in GPa) and wet apparent density (ρ in g/cm³)#

	Cadavers		*Specimens*	$E = a\rho + b$			$E = a\rho^b$			
Tissue Source	*Number*	*Age*	*Number*	a	b	r^2	a	b	r^2	*Source*
Proximal Tibia*	9	59–82	121	1.207	-0.0797	0.60	1.401	1.43	0.66	[19]
Proximal Tibia†	3	52–67	75	4.360	-0.0412	0.86	4.606	1.07	0.86	[20]
Proximal Femur††	4	25–82	49	—	—	—	1.310	1.40	0.91	[21]
Lumbar Spine**	3	70–84	199	0.160	-0.007	0.54	0.479	1.94	0.70	[22]

* Compressive loading of human trabecular bone specimens loaded at 'low' strain rates (≤ 1.0/sec) and taken from a range of anatomic sites.
** Originally reported dry densities have been converted to wet densities.
† Ultrasound was used to measure the elastic properties.
†† Specimens oriented along femoral neck axis.

Table A2.3 Linear and power-law regressions between ultimate strength (σ in MPa) and wet apparent density (ρ in g/cm^3)#

	Cadavers		*Specimens*	$\sigma = a\rho + b$			$\sigma = a\,\rho^b$			
Tissue Source	*Number*	*Age*	*Number*	a	b	r^2	a	b	r^2	*Source*
Proximal Tibia*	10	60–83	94	19.2	-1.60	0.78	25.6	1.60	0.82	[19]
Proximal Femur†	4	25–82	49	—	—	—	25.0	1.80	0.93	[21]
Lumbar Spine**	3	70–84	199	13.4	-0.97	0.55	56.9	2.30	0.60	[22]

* For compressive loading of human trabecular bone specimens loaded at 'low' strain rates (≤ 1.0/sec) and taken from a range of anatomic sites.
** Originally reported dry densities have been converted to wet densities using y = 1.86x
† Ultrasound was used to measure the elastic properties.
(Note: A dash represents that no data were reported.)

on anatomic site from which the specimens are obtained. Similarly, strength values can also be in error [39], and failure strain data are also suspect [40] because of the confounding effect of the artifactual 'toe' [41] in the initial portion of the stress–strain curve. Thus, *in vivo* values of most of the above mechanical properties must be extrapolated carefully from the available *in vitro* data. Furthermore, inter-study comparisons of the *in vitro* data should address the confounding effects of these testing artifacts.

ADDITIONAL READING

Cowin S.C. (1989) *Bone Mechanics*, CRC Press, Boca Raton.

Presents an excellent treatment (p. 129ff) of the structure–function relationships for trabecular bone using the principles of continuum mechanics and quantitative stereology.

Gibson L.J. (1985) The mechanical behavior of cancellous bone. *J. Biomech.*, **18**, 317–328.

Contains a theoretical analysis of some possible underlying deformation and failure mechanisms of individual trabeculae, based upon analogies to cellular solids.

Goldstein S.A. (1987) The mechanical properties of trabecular bone: Dependence on anatomic location and function. *J. Biomech.*, **20**, 1055–1061.

Keaveny T.M. and Hayes W.C. (1993) A 20-year perspective on the mechanical properties of trabecular bone. *J. Biomech. Eng*, **15**, 534–542.

These comprehensive articles provide a more general survey of properties than presented above and include results derived from animal bone, as well as data on the mechanical behavior of individual trabeculae. In the absence of human data, data from animal studies can be used, although extrapolation of behavior from differing anatomic sites must be done with caution.

REFERENCES

1. Mosekilde, L. (1988) Age-related changes in vertebral trabecular bone architecture – Assessed by a new model. *Bone*, **9**, 247–250.
2. Mosekilde, L., Bentzen, S.M., Ortoft, G. *et al.* (1989) The predictive value of quantitative computed tomography for vertebral body compressive strength and ash density. *Bone*, **10**, 465–470.
3. Kuhn, J.L., Goldstein, S.A., Feldkamp, L.A. *et al.* (1990) Evaluation of a micro-computed tomography system to study trabecular bone structure. *J. Orthop. Res.*, **8**, 833–842.
4. Galante, J., Rostoker, W. and Ray, R.D. (1970) Physical properties of trabecular bone. *Calcif. Tissue Res.*, **5**, 236–246.
5. Ashman, R.B. and Rho, J.Y. (1988) Elastic modulus of trabecular bone material. *J. Biomech.*, **21**, 177–181.
6. Linde, F., Hvid, I. and Pongsoipetch, B. (1989) Energy absorptive properties of human trabecular bone specimens during axial compression. *J. Orthop. Res.*, **7**, 432–439

7. Rohlmann, A., Zilch, H., Bergman, G. *et al.* (1980) Material properties of femoral cancellous bone in axial loading. Part I: Time independent properties. *Arch Orthop. Trauma Surg.*, **97**, 95–102.
8 Mosekilde, L., Mosekilde, L. and Danielsen, C.C. (1987) Biomechanical competence of vertebral trabecular bone in relation to ash density and age in normal individuals. *Bone*, **8**, 79–85.
9. Hansson, T.H., Keller, T.S. and Panjabi, M.M. (1987) A study of the compressive properties of lumbar vertebral trabeculae: effects of tissue characteristics. *Spine*, **12**, 56–62.
10. Fyhrie, D.P., Fazalari, N.L., Goulet, R. *et al.* (1993) Direct calculation of the surface-to-volume ratio for human cancellous bone. *J. Biomech.*, **26**, 955–967.
11. Gong, J.K., Arnold, J.S. and Cohn, S.H. (1964) Composition of trabecular and cortical bone. *Anat. Rec.*, **149**, 325–332.
12. Goldstein, S.A., Wilson, D.L., Sonstegard, D.A. *et al.* (1983) The mechanical properties of human tibial trabecular bone as a function of metaphyseal location. *J. Biomech.*, **16**, 965–969.
13. Townsend, P.R., Raux, P. and Rose, R.M. (1975) The distribution and anisotropy of the stiffness of cancellous bone in the human patella. *J. Biomech.*, **8**, 363–367.
14. Linde, F., Pongsoipetch, B., Frich, L.H. *et al.* (1990) Three-axial strain controlled testing applied to bone specimens from the proximal tibial epiphysis. *J. Biomech.*, **23**, 1167–1172.
15. Ciarelli, M.J., Goldstein, S.A., Kuhn, J.L. *et al.* (1991) Evaluation of orthogonal mechanical properties and density of human trabecular bone from the major metaphyseal regions with materials testing and computed tomography. *J. Orthop. Res.*, **9**, 674–682.
16. Goulet, R.W., Goldstein, S.A., Ciarelli, M.J. *et al.* (1994) The relationship between the structural and orthogonal compressive properties of trabecular bone. *J. Biomech.*, **27**, 375–389.
17. Pugh, J.W., Radin, E.L. and Rose, R.M. (1974) Quantitative studies of human subchondral cancellous bone. Its relationship to the state of its overlying cartilage. *J. Bone Joint Surg.*, **56A**, 313–321.
18. Hipp, J.A., Rosenberg, A.E. and Hayes, W.C. (1992) Mechanical properties of trabecular bone within and adjacent to osseous metastases. *J. Bone Miner. Res.*, **7**, 1165–1171.
19. Hvid, I., Bentzen, S.M., Linde, F. *et al.* (1989) X-ray quantitative computed tomography: The relations to physical properties of proximal tibial trabecular bone specimens. *J. Biomech.*, **22**, 837–844.
20. Ashman, R.B., Rho, J.Y. and Turner, C.H. (1989) Anatomical variation of orthotropic elastic moduli of the proximal human tibia. *J. Biomech.*, **22**, 895–900.
21. Lotz, J.C., Gerhart, T.N. and Hayes, W.C. (1990) Mechanical properties of trabecular bone from the proximal femur: A quantitative CT study. *J. Comput. Assist. Tomogr.*, **14**, 107–114.
22. Keller, T.S. (1994) Predicting the compressive mechanical behavior of bone. *J. Biomech.*, **27**, 1159–1168.
23. McElhaney, J., Fogle, J., Melvin, J. *et al.* (1970) Mechanical properties of cranial bone. *J. Biomech.*, **3**, 495–511.

24. Gilbert, J.A., Maxwell, G.M., McElhaney, J.H. *et al.* (1984) A system to measure the forces and moments at the knee and hip during level walking. *J. Orthop. Res.*, **2**, 281–288.
25. Klever, F., Klumpert, R., Horenberg, J. *et al.* (1985) Global mechanical properties of trabecular bone: experimental determination and prediction from a structural model. In *Biomechanics: Current Interdisciplinary Research*, 167–172, Ed. Perren S.M. and Schneider E.; Martinus Nijhoff, Dordrecht.
26. Snyder, B. (1991) *Anisotropic Structure–Property Relations for Trabecular Bone*. Ph.D. Dissertation, University of Pennsylvania, Philadelphia, PA.
27. Hvid, I., Jensen, N.C., Bunger, C. *et al.* (1985) Bone mineral assay: its relation to the mechanical strength of cancellous bone. *Eng. Med.*, **14**, 79–83.
28. Rohl, L., Larsen, E., Linde, F. *et al.* (1991) Tensile and compressive properties of cancellous bone. *J. Biomech.*, **24**, 1143–1149.
29. Carter, D.R., Schwab, G.H. and Spengler, D.M. (1980) Tensile fracture of cancellous bone. *Acta Orthop. Scand.*, **51**, 733–741.
30. Carter, D.R. and Hayes, W.C. (1977) The compressive behavior of bone as a two-phase porous structure. *J. Bone Joint Surg.*, **59A**, 954–962.
31. Linde, F., Norgaard, P., Hvid, I. *et al.* (1991) Mechanical properties of trabecular bone. Dependency on strain rate. *J. Biomech.*, **24**, 803–809.
32. Ochoa, J.A., Sanders, A.P., Heck, D.A. *et al.* (1991) Stiffening of the femoral head due to inter-trabecular fluid and intraosseous pressure. *J. Biomech. Eng.*, **113**, 259–262.
33. Zilch, H., Rohlmann, A., Bergmann, G. *et al.* (1980) Material properties of femoral cancellous bone in axial loading. Part II: Time dependent properties. *Arch. Orthop. Trauma. Surg.*, **97**, 257–262.
34. Deligianni, D.D., Maris, A. and Missirlis, Y.F. (1994) Stress relaxation behaviour of trabecular bone specimens. *J. Biomech.*, **27**, 1469–1476.
35. Linde, F., Hvid, I. and Madsen, F. (1992) The effect of specimen geometry on the mechanical behaviour of trabecular bone specimens. *J. Biomech.*, **25**, 359–368. 439.
36. Keaveny, T.M., Borchers, R.E., Gibson, L.J. *et al.* (1993) Theoretical analysis of the experimental artifact in trabecular bone compressive modulus. *J. Biomech.*, **26**, 599–607.
37. Zhu, M., Keller, T.S. and Spengler, D.M. (1994) Effects of specimen load-bearing and free surface layers on the compressive mechanical properties of cellular materials. *J. Biomech.*, **27**, 57–66.
38. Odgaard, A. and Linde, F. (1991) The underestimation of Young's modulus in compressive testing of cancellous bone specimens. *J. Biomech.*, **24**, 691–698.
39. Keaveny, T.M., Borchers, R.E., Gibson, L.J. *et al.* (1993) Trabecular bone modulus and strength can depend on specimen geometry. *J. Biomech.*, **26**, 991–1000.
40. Turner, C.H. (1989) Yield behavior of bovine cancellous bone. *J. Biomech. Eng.*, **111**, 256–260.
41. Keaveny, T.M., Guo, X.E., Wachtel, E.F. *et al.* (1994) Trabecular bone exhibits fully linear elastic behavior and yields at low strains. *J. Biomech.*, **27**, 1127–1136.

A3 Dentin and enamel

K.E. Healy

A3.1 INTRODUCTION

A3.1.1 Structure of human dentition:

The permanent adult human dentition normally consists of 32 teeth, of which 16 are located in the mandible and 16 in the maxilla. There are 4 incisors, 2 canines, 4 premolars and 6 molars for the upper and lower dentition. The incisors are used for cutting food, the canines for tearing, the premolars for grasping, and the molars for grinding (i.e., masticating). There is a generic heterogeneous structure for these teeth, where enamel forms an exterior layer over the underlying dentin. From the cervix to the apex of the root, the exterior of the dentin is covered by cementum to which the periodontal ligament attaches the tooth to alveolar bone. Dental enamel is dense, highly mineralized, hard, and brittle. It contains prism-like structures that span from the enamel surface to the junction of enamel and dentin, the dentino-enamel junction (DEJ). The prisms are comprised of hydroxyapatite crystallites and contain very little organic matrix. These properties make dental enamel an excellent material for cutting and masticating food (i.e., processes that involve friction and wear). In contrast, dentin is not as hard as enamel, but it is tougher. Dentin is a heterogeneous material and can be thought of as a composite structure containing four major components: dentin matrix; dentinal tubules; mineral (i.e., carbonate containing hydroxyapatite); and, dentinal fluid. The dentinal tubules (~45 000 per mm^2) are formed during development of the dentin matrix and are distributed throughout the dentin matrix in a somewhat uniform manner. The dentin matrix mineralizes in an anisotropic fashion, where a highly mineralized tissue, peritubular dentin,

Handbook of Biomaterial Properties. Edited by J. Black and G. Hastings. Published in 1998 by Chapman & Hall, London. ISBN 0 412 60330 6.

surrounds the dentinal tubules. The mineralized tissue between the dentinal tubules and peritubular dentin is referred to as intertubular dentin. Histological examination has revealed that intertubular dentin is less mineralized than peritubular dentin. Furthermore, the matrix and mineral content of root dentin is different from coronal dentin. A good review of the structure of teeth can be found in Waters [1].

A3.2 COMPOSITION

Table A3.1 Basic Constituents of Human Dentin and Enamel*

	Enamel		*Dentin*	
	Weight %	*Volume %*	*Weight %*	*Volume %*
Mineral (density, 3000 kg m^{-3})	96	90	70	50
Organic (density, 1400 kg m^{-3})	1	2	20	30
Water (density, 1000 kg m^{-3})	3	8	10	20

* Adapted from [1–3].

Table A3.2 Major Elemental Composition of Surface and Bulk Dental Enamel

	Enamel Mean wt% (range or standard deviation, ±)	*Dentin Mean wt% (range or standard deviation, ±)*	*Source, Comments*
Ca	37.4 ± 1.0	—	[4]#
	37.1 ± 0.2 (26.7–47.9)	26.9 ± 0.2 (21.8–31.3)	[5]#
	36.3 ± 0.1 (27.7–42.0)	27.6 ± 0.1 (24.7–31.5)	[5]‡
P	17.8 ± 0.2	13.5 ± 0.1	[5]●, age >25yrs
	17.68 ± 0.2		[6]¤
Na	0.72 ± 0.008 (0.42–1.03)	0.72 ± 0.008 (0.26–0.87)	[5]#
	0.72 ± 0.008 (0.49–0.88)	0.64 ± 0.001 (0.55–0.75)	[5]‡
Cl	0.28 ± 0.01	0.05 ± 0.004	[5]#, age >25yrs
	0.32 ± 0.01	0.072 ± 0.022	[7]#
K	0.026 ± 0.001	0.02 ± 0.001	[5]‡, age <25yrs
Mg	0.39 ± 0.02 (0.13–0.77)	0.74 ± 0.02 (0.25–0.94)	[5]#
	0.32 ± 0.004 (0.24–0.48)	0.76 ± 0.004 (0.58–0.89)	[5]‡
CO_3	3.2 (2.4–4.2)	4.6 (4–5)	[2,3]†

Neutron activated gamma-ray spectrometric analysis.
‡ Atomic absorption spectrophotometry.
● Colorimetic assay.
† Average compiled from the literature.
* Neutron activated gamma-ray spectrometric analysis (Na, Cl, Al, Mn, Ca, and P), atomic absorption spectrophotometry (K, Mg, Zn, Cu, and Fe), or a fluoride-specific electrode (F).
¤ Atomic absorption spectrophotometry (Ca), and colorimetric method (P).

Table A3.3 Trace Elemental Composition of Surface and Bulk Dental Enamel

		Surface Enamel		*Whole Enamel*		
	At.#	*Mean (range)* μg/g	*Median* μg/g	*Mean (range)* μg/g	*Median* μg/g	*Source, comments*
S	16			281 (530–130)	270	[8]†,[9]‡
F	9	752 (1948–25)	666	293 (730–95)	200	[8]†,[9]‡
				123.8 ± 7.9		[10]◊
Zn	30	893 (5400–61)	576	199 (400–91)	190	[8]†,[9]‡
				276 ± 106		[4]#
				263.42 ± 14.8		[10]◊
Mg	12	745 (3600–115)	576	1,670 (3,000–470)	1,550	[8]†,[9]‡
Al	13	343 (2304–16)	202	12.5 (70–1.5)	5.6	[8]†,[9]‡
Sr	38	204 (7632–9)	36	81 (280–26)	56	[8]†,[9]‡
				93.5 ± 21.9		[4]#
				111.19 ± 9.86		[10]◊
Fe	26	138 (1404–18)	68	4.4 (21–0.8)	2.6	[8]†,[9]‡
				2.77		[7]*
Si	14	70 (504–1.3)	40			[8]†,[9]‡
Mn	25	59 (468–2.6)	33	0.28 (0.64–0.08)	0.26	[8]†,[9]‡
				0.54 ± 0.08		[4]#
				0.59 ± 0.04		[10]◊
Ag	47	32 (396–0.2)	2	0.35 (1.3–0.03)	0.16	[8]†,[9]‡
				0.56 ± 0.29		[10]◊
Pb	82	24 (79–1.2)	18	3.6 (6.5–1.3)	3.6	[8]†,[9]‡
Ni	28	23 (270–0.4)	9			[8]†,[9]‡
Ba	56	22 (432–0.8)	7	4.2 (13–0.8)	3.4	[8]†,[9]‡
Se	34	18 (72–2.9)	16	0.27 (0.5–0.12)	0.22	[8]†,[9]‡
Li	3	14 (58–0.3)	10	1.13 (3.4–0.23)	0.93	[8]†,[9]‡
Sb	51	8 (90–0)	3	0.13 (0.34–0.02)	0.11	[8]†,[9]‡
Ga	31	6 (32–0)	5			[8]†,[9]‡
Sn	50	9.3 (72–0.9)	5.8	0.21 (0.92–0.03)	0.14	[8]†,[9]‡
Ge	32	7.6 (39.6–0.5)	4.0			[8]†,[9]‡
B	5	5.3 (13.0–0.8)	3.6	5.0 (39–0.5)	2.4	[8]†,[9]‡
Cu	29			4.20 (81–0.1)	0.45	[8]†,[9]‡
				0.26 ± 0.11		[4]#
				1.38		[7]*
Br	35	3.1 (14.0–0.4)	4.1	1.12 (2.6–0.32)	0.93	[8]†,[9]‡
				4.6 ± 1.1		[4]#
Cd	48	2.7 (7.6–0.6)	1.8	0.51 (2.4–0.03)	0.22	[8]†,[9]‡
Y	39	1.8 (9.3–0)	0.9	0.007 (0.17–<0.01)	<0.01	[8]†,[9]‡
Ti	22	1.6 (24.5–0.1)	0.6	0.19 (4.4–<0.1)	<0.1	[8]†,[9]‡
V	23	1.4 (14.4–0.1)	0.5	0.017 (0.03–0.01)	0.02	[8]†,[9]‡
La	57	1.4 (7.2–0)	0.8			[8]†,[9]‡
Be	4	1.3 (6.1–0)	1.2			[8]†,[9]‡
Cr	24	1.1 (4.7–0.2)	0.7	3.2 (18–0.1)	1.5	[8]†,[9]‡
				1.02 ± 0.51		[10]◊

Table A3.3 *Continued*

	At.#	Surface Enamel Mean (range) μg/g	Surface Enamel Median μg/g	Whole Enamel Mean (range) μg/g	Whole Enamel Median μg/g	Source, comments
Rb	37	0.6 (4.0–0.1)	0.4	0.39 (0.87–0.17)	0.32	[8]†,[9]‡
Zr	40	0.6 (1.9–0)	0.3	0.1 (0.57–<0.02)	0.07	[8]†,[9]‡
Ce	58	0.6 (6.1–0)	0	0.07 (1.9–0.02)	0.07	[8]†,[9]‡
W	74			0.24 ± 0.12		[8]†,[9]‡
Co	27	0.2 (2.7–0)	0.1			[8]†,[9]‡
				0.13 ± 0.13		[10]◊
Pr	59	0.2 (4.7–0)	0	0.027 (0.07–<0.01)	0.03	[8]†,[9]‡
Cs	55	0.1 (1.9–0)	0	0.04 (0.1–<0.02)	0.04	[8]†,[9]‡
Mo	42	0.1 (0.5–0.04)	0.04	7.2 (39–0.7)	6.3	[8]†,[9]‡
I	53	0.05 (4.7–0)	0.05	0.036 (0.07–0.01)	0.03	[8]†,[9]‡
Bi	83	0.001 (0.04–0)	0	0.006 (0.07–<0.02)	0.02	[8]†,[9]‡
Nd	60	0.045 (0.09–<0.02)	0.05			[8]†,[9]‡
Nb	41			0.28 (0.76–<0.1)	0.24	[8]†,[9]‡
Au	79			0.02 ± 0.01		[4]#

‡ Whole enamel from premolars of young patients (age<20 yrs), determined by spark source mass spectroscopy.
† Surface enamel (depth of analysis 42 ± 8.5 μm) from premolars of young patients (age<20 yrs), determined by spark source mass spectroscopy.
# Bulk enamel from premolars of 14–16 yrs male and female patients, selected population of Stockholm Sweden, determined by neutron activated gamma-ray spectrometric analysis. Standard deviation, ±.
◊ Neutron activated gamma-ray spectrometric analysis.
* Neutron activated gamma-ray spectrometric analysis (Na, Cl, Al, Mn, Ca, and P), atomic absorption spectrophotometry (K, Mg, Zn, Cu, and Fe), or a fluoride-specific electrode (F).

Table A3.4 Significant Differences in Trace Element Composition of Whole Human Enamel for High and Low Caries Populations†

	At.#	High Caries (Mean ± SE), μg/g	Low Caries (Mean ± SE), μg/g	Source
F	9	82.1 ± 7.99	125.7 ± 11.23	[11]
Sr	38	104.1 ± 9.14	184.0 ± 14.68	[11]
Mn	25	1.57 ± 0.24	0.87 ± 0.15	[12]
Zr	40	0.27 ± 0.1	0.16 ± 0.09	[11]
Cu	26	0.71 ± 0.2	0.17 ± 0.04	[12]

† Determined by spark source mass spectroscopy

Table A3.5 Ca/P Molar Ratio of Human Enamel and Dentin

Enamel Ca/P molar ratio	*Dentin Ca/P molar ratio*	*Source, comments*
1.58		[4]#
1.61	1.54	[5]†, ●, age >25 yrs
1.58	1.58	[5]*, ●, age >25 yrs
1.65		[13]**
1.64		[6]¤
	1.61	[14]**

Neutron activated gamma-ray spectrometric analysis.
† Ca determined by neutron activated gamma-ray spectrometric analysis
* Ca determined by atomic absorption spectrophotometry
● P determined by colorimetic assay.
** Determined by energy dispersive X-ray analysis.
¤ Determined by atomic absorption spectrophotometry (Ca), and by the colorimetric method (P).

Table A3.6 Crystallite Size and Lattice Parameters of the Apatite in Human Enamel and Dentin*

	a-axis (nm)	*c-axis (nm)*	*Width (nm)*	*Thickness (nm)*	*Source, Comments*
Enamel					
	0.9445	0.6885			[2]#
	0.9440	0.6872			[15]†
	0.9441	0.6880	68.4 ± 3.4	26.3 ± 2.2	[6]†,● ± S.D.
	0.9446	0.6886			[16]†
			68.3 ± 13.4	26.3 ± 2.19	[17]‡,● ± S.E.
Dentin					
	0.9434 ± 0.0007	0.6868 ± 0.0009			[18]‡
			29.6 ± 3.7	3.2 ± 0.5	[19]●, intertubular dentin
			36.55 ± 1.45	10.33 ± 7.91	[20]●, mixed carious and sound dentin

* Asymmetric hexagonal crystal with the thickness of the crystal less than the width.
† X-ray diffraction method of determination.
● High resolution transmission electron microscopy.
Data from [2], average compiled from the literature.

Table A3.7 Elastic Moduli and Viscoelastic Properties of Human Dentin and Enamel

	Incisors	*Canine*	*Pre-molars*	*Molars*	*Source, Comments*
E: Dentin					
				11.0 (5.8)	[21]t,†,‡
	13 (4)	14 (6)	14 (0.7)	12 (2)	[22]Crown, c,†
	9.7 (2)	12 (3)	9.0 (2)	7.6 (3)	[22]Root, c,†
				10.16	[23]b,‖
				10.87	[23] b,dehyd., ‖
				9.49	[23] b, re-hyd, ‖
E: Enamel					
				84.3 (8.9)	[24]Cusp, c, ‖
				77.9 (4.8)	[24]Side, c, ‖
		48 (6)		46 (5)	[22]Cusp, c,‡
		33 (2)		32 (4)	[22]Axial (side), c, ^
				9.7 (3)	[22]Axial (side), c, ‖
				12 (3)	[22]Occlusal, c, ‖
$E_r(\infty)$: Dentin					
				12	[25]c, constant strain, hydrated,^,‡
$H_1(t)$: Dentin					
				0.38 (0.136)	[25] c, constant strain, hydrated,^,‡

E: modulus of elasticity (GPa); E_r (∞): relaxed modulus (GPa); $H_1(t)$: distribution of relaxation times (GPa); c: compression; t: tension; b: three-point bending.
‖ Applied load approximately parallel to either the long axis of the enamel rods or dentinal tubules.
^Applied load approximately perpendicular to either the long axis of the enamel rods or dentinal tubules.
† Applied load with respect to either the long axis of the enamel rods or dentinal tubules was variable.
‡ Type of tooth unknown or various teeth used for measurement; data are tabulated under molar.
Note: standard deviations are given in parentheses.

Table A3.8 Mechanical Properties of Human Enamel

	Incisors	*Canine*	*Pre-molars*	*Molars*	*Source, comments*
Stress at Proportional Limit (MPa)				353 (83)	[24]Cusp, c, ∥
				336 (61)	[24]Axial(side), c, ∥
		194 (19)		224 (26)	[22]Cusp, c,†
		183 (12)		186.2 (17)	[22]Axial (side), c, ˆ
				70.3 (22)	[22]Axial (side), c, ∥
				98.6 (26)	[22]Occlusal, c, ∥
		91.0 (10)			[22]Incisal edge, c,†
Tensile Strength (MPa)				10 (2.6)	[26]†
Compressive Strength (MPa)				384 (92)	[24]Cusp, c, ∥
				372 (56)	[24]Axial (side), c, ∥
		288 (48)		261 (41)	[22]Cusp, c,†
		253(35)		239 (30)	[22]Axial (side), c, ˆ
				94.5 (32)	[22]Axial (side), c, ∥
				127 (30)	[22]Occlusal, c, ∥
		220 (13)			[22]Incisal edge, c,†

c: compression; hyd: hydrated; dehyd: dehydrated; re-hyd: re-hydrated.
∥ Fracture or applied load approximately parallel to the long axis of the enamel rods.
ˆ Fracture or applied load approximately perpendicular to the long axis of the enamel rods.
† Applied load with respect to either the long axis of the enamel rods or dentinal tubules was variable.
‡ Type of tooth unknown or various teeth used for measurement; data are tabulated under molar.
Note: standard deviations are given in parentheses.

Table A3.9 Mechanical Properties of Human Dentin

	Incisors	*Canine*	*Pre-molars*	*Molars*	*Comments*
Stress at				167 (20.0)	[24]c
Proportional	124 (26)	140 (15)	146 (17)	148 (21)	[22]c
Limit (MPa)	86 (24)	112 (34)	110 (38)	108 (39)	[22]c
				110.5 (22.6)	[23]b, hyd., ‖
				167.3 (37.5)	[23]b, dehyd, ‖
				103.1 (16.8)	[23]b, re-hyd, ‖
				158 (32)	[17]
				154 (23)	[17]
Tensile				52 (10)	[26]hyd,†,‡
Strength				37.3 (13.6)	[23]hyd, ‖
(MPa)				34.5 (11.1)	[23]dehyd, ‖
				37.3 (9.0)	[23]re-hyd, ‖
				39.3 (7.4)	[21]hyd,†,‡
Compressive				297 (24.8)	[24]Crown
Strength	232 (21)	276 (72)	248 (10)	305 (59)	[22]Crown
(MPa)	233 (66)	217 (26)	231 (38)	250 (60)	[22]Root
				295 (21)	[23]Crown,‡
				251 (30)	[23]Crown,‡
Shear Strength (MPa)				134 (4.5)	[27]Oil, Cervical root, ^,‡
Flexural				165.6 (36.1)	[23]hyd, ‖
Strength				167.3 (37.5)	[23]dehyd, ‖
(MPa)				162.5 (25.4)	[23]re-hyd, ‖

hyd: hydrated; dehyd: dehydrated; re-hyd: re-hydrated
‖ Applied load approximately parallel to the long axis of the dentinal tubules
* Applied load approximately perpendicular to the long axis of the dentinal tubules;
‡ Type of tooth unknown or various teeth used for measurement; data are tabulated under molar;
† Applied load with respect to either the long axis of the dentinal tubules was variable.
‡ 95% confidence intervals.
Note: standard deviations are given in parentheses.

Table A3.10 Toughness, Fracture Toughness, and Work of Fracture of Human Dentin and Enamel

	Incisors	*Canine*	*Pre-molars*	*Molars*	*Source, comments*
Fracture Toughness, K_c ($MNm^{-3/2}$)					
					[28]*
Enamel	0.97(0.09)	1.00(0.23)			Maxillary, cervical,†
	1.27(0.09)			0.7(0.08)	Mandibular, cervical,†
Toughness (MJm^{-3})					
Dentin				62.7 (6.2)†	[27] Root, shear, oil storage, ˆ,‡
				2.4 (1.1)	[17]Tension, crown, hydr., ‖
Work of Fracture (10^2 Jm^{-2})					
Dentine			2.7 (1.6)		[29] ˆ
			5.5 (1.7)		[29] ‖
Enamel			1.9(0.56)		[29] ˆ
			0.13(.065)		[29] ‖

‖ Applied load approximately parallel to either the long axis of the enamel rods or dentinal tubules.
ˆ Applied load approximately perpendicular to either the long axis of the enamel rods or dentinal tubules.
† Applied load with respect to either the long axis of the enamel rods or dentinal tubules was variable.
‡ Type of tooth unknown or various teeth used for measurement; data are tabulated under molar.
* Microindentation method used. Load was 500 g with a Vickers' indenter.
Note: standard deviations are given in parentheses.

Table A3.11 Hardness of Fracture of Human Dentin and Enamel (see notes for units)

	Incisor	*Pre-molar*	*Molar*	*Source, comments*
Enamel	365 (35)			[30] >90% incisors,®,†
			393 (50)	[30]‡, molars and premolars,®,†
			385 (5.8)	[31]⊗,†,‡
		367 (17)		[32] ||,⊗, incisors, premolars
		327 (34)		[32]ˆ,⊗, incisors, premolars
Dentin				
.			25–81.7	[33]Δ, ||, [34][a]
			97.8	[33]a, calculated for zero tubule density
			44.5–80.9	[14]◊, ||, [34][a]
			100	[14]a, calculated for zero tubule density
			75 (0.8)	[31]⊗,†,‡

[a] Inverse correlation between hardness and dentinal tubule density.
|| Applied load approximately parallel to either the long axis of the enamel rods or dentinal tubules.
ˆ Applied load approximately perpendicular to either the long axis of the enamel rods or dentinal tubules.
† Applied load with respect to either the long axis of the enamel rods or dentinal tubules was variable.
‡ Type of tooth unknown or various teeth used for measurement; data are tabulated under molar.
* Microindentation method used. Load was 500 g with a Vickers' indenter.
® Knoop hardness test using 500 g load.
⊗ Knoop microhardness test using 50 g load.
Δ Knoop microhardness test using 100 g load.
◊ Microindentation method used. Load was 50 g with a Vickers' indenter.

Table A3.12 Permeability[a] of Human Dentin

Periphery ($\mu l\ cm^{-2}\ min^{-1}$)	*Center ($\mu l\ cm^{-2}\ min^{-1}$)*	*Source, comments*
36.4 (13.1)‡	14.3 (7.0)†	[33], unerupted third molars,

[a] Fluid filtration rate.
‡ Sound human dentin, average of 4 samples, 4 readings per sample.
† Sound human dentin, average of 4 samples, 1 reading per sample.

Table A3.13 Wetability of Human Enamel

Liquid	*Surface Tension, γLV (dynes/cm)*	*Contact Angle, θ (deg)* *In situ enamel*	*Ground enamel*	*Source Comments*
Polar				
Water	72.4 [35]	25.4 [36]†		
	72.8	36		[37]
	72.6		40.0 (0.1)	[38]* n=330
Glycerol	63.7 [35]	44.7 [36]†		
	63.4	55		[37]
	63.4		45.6 (0.2)	[38]* n=50
Formamide	58.5 [35]	28.0 [35]†		
	58.2	24		[36]
	58.2		37.6 (0.1)	[37]* n=50
Thiodiglycol	53.5 [34]	30.8 [36]†		
	54.0	43		[37]
	54.0		27.6 (0.2)	[38]* n=60
Non-polar				
Methylene iodide	51.7 [35]	48.6 [36]†		
	50.8	50		[37]
	50.8		38.1 (0.1)	[38] n=50
S-Tetrabromoethane	49.8 [35]	38.3 [36]†		
	47.5	40		[38]
1-Bromonaphthalene	44.6	34		[38]*, n=50
	44.6		16.1 (0.1)	
o-Dibromobenzene	42.0	22		[37]
Propylene carbonate	41.8 [35]	31.8 [36]†		
1-Methyl-naphthalene	38.7	20		[36]
Dicyclohexyl	32.7 [35]	12.2-spread		[37]
	33.0	7		[36]†
n-Hexadecane	27.6 [35]	spreading		[37]
	27.7	spreading		[36]†

* Plane ground enamel surfaces, measurements from 46 erupted and unerupted teeth, mixed location (molars, premolars, incisors). Parentheses: standard error

†: *in situ* contact angle measurements on human enamel, average of mean values for 4 teeth (maxillary or mandibular incisors).

Table A3.14 Wetability of Human Dentin [38]

Liquid	*Surface Tension, γ_{LV} (dynes/cm)*	*Ground Dentin Contact Angle, θ (deg)*	*Comments*
Polar			
Water	72.6	45.3 (0.2)	*, n=100
Glycerol	63.4	44.6 (0.1)	*, n=50
Formamide	58.2	37.6 (0.2)	*, n=50
Thiodiglycol	54.0	33.6 (0.3)	*, n=50
Non-polar			
Methylene iodide	50.8	36.7 (0.3)	*, n=50
1-bromo-naphthalene	49.8	16.8 (0.2)	*, n=50

* Plane ground dentin surfaces, measurements from 46 erupted and unerupted teeth, mixed location (molars, premolars, incisors). Parentheses: standard error.

Table A3.15 Critical Surface Tensions (γ_c) of Human Enamel and Dentin

	Critical Surface Tension, γ_c (dynes cm^{-1})	*Source, Comments*
Enamel		
Ground surface	46.1 (40.0 - 55.6)[a]	[38]*, calculated from polar and non-polar liquids
In situ enamel, γ_c^p	45.3 ± 70.2[b]	[39]Δ, calculated from polar liquids,
In situ enamel, γ_c^d	32.9 ± 4.7	[38]Δ, calculated from non-polar liquids
In situ enamel, γ_c^d	32	[37]†, calculated from non-polar liquids
Dentin		
	45.1 (40.7 - 51.1)[a]	[38]*, calculated from polar and non-polar liquids

[a] Range of values from different test liquids.
[b] Standard deviation.
* Plane ground dentin surfaces, measurements from 46 erupted and unerupted teeth, mixed location (molars, premolars, incisors). Parentheses: standard error.
Δ In situ measurements from 76 test subjects: 29 female and 47 male. Measurements made on teeth with intact pellicle (i.e., biofilm). γ_c^p only calculated from glycerol and thiodiglycol.
† Average of 4 teeth from 2 subjects. γ_c^d calculated from non-polar liquids.

A3.3 FINAL COMMENTS

The quality of data presented can be inferred from the standard deviations or standard error associated with the mean values. In some cases the error can be attributed to either small sample populations or specimen preparation. Where possible, either the number of specimens used or the number of replications of a measurement was reported. The reader should use this information as a guideline of the quality of data. When data are reported for small sample populations, then these data were usually the only source for a given physical property. In review of the literature, specimen preparation appears to have had the most influence on the precision and accuracy of data. Sample collection and storage conditions (e.g., dehydration, crosslinking agents, exogenous contamination) need to be taken into consideration when utilizing the information tabulated. Additional sources of error are dependent on the analytical technique or test method used to make the measurement. It is more difficult to discern the influence of the instrumentation on the reliability of the measurements. However, confidence of the accuracy was judged based on the use of adequate control samples with known physical properties (e.g., correction of mechanical data). In light of these comments, data in the literature were deemed most accurate and appropriate for this handbook when the following conditions were met: the sample population was large; non-destructive specimen preparation and storage conditions were used; and, multiple replications of measurements on a single sample were performed.

There are significant omissions in the data available in the literature. Most notable, is the lack of quantitative analysis of the organic phase of dentin and enamel, and determination of the viscoelastic properties of dentin. The lack of data is attributed to the technical difficulty required to make such measurements and the heterogeneous nature of the dentin, which imparts large variations in these data depending on anatomical location. Other significance absences are the lack of electrical and thermal properties. Finally, vacancies in the tables provided demonstrate omissions in available data.

ADDITIONAL READING

Carter, J.M., Sorensen, S.E., Johnson, R.R., Teitelbaum, R.L. and Levine, M.S. (1983) Punch Shear Testing of Extracted Vital and Endodontically Treated Teeth. *J. Biomechanics* **16(10)**, 841–848.

Utilized a miniature punch shear apparatus to determine shear strength and toughness perpendicular to the direction of dentinal tubules. Dentin harvested from the cemento–enamel junction to one-third the distance to the root apex. Strengths: novel measurements, precise measurements, defined specimen location, defined orientation of testing. Limitations: tooth type not defined for 'constrained' tests, teeth stored in mineral oil prior to testing.

Driessens, F.C.M., and Verbeeck, R.M.H. (1990a) The Mineral in Tooth Enamel and Dental Carries. In *Biominerals*, F.C.M and Verbeeck, R.M.H. (eds), CRC Press, Boca Raton, Florida, pp. 105–161.

Driessens, F.C.M., and Verbeeck, R.M.H. (1990b) Dentin, Its Mineral and Caries, In *Biominerals*, F.C.M and Verbeeck, R.M.H. (eds), CRC Press, Boca Raton, Florida, pp. 163–178.

An authoritative text on biominerals with an excellent review of the properties of enamel and dentin. An excellent supplement to this handbook.

Glantz, P-O. (1969) On Wetability and Adhesiveness. *Odontologisk Revy*, **20 supp. 17**, 1–132.

Comprehensive assessment of the wetability of human enamel and dentin. Strengths include using multiple probe liquids on numerous teeth.

Korostoff, E., Pollack, S.R., and Duncanson, M.G. (1975) Viscoelastic Properties of Human Dentin. *J. Biomedical Materials Res.*, **9**, 661–674.

Measured some viscoelastic properties of human radicular dentin under constant strain. Linear viscoelastic theory applied. Strengths: unique examination of viscoelastic properties, defined orientation of dentinal tubules, storage conditions and testing environment well controlled. Limitations: large scatter in $H_1(t)$, mixed data for different teeth.

Marshall, G.W. (1993) Dentin: Microstructure and Characterization. *Quintessence International*, **24(9)**, 606–616.

A Review of the microstructure and characterization of dentin.

Waters, N.E. (1980) Some Mechanical and Physical Properties of Teeth. *Symposia of the Society for Experimental Biology*, **34**, 99–135.

Concise review of mechanical and physical properties of teeth. Good paper for anatomy of enamel and dentin.

REFERENCES

1. Waters, N.E. (1980) Some mechanical and physical properties of teeth. *Symp. Soc. Exp. Biol.*, **34,** 99–135.
2. Driessens, F.C.M. and Verbeeck, R.M.H. (1990) The mineral in tooth enamel and dental caries. In: *Biominerals*, F.C.M. and Verbeeck, R.M.H. (eds), CRC Press, Boca Raton, Florida, pp. 105–161.
3. Driessens, F.C.M. and Verbeeck, R.M.H. (1990) Dentin, its mineral and caries, In: *Biominerals*, Driessens, F.C.M. and Verbeeck, R.M.H. (eds), CRC Press, Boca Raton, Florida, pp. 163–178.
4. Söremark, R. and Samsahl, K. (1961) Gamma-ray spectrometric analysis of elements in normal human enamel. *Arch. Oral. Bio., Special Suppl.*, **6,** 275–283.
5. Derise, N.L., Ritchey, S.J. and Furr, A.K. (1974) Mineral composition of normal human enamel and dentin and the relation of composition to dental caries: I Macrominerals and comparison of methods of analyses. *J. Dental Res.*, **53(4),** 847–852.
6. LeGeros, R.Z., Silverstone, L.M., Daculsi, G. *et al.* (1983) *In vitro* caries-like lesion formation in F-containing tooth enamel. *J. Dental Res.*, **62(2),** 138–144.
7. Lakomaa, E-L. and Rytömaa, I. (1977) Mineral composition of enamel and dentin of primary and permanent teeth in Finland. *Scand. J. Dent. Res.*, **85,** 89–95.
8. Cutress, T.W. (1979) A preliminary study of the microelement composition of the outer layer of dental enamel. *Caries Res.*, **13,** 73–79.
9. Losee, F.L., Cutress, T.W. and Brown, R. (1974) Natural elements of the periodic table in human dental enamel. *Caries Res.*, **8,** 123–134.

10. Retief, D.H., Cleaton-Jones, P.E., Turkstra, J. *et al.* (1971) The quantitative analysis of sixteen elements in normal human enamel and dentine by neutron activation analysis and high-resolution gamma-spectrometry. *Arch. Oral Bio.*, **16,** 1257–1267.
11. Curzon, M.E.J. and Losee, F.L. (1977) Dental caries and trace element composition of whole human enamel: Eastern United States. *J. Amer. Dental Assoc.*, **94,** 1146–1150.
12. Curzon, M.E.J. and Losee, F.L. (1978) Dental caries and trace element composition of whole human enamel: Western United States. *J. Amer. Dental Assoc.*, **96,** 819–822.
13. Kodaka, T., Debari, K., Yamada, M. *et al.* (1992) Correlation between microhardness and mineral content in sound human enamel. *Caries Res.*, **26,** 139–141.
14. Panighi, M. and G'Sell, C. (1992) Influence of calcium concentration on the dentin wetability of an adhesive. *J. Biomed. Mater. Res.*, **26,** 1081–1089.
15. Holcomb, D.W. and Young, R.A. (1980) Thermal decomposition of human tooth enamel. *Calcif. Tiss. Intern.*, **31,** 189–201
16. Sakae, T. (1988) X-Ray diffraction and thermal studies of crystals from the outer and inner layers of human dental enamel. *Archs. Oral Bio.*, **33(10),** 707–713.
17. Huang, T.-J.G., Schilder, H. and Nathanson, D. (1992) Effects of moisture content and endodontic treatment on some mechanical properties of human dentin. *J. Endodontics*, **18(5),** 209–215
17. Kerebel, B, Daculsi, G. and Kerebel, L.M. (1979) Ultrastructure studies of enamel crystallites. *J. Dental Res.*, **58(B),** 844–851.
18. Jervøe, P. and Madsen, H.E.L. (1974) Calcium phosphates with apatite structure. I. Precipitation at different temperatures. *Acta Chem. Scand.*, **A28,** 477–481.
19. Daculsi, G., Kerebel, B. and Verbaere, A (1978). (Méthode de mesure des cristaux d'apatite de la dentine humanie en microscopie électronique en transmission de Haute Résolution)(Fr.)(Method of measurement of apatite crystals in human dentin by high resolution transmission electron microscopy), *Comptes Rendu Acad. Sci. Paris*, Sér. D., **286,** 1439.
20. Voegel, J.C. and Frank, R.M. (1977) Ultrastructural study of apatite crystal dissolution in human dentine and bone. *Jour. Biol. Buccale*, **5,** 181–194.
21. Lehman, M.L. (1963) Tensile strength of human dentin. *J. Dent. Res.*, **46(1),** 197–201.
22. Stanford, J.W., Weigel, K.V., Paffenbarger, G.C. *et al.* (1960) Compressive properties of hard tooth tissues and some restorative materials. *J. American Dental Assoc.*, **60,** 746–756.
23. Jameson, M.W., Hood, J.A.A. and Tidmarsh, B.G. (1993) The effects of dehydration and rehydration on some mechanical properties of human dentine. *J. Biomech.*, **26(9),** 1055–1065.
24. Craig, R.G., Peyton, F.A. and Johnson, D.W. (1961) Compressive properties of enamel, dental cements, and gold. *J. Dent. Res.*, **40(5),** 936–945.
25. Korostoff, E., Pollack, S.R. and Duncanson, M.G. (1975) Viscoelastic properties of human dentin. *J. Biomed. Mater. Res.*, **9,** 661–674.
26. Bowen, R.L. and Rodriguez, M.S. (1962) Tensile strength and modulus of elasticity of Tooth Structure and Several Restorative Materials. *J. American Dental Assoc.*, **64,** 378–387.

27. Carter, J.M., Sorensen, S.E., Johnson, R.R., *et al.* (1983) Punch shear testing of extracted vital and endodontically treated teeth. *J. Biomech.*, **16(10),** 841–848.
28. Hassan, R., Caputo, A.A. and Bunshah, R.F. (1981) Fracture toughness of human enamel. *J. Dent. Res.*, **60(4),** 820–827.
29. Rasmussen, S.T., Patchin, R.E., Scott, D.B. *et al.* (1976) Fracture properties of human enamel and dentin. *J. Dent. Res.*, **55(1),** 154–164.
30. Caldwell, R.C., Muntz, M.L., Gilmore, R.W. *et al.* (1957) Microhardness studies of intact surface enamel. *J. Dent. Res.*, **36(5),** 732–738.
31. Remizov, S.M., Prujansky, L.Y. and Matveevsky, R.M. (1991) Wear resistance and microhardness of human teeth. *Proc. Inst. Mech. Eng., Part H: J. Eng. in Med.*, **205(3),** 201–202.
32. Davidson, C.L., Hoekstra, I.S. and Arends, J. (1974) Microhardness of sound, decalcified and etched tooth enamel related to the calcium content. *Caries Res.*, **8,** 135–144.
33. Pashley, D.H., Andringa, H.J., Derkson, G.D. *et al.* (1987) Regional variability in the permeability of human dentin. *Arch. Oral Biol.*, **32(7),** 519–523.
34. Pashley, D.H., Okabe, A. and Parham, P. (1985) The Relationship between dentin microhardness and tubule density. *Endod. Dent. Traumatol.*, **1,** 176–179.
35. Baier, R.E. and Zisman, W.A. (1975) Wetting properties of collagen and gelatin surfaces, *in* 'Applied Chemistry at Protein Interfaces', vol. 145, Advances in Chemistry series (ed. R.F. Gould), American Chemical Society, Washington DC, pp. 155–174.
36. Jendresen, M.D., Baier, R.E. and Glantz, P-O. (1984) Contact angles in a biological setting: Measurements in the human oral cavity. *J. Coll. Interface Sci.*, **100(1),** 233–238.
37. Baier, R.E. (1973) Occurrence, nature, and extent of cohesive and adhesive forces in dental integuments. in: *Surface Chemistry and Dental Integument's.* Lasslo, A. and Quintana, R.P. (eds), Thomas, Springfield, IL pp. 337–391.
38. Glantz, P-O. (1969) On wetability and adhesiveness. *Odontologisk Revy*, **20 supp. 17,** 1–132.
39. Jendresen, M.D. and Glantz, P-O. (1980) Clinical adhesiveness of the tooth surface. *Acta Odontol. Scand.*, **38,** 379–383.

B1 Cartilage

J.R. Parsons

B1.1 INTRODUCTION

B1.1.1 Articular cartilage

Articular or hyaline cartilage forms the bearing surfaces of the movable joints of the body. Hyaline cartilage also exists in tissues of the larynx, tracheal tube rings, rib and costral cartilage, nasal septum and in the growth plates of long bones. As a bearing surface, this tough, resilient tissue displays exceptional mechanical and tribologic properties due exclusively to the unique interaction of the constituents of the tissue extracellular matrix. Usually, the phenotypic cells (chondrocytes) of cartilage make up less than 10% of the total volume of the tissue and have not been considered to contribute to the mechanical properties of the tissue. The extracellular matrix consists of a tight collagen fiber network which contains and constrains a highly hydrophilic gel of aggregated proteoglycan macromolecules. Collagen accounts for approximately 50% of the dry weight of the tissue, the remainder being proteoglycans and cellular material. In the fully hydrated state, water contributes 60% to 80% of the wet weight of the tissue. Mechanically, intact normal articular cartilage behaves as a linear viscoelastic solid. This behavior is the result of viscous drag of fluid through the tissue in concert with the intrinsic properties of the extracellular matrix. Further, fluid exudation across the cartilage surface in response to physiologic loading is thought to play a significant role in the lubrication of joints. The importance of articular cartilage as a bearing surface has led to extensive mechanical and tribologic studies of this tissue.

Handbook of Biomaterial Properties. Edited by J. Black and G. Hastings.
Published in 1998 by Chapman & Hall, London. ISBN 0 412 60330 6.

B1.1.2 Fibrocartilage

Fibrocartilage contains a higher dry weight percentage of collagen and less proteoglycan than does articular cartilage. Consequently, in the hydrated state, fibrocartilage contains less water. Fibrocartilage is generally considered to be tougher and somewhat less resilient than articular cartilage. In humans, fibrocartilage is found in the meniscus of the knee joint, the annulus fibrosus of the intervertebral disc and in the tempero-mandibular joint. The mechanical behavior of fibrocartilage has not been studied to the extent of articular cartilage; however, it is not as satisfactory a load bearing material.

B1.1.3 Elastic cartilage

Elastic cartilage is more elastic and resilient in nature than is either hyaline or fibrocartilage. This is the result of lower collagen content coupled with the presence of elastin fibers. Elastic cartilage is found in the human epiglottis, external ear structures and eustachian tube. As elastic cartilage is not a major structural component of the musculoskeletal system, the mechanical properties of this tissue have been largely ignored.

B1.2 COMPOSITION

Table B1.1 Cartilage Composition

	Water (wt%)	*Organic (wt%)*	*Source*
Articular Cartilage	60–80	20–40	[1]
Type II Collagen	—	15–20	
Other collagen	—	<2	
Proteoglycan	—	10	
Fibrocartilage	74	26	[2]
Type I Collagen	—	20	
Other collagen	—	<1	
Proteoglycan		<1	

B1.3 MECHANICAL PROPERTIES OF ARTICULAR CARTILAGE

B1.3.1 Compression (Table B1.2)

Compressive cartilage properties have often been examined using creep indentation, confined compression or free/unconfined compression methods. Indentation techniques permit in situ testing without the necessity of

Table B1.2 Compressive Properties of Articular Cartilage

Location	*Value (MPa)*	*Source*
	Unrelaxed (initial):	
	Creep modulus (indentation):	
Femoral head	1.9–14.4	[7]
	Young's modulus (indentation):	
Patella	2.25	[8]
	Young's Modulus (confined compression):	
Tibial plateau	5.1–7.9*	[9]
	11.6*	[6]
	Bulk Modulus (confined compression):	
Tibial plateau	31–56	[9]
	25*	[6]
	Young's Modulus (unconfined compression):	
Various	8.4–15.3	[7]
	Relaxed (equilibrium):	
	Aggregate modulus (Indentation):	
Patella	0.3–0.6	[4]
	0.3–1.5	[10]
Femoral condyle	0.4–1.0	[10]
	0.5–0.7	[11]
Carpo-metacarpal joint	0.4–0.8	[12]
	Young's modulus (confined compression):	
Patella	0.7	[8]
Tibial plateau	0.7*	[6]
	Bulk modulus (confined compression):	
Tibial plateau	9.1*	[6]

* Calculated from other measurements.

special specimen preparation as with tensile testing. However, the extraction of intrinsic mechanical parameters from creep indentation data is analytically complex [3, 4]. Confined compression or unconfined compression tests require preparation of cylindrical cored specimens of tissue and underlying bone. With unconfined compression, the free draining tissue edges and low aspect ratio, layered nature of the test specimen may introduce error. Compression of a laterally confined specimen by a porous plunger produces uniaxial deformation and fluid flow. Confined compression creep data has been analyzed to yield an aggregate equilibrium compressive modulus and permeability coefficient [5] and uniaxial creep compliance [6].

B1.3.2 Tensile (Table B1.3)

Tensile properties for human articular have been determined by cutting standard tensile specimens from the cartilage surface and performing constant strain rate, creep or stress relaxation tensile tests. Test results are strongly influenced by collagen volume fraction and orientation and

Table B1.3 Tensile Properties of Articular Cartilage

Location	*Value (MPa)**	*Source*
	Relaxed (equilibrium):	
	Young's modulus:	[13]
Femoral condyle,		
Surface zone	10.5	
Subsurface zone	5.5	
Middle zone	3.7	
	Unrelaxed (100%/min):	
	Young's modulus:	[7]
Femoral condyle,		
Surface zone	200–400	
Middle zone	40–175	
	Strength:	[7]
Femoral condyle,		
Surface zone	20–35	
Middle zone	11–25	

* All measurements parallel to collagen direction.

are largely insensitive to proteoglycan content [7] Collagen volume fraction and orientation is highest in the cartilage surface layer. Collagen content and orientation diminishes in subsequent lower layers.

B1.3.3 Shear (Table B1.4)

Shear properties for articular cartilage have been determined through torsional creep, stress relaxation and torsional dynamic tests of excised cartilage disks. Creep and dynamic shearing of rectangular cartilage specimens between plates has been conducted on animal tissue (usually bovine) but not human tissue. When torsional shear strains remain small, the observed shear properties are flow independent. That is, under small strain conditions, fluid flow is negligible and viscoelastic behavior can be attributed strictly to the collagen/proteoglycan extracellular matrix.

Table B1.4 Shear Properties of Articular Cartilage

Location	*Value (MPa)*	*Source*
	Relaxed (equilibrium):	
	Shear modulus:	
Patella,		
Middle zone	0.25	[14]
Tibial plateau	2.6	[6]
	Unrelaxed (initial):	
	Shear modulus:	
Tibial plateau	4.1	[6]
	5.1–7.9	[9]

B1.3.4 Poisson's ratio

Poisson's ratio has been calculated directly from tensile tests (ν = 0.37–0.50) [10] and indirectly from torsional shear and confined compression creep data (ν = 0.37–0.47) [6, 9]. More recently, the relationship between Poisson's ratio, n, aggregate modulus, Ha, and permeability, k, have been established for cartilage indentation testing based on biphasic (fluid and porous solid) constitutive theory [15]. Using a complex numerical solution and curve fitting scheme, Poisson's ratio can be extracted from indentation data, resulting in values of ν = 0.00–0.30 [11, 12, 16]. However, care must be exercised in interpreting such indirect measures of Poisson's ratio as unexpected results can arise; e.g. ν = 0.0.

B1.3.5 Permeability

The porous solid matrix of articular cartilage permits the movement of interstitial water in response to a pressure gradient. Flow of water through and across the tissue is largely responsible for the viscoelastic character of cartilage. Flow is related to tissue permeability through the hydraulic permeability coefficient, k, as defined by Darcy's law. The permeability coefficient has been measured in flow chambers where a known pressure gradient produces flow across a cartilage layer of known thickness and area (k = 4.0 - 17.0 $\times$ 10^{-16} m^4/Ns)[7]. However, such experiments have demonstrated significant decreases in permeability coefficient with increasing pressure gradient, increasing compressive tissue strain and with increasing proteoglycan content. Evoking biphasic constitutive theory with numerical solutions and/or curve fitting routines permits an indirect determination of the permeability coefficient from confined compression creep data and creep indentation data (k = 5.2 - 21.7 $\times$ 10^{-16} m^4/Ns)[11,12].

B1.3.6 Articular cartilage tribologic properties

Healthy articular cartilage has remarkable tribologic properties. Under high load conditions the tissue displays extremely low frictional coefficients and virtually undetectable wear. The dynamic coefficient of friction, μ_d, has been measured in whole joints using Stanton pendulum or other pendulum techniques where the joint forms the pendulum pivot (μ_d = 0.015–0.04)[17–19]. The coefficients of friction of cartilage plugs bearing on other materials has been determined for human and animal tissue but these sorts of experiments have little relevance for actual in situ cartilage behavior and are not reported here.

The lubrication of articular cartilage remains a subject of continuing debate and no one lubrication mechanism can be clearly identified. Both fluid film and boundary lubrication are thought to play primary roles in joint lubrication and the dominance of one or the other probably depends on loading and velocity conditions. Further as cartilage is a relatively soft viscoelastic material, elastohydrodynamics may discourage fluid film breakdown and thus promote hydrodynamic lubrication. Exudation of fluid across the cartilage surface in response to an advancing load has also been suggested to aid lubrication.

No reliable wear tests have been performed on human articular cartilage bearing surfaces under physiologic conditions.

B1.4 FIBROCARTILAGE MECHANICAL PROPERTIES

Human fibrocartilage tensile mechanical properties have been determined by cutting standard tensile specimens either from the knee meniscus or from single or multiple lamella from the annulus fibrosus and performing constant strain rate tensile tests. Test results are strongly influenced by collagen volume fraction and orientation and are largely insensitive to proteoglycan content. Annulus fibrosus has also been tested in confined compression, permitting derivation of an aggregate compressive modulus and permeability. Data are reported in Section B2.

B1.5 ELASTIC CARTILAGE MECHANICAL PROPERTIES

No reliable data are available for human tissue.

ADDITIONAL READING

Freeman, MAR (ed.) (1979) *Adult Articular Cartilage*, 2nd ed., Pitman Medical Publishing Co, Kent, UK.

Although now somewhat out of date, this classic text forms the basis for current thinking on cartilage biochemistry, physiochemistry, biomechanics and tribology. The volume of original data, found nowhere else, is truly impressive.

Mow V.C., Holmes, M.H. and Lai, W.M. (1984): Fluid transport and mechanical properties of articular cartilage. A review. *J. Biomech.*, 17:377–394.

This survey article provides an historical perspective of cartilage mechanics research and leads the reader through the modern biphasic theory of cartilage mechanics at the material level. References provided are particularly useful in developing a bibliography of the important classic studies in this field.

Mow, V.C. and Ratcliffe, A (eds)(1993): *Structure and Function of Articular Cartilage*, CRC Press, Boca Raton.

This up-to-date monograph is perhaps the best current work on the subject. Details from many of the references in this section (below) can be found in the section on cartilage biomechanics.

REFERENCES

1. Maroudas, A. (1979) Physiochemical properties of articular cartilage. in *Adult Articular Cartilage*, 2nd ed., M.A.R. Freeman (ed.), Pitman Medical Publishing Co, Kent, UK, pp. 215–290.
2. Fithian, D.C., Kelly, M.A. and Mow, V.C. (1990) Material properties and structure–function relationships in the menisci. *Clin. Orthop. Rel. Res.*, **252,** 19–31.
3. Mak, A., Lai, W.M. and Mow, V.C. (1987) Biphasic indentation of articular cartilage: Part I, Theoretical analysis. *J. Biomech.*, **20,** 703–714.
4. Mow, V., Gibbs, M.C. and Lai, W.M., *et al.* (1989) Biphasic indentation of articular cartilage: Part II, A numerical algorithm and experimental study. *J. Biomech.*, **22,** 853–861.
5. Mow, V., Kuei, S.C. and Lai, W.M. (1980) Biphasic creep and stress relaxation of articular cartilage in compression: Theory and experiments. *J. Biomech, Eng.*, **102,** 73–84.
6. Hayes, W. and Mockros, L.F. (1971) Viscoelastic properties of human articular cartilage. *J. Appl. Physiol.*, **31,** 562–568.
7. Kempson, G. (1979) Mechanical properties of articular cartilage. In *Adult Articular Cartilage*, 2nd ed., Freeman M.A.R., Editor, Pitman Medical Publishing Co. Ltd., Kent, England, pp. 333–414.
8. Sokoloff, L. (1966) Elasticity of aging cartilage. *Fed. Proc.*, **25,** 1089–1095.
9. Hori, R. and Mockros, L.F. (1976) Indentation tests of human articular cartilage. *J. Biomech.*, **9,** 259–268.
10. Armstrong, C. and Mow, V.C. (1982) Variations in the intrinsic mechanical properties of human articular cartilage with age, degeneration and water content. *J. Bone Joint Surg.*, **64A,** 88–94.
11. Athanasiou, K., Rosenwasser, M.P., and Buckwalter, J.A., *et al.* (1991) Interspecies comparison of in situ intrinsic mechanical properties of distal femoral cartilage. *J. Orthop. Res.*, **9,** 330–340.
12. Ateshian, G., Gardner, J.R., Saed-Nejad, F. *et al.* (1993) Material properties and biochemical composition of thumb carpometacarpal joint cartilage. *Trans. Orthop. Res. Soc.*, **18,** 323.
13. Akizuki, S., Mow, V.C. and Muller, F., *et al.* (1986) Tensile properties of human knee joint cartilage: Part I, Influence of ionic concentrations, weight bearing and fibrillation on the tensile modulus. *J. Orthop. Res.*, **4,** 379–392.
14. Zhu, W., Lai, W.M. and Mow, V.C. (1986) Intrinsic quasilinear viscoelastic behavior of the extracellular matrix of cartilage. *Trans. Orthop. Res. Soc.*, **11,** 407.
15. Mak, A. (1986) The apparent viscoelastic behavior of articular cartilage – The contributions from the intrinsic matrix viscoelasticity and interstitial fluid flows. *J. Biomech. Eng.*, **108,** 123–130.
16. Akizuki, S., Mow, V.C., Lai, W.M., *et al.* (1986) Topographical variation of the biphasic indentation properties of human tibial plateau cartilage. *Trans. Orthop. Res. Soc.*, **11,** 406.
17. Charnley, J. (1960) The lubrication of animal joints in relation to surgical reconstructions by arthroplasty. *Ann. Rheum. Dis.*, **19,** 10–19.

18. Little, J., Freeman, M.A.R., and Swanson, S.V. (1969) Experience on friction in the human joint. In *Lubrication and Wear in Joints*, Wright V., Editor, Sector Publishing, London, UK., pp. 110–114.
19. Unsworth, A., Dawson, D. and Wright, V. (1975) Some new evidence on human joint lubrication. *Ann. Rheum. Dis.*, **34,** 277–285.

B2 Fibrocartilage

V.M. Gharpuray

B2.1 INTRODUCTION

The human menisci and intervertebral discs perform several important mechanical functions in the human body. The ability to perform these functions and consequently their intrinsic biomechanical properties are dependent on the interaction of the constituents of these structures. Both the menisci and intervertebral discs have a fibrocartilaginous structure that consists of two distinct phases: a fluid phase consisting of mainly water and dissolved electrolytes, and a solid phase composed of highly oriented collagen fibers, cells, proteoglycans and other proteins. As with all other biological materials, both menisci and discs exhibit non-linear viscoelastic and anisotropic properties. The non-linear stiffness or elasticity of the structure is imparted by the collagen fibers and to a lesser extent by osmotic pressures within the tissue which are generated by the degree of hydration [1, 2]. The viscoelastic or energy dissipation properties are a result of fluid flow within and through the structures and also of molecular relaxation effects from the motion of long chains of collagen and proteoglycans [3]. Anisotropy is a consequence of the orientation and concentration of collagen fibers within the proteoglycan gel.

B2.2 STRUCTURE AND COMPOSITION

A normal adult human knee contains two menisci – the lateral and the medial, whose average lengths are 38 and 45 mm, and average volumes are 2.9 and 3.45 cm^3 respectively [4]. At the femoral articulating surface

Handbook of Biomaterial Properties. Edited by J. Black and G. Hastings.
Published in 1998 by Chapman & Hall, London. ISBN 0 412 60330 6.

of each meniscus, for a depth of approximately 100 μm, fine collagen fibrils (mainly Type II) are randomly oriented to form a woven mesh [5, 6]. Beneath this surface layer, larger rope-like bundles (approximately 100 μm in diameter) of Type I collagen are arranged predominantly in the circumferential direction. In the posterior half of the medial meniscus however, the fibers are not as highly oriented [6, 7]. A few radial fibers may also be seen interspersed within the circumferential fibers [6–8]. At the tibial surface is another articulating layer, in which the principal orientation of the fibers is radial.

Collagen and other proteins make up the organic content of the meniscus, while dissolved electrolytes make up the inorganic content (which is negligibly small). The collagen is primarily Type I (98%) with small amounts of Type II, III and Type V [9], and comprises up to 25% of the wet weight and 90% of the dry weight in human material (Table B2.1). 10% of the dry weight and up to 2% of the wet weight are due to non-collagenous proteins, which consist predominantly of proteoglycans, and smaller amounts of structural glycoproteins, cell membrane bound receptors and intercalated membrane glycoproteins. These proportions do not appear to vary with location in the menisci [10].

There are 23, approximately cylindrical, intervertebral discs in the human spine that account for 20–30% of its overall length [13]. The cross sectional shape varies with level: roughly elliptical, rounded triangular and kidney shaped in the cervical, thoracic and lumbar regions respectively [14]. The cross sectional shape is sometimes quantified by a shape index (S) defined by $S = 4\pi A/C^2$ where A = cross sectional area, and C = circumference of the cross section (Table B2.2). Most discs are wedge-shaped in sagittal section with the anterior height greater that the posterior height. The cross sectional area increases with level such that lumbar discs are larger than cervical discs.

The intervertebral disc contains two distinct regions, the nucleus pulposus and the annulus fibrosus. The nucleus occupies about 50% of the volume of the disc, and contains mostly water and small amounts of randomly oriented collagen fibers, cells and non-collagenous proteins [19]. The annulus is a tough ring-like structure that surrounds the nucleus. Highly oriented collagen fibers (primarily Types I and II) form a laminate structure in the annulus, with approximately 20–25 laminae oriented alternately at

Table B2.1 Composition of the menisci

Wet weight			*Dry weight*	
Water	Collagen	NCP*	Collagen	NCP
60–70%[a]	15–25%[a]	1–2%[a]	70–90%[a,b]	8–20%[b,c‡]

* NCP = non-collagenous proteins; ‡ 21.9% in neonates decreasing to 8.1% between 30–70 years. a: [8];b: [11];c: [12].

Table B2.2 Shape and size of the adult intervertebral disc

Disc Level	*Shape Index (S^a)*	*Posterior/Anterior Height[a]*	*Cross Sectional Area (mm^2)*	*Height (mm)*
L5-S1	0.885	0.35		
L4-L5	0.897	0.51	1714[b]	11–12[b,c]
L3-L4	0.866	0.55	1662[b]	10.4[b]
L2-L3	0.866	0.61	1859[b]	9.75[b]
L1-L2	0.825	0.68	1640[b]	8.83[b]
T12-L1	0.844	0.75		
T11-T12	0.856	0.80		
T10-T11	0.885	1.11		
T9-T10	0.879	0.74		
T8-T9	0.919	0.88		4–6[c]
T7-T8	0.878	0.81		
T6-T7	0.898	0.84		
T5-T6	0.935	1.07		
T4-T5	0.868	0.97		
T3-T4	0.836	0.72		
T2-T3	0.870	0.74		
T1-T2	0.815	0.76		
C7-T1	0.785	0.62	1292*	6.00[d]
C6-C7	0.708	0.82	1152*	5.67[d]
C5-C6	0.828	0.44	949*	5.50[d]
C4-C5	0.825	0.47	892*	5.25[d]
C3-C4	0.870	0.50	827*	5.00[d]
C2-C3	0.893	0.56	732*	4.75[d]

* Computed from data in [18]. a: [13];b: [15,16];c: [17];d: [18].

approximately +(60–70)° and -(60–70)° to the spinal axis [14, 20, 21]). Type IX collagen is believed to cross link the Types I and II fibers, and provide some resistance to circumferential tears. Collagen content and fiber orientation is highest in the outermost layers, and both decrease as the nucleus is approached from the periphery of the disc (Table B2.3) The water content in the disc varies with position in the disc: it is highest in the nucleus and lowest in the outermost layers of the annulus [22, 23]. It has also been shown that the water content varies with circumferential position [4], and is higher in the posterior of the disc. The nucleus loses water and becomes more fibrous and desiccated with age, causing the boundary between the annulus and the nucleus to become less clear [19, 23].

Table B2.3 Composition of the intervertebral disc in young adults

Tissue	*Water Content %*	*Collagen Content %*
Nucleus Pulposus	85–95[a]	2–5[b]
Annulus Fibrosus	85 (innermost layer)	5 (innermost layer)
	65 (outermost layer)	21 (outermost layer)

a: [23]; b: [24].

B2.3 HYDRAULIC PERMEABILITY AND DRAG COEFFICIENTS

Experimental data suggest that water is capable of flowing through both meniscal and discal tissues, and is dependent on a material property of the tissue called hydraulic permeability [25], which may be modeled by Darcy's Law as:

$$Q = k \frac{A \, \Delta P}{h} \tag{B2.1}$$

where k = hydraulic permeability coefficient of the tissue; Q = volume rate of fluid flow; A = area across which fluid flow occurs; h = thickness of the tissue; and ΔP = pressure gradient across the thickness h that causes fluid flow.

The diffusive drag coefficient K is related to the permeability coefficient by

$$K = \frac{(\phi^f)^2}{k} \tag{B2.2}$$

where ϕf is the porosity of the tissue and is defined as the ratio of interstitial fluid volume to total tissue volume.

For human meniscal (annulus) tissue, k, the permeability is 2.5×10^{-16} m^4/Ns [22], about one third of that reported for bovine tissue: 8.1×10^{-16} m^4/Ns [26]. There is no significant variation in the permeability coefficient with location of the specimen. The porosity (ϕf) of both tissues is approximately 0.75, and therefore the drag coefficient, K, is very high and ranges from 10^{14} to 10^{15} Ns/m^4.

B2.4 ELASTIC PROPERTIES

Under quasi-static loading, or in conditions under which 'short-term' loading responses are expected to occur [27], both meniscal and discal tissues may be modeled as linear elastic and orthotropic. Under a constant load rate, the non-linear behavior may be described by an exponential stress–strain relationship given by

$$\sigma = A[e^{B\epsilon} - 1] \tag{B2.3}$$

where A and B are constants for the given material. The constant B is proportional to the tangent modulus (i.e., $d\sigma/d\epsilon$), and sometimes a third constant C is defined as $C = A*B$, and is the tangent modulus as $\sigma \rightarrow 0$ [8].

The macroscopic tensile strength of the entire meniscus was studied by Mathur *et al.* [4] by gripping the horns of the meniscus, and stretching it to failure. The results suggested that the medial meniscus was significantly weaker than the lateral meniscus (ultimate loads of 247 N and 329 N respectively), and that the mode of failure was not by transverse cracking, but predominantly by oblique (medial) or spiral (lateral) tearing.

Strength and modulus of the meniscus vary with different locations and with different orientations of the specimen due to structural and compositional changes (Table B2.4). For loading parallel to the fibers, it appears that the meniscus may be stronger in the anterior location, and that the lateral meniscus may be stronger than the medial meniscus. This may be explained in part by the fact that the fiber orientation is more random in the posterior part of the medial meniscus.

A similar trend is seen in the tensile modulus of meniscal specimens oriented parallel to the circumferential direction (Table B.2.5), and if a power law is used as the constitutive equation (equation B2.3), the coefficients A and C show an identical pattern [7, 10, 28].

The properties of intervertebral discs are more complex than those of the menisci, since properties vary with disc level, and discs must withstand loads and moments in three orthogonal directions. (Table B2.6).

As with the meniscus, strength and modulus of discal tissue vary with location and orientation of the specimen (Table B2.7). Lin *et al.* [15, 16] have however shown that elastic moduli of annular specimens are independent of disc level.

Table B2.4 Tensile strength of meniscal tissue (MPa)[a,*]

		Location		
Meniscus	*Orientation†*	*Anterior*	*Central*	*Posterior*
Lateral	Parallel	10.37	6.31	6.87
	Perpendicular	0.80	0.88	0.54
Medial	Parallel	—	3.36	5.86
	Perpendicular	—	0.85	1.23

a: Averaged from data in [6].
* Tissues were fixed in formalin before testing.
† Either parallel or perpendicular to the circumferential direction.

Table B2.5 Non-linear parameters and tensile modulus of menisci

Meniscus	*Location*	*A*	*B*	*C*	*Tensile modulusa (MPa)*
Medial	Anterior	1.6	28.4	42.4	159.6
	Central	0.9	27.3	23.7	93.2
	Posterior	1.4	20.1	25.2	110.2
Lateral	Anterior	1.4	28.8	30.2	159.1
	Central	2.1	31.9	55.7	228.8
	Posterior	3.2	27.5	67.5	294.1

a: Slope of the stress–strain curve in the linear portion after the toe region.

Table B2.6 Mechanical properties of the intervertebral disc

Loading mode	Level	Strength (N)	Stiffness (N/mm or Nm/rad) Initiala	Averageb	Finalc
Compression	L5-S1	5574[d]	1448[d]		3511[d]
	L4-L5	5128[d]	306[d], 413[e]		2405[d], 721[e]
	L3-L4	5351[d]	1352[d]		2756[d]
	L2-L3	4905[d]	439[d], 461[e]		3160[d], 997[e]
	L1-L2				
Flexion	Lumbar		46[f]		8451[f]
Extension	Lumbar		74[f]		
Lateral bending	Lumbar		64[f]		704[f]
Axial torsion	Lumbar		157[f]		604[f]
Compression	Lumbar			800[g]	
Posterior shear	Lumbar		102[g]		148[g]
Anterior shear	Lumbar		91[g]		123[g]
Lateral shear	Lumbar		113[g]		169[g]

a: Slope of the toe region of the load displacement curve.
b: Average slope of the load displacement curve.
c: Slope of the load displacement curve excluding the toe region.
d: [29]; e: [30]; f: [31]; g: [32].

Table B2.7 Mechanical properties of the annulus fibrosus

Property	Specimen orientation	Layer Location Average	Inner	Middle	Outer
Tensile Modulus	Horizontal	3.54[c]			
	Parallel to fibers	3.41			410[a]
	Perpendicular to lamellae				0.16[b]
Ultimate stress	Horizontal				
	Parallel to fibers				110[a]
	Perpendicular to lamellae				0.187[b]

a: MPa, Specimen 2×2.5 mm cross section, 6.5 mm length [33].
b: MPa, Specimen 7.5×2.5 mm cross section, 4.5 mm length [33].
c: N/mm, Specimen 2×1.5 mm cross section, 15–25 mm length [34].

B2.5 VISCOELASTIC BEHAVIOR

Finally, the rate dependent properties are usually modeled by a three-parameter solid which consists of a spring (m_2) and a dashpot (h) in parallel connected to another spring (m_1) in series. Viscoelastic properties may also be expressed in terms of the dynamic modulus G*. A sinusoidal displacement of the form $u = u_o\, e^{i\omega t}$ is applied to the specimen (this is usually a torsional strain), and the resulting force response $F = F_o\, e^{i\omega t + \delta}$ is measured. Here φ = circular frequency, $i = \sqrt{(-1)}$ and δ

is the phase angle shift between the applied displacement and the measured force. The dynamic modulus is than obtained as

$$G^* = \frac{F}{u} = \frac{F_o}{u_o} e^{i\delta} = G' + iG'' \tag{B2.4}$$

where G′ and G″ are the loss and storage moduli respectively. In some cases, it may be more convenient to express viscoelastic properties in terms of the magnitude of the dynamic shear modulus and the phase angle shift as

$$|G|^* = \sqrt{(G'^2 + G''^2)}; \quad \delta = \tan^{-1}\left(\frac{G''}{G'}\right) \tag{B2.5}$$

The anisotropic viscoelastic properties in shear of the meniscus have been determined by subjecting discs of meniscal tissue to sinusoidal torsional loading [35](Table B2.8). The specimens were cut in the three directions of orthotropic symmetry, i.e. circumferential, axial and radial. A definite correlation is seen with the orientation of the fibers and both the magnitude of the dynamic modulus |G*| and the phase angle δ.

Table B2.8 Viscoelastic properties of meniscal tissue

Specimen orientation	*|G*| (MPa)*	*δ (degrees)*
Circumferential	36.8	16.7
Axial	29.8	19.4
Radial	21.4	20.8

The viscoelastic properties of the human intervertebral disc have been modeled [36, 37] using the three-parameter solid. The parameters were obtained by fitting experimentally obtained creep curves to analytical equations using linear regression (Table B2.9).

Table B2.9 Viscoelastic properties of the intervertebral disc* [36,37]

m_1 *(MPa)*	m_2 *(MPa)*	*h (GPas)*
10–13	13–40	65–280

* Ranges.

B2.6 DISCUSSION

Since it is nearly impossible to carry out meaningful experiments *in vivo* on the human disc or meniscus, the properties reported above have been obtained from cadaveric tissue. Test specimens were obtained from autopsy material (10–48 hours after death), and were either tested immediately or stored frozen for varying periods of time before testing. Statistical analyses of these data show high standard deviations and errors that are caused by a number of factors. Changes in water content (which may be a consequence of aging and degeneration, diurnal changes or surgical interventions) cause a subsequent change in mechanical properties. Further, it has been well documented that the mechanical properties of collagenous tissues change with storage medium, storage temperature, time after death and 'preconditioning' state [38, 39]. Both the disc and the meniscus contain highly oriented collagen fibers, and location and orientation of the test specimen can cause significant changes in the test results. Additional factors such as sex, diet, and level of activity also play a relatively minor role in this variation.

ADDITIONAL READING

Ghosh, P. (ed.) (1988) *The Biology of the Intervertebral Disc*, Vol I and II, CRC Press, Boca Raton.

One of the most comprehensive texts available about the intervertebral disc. It is written from the biological perspective, and contains exhaustive information about each component of the disc. Volume I includes chapters on disc structure and development, vasculature, innervation, collagen and non-collagenous proteins. Volume II contains information on nutrition and metabolism, mechanics, pathology and disease states.

Mow, V.C., Arnoczky, S.P. and Jackson, D.W. (1992) *Knee Meniscus: Basic and Clinical Foundations*. Raven Press, New York.

This monograph is designed to serve as a comprehensive reference for clinicians and researchers interested in the meniscus. It includes chapters on gross anatomy, structure and function of the menisci and their mechanical behavior, pathological disorders, clinical and surgical methods of treatment and meniscal disorders.

Mow, V.C. and Hayes, W.C. (1991) *Basic Orthopaedic Biomechanics*, Raven Press, New York.

This book is aimed at teaching senior engineering students or orthopaedic residents the fundamental principles of biomechanics of the musculoskeletal system. The book contains several chapters on the mechanics of joints, and the properties and functions of joint tissues. The chapter devoted to articular cartilage and the meniscus includes a review of collagen-proteoglycan interactions, and how these directly affect the mechanical behavior of the tissue. The biphasic and the triphasic theories for the viscoelastic properties are also discussed.

White, A.A. and Panjabi, M.M., (1990) *Clinical Biomechanics of the Spine*, J.B. Lippincott Company, Philadelphia.

An excellent reference book for an engineer or a physician interested in the spine. Each topic is written from the viewpoint of a biomechanician and the topics covered include kinetics and kinematics of vertebral joints, pathological disorders of the spine and their surgical management. Chapter 1 contains an introductory section on the intervertebral disc that describes its structure, function and biomechanics.

REFERENCES

1. Armstrong, C.G. and Mow, V.C. (1982) Variations in the intrinsic mechanical properties of human articular cartilage with age, degeneration and water content. *J. Bone Joint Surg.*, **64A,** 88–94.
2. Mow, V.C., Holmes, M.H. and Lai, W.M. (1984) Fluid transport and mechanical properties of articular cartilage: A review. *J. Biomech.*, **102,** 73–84.
3. Hayes, W.C. and Bodine, A.J. (1978) Flow independent viscoelastic properties of articular cartilage matrix. *J. Biomech.*, **11,** 407–419.
4. Mathur, P.D., McDonald, J.R. and Ghormley, R.K. (1949) A study of the tensile strength of the menisci of the knee. *J. Bone Joint Surg.*, **32A,** 650–654.
5. Aspden, R.M., Yarker, Y.E. and Hukins, D.W.L. (1985) Collagen Orientations in the meniscus of the knee joint. *J. Anat.*, **140,** 371–380.
6. Bullough, P.G., Munuera, L., Murphy, J. and Weinstein, A.M. (1970) The strength of the menisci of the knee as it relates to their fine structure. *J. Bone Joint Surg.*, **52B,** 564–570.
7. Fithian, D.C., Kelly, M.A. and Mow, V.C. (1990) Material properties and structure-function relationships in the menisci. *Clin. Orthop. Rel. Res.*, **252,** 19–31.
8. Mow, V.C., Zhu, W. and Ratcliffe, A. (1991) Structure and function of articular cartilage and meniscus, in *Basic Orthopaedic Biomechanics*, (eds V.C. Mow and W.C. Hayes), Raven Press, New York, pp. 143–198.
9. Eyre, D.R. and Wu, J.J. (1983) Collagen of fibrocartilage: A distinctive molecular phenotype in bovine meniscus. *F. E. B. S. Letters*, **158,** 265–270.
10. Fithian, D.C., Zhu, W.B., Ratcliffe, A., Kelly, M.A. and Mow, V.C. (1989b) Exponential law representation of tensile properties of human meniscus. *Proceedings of the Institute of Mechanical Engineers. The Changing Role of Orthopaedics*, Mechanical Engineering Publications Limited, London. pp. 85–90
11. Ghosh, P. and Taylor, T.K.F. (1987) The knee joint meniscus: A fibrocartilage of some distinction. *Clin. Orthop. Rel. Res.*, **224,** 52–63.
12. Ingman, A.M., Ghosh, P. and Taylor, T.K.F. (1974) Variation of collagenous and non-collagenous proteins of human knee joint menisci with age and degeneration. *Gerontology*, **20,** 212–223.
13. Pooni, J.S., Hukins, D.W.L., Harris, P.F., Hilton, R.C. and Davies, K.E. (1986) Comparison of the structure of human intervertebral discs in the cervical, thoracic and lumbar regions of the spine. *Surg. Radiol. Anat.*, **8,** 175–182.
14. Hirsch, C., Inglemark, B-H. and Miller, M. (1963) The anatomical basis of back pain. *Acta Orthop. Scand.*, **33**, 2–17.
15. Lin, H.S., Liu, Y.K. and Adams, K.H. (1978) Mechanical response of the lumbar intervertebral joint under physiological (complex) loading. *J. Bone Joint Surg.*, **60A,** 41–55.
16. Lin, H.S., Liu, Y.K., Ray, G. and Nikravesh, P. (1978) System identification for material properties of the intervertebral joint. *J. Biomech.*, **11,** 1–14.
17. Taylor, J.R. (1975) Growth of human intervertebral discs and vertebral bodies. *J. Anat.*, **120,** 49–68.
18. Panjabi, M.M., Summers, D.J., Pelker, R.R., Videman, T., Friedlander, G.E. and Southwick, W.O. (1986) Three-dimensional load-displacement curves due to forces on the cervical spine. *J. Ortho. Res.*, **4,** 152–161.

19. Inoue, H. (1981) Three-dimensional architecture of lumbar intervertebral discs. *Spine*, **6,** 139–146.
20. Panagiotacopulos, N.D., Knauss, W.G. and Bloch, R. (1979) On the mechanical properties of human intervertebral disc materials. *Biorheology*, **16,** 317–330.
21. Marchand, F. and Ahmed, A.M. (1988) Investigation of the laminate structure of lumbar disc annulus fibrosus. *Trans. Orthop. Res. Soc.*, **13,** 271.
22. Best B.A., Guilak, F., Setton, L.A., Zhu, W., Saed-Nejad, F., Ratcliffe, A., Weidenbaum, M. and Mow, V.C. (1994) Compressive mechanical properties of the human annulus fibrosus and their relationship to biochemical composition. *Spine*, **19,** 212–221.
23. Gower, W.E. and Pedrini, V. (1969) Age-related variations in protein-polysaccharide from human nucleus pulposus, annulus fibrosus and costal cartilage. *J. Bone Joint Surg.*, **51A,** 1154–1162.
24. Lyons, G., Eisenstein, S.M. and Sweet, M.B.E. (1981) Biochemical changes in intervertebral disc degeneration, *Biophysics Acta*, **673,** 443.
25. Lai, W.M. and Mow, V.C. (1980) Drag-induced compression of articular cartilage during a permeation experiment. *Biorheology*, **17,** 111–123.
26. Proctor, C.S., Schmidt, M.B., Whipple, R.R., Kelly, M.A. and Mow, V.C. (1989) Material Properties of the normal medial bovine meniscus. *J. Ortho. Res.*, **7,** 771–782.
27. Eberhardt, A.W., Keer, L.M., Lewis, J.L. and Vithoontien, V. (1990) An analytical model of joint contact. *J. Biomech. Eng.*, **112,** 407–413.
28. Fithian D.C., Schmidt, M.B., Ratcliffe, A. and Mow, V.C. (1989a) Human meniscus tensile properties: Regional variation and biochemical correlation. *Trans. Orthop. Res. Soc.*, **14,** 205.
29. Brown, T., Hansen, R.J. and Torra, A.J. (1957) Some mechanical tests on the lumbosacral spine with particular reference to the intervertebral discs. *J. Bone Joint Surg.*, **39A,** 1135–1164.
30. Hirsch, C. and Nachemson, A. (1954) New observations on the mechanical behavior of the lumbar discs. *Acta Orthop. Scand.*, **23,** 254–283.
31. Schultz, A.B., Warwick, D.N., Berkson, M.H. and Nachemson, A.L. (1979) Mechanical properties of human lumbar spine motion segments Part I. *J. Biomech. Eng.*, **101,** 46–52.
32. Berkson, M.H., Nachemson, A. and Schultz, A.B. (1979) Mechanical properties of human lumbar spine motion segments Part I. *J. Biomech. Eng.*, **101,** 53–57.
33. Marchand, F. and Ahmed, A.M. (1989) Mechanical properties and failure mechanisms of the lumbar disc annulus. *Trans. Orthop. Res. Soc.*, **14,** 355.
34. Galante, J.O. (1967) Tensile properties of the human lumbar annulus fibrosus. *Acta Orthop. Scand.*, (Suppl. 100), 1–91.
35. Chern, K.Y., Zhu, W.B. and Mow, V.C. (1989) Anisotropic viscoelastic shear properties of meniscus. *Adv. Bioeng.*, **BED-15,** 105–106.
36. Burns, M.L. *et al.* (1984) Analysis of compressive creep behavior of the vertebral unit subjected to uniform axial loading using exact parametric solution equations of Kelvin solid models Part I. *J. Biomech.*, **17,** 113–130.
37. Kazarian, L.E. and Kaleps, I. (1979) Mechanical and physical properties of the human intervertebral joint. Technical Report AMRL-TR-79-3, Aerospace Medical Research Laboratory, Wright Patterson Air Force Base, OH

38. Black, J. (1976) Dead or alive: The problem of *in vitro* tissue mechanics. *J. Biomed. Mats. Res.*, **10,** 377–389.
39. Black, J. (1984) Tissue properties: Relation of *in vitro* studies to *in vivo* behavior, in *Natural and Living Biomaterials*, Ed. G.W. Hastings and P. Ducheyne, CRC Press, Boca Raton, pp. 5–26.

Ligament, tendon and fascia — B3

S. L-Y. Woo and R.E. Levine

B3.1 INTRODUCTION

Ligament, tendon, and fascia are soft tissues composed primarily of collagen fibers. In ligaments and tendons these fibers are organized into roughly parallel bundles to transmit tensile forces between two bones (ligament) or between muscle and bone (tendon). In tendons the bundles are nearly all oriented along the long axis, whereas in ligaments, typically shorter than tendons, the bundles are also generally organized except for bends and twists at insertion sites to bone, e.g. the anterior cruciate ligament in the knee [1]. Fascia, on the other hand, is a sheet of fibrous tissue which encloses muscle. In the leg, fascia lata encompasses the entire thigh musculature and becomes thicker as it progresses distally [2].

An extensive compilation of mechanical properties of human ligament, tendon and fascia was published in 1970 by Yamada in *Strength of Biological Materials* [3]. Since then, numerous studies of the connective tissue in human joints has been published. The data presented in this review are from studies conducted since 1970 and are limited to mechanical (or material) properties determined from uniaxial tensile tests. Samples of tendons and ligaments are usually gripped by their muscle or bone ends. The tensile test yields a load–elongation curve representing the structural properties of a bone-ligament-bone (or muscle-tendon-bone) complex. The area of a transverse section of the tissue sample (cross-sectional area), generally assumed to be constant along the sample length, is used to convert load to stress. Strain in the direction of loading is calculated as a change in length divided by an initial gauge length. The initial gauge length is taken to be either the initial length of the test

Handbook of Biomaterial Properties. Edited by J. Black and G. Hastings.
Published in 1998 by Chapman & Hall, London. ISBN 0 412 60330 6.

specimen from one clamp to the other (grip-to-grip length) or a smaller gauge length marked with dye on the midportion of the tissue (direct). From the stress-strain curve, the modulus, ultimate tensile strength (UTS), strain at UTS, and strain energy density are calculated [1].

Although tendons and ligaments are often tested as composite bone-ligament-bone and muscle-tendon-bone complexes for ease of gripping, the maximum load, stiffness and elongation values represent the average properties of a composite, and vary depending on the material behavior of the bone, and the size, shape, and orientation of the test specimen [4]. Due to the complex geometry of human ligament, tendon, and fascia, uniform loading across a specimen during a tensile test may not always be possible. Thus, while some studies tested the entire ligament or tendon [5–7], other studies partitioned the ligaments and tendons [8–24] such that distinct bundles could be tested with a more uniform stress distributions throughout the tissue during a tensile test. In the case of fascia, samples are obtained by cutting out a rectangular bands from the fascia sheet for testing [11].

Tables B3.1 and B3.2 list the mechanical properties of human ligaments, tendons, and fascia from various joints. For those tissues that were either

Table B3.1 Mechanical properties of lower limb ligaments, tendons and fascia

Tissue	*Modulus (MPa)*	*Ultimate tensile strength (MPa)*	*Strain at ultimate tensile strength (%)*	*Strain energy density (MPa)*	*Source*
Knee					
Ligament					
Ant. cruciate	65–541	13–46	9–44	1–3	[11, 24, 25]
Pos. cruciate	109–413	24–36	10–29	2–3	[6 20, 24]
Tendon					
Patellar	143–660	24–69	14–27	4–5	[8, 9, 11, 13, 17]
Ankle					
Ligament					
Lat. collateral	216–512	24–46	13–17	na	[7]
Med. collateral	54–321	16–34	10–33	na	[7, 21]
Tendon					
Achilles	65	24–61	24–59	na	[26, 27]
Palmaris longus	2310±620	91±15	na	na	[21]
Other					
Tendon					
Semitendinosus	362±22	89±5	52±3	23±1	[11]
Gracilis	613±41	112±4	34±2	18±2	[11]
Fascia					
Tibial	283±132	14±4	na	na	[28]
Fascia lata	150–571	30–105	27–29	13±2 [11]	[11, 26, 27, 29]

Notes: Ant.: anterior; Pos.: posterior; Med.: medial; Lat.: lateral, Long.: longus; Semitend.: semitendenosis; na: not available.

Table B3.2 Mechanical properties of upper limb and trunk ligaments and associated tissues

Tissue	*Modulus (MPa)*	*Ultimate tensile strength (MPa)*	*Strain at ultimate tensile strength (%)*	*Source*
Shoulder				
Ligament				
Inf. glenohum.	30–42	5–6	8–15	[30]
Capsule	32–67	8–21	na	[16]
Spine				
Ligament				
Pos. long.	na	21–28	11–44	[6, 19]
Liga. flavum	na	1–15	21–102	[6, 19]
Ant. long.	286–724	8–37	10–57	[6, 18, 19]
Supraspinal	na	9–16	39–115	[6, 19]
Interspinal	na	2–9	39–120	[6, 19]
Intertransverse	na	51±1.4	16.5±0.7	[6]
Forearm				
Ligament				
Carpal joint	23–119	na	na	[22]
Palmar radioul.	39±18	5.7±1.7	51±24	[23]
Dorsal radiolul.	52±33	8±5	61±29	[23]
Interosseous membrane	528±82	43±1.4	10±2	[10]

Notes: Ant.: anterior; Inf.; inferior; Long.: longitudinal; Radioul.: radioulnar; Glenohum.: glenohumoral; na: not available.

partitioned into separate bundles and/or that were tested in multiple studies, the mechanical properties are given as a range of values. Data determined for one specimen bundle or measured in one study are given as mean ± one standard deviation.

A variety of factors contribute to the quality of biomechanical data [1], including donor age [4, 17, 25, 27, 31], donor gender, storage method, test environment [15], orientation of tissue during testing [4], rate of loading [9], and accuracy of measuring devices [11, 32]. Errors in mechanical property measurements may be due to the use of a grip-to-grip gauge length [5, 7–9, 12–16, 19–26], rather than a midsubstance gauge length [10, 11, 17, 18, 30, 32], for strain measurement, due to nonuniform elongation along the specimen length. Another source of error may be the cross-sectional area measurement methods which contact, or deform, the tissue surface [5, 7–9, 11–13, 15, 16, 18, 19, 20–23, 25]. A comparative study by Woo *et al.* [33] demonstrated that measurements made with two contact methods, digital calipers and a constant pressure area micrometer, were 16% and 20% smaller, respectively, than those measured by a non-contact laser micrometer system. Further discussion of the strengths and weaknesses of those studies referenced in the tables are included in the annotated bibliography.

B3.2 DISCUSSION

The use of tendon, ligament, and fascia as allografts or autografts motivate the investigation of their biomechanical properties. One-dimensional, static properties such as the ultimate tensile strength, modulus, strain, and strain energy density values shown in Tables B3.1 and B3.2 are useful for comparing different candidates for replacement tissue. However, other biomechanical characterizations of human connective tissue are available in the literature. Several experimental studies have examined the time- and history-dependent, or viscoelastic, properties of human ligament and tendon [15, 17, 28, 31, 34, 35] to help predict tissue behavior after long periods of use. Mathematical models have also been used to describe short-term behavior observed in experiments [36, 37] and to predict long-term behavior [17, 34, 36–38]. Various mathematical models of ligaments and tendons have been described by Woo *et al.* [38], including a description of the quasi-linear viscoelasticity (QLV) theory, a commonly used viscoelastic model of ligaments and tendons. Other studies have examined how certain biomechanical properties vary throughout the tissue [14, 18, 32, 39]. Future studies must recognize that human ligament, tendon, and fascia are three-dimensional, anisotropic, nonhomogenous, composite materials which are subject to complex, dynamic loads. Successful replacement of these tissues depends on accurate replication of their static and dynamic mechanical properties.

ADDITIONAL READING

Blevins F.T., Hecker A.T., Bigler G.T., *et al.* (1994) The effects of donor age and strain rate on the biomechanical properties of bone-patellar tendon-bone allografts. *American Journal of Sports Medicine*, **22**(3), 328–33.

Patellar tendons from donors ranging in age from 17 to 54 years were tested at either 10% or 100% elongation per second, to examine effects of donor and strain rate on tensile properties. A pressure micrometer was used to measure cross-sectional area and the initial length of the tendon (from patellar to tibial insertion site) was used for strain measurements. Specimens were kept moist with a saline spray during tensile testing. Medial, lateral, and sometimes central portions were taken from 25 donors; regional differences across the tendon were not considered.

Butler D.L., Grood E.S., Noyes F.R., *et al.* (1984) Effects of structure and strain measurement technique on the material properties of young human tendons and fascia. *Journal of Biomechanics*, **17**(8), 579–96.

This study compares mechanical properties between different tissue structures as well as analyzing the effect of strain measurement technique on tissue modulus. A diverse number of analysis techniques were employed including light microscopy, scanning electron microscopy, and tensile testing. Surface strain was measured using high-speed filming. A constant pressure micrometer was used to measure cross-sectional area. Specimens were tensile tested at 100%/second at room temperature and humidity. Data are given as mean ± SEM (standard error of the mean) rather than standard deviation.

Hurschler C., Vanderby R. Jr., Martinez D.A., *et al.* (1994) Mechanical and biochemical analyses of tibial compartment fascia in chronic compartment syndrome. *Annals of Biomedical Engineering*, **22**(3), 272–9.

This study was the first to report mechanical properties of tibial compartment fascia in humans. Fascia specimens were tested in directions along a visible fiber orientation (axial) and perpendicular to the fibers (transverse). Cross-sectional area was measured using a caliper and surface strain was measured from video analysis of stain markers on the tissue surface. Specimens were subject to stress relaxation tests as well as as load-to-failure tests conducted at 20 mm/second at room temperature and humidity.

Neumann P., Keller T.S., Ekstrom L., *et al.* (1992) Mechanical properties of the human lumbar anterior longitudinal ligament. *Journal of Biomechanics*, **25**(10), 1185–94.

A motion analysis system was used to measure the distribution of surface strain along the anterior longitudinal ligament. Calipers were used to measure specimen thickness and width for calculating cross sectional area. Specimens were tensile tested to failure at a displacement rate of 2.5 mm/second at room temperature and humidity. Although a strain distribution was measured, area was assumed to be constant along the ligament length.

REFERENCES

1. Woo, S.L-Y., An, K-N., Arnoczky, S.P., *et al.* (1994) Anatomy, Biology, and Biomechanics of Tendon, Ligament, and Meniscus, in *Orthopaedic Basic Science*, (eds S.R. Simon), American Academy of Orthopaedic Surgeons, pp. 45–87.
2. Fox, J.M. (1986) Injuries to the thigh, in *The Lower Extremity and Spine in Sports Medicine*, (eds J.A. Nicholas and E.B. Hershman), The C. V. Mosby Company, St Louis, pp. 1087–1117.
3. Yamada, H. (1970) Mechanical properties of ligament, tendon, and fascia, in *Strength of Biological Materials*, (eds F.G. Evans), The Williams & Wilkins Co., Baltimore, pp. 92–105.
4. Woo, S.L., Hollis, J.M., Adams, D.J., *et al.* (1991) Tensile properties of the human femur-anterior cruciate ligament-tibia complex. The effects of specimen age and orientation. *American Journal of Sports Medicine*, **19**(3), 217–25.
5. Chazal, J., Tanguy, A., Bourges, M., *et al.* (1985) Biomechanical properties of spinal ligaments and a histological study of the supraspinal ligament in traction. *Journal of Biomechanics*, **18**(3), 167–76.
6. Prietto, M.P., Bain, J.R., Stonebrook, S.N., *et al.* (1988) Tensile strength of the human posterior cruciate ligament (PCL). *Transactions of the Orthopaedic Research Society*, **13,** 195.
7. Siegler, S., Block, J. and Schneck, C.D. (1988) The mechanical characteristics of the collateral ligaments of the human ankle joint. *Foot & Ankle*, **8**(5), 234–42.

8. Bechtold, J.E., Eastlund, D.T., Butts, M.K., *et al.* (1994) The effects of freeze-drying and ethylene oxide sterilization on the mechanical properties of human patellar tendon. *American Journal of Sports Medicine*, **22**(4), 562–6.
9. Blevins, F.T., Hecker, A.T., Bigler, G.T., *et al.* (1994) The effects of donor age and strain rate on the biomechanical properties of bone-patellar tendon-bone allografts. *American Journal of Sports Medicine*, **22**(3), 328–33.
10. Boardman, N.D., Pfaeffle, H.J., Grewal, R., *et al.* (1995) Tensile properties of the interosseous membrane of the human forearm. *Transactions of the Orthopaedic Research Society*, **20,** 629.
11. Butler, D.L., Grood, E.S., Noyes, F.R., *et al.* (1984) Effects of structure and strain measurement technique on the material properties of young human tendons and fascia. *Journal of Biomechanics*, **17**(8), 579–96.
12. Butler, D.L., Guan, Y., Kay, M.D., *et al.* (1992) Location-dependent variations in the material properties of the anterior cruciate ligament. *Journal of Biomechanics*, **25**(5), 511–8.
13. Butler, D.L., Kay, M.D. and Stouffer, D.C. (1986) Comparison of material properties in fascicle-bone units from human patellar tendon and knee ligaments. *Journal of Biomechanics*, **19**(6), 425–32.
14. Chun, K.J., Butler, D.L., Bukovec, D.B., *et al.* (1989) Spatial variation in material properties in fascicle-bone units from human patellar tendon. *Transactions of the Orthopaedic Research Society*, **14,** 214.
15. Haut, R.C. and Powlison, A.C. (1990) The effects of test environment and cyclic stretching on the failure properties of human patellar tendons. *Journal of Orthopaedic Research*, **8**(4), 532–40.
16. Itoi, E., Grabowski J., Morrey, B.F., *et al.* (1993) Capsular properties of the shoulder. *Tohoku J. Exp. Med.*, **171,** 203–10.
17. Johnson, G.A., Tramaglini, D.M., Levine, R.E., *et al.* (1994) Tensile and viscoelastic properties of human patellar tendon. *Journal of Orthopaedic Research*, **12**(6), 796–803.
18. Neumann, P., Keller, T.S., Ekstrom, L., *et al.* (1992) Mechanical properties of the human lumbar anterior longitudinal ligament. *Journal of Biomechanics*, **25**(10), 1185–94.
19. Pintar, F.A., Yoganandan, N., Myers, T., *et al.* (1992) Biomechanical properties of human lumbar spine ligaments. *Journal of Biomechanics*, **25**(11), 1351–6.
20. Race, A. and Amis, A.A. (1994) The mechanical properties of the two bundles of the human posterior cruciate ligament. *Journal of Biomechanics*, **27**(1), 13–24.
21. Regan, W.D., Korinek, S.L., Morrey, B.F., *et al.* (1991) Biomechanical study of ligaments around the elbow joint. *Clinical Orthopaedics & Related Research*, **271,** 170–9.
22. Salvelberg, H.H.C.M., Kooloos, J.G.M., Huiskes, R., *et al.* (1992) Stiffness of the ligaments of the human wrist joint. *Journal of Biomechanics*, **25**(4), 369–376.
23. Schuind, F., An, K.N., Berglund, L., *et al.* (1991) The distal radioulnar ligaments: a biomechanical study. *Journal of Hand Surgery – American Volume*, **16**(6), 1106–14.
24. Sheh, M., Butler, D.L and Stouffer, D.C. (1986) Mechanical and structural properties of the human cruciate ligaments and patellar tendon. *Transactions of the Orthopaedic Research Society*, **11,** 236.

25. Noyes, F.R. and Grood, E.S. (1976) The strength of the anterior cruciate ligament in humans and rhesus monkeys. *Journal of Bone and Joint Surgery*, **58-A**(8), 1074–1082.
26. France, E.P., Paulos, L.E., Rosenberg, T.D., *et al.* (1988) The biomechanics of anterior cruciate allografts, in *Prosthetic Ligament Reconstruction of the Knee* (eds M.J. Friedman and R.D. Ferkel), W.B. Saunders Company, Philadelphia, pp. 180–5.
27. Paulos, L.E., France, E.P., Rosenberg, T.D., *et al.* (1987) Comparative material properties of allograft tissues for ligament replacement: effects of type, age, sterilization and preservation. *Transactions of the Orthopaedic Research Society*, **12,** 129.
28. Hurschler, C., Vanderby, R. Jr., Martinez, D.A., *et al.* (1994) Mechanical and biochemical analyses of tibial compartment fascia in chronic compartment syndrome. *Annals of Biomedical Engineering*, **22**(3), 272–9.
29. Butler, D.L., Noyes, F.R., Walz, K.A., *et al.* (1987) Biomechanics of human knee ligament allograft treatment. *Transactions of the Orthopaedic Research Society*, **12,** 128.
30. Bigliani, L.U., Pollock, R.G., Soslowsky, L.J., *et al.* (1992) Tensile properties of the inferior glenohumeral ligament. *Journal of Orthopaedic Research*, **10**(2), 187–97.
31. Hubbard, R.P. and Soutas-Little, R.W. (1984) Mechanical properties of human tendon and their age dependence. *Journal of Biomechanical Engineering*, **106**(2), 144–50.
32. Noyes, F.R., Butler, D.L., Grood, E.S., *et al.* (1984) Biomechanical analysis of human ligament grafts used in knee-ligament repairs and reconstructions. *Journal of Bone & Joint Surgery*, **66-A**(3), 344–52.
33. Woo, S.L-Y., Danto, M.I., Ohland, K.J., *et al.* (1990) The use of a laser micrometer system to determine the cross-sectional shape and area of ligaments: A comparative study with two existing methods. *Journal of Biomechanical Engineering*, **112,** 426–431.
34. Lyon, R.M., Lin, H.C., Kwan, M.K-W., *et al.* (1988) Stress relaxation of the anterior cruciate ligament (ACL) and the patellar tendon (PT). *Transactions of the Orthopaedic Research Society*, **13,** 81.
35. Schwerdt, H., Constantinesco, A. and Chambron, J. (1980) Dynamic viscoelastic behavior of the human tendon *in vitro*. *Journal of Biomechanics*, **13,** 913–922.
36. Arms, S.W. and Butler, D.L. (1989) Cruciate ligament fiber bundle recruitment: A mathematical model. *Transactions of the Orthopaedic Research Society*, **14,** 190.
37. Chun, K.J., Butler, D.L., Stouffer D.C., *et al.* (1988) Stress-strain relationships in fascicle-bone units from human patellar tendon and knee ligaments. *Transactions of the Orthopaedic Research Society*, **13,** 82.
38. Woo, S.L-Y., Johnson, G.A., and Smith, B.A. (1993) Mathematical modeling of ligaments and tendons. *Journal of Biomechanical Engineering*, **115,** 468–473.
39. Butler, D.L., Sheh, M.Y., Stouffer, D.C., *et al.* (1990) Surface strain variation in human patellar tendon and knee cruciate ligaments. *Journal of Biomechanical Engineering*, **112,** 38–45.

B4 Skin and muscle*

A.F.T. Mak and M. Zhang

B4.1 INTRODUCTION

Early studies [11] of the material properties of human skin and muscle are largely suspect due to problems of inappropriate tissue handling, preservation and specimen preparation. Recent efforts have focused on methods which can determine properties in situ in living individuals or on very freshly excised tissues. Among the *in vivo* testing methodologies, indentation has proven to be the most popular, although it sums up the contributions of various tissue layers [1, 3, 4, 6, 7, 9]. The load–displacement curve obtained during indentation depends in decreasing degree upon each of the tissues beneath the indentor. The derived properties, in addition, can be expected to vary with anatomical site, subject age and external environmental conditions (temperature, relative humidity, etc.). Additional results have been obtained *in vivo* through the use of Doppler ultrasound techniques [2, 5].

B4.2 IN-VIVO MECHANICAL PROPERTIES

B4.2.1 Doppler Results

Krouskop *et al.* [5, 8] applied Doppler ultrasound techniques to measure the point-to-point biomechanical property of the human skin and subcutaneous musculatures. Tests of the forearms and legs suggested that the elastic moduli are strongly dependent on the contraction status of the muscles. A 16-fold increase (from 6.2 kPa to 109 kPa) in the modulus

* Data are provided from indentation and ultrasound measurement techniques only.

Handbook of Biomaterial Properties. Edited by J. Black and G. Hastings.
Published in 1998 by Chapman & Hall, London. ISBN 0 412 60330 6.

was reported at a 10% strain as muscle contraction changed from minimal to maximum. Malinauskas *et al.* [5] used the same technique to examine the stump tissues of above-knee amputees and found that the average modulus was significantly higher in posterior tissues than in other locations (Table B4.1). They found, additionally, that superficial tissues were stiffer than deeper structures. Note that the ages and sex of the subjects of these two studies [2, 5] were not reported.

Table B4.1 Apparent Elastic Moduli of Relaxed Above Knee Tissues [5]*

Anatomical Location	*Elastic Modulus (kPa)(std dev.)*
Anterior	57.9 (31.1)
Lateral	53.2 (30.5)
Posterior	141.4 (79.1)
Medial	72.3 (45.5)
Superficial	117.6 (63.0)
Underlying	59.1 (74.0)

* Determined by Doppler ultrasonic techniques.

B4.2.2 Indentation results

Ziegert and Lewis [9] measured the *in vivo* indentation properties of the soft tissues covering the anterior-medial tibiae. A preload of 22.4 N was used with indentors of 6 to 25 mm in diameter. The observed load displacement relationship were essentially linearly elastic. The structural stiffness was noted to vary by up to 70% between sites in one individual and up to 300% between individuals. Unfortunately, the thicknesses of overlying tissues were not determined at the different sites for the individuals studied.

Lanir *et al.* [3] measured the *in vivo* indentation behavior of human forehead skin with pressures up to 5 kPa. The observed behavior was linearly elastic and calculated stiffnesses were 4 to 12 kPa.

Bader and Bowker [1] studied the *in vivo* indentation properties of soft tissues on the anterior aspects of human forearms and thighs by applying constant pressures of 11.7 and 7 kPa respectively. Tissue thickness was measured by using a skinfold caliper and Poisson's rato was assumed to be 0.3. With these data, the stiffness of forearm and thigh tissue were calculated to be, respectively, 1.99 and 1.51 kPa.

Vannah and Chlidress [7] applied similar techniques to measure the human calf, but confined the limb within a shell. They noted that stress relaxation occurred within one second of load application and no preconditioning effect was noted. Torres-Morenos *et al.* [6] performed a similar study, working through ports in quadrilateral sockets of three above-knee amputees. However, they found the mechanical properties of the tissues to be significantly non-linear, with site and rate dependencies, as well as being strongly influenced by muscular activity.

Mak *et al.* [4] (Table B4.2) measured the *in-vivo* indentation properties of the below knee tissues of young adults (N=6) between the ages of 25 and 35. A 4 mm diameter indentor was used, with a final indentation of about 5 mm. The fixed indentation was then maintained for 2–3 seconds to observe the difference between initial and relaxed (equilibrium) properties. The tests were done with the knee in 20° of flexion and were repeated with and without muscular contraction. The Poisson's ratio was assumed to be 0.5 for initial measurements and 0.45 for relaxed (equilibrium) measurements.

Table B4.2 Initial and Relaxed Elastic Moduli of Tissues Around Proximal Human Tibiae [4]*

Anatomical Location	*Initial Elastic Modulus (E_{in}) (kPa)(std dev.)*	*Relaxed Elastic Modulus (E_{eq}) (kPa)(std dev.)*
Medial		
Relaxed	102.6 (8.6)	99.8 (9.2)
Contracted	147.3** (15.8)	142.9** (16.7)
Con./Relax.	1.44	1.43
Lateral†		
Relaxed	132.9 (7.2)	130.1 (7.9)
Contracted	194.3** (24,7)	188.4** (23.0)
Con./Relax.	1.46	1.45

* By indentation; ** Different from relaxed (p <0.001); † Between tibia and fibula.

ADDITIONAL READING

Bader, D.L. and Bowker, P. (1983) Mechanical characteristics of skin and underlying tissues *in vivo*. *Biomaterials*, **4**, 305–8

This paper describes an indentation experiment to investigate *in vivo* the bulk mechanical properties of the composite of skin and underlying tissues on the anterior aspects of human forearms and thighs by applying constant pressures. Significant variations in tissue stiffness with sex, age and body site were also demonstrated.

Malinauskas, M., Krouskop, T.A. and Barry, P.A. (1989) Noninvasive measurement of the stiffness of tissue in the above-knee amputation limb. *J. Rehab. Res. Dev.*, **26**(3), 45–52

The paper reports a noninvasive technique to measure the mechanical properties of the bulk soft tissues by a pulsed ultrasonic Doppler system. An ultrasonic transducer was used to measure internal displacement resulting from external acoustical perturbations. Measurements were made at four sites of 8 above-knee residual limbs. The Young's moduli were found in a range of 53–141 kPa. Superficial tissue had a significantly higher modulus than the tissue beneath.

The repeatability test indicated an acceptable repeatibility. An improved device can possibly be a useful tool in prosthetic fitting and CAD socket design.

Rab, G.T. (1994) Muscle, in *Human Walking* (2nd ed.) (eds J. Rose, J.C. Gamble), Williams & Wilkins, Baltimore, pp. 101–122.

A concise description of the active properties of muscle tissue, with direct application to the development of forces within the human gait cycle.

Reynolds, D. and Lord, L. (1992) Interface load for computer-aided design of below-knee prosthetic sockets. *Med. & Biol. Eng. & Comput.*, **30**, 419–426.

The authors investigated the bulk tissue behaviour of the below-knee amputee's residual limb. An assessment of Young's modulus was made by matching the indentation experimental curves with the curves produced by the finite element modelling of the indentation into a layer of tissue with idealized mechanical properties. *In vivo* tests, conducted at four sites of a below-knee amputee's limb (patella tendon, popliteal, and anterolateral regions) found the local moduli to be 145, 50, 50 and 120 kPa respectively. The effect of muscle tension on the measured indentation response was also investigated. The results showed that the stiffness increased with muscle contraction.

REFERENCES

1. Bader, D.L. and Bowker, P. (1983) Mechanical characteristics of skin and underlying tissues *in vivo*. *Biomaterials,* **4,** 305–8.
2. Krouskop, T.A., Dougherty. D.R. and Vonson, F.S. (1987) A pulsed Doppler ultrasonic system for making noninvasive measurements of the mechanical properties of soft tissue. *J. Rehab. Res. Dev.*, **24**(1), 1–8.
3. Lanir, Y., Dikstein, S., Hartzshtark, A., *et al.* (1990) In-vivo indentation of human skin. *Trans. ASME (J. Biomech. Eng.)*, **112,** 63–69.
4. Mak, A.F.T., Liu, G.H.W. and Lee, S.Y. (1994) Biomechanical assessment of below-knee residual limb tissue, *J. Rehab. Res. Dev.*, **31**, 188–198.
5. Malinauskas, M., Krouskop, T.A. and Barry, P.A. (4) (1989) Noninvasive measurement of the stiffness of tissue in the above-knee amputation limb. *J. Rehab. Res. Dev.*, **26**(3), 45–52.
6. Torres-Morenos, R., Solomonidis, S.E. and Jones, D. (1992) Geometric and mechanical characteristics of the above-knee residual limb. *Proc. 7th. World Cong. Int. Soc. Prosthetics Orthotics*, pp. 149.
7. Vannah, W.M. and Chlidress, D.S. (1988) An investigation of the three dimensional mechanical response of bulk muscular tissue: Experimental methods and results, in *Computational Methods in Bioengineering* (eds R.L. Spilker and B.R. Simon), Amer. Soc. Mech. Eng., New York, pp. 493–503.
8. Yamada, H. (1970) (ed. F.G. Evans) *Strength of Biological Tissues*, Williams & Wilkins, Baltimore.
9. Ziegert, J.C. and Lewis, J.L. (1978) In-vivo mechanical properties of soft tissue covering bony prominence, *Trans ASME (J. Biomech. Eng.)*, **100**, 194–201.

B5 Brain tissues

S.S. Margulies and D.F. Meaney

B5.1 INTRODUCTION

The brain is organized into the cerebrum, brain stem, and cerebellum. The cerebrum consists of two cerebral hemispheres, basal ganglia, and the diencephalon. The hemispheres contain the cerebral cortex and underlying white matter, and are associated with higher order functioning, including memory, cognition, and fine motor control. The basal ganglia, contained within the hemispheres, controls gross motor function. The diencephalon is much smaller than the cerebrum, contains the thalamus and hypothalamus, and is associated with relaying sensory information and controlling the autonomic nervous system. The brainstem contains the mesencephalon, pons and the medulla oblangata. The smallest segment of the brain, the mesencephalon, is located below the diencephalon and is thought to play a role in consciousness. Muscle activation, tone and equilibrium is controlled in the pons and cerebellum located below the mesencephalon, and respiratory and cardiac processes are governed by the medulla oblongata, located directly beneath the pons.

The brain contains grey matter and white matter substances that are easily distinguished upon gross examination. Grey matter contains a densely packed network of neural cell bodies and associated glial cells, whereas white matter contains myelinated axonal tracts, relatively few neuronal cell bodies, and a supporting environment of glial cells. The entire brain is surrounded by cerebrospinal fluid contained within an extensive ventricular system that occupies approximately one-tenth of the total brain volume. The ventricular system supports the brain as well as the spinal cord, and provides nutrients to and removes waste products from the central nervous system.

Handbook of Biomaterial Properties. Edited by J. Black and G. Hastings.
Published in 1998 by Chapman & Hall, London. ISBN 0 412 60330 6.

Understanding the response of the complex brain structure to thermal, electrical, or mechanical stimuli necessitates a thorough investigation of the physical properties of each brain component. This task is still in its infancy, and therefore the material cited in this chapter is accompanied by several caveats. First, most properties cited are for whole brain. However, where available, properties of the white matter, gray matter, cerebrum, cerebellum, and brainstem are noted. Second, extensive studies have been conducted on brain tissue from a broad range of species. To provide the reader with information most similar to human tissue, only primate data (nonhuman and human) have been included. Exceptions occur only when there is no primate data available, and are noted. Finally, because the brain is a highly perfused organ and its properties may differ between *in vivo* and *in vitro* conditions, and with the post mortem time period before testing. To facilitate comparison between tests, information regarding *in vivo/in vitro* conditions, post mortem time, and test procedure is included with the data.

B5.2 COMPOSITION

Table B5.1 Brain Tissue Composition

	Water (wt%)	*Ash (wt%)*	*Lipid (wt%)*	*Protein (wt%)*
Whole brain	76.3–78.5 (77.4)	1.4–2 (1.5)	9–17	8–12
Grey matter	83–86	1.5	5.3	8–12
White matter	68–77	1.4	18	11–12

Approximate overall ranges given. Values in parentheses indicate averages.
Source: [1–3].

B5.2.1 Mass [2]

Adult male whole brain (20–30 yr): 1400 g
(cerebrum 1200 g, cerebellum, 150 g)
Adult female whole brain (20–30 yr): 1200 g
Adult male whole brain (90 yr): 1161 g

B5.2.2 Dimensions and shape [2]

The adult brain with the brain stem is approximately half an ellipsoid.

Diameter:	Vertical	Transverse	Anteroposterior
Male:	13 cm	14 cm	16.5 cm
Female:	12.5 cm	13 cm	15.5 cm

B5.2.3 Density (adult) in kg/m^3

Brain	1030–1041	[2]
Grey matter	1039	[1, 3]
White matter	1043	[1, 3]

B5.3 MECHANICAL PROPERTIES

B5.3.1 Bulk modulus

Excised brain samples: 2.1×10^6 kPa (independent of frequency) [4].

B5.3.2 Poisson's ratio

Using the relationship $\nu = (3K - E)/6K$
where K is the bulk modulus and E is the elastic modulus, and considering that K is 4–5 orders of magnitude larger than E, brain is approximated as an incompressible material (ν=0.5) [5].

B5.3.3 Elastic and shear moduli

See Table B5.2.

B5.3.4 Creep modulus

See Table B5.3.

Table B5.2 Elastic Modulus and Shear Modulus of Normal Brain at 37°C (typical values, not averages)

Testing technique	*Species (post mortuum time)*	*Frequency (Hz)*	*Analysis format*	*Results (kPa)*	G_1 *(kPa)*	G_2 *(kPa)*	*Source*
Free vibration	Rhesus monkey (15 min)	31	$E^* = E_1 + i E_2$	$E_1 = 91.2$ $E_2 + 53.9$	30.3	18.0	[6]
Free vibration	Human (6–12 hr)	34	$E^* = E_1 + i E_2$	$E_1 = 66.8$ $E_2 = 26.3$	22.3	8.7	[6]
Harmonic shear	Human white matter (10–62 hr)	9–10	$G^* = G_1 + i G_2$	Min: $G^* = 0.75 + i\,0.3$ Max $G^* = 1.41 + i\,0.6$	0.75-1.41	0.3–0.6	[7]
Driving point impedançe	Rhesus (*in vivo*)	80	Theoretical approx of data $G^* = G_1 + i G_2$	$G_1 = 19.6$ $G_2 = 11.2$	19.6	11.2	[7,8]
Quasi-static expansion of balloon within tissue	Rhesus monkey live (in vivo) dead (5–45 min) fixed (formaldehyde)	0	Static elastic Modulus, E_1	$E_1 = 10$–60 live and dead $E_1 = 40$–120 fixed	10–60		[9]
Sudden acceleration of a cylinder filled with tissue	Human	(acceleration duration ≈ 17.5 ms.)	compare tissue displacement with that of a Voigt solid cylinder	Shear modulus G=1.17–2.19 kPa (average=1.7) Kinematic viscosity ν = 14–124 cm^2/s (average=89)	1.7		[10] (Tissue temp unknown)
Harmonic shear	Human (<3 hr)	5–350	$G^* = G_1 + i G_2$	G_1 G_2	7.6–33.9	2.76–81.4	[11]
		5		7.6 2.8			
		15		8.4 3.5			
		35		11.7 5.2			
		85		19.3 13.4			
		105		21.4 18.0			
		225		29.0 45.9			
		350		33.9 81.4			

Table B5.2 *Continued*

Testing technique	*Species (post mortuum time)*	*Frequency (Hz)*	*Analysis format*	*Results (kPa)*		*G_1 (kPa)*	*G_2 (kPa)*	*Source*
Harmonic shear	Human (<3 hr)		$G^* = G_1 + i\ G_2$	G_1	G_2			[11]
	Grey matter	2–10						
	Axis 1			10.6	1.5			
	Axis 2			6.3	1.5			
	Axis 3			4.1	1.4			
	average			7.0	1.5	7.0	1.5	
	white matter	2–10						
	Axis 1			7.7	2.6			
	Axis 2			7.0	3.2			
	Axis 3			7.3	3.5			
	average			7.3	3.1	7.3	3.1	

* Assumed tissue is incompressible (ν=0.5), therefore $G^* = E^*/3$.

Table B5.3 Creep Modulus of Normal Brain at 37°C (typical values, not averages)

*Testing technique**	*Species*	*Model*	*Results*	*Source*
Compression	Rhesus monkey (15 min)	$J(t) = C_1 + C_2 \ln(t)$	$C_1 = 2.97\ kPa^{-1}$ $C_2 = 0.18\ kPa^{-1}$ $t > 0.1\ s$	[6]
Compression	Human (6–12 hr)	$J(t) = C_1 - C_2 \ln(t)$	$C_1 = 2.45\ kPa^{-1}$ $C_2 = 0.18\ kPa^{-1}$ $t > 0.1\ s$	[6]
Compression	Human (6–12 hr)	Nonlinear solid $\epsilon(t) = \frac{\sigma_0 e^{-\mu t}}{K_2} + \left(\frac{\sigma_0}{K_1} + \frac{(K_2^2 + 4\sigma_0 K_3)^{1/2}}{2K_3} - \frac{K_2}{2K_3}\right) \cdot (1 - e^{-\mu t})$ where $\mu = K_2/C_1$	$K_1 = 25.77\ kPa$ $K_2 = 20.46\ kPa$, $K_3 = 104.04\ kPa$ $C_1 = 651.8\ kPa\ s$ $\sigma_0 = 3.44, 4.82, 6.89\ kPa$	[12]
Compression	Human (6–12 hr)	Nonlinear fluid $\epsilon(t) = \frac{\sigma_0}{K_2} + \frac{C_1 C_2}{2K_1 C_3} - \frac{C_1(C_2^2 + 4\sigma_0 C_3)^{1/2}}{2K_1 C_3}$ $+ \frac{1}{2C_3}\left[(C_2^2 + 4\sigma_0 C_3)^{1/2} - C_2\right]\left(t + \frac{C_1}{K_1} e^{-\mu t}\right)$ $+ \frac{\sigma_0}{K_1} \cdot \left[1 + \frac{C_1}{C_2}\right](1 - e^{-\mu t})$	$K_1 = 74.41\ kPa$ $K_2 = 20.67\ kPa$ $C_1 = 1266.38\ kPa$ $C_2 = 36599.7\ kPa\ s$ $C_3 = 1.38\ kPa\ s^2$ $\sigma_0 = 3.44, 4.82, 6.89\ kPa$	[12]

Table B5.3 *Continued*

*Testing technique**	*Species*	*Model*	*Results*	*Source*
Compression	Human (6–12 hr)	Hyperelastic with material dissipation $\frac{\sigma_{11}}{2C_1} = \left[\lambda^2 - \frac{1}{\lambda}\right]\left[1 + \frac{C_2}{C_1 \lambda}\right] + \frac{B_1}{C_1} \frac{\dot{\lambda}}{\lambda^3} \cdot [\lambda^2 - 6\lambda^3 + 1]$	$C_1 = 6.89$ kPa $C_2 = 17.23$ kPa $B_1 = 0.55$ kPa s^2 λ = stretch ratio $\dot{\lambda}$ = stretch rate	[12]
Fluid infusion	Cat	Poroelastic $\frac{\partial e}{\partial t} = \kappa(2G + \lambda)\nabla^2 e$ G = shear modulus λ = Lame constant κ = permeability	*Grey matter* G= 2 kPa $\lambda = 90$ kPa $\kappa = 7.5 \times 10^{-9}$ kPa-m^2/s *White matter* G = 0.9 kPa $\lambda = 40$ kPa $\kappa = 5 \times 10^{-9}$ kPa-m^2/s	[13]

* All tests consisted of a load applied rapidly and then held constant.

B5.4 ELECTRICAL PROPERTIES

(no primate data available)

B5.4.1 Electrical conductivity temperature coefficient [14]

Cow and pig whole brain $(\Delta\sigma/\sigma)/\Delta T = 3.2\ °C^{-1}$.

Table B5.4 Electrical conductivity of brain tissues

	Temp (°C)	*Conductivity (s) (mS/cm)*	*Species*	*Source*
Whole brain	37	1.7	cow, pig	[14]
Cerebrum	39	1.38–1.92	rabbit	[15]
Cerebellum	39	1.17–1.64	rabbit	[15]
Cortex	body	3.1	rabbit	[16]
Cortex	37	4.5	cat	[17]
White matter	body	1.0	rabbit	[18]
White matter	37	2.9	cat	[17]

B5.5 THERMAL PROPERITES

Table B5.5 Thermal properties of normal, unperfused human brain tissue

	Temp (°C)	*Conductivity, (W/m°K)*	*Diffusivity, ($cm^2/s \times 10^3$)*	*Specific heat, (J/g °K)*	*Source*
Whole brain	5–20	0.528	1.38 ± 0.11	—	[19]
Whole brain	37	0.503–0.576	–	—	[20]
Cortex	37	0.515	1.47	—	[21]
	5–20	0.565	1.43 ± 0.09	3.68	[19]
White matter	5–20	0.565	1.34 ± 0.10	3.60	[19]

Values A–B indicate approximate range, values A ± B indicate mean ± standard deviation.

B5.6 DIFFUSION PROPERTIES

5.6.1 Sucrose (feline brain) [22]

D ~ $3.2\text{-}3.8 \times 10^{-6}$ cm^2/sec matter
~ $1.3 - 1.9 \times 10^{-6}$ cm^2/sec white matter

B5.6.2 Small ions [23]

D ~ 8.6×10^{-6} cm^2/sec

5.6.3 Large molecules (>150 angstrom): [23]

Hindered diffusion occurs

B5.7 COMMENTS

The list of primate brain tissue properties presented in this chapter highlights the numerous areas where data are either unavailable or largely incomplete. With a renewal of interest in modeling the normal and pathological response of the brain to various stimuli, it is possible that some of the missing tissue property data will be generated in the near future. Investigators should be cautioned, however, that because brain tissue properties vary with environmental factors, measurements made under unphysiologic conditions may differ from those of living tissue. As an example, the brain is highly vascularized, and the role of blood flow, volume, and pressure on tissue behavior remains to be determined.

The caution exercised by the experimentalist in generating new data should be matched by sound skepticism on the part of the investigators who are developing analytical or computational models of brain functional and structural response. Although the ability to calculate detailed responses has improved greatly in the past decade, these sophisticated models are limited by the available experimental data used to develop and validate the models. To create a realistic representation of normal or pathological response of the brain, it is essential that the model parameters be based on measured tissue properties and that any conclusions drawn from the models be validated with measured response data. Therefore, it is clear that future experimental studies are needed to determine the properties and response of living primate brain tissue.

ADDITIONAL READING

Cooney, D.O. (1976) *Biomedical Engineering Principles: An introduction to fluid, heat and mass transfer processes*, Marcel Dekker, New York.

Provides more detailed examples in bioheat transfer and pharmacokinetics which may be useful in modeling heat and mass transfer in the brain parenchyma.

Fung, Y.C. (1993) *Biomechanics: Mechanical properties of living tissues*, 2nd ed., Springer-Verlag, New York.

Fung, Y.C. (1990) *Biomechanics: Motion, flow, stress and growth*, Springer-Verlag, New York.

Fung, Y.C. (1965) *Foundations of Solid Mechanics*, Prentice Hall, Englewood Cliffs.

These works describe both basic principles of mechanics and their specific applications in biomechanics. A review of the constitutive property relationships for biological tissues included throughout these texts may be particularly helpful for applying the material-property information listed previously.

Lih, M.L. (1975) *Transport Phenomena in Medicine and Biology*, John Wiley & Sons, New York.

A concise review of the principles used in modeling the transport phenomena in several biological systems including examples of heat and mass transfer.

Nolte, J. (1988) *The Human Brain*, 2nd. ed., C.V. Mosby, St Louis

Provides a more detailed review of the structure and function of the different brain regions.

REFERENCES

1. Duck, F.A. (1990) *Physical Properties of Tissue*, Academic Press, New York.
2. ICRP (1975) *Report of the Task Group on Reference Man*, ICRP Publication 23, International Commission on Radiological Protection, Pergamon Press, Oxford, pp. 212–215; 280–281.
3. Woodard, H.Q. and White, D.R. (1986) The composition of body tissues. *Brit. J. Radiol.*, **59,** 1209–1219.
4. McElhaney, J.H., Roberts, V.L. and Hilyard, J.F. (1976) *Handbook of Human Tolerance*, Japanese Automobile Research Institute, Tokyo, pp. 151.
5. Fung, Y.C. (1993) *Biomechanics: Mechanical properties of living tissues*, 2nd ed., Springer-Verlag, New York.
6. Galford, J.E. and McElhaney, J.H. (1970) A viscoelastic study of scalp, brain, and dura. *J. Biomech.*, **3,** 211–221.
7. Fallenstein, G.T., Hulce, V.D. and Melvin, J.W. (1969) Dynamic mechanical properties of human brain tissue. *J. Biomech.*, **2,** 217-226.
8. Wang, H.C. and Wineman, A.S. (1972) A mathematical model for the determination of viscoelastic behavior of brain in vivo – I: Oscillatory response. *J. Biomech.*, **5,** 431–446.
9. Metz, H., McElhaney, J. and Ommaya, A.K. (1970) A comparison of the elasticity of live, dead, and fixed brain tissue. *J. Biomech.*, **3,** 453–458.
10. Ljung, C. (1975) A model for brain deformation due to rotation of the skull. *J. Biomech.*, **8,** 263–274.
11. Shuck, L.Z. and Advani, S.H. (1972) Rheological response of human brain tissue in shear. *J. Basic Eng., Trans ASME*, **94,** 905–911.
12. Pamidi, M. and Advani, S. (1978) Nonlinear constitutive relations for human brain tissue. *J. Biomech. Eng.*, **100,** 44–48.
13. Basser, P. (1992) Interstitial pressure, volume and flow during infusion into brain tissue. *Microvascular Res.*, **44,** 143–165.
14. Osswald, K. (1937), (Measurement of the conductivity and dielectric constants of biological tissues and liquids by microwave) (Ger.) Messung der Leitfahigkeit und Dielektrizitatkonstante biologischer gewebe und Flussigkeiten bei kurzen Wellen. *Hochfrequentz Tech. Elektroakustik*, **49,** 40–49.
15. Crile, G.W., Hosmer, H.R. and Rowland, A.F. (1922) The electrical conductivity of animal tissues under normal and pathological conditions. *Am. J. Physiol.*, **60,** 59–106.
16. Ranck, J.B. and Be Merit, S.L. (1963) Specific impedance of rabbit cerebral cortex. *Exp. Neurol.*, **7** 144–152.

17. Freygang, W.H. and Landaw, W.M. (1955) Some relations between resistivity and electrical activity in the cerebral cortex of the cat. *J. Cell. Comp. Physiol.*, **45,** 377–392.
18. van Harreveld, A., Murphy, T. and Nobel, K.W. (1963) Specific impedance of rabbit's cortical tissue. *Am. J. Physiol.*, **205,** 203–207.
19. Cooper, T.E. and Trezek, G.J. (1972) A probe technique for determining thermal conductivity of tissue. *J. Heat Transfer, Trans. ASME*, **94,** 133–140.
20. Bowman, H.F. (1981) Heat transfer and thermal dosimetry. *J. Microwave Power*, **16,** 121–133.
21. Valvano, J.W., Cochran, J.R. and Diller, K.R. (1985) Thermal conductivity and diffusivity of biomaterial measured with self-heating thermistors. *Int. J. Thermophys.*, **6,** 301–311.
22. Rosenberg, G.A., Kyner, W.T. and Estrada, E. (1980) Bulk flow of brain interstitial fluid under normal and hypermolar conditions. *Am. J. Physiol.*, **238,** f42–f49.
23 Nicholson, C. (1985) Diffusion from an injected volume of substance in brain tissue with arbitrary volume fraction and tortuosity. *Brain Research*, **333,** 325–329.

Arteries, veins and lymphatic vessels

B6

X. Deng and R. Guidoin

B6.1 INTRODUCTION

Blood and lymphatic vessels are soft tissues with densities which exhibit nonlinear stress–strain relationships [1]. The walls of blood and lymphatic vessels show not only elastic [2, 3] or pseudoelastic [4] behavior, but also possess distinctive inelastic character [5, 6] as well, including viscosity, creep, stress relaxation and pressure–diameter hysteresis. The mechanical properties of these vessels depend largely on the constituents of their walls, especially the collagen, elastin, and vascular smooth muscle content. In general, the walls of blood and lymphatic vessels are anisotropic. Moreover, their properties are affected by age and disease state. This section presents the data concerning the characteristic dimensions of arterial tree and venous system; the constituents and mechanical properties of the vessel walls. Water permeability or hydraulic conductivity of blood vessel walls have been also included, because this transport property of blood vessel wall is believed to be important both in nourishing the vessel walls and in affecting development of atherosclerosis [7–9].

The data are collected primarily from human tissue but animal results are also included in places for completeness. Among the three kinds of vessels, the arterial wall has been extensively investigated while studies of lymphatic vessels are very rare.

Handbook of Biomaterial Properties. Edited by J. Black and G. Hastings.
Published in 1998 by Chapman & Hall, London. ISBN 0 412 60330 6.

B6.2 MORPHOMETRY OF THE ARTERIAL TREE AND VENOUS SYSTEM

Detailed measurements of the number and size of blood vessels in the living body are very difficult to perform, so reliable information is scarce. Moreover, data collected on vessels in one tissue or organ are not applicable to another. Thus one should be cautious in using morphometric data; only the data for large vessels are reliable.

The aorta is tapered, but most other arteries can be considered to have a constant diameter between branches. The rate of taper varies from individual to individual, presumably, between species. However, in the dog, the change of aortic cross sectional area can be described by the exponential equation:

$$A = A_o e^{(-\beta x/R_0)} \quad \text{(B6.1)}$$

where A is the cross sectional area of the aorta, A_o and R_o are the respective cross sectional area and radius at the upstream site, x is the distance from the upstream site, and β a taper factor, which varies between 0.02 and 0.05 [10]. In man, the taper is found not to be as smooth as implied by the above equation; thus values of β are unavailable.

Morphometric and related data are given in Tables B6.1, B6.2 and B6.3.

B6.3 CONSTITUENTS OF THE ARTERIAL WALL

B6.3.1 Normal arterial wall

The main constituents of normal human arterial tissues from young adult subjects (20–39 years) are listed in Table B6.4 [20]. The major part of the

Table B6.1 Morphometric and Related Properties of the Human Systemic Circulation*

Vessel	*Diameter (mm)*	*Wall thickness (mm)*	*Length (cm)*	*Blood velocity (cm/sec)*	*Reynolds number*
Ascending aorta	32	1.6	5–5.5	63	3600–5800
Arch of aorta	25–30		4–5		
Thoracic aorta	20	1.2	16	27	1200–1500
Abdominal aorta	17–20	0.9	15		
Femoral artery	8	0.5	32		
Carotid artery	9	0.75	18		
Radial artery	4	0.35	23		
Large artery	2–6			20–50	110–850
Capillaries	0.005–0.01			0.05–0.1	0.0007–0.003
Large veins	5–10			15–20	210–570
Vena cava	20			11–16	630–900

* Source [11–17]. Note: The Reynolds numbers were calculated assuming a value for the viscosity of the blood of 0.035 poise.

Table B6.2 Morphometrics of the Pulmonary Arterial System*

Zone	*Number of branches*	*Diameter (mm)*	*Length (mm)*
Proximal	1.000	30.000	90.50
	3.000	14.830	32.00
	8.000	8.060	10.90
	2.000×10	5.820	20.70
	6.600×10	3.650	17.90
	2.030×10^2	2.090	10.50
	6.750×10^2	1.330	6.60
	2.290×10^3	0.850	4.69
Intermediate	5.861×10^3	0.525	3.16
	1.756×10^4	0.351	2.10
	5.255×10^4	0.224	1.38
	1.574×10^5	0.138	0.91
Distal	4.713×10^5	0.086	0.65
	1.411×10^6	0.054	0.44
	4.226×10^6	0.034	0.29
	1.266×10^7	0.021	0.20
	3.000×10^8	0.013	0.13

* Source: Adapted from [18].
Note: The data were obtained from a 32-year-old woman who had been free of respiratory disease and died of uremia. For the purpose of description, the pulmonary arterial tree was divided into three zones.

dry matter in the arterial wall consists of proteins such as elastin and collagen. Because the importance of elastin and collagen in the mechanical properties of arterial wall, the composition of media and adventitial layers in terms of collagen, elastin, smooth muscle and ground substance is listed in Table B6.5 for three different arterial tissues [1]. The collagen in adventitia and media is mostly Type III, some Type I, and a trace of Type V while the collagen of the basal lamina is Type IV [1].

Table B6.6 lists the constituents of additional arteries (canine), and the the ratio of collagen to elastin [21].

Composition changes of arterial tissues with age

The composition of normal human arterial tissues is altered with age in many aspects. Table B6.7 lists the observed changes in human aorta, pulmonary and femoral arteries [20]. There is a tendency that both the dry matter and nitrogen content of arterial tissues decreases with age. However, the relative quantity of collagen [22] and elastin [23, 24] in the arterial wall remains almost unchanged with age. Below the age of 39, the wall of human thoracic aorta has 32.1 ± 5.5% elastin, between the age 40–69, the wall contains 34.4 ± 9.3%, and from 70–89, the elastin content is 36.5 ± 10.1 [24].

Table B6.3 Morphometric and Related Properties of the Canine Systemic Circulation*†

Site	*Ascending aorta*	*Descending aorta*	*Abdominal aorta*	*Femoral artery*	*Carotid artery*	*Arteriole*	*Capillary*	*Venule*	*Vena cava, inferior*	*Pulmonary artery, main*
Internal diameter, d_i (cm)	1.5 (1.0–2.4)	1.3 (0.8–1.8)	0.9 (0.5–1.2)	0.4 (0.2–0.8)	0.5 (0.2–0.8)	5×10^{-3} ($1–8 \times 10^{-3}$)	6×10^{-4} ($4–8 \times 10^{-4}$)	4×10^{-3} ($1–7.5 \times 10^{-3}$)	1.0 (0.6–1.5)	1.7 (1.0–2.0)
Wall thickness, h (cm)	0.065 (0.05–0.08)	—	0.05 (0.04–0.06)	0.04 (0.02–0.06)	0.03 (0.02–0.04)	2×10^{-3}	1×10^{-4}	2×10^{-4}	0.015 (0.01–0.02)	0.02 (0.01–0.03)
h/d_i	0.07 (0.055–0.084)	—	0.06 (0.04–0.09)	0.07 (0.055–0.11)	0.08 (0.053–0.095)	0.4	0.17	0.05	0.015	0.01
In vivo length (cm)	5	20	15	10	15 (10–20)	0.15 (0.1–0.2)	0.06 (0.02–0.1)	0.15 (0.1–0.2)	30 (20–40)	3.5 (3–4)
Cross-section area (cm^2)	2	1.3	0.6	0.2	0.2	2×10^{-5}	3×10^{-7}	2×10^{-5}	0.8	2.3
Total vascular cross-section at each level (cm^2)	2	2	2	3	3	125	600	570	3.0	2.3
Blood velocity (peak) (ms^{-1})	1.2 (0.4–2.9)	1.05 (0.25–2.5)	0.55 (0.5–0.6)	1.0 (1.0–1.2)	—	0.75	0.07	0.35	0.25 (0.15–0.4)	0.7
Blood velocity (mean) (ms^{-1})	0.2 (0.1–0.4)	0.2 (0.1–0.4)	0.15 (0.08–0.2)	0.1 (0.1–0.15)	—	($5–10 \times 10^{-3}$)	$2–17 \times 10^{-4}$	$2–5 \times 10^{-3}$	—	0.15 (0.06–0.28)
Peak Reynolds number, $\hat{R}e$	4500	3400	1250	1000	—	0.09	0.001	0.035	700	3000

* Source: Adapted from [19].

† Normal values for canine cardiovascular parameters. An approximate average value, and then the range, is given where possible. All values are for the dog except those for arteriole, capillary, and venule, which have only been measured in smaller mammals.

Table B6.4 Composition of Normal Arterial Tissue*

	Components	*Aorta (human)*	*Femoral artery (human)*	*Brachial artery (human)*
Organic	Dry matter	28.0†	25.3	26.3
	Nitrogen	4.1	3.5	—
	Total lipids	1.680	—	—
	Cholesterol	0.290	0.135	0.185
Inorganic	Total ash	0.730	0.675	0.670
	Calcium	0.070	0.147	0.144
	Total PO_4	0.375	—	—

* Source: Adapted from [20].
† Values are expressed in percentage of wet tissue weight.

Table B6.5 Composition of Human Arteries at *In Vivo* Blood Pressure

	Thoracic aorta	*Plantar artery*	*Pulmonary artery*
Media			
Smooth muscle	33.5 ± 10.4†	60.5 ± 6.5	46.4 ± 7.7
Ground substance	5.6 ± 6.7	26.4 ± 6.4	17.2 ± 8.6
Elastin	24.3 ± 7.7	1.3 ± 1.1	9.0 ± 3.2
Collagen	36.8 ± 10.2	11.9 ± 8.4	27.4 ± 13.2
Adventitia			
Collagen	77.7 ± 14.1	63.9 ± 9.7	63.0 ± 8.5
Ground substance	10.6 ± 10.4	24.7 ± 2.6	25.1 ± 8.3
Fibroblasts	9.4 ± 11.0	11.4 ± 2.6	10.4 ± 6.1
Elastin	2.4 ± 3.2	0	1.5 ± 1.5

* Source: Adapted from [1].
† (Mean ± S.D.)

Changes in elastin and collagen content due to hypertension

Experimental observation by Wolinsky [25] showed that the absolute amounts of both elastin and collagen contents increased in hypertensive rats; however, the percentage of these elements remained essentially constant (Table B6.8)

Changes in elastin and collagen content due to atherosclerosis

Table B6.9 lists the changes in elastin and collagen contents of canine carotid and iliac arteries due to dietary atherosclerosis [26]. In the iliac site the ratio of collagen to elastin was increased, while the ratio in the carotid site was decreased.

Table B6.6 Arterial Wall Constituents, and Ratio of Collagen to Elastin*

		Percentage of wet tissue		*Percentage of dry defatted tissue*			C
Artery	*n*†	H_2O	*Extracted fat+*H_2O	*Collagen*	*Elastin*	*Collagen+elastin*	E
Coronary	9	63.2 ± 1.0‡	71.5 ± 1.4	47.9 ± 2.6	15.6 ± 0.7	63.5 ± 2.7	3.12 ± 0.21
Aorta, ascending	9	73.8 ± 0.6	74.0 ± 0.5	19.6 ± 1.2	41.1 ± 2.1	60.7 ± 2.2	0.49 ± 0.04
Carotid	6	71.1 ± 0.1	71.2 ± 0.1	50.7 ± 2.1	20.1 ± 1.0	70.8 ± 2.5	2.55 ± 0.13
Aorta, abdominal	10	70.4 ± 0.4	70.8 ± 0.3	45.5 ± 1.7	30.1 ± 1.7	75.6 ± 1.8	1.58 ± 0.15
Cranial mesenteric, proximal	10	70.8 ± 0.5	71.6 ± 0.4	38.1 ± 1.7	26.5 ± 1.7	64.6 ± 1.8	1.51 ± 0.15
Cranial mesenteric, distal	9	71.4 ± 0.4	72.0 ± 0.4	37.4 ± 1.4	22.4 ± 1.5	59.8 ± 1.6	1.72 ± 0.11
Cranial mesenteric, branches	10	69.5 ± 0.6	73.1 ± 0.7	36.1 ± 1.5	21.8 ± 0.9	57.9 ± 1.7	1.69 ± 0.10
Renal	9	70.4 ± 0.7	70.8 ± 0.7	42.6 ± 1.6	18.7 ± 1.8	61.3 ± 2.1	2.46 ± 0.27
Femoral	10	68.0 ± 0.3	68.1 ± 0.3	44.5 ± 1.4	24.5 ± 1.6	69.0 ± 2.1	1.89 ± 0.14

* Source: [21] by permission.
† Number of specimens.
‡ Specimens slightly dehydrated owing to unavoidably long dissection. Mean ± standard deviation. All percentage values refer to w/w.

Table B6.7 Variation of Normal Human Arterial Tissue Composition with Age*

Age group (years)	*Aorta*								
	Dry matter	*Nitro-gen*	*Total lipids*	*Choles-terol*	*Total ash*	*Cal-cium*	*Total PO_4*	*Acid-soluble PO_4*	*Potas-sium*
10–19	29.5†	4.38	1.23	0.15	—	0.03	0.25	0.16	0.055
30–39	28.5	4.03	1.75	0.28	0.81	0.09	0.40	0.29	0.040
50–59	28.0	3.67	1.90	0.48	1.55	0.21	0.54	0.41	0.039
70–79	28.0	3.38	—	0.71	2.80	0.39	—	—	0.033

Age group (years)	*Pulmonary artery*					*Femoral artery*				
	Dry matter	*Nitro-gen*	*Choles-terol*	*Cal-cium*	*Potas-ium*	*Dry matter*	*Nitro gen*	*Choles-terol*	*Total ash*	*Cal-cium*
10–19	26.5	3.91	0.12	0.025	0.033	26.9	3.84	0.11	0.59	0.14
30–39	25.7	3.71	0.17	0.028	0.031	24.4	3.30	0.15	0.71	0.18
50–59	24.9	3.45	0.22	0.027	0.026	22.8	2.83	0.23	1.15	0.40
70–79	23.0	3.25	—	0.060	0.025	25.3	2.90	0.55	3.17	1.07

* Source: Adapted from [20]; see for additional age group values.
† Values expressed in percentage of wet tissue weight.

Table B6.8 Effect of Hypertension on Composition of Arteries*

Group	*N‡*	*dry wt (mg)*	*Elastin (E)*		*Collagen (C)*		*E and C*
			Wt(mg)	*(% total wt)*	*WT(mg)*	*(% total wt)*	*(% total wt)*
III C†	2	5.25	1.76	33.5	0.69	13.1	46.6
		5.58	2.20	39.0	0.83	14.3	53.3
III H†	2	7.00	2.86	41.6	1.44	20.6	62.2
		6.50	2.78	42.8	1.06	16.3	59.1
II C	2	4.96	2.23	44.9	0.72	14.5	59.4
		5.26	2.14	40.6	0.68	12.8	53.4
II H	2	8.12	2.94	36.2	1.68	20.7	56.9
		7.50	2.70	36.0	1.52	20.3	56.3
I C	2	4.36	1.91	43.8	1.12	25.7	69.5
		5.56	2.09	37.6	1.24	22.3	59.9
I H	2	8.88	3.08	34.7	2.08	23.4	58.1
		10.89	3.50	32.1	2.33	21.4	53.5
		P<0.01#	P<0.001	P>0.2	P<0.01	P=0.2	P>0.8

* Source: [25] by permission: †: N = number of animals (rats); C = normotensive; H - hypertensive. #: Normotensive vs. hypertensive

Table B6.9 Effect of Atherosclerosis on Comparison of Arteries*

Site	*H_2O (g/kg wet wt)*	*Collagen (% dry wt)*	*Elastin (% dry wt)*	*Collegen + Elastin (% dry wt)*	*Collegen Elastin*
Carotid					
Control (n = 11)	740±3†	50.6±0.8	28.0±0.3	78.6±0.8	1.81±0.04
Diet (n = 7)	764±7##	49.8±1.6	33.1±1.3##	84.2±1.9##	1.61±0.07#
Iliac					
Control (n = 16)	742±3	46.2±0.6	33.0±0.7	79.2±1.1	1.41±0.03
Diet (n = 5)	724±6##	37.8±2.0	25.1±1.2##	66.0±2.3##	1.49±0.02#

* Source: [26] by permission; canine subjects.
† means ± SE.
Significantly different, P < 0.01; # Significantly different, P < 0.05.

B6.4 CONSTITUENTS OF THE VENOUS WALL

B6.4.1 Normal venous wall

The main constituents of normal human venous tissue are listed in Table B6.10.

Table B6.10 Composition of Normal Human Venous Tissue*

	Femoral vein	*Vena cava, inferior*
Dry matter	28.0†	26.1
Nitrogen	4.08	—
Cholesterol	0.076	0.083
Total ash	0.590	—
Calcium	0.058	0.012
Potassium	—	0.065

* Source: adapted from [27].
† Percentage of wet tissue weight.

B6.4.2 Changes with age in composition of normal venous tissues

The changes with age in the composition of normal venous vessels are listed in Table B6.11.

B6.5 MECHANICAL PROPERTIES OF ARTERIES

The blood vessel wall consists of three layers: the intima, media, and adventitia. The intima contains mainly the endothelial cells that contribute little to the strength of the blood vessels. The media and the adventitia

Table B6.11 Composition of Normal Human Venous Tissue*

		Femoral vein			
Age group	*Dry matter*	*Nitrogen*	*Cholesterol*	*Total ash*	*Calcium*
0–9	31.1†	4.63	0.058	0.525	0.051
20–29	27.4	3.88	0.071	0.586	0.053
40–49	24.7	3.34	0.064	0.542	0.065
60–69	23.2	3.06	0.087	0.555	0.075
70–79	21.8	2.92	0.087	0.600	0.083
		Vena cava, inferior			
Age group	*Dry matter*	*Nitrogen*	*Cholesterol*	*Calcium*	*Potassium*
0–9	30.9	—	—	—	—
20–29	26.8	—	0.082	0.011	0.072
40–49	24.5	—	0.091	0.011	0.053
60–69	21.7	—	0.097	0.010	0.048
70–79	22.7	—	0.097	0.011	0.048

* Source: [27] by permission.; see source for additional age groups.
† Percentage of wet tissue weight.

contain smooth muscle cells, elastin and collagen. Elastin is the most 'linearly' elastic biosolid material known. Unlike elastin, collagen does not obey Hooke's Law. However, collagen is the main load carrying element of blood vessels. Table B6.12 lists the mechanical properties of tissues composing the blood vessel wall.

B6.5.1 Static mechanical properties of arteries

Studies of arterial wall mechanics have clearly established the anisotropic nature of arteries [1, 29, 30]. *In vivo* pressurized arteries are deformed simultaneously in all directions. But, experimental studies [31] have demonstrated that arteries deform orthotropically. Therefore, arterial deformations may be examined in three orthogonal directions, namely, the longitudinal, circumferential, and radial directions. There are nine

Table B6.12 Mechanical Properties of Layers of the Vascular Wall*

Material	*Young's modulus (dynes/cm²)*	*Relative extensibility[a] (cm)*	*Maximum extension (%)*	*Tensile strength (dynes/cm²)*
Elastin	3 to 6×10^6	10	100–220	3.6×10^6 to 4.4×10^7
Collagen	1×10^9 to 2.9×10^{10}	0.03	5.50	5×10^7 to 5×10^9
Smooth muscle				
Relaxed	6×10^4	—	300	—
Contracted	1×10^5 to 12.7×10^6	2.3	300	—

* Source: Adapted from [28]; Fiber 10 cm in length, 1 mm² cross section, sustaining a load of 30 g.

elastic parameters: the three elastic moduli, E_θ, E_z and E_r; and six Poisson's ratios, $\sigma_{r\theta}$, $\sigma_{\theta r}$, $\sigma_{z\theta}$, $\sigma_{\theta z}$, σ_{rz} and σ_{zr}. As far as hemodynamics is concerned, however, among the three elastic moduli the circumferential one is most important.

The cicumferential elastic modulus is termed the incremental modulus and determined by the following equation (B6.2):

$$E_\theta = \frac{\Delta p_i \, 2(1 - \sigma^2)R_o \, R_i^2}{\Delta R_o \, (R_o^2 - R_i^2)} \qquad \text{(B6.2)}$$

where Δp_i is the transmural pressure increment, R_o and R_i are the respective external and internal diameter of the vessel, ΔR_o is the change in the external diameter due to Δp_i, and σ the Poisson's ratio (the ratio of transverse strain to longitudinal strain). The detailed technique for measuring the circumferential incremental elastic modulus of the arteries was described by Bergel [32].

Table B6.13 presents the circumferential incremental elastic modulus of human arterial walls from young adults (≤ 35 years) at a transmural pressure of 100 mmHg.

Experimental data by Bader [34] demonstrated that the circumferential elastic modulus of human thoracic aorta increased almost linearly with age. Table B6.14 gives the variation with age in the elastic moduli for human thoracic and abdominal aorta at a pressure of 100 mmHg.

It should be mentioned that all the circumferential elastic moduli given in Table B6.14 are based on the assumption of a Poisson's ratio of 0.5. This is not strictly true when large strains are considered [36]. Patel *et al.* [37] measured Poisson's ratios for the aorta in living dogs at a transmural pressure of about 110 mmHg, as well as the circumferential, longitudinal and radial incremental elastic moduli and determined that individual values vary between 0.29 and 0.71.

Table B6.13 Elastic Modulus of Human Arteries*

Arterial segment	E_θ *(×10⁶ dynes/cm²)*
Thoracic aorta	4.0–10
Abdominal aorta	4.0–15
Iliac artery	8.0–40
Femoral artery	12–40
Carotid artery	3.0–8.0

* Source: Adapted from [33,34]; young subjects (≤ 30 years) at a transmural pressure of 100 mmHg.
Note: The circumferential elastic moduli were calculated assuming that the arterial walls have a Poisson's ratio (the ratio of transverse to longitudinal strain) of 0.5.

Table B6.14 Hydrodynamic Properties of the Aorta*

		Thoracic aorta	
Age (yrs)	*Z_o (mmHgS cm^3)*	*Vp (m/s)*	*E_o† (10^6 N/m^2)*
30–39	0.13	5.8	0.56
40–49	0.17	7.4	0.8
50–59	0.19	9.0	1.13
60–69	0.19	10.0	1.25
70–79	0.22	12.4	1.87
80–89	0.22	13.6	2.2
		Abdominal aorta	
Age (yrs)	*Z_o (mmHgS cm^3)*	*Vp (m/s)*	*E_o† (10^6 N/m^2)*
30–39	0.31	7.9	0.8
40–49	0.53	10.5	1.22
50–59	0.53	11.4	1.3
60–69	0.51	12.0	1.5
70–79	0.68	14.5	1.75

* Adapted from [35] by permission;
† Poisson's ratio of arterial wall assumed to be 0.5.

B6.5.2 Compliance, pressure cross-sectional area relationship, and retraction

By measuring the static elastic properties of human thoracic and abdominal aortas *in vitro*, Langewouters *et al.* [35] proposed the following empirical relationship between the cross-sectional area of the lumen (A) and the pressure in the vessel (p):

$$A(p) = A_m \left\{ \frac{1}{2} + \frac{1}{\pi} \tan^{-1} \left(\frac{p - p_o}{p_1} \right) \right\} \qquad (B6.3)$$

in which A_m, p_o and p_1 are three independent parameters that are defined in Equation (B6.4) below.

Another important mechanical property of blood vessels in the compliance. Langewouters *et al.* [35] defined the 'static' compliance as the derivative of equation (B6.3) with respect to pressure

$$C(p) = \frac{C_m}{1 + \left(\frac{p - p_o}{p_1} \right)^2} \; ; \; C_m = \frac{A_m}{\pi \, p_1} \qquad (B6.4)$$

where C_m and A_m are the maximum compliance and the maximum cross-sectional area of the vessel, respectively; p_o is the pressure at which aortic compliance reaches its maximum; and p_1 is the half-width pressure, i.e. at $p_o \pm p_1$, aortic compliance is equal to $C_m/2$. According to Langewouters *et al.* [35], the 'static' compliance values of human thoracic aorta at 100 mmHg range from 1.9 to 17 × 10^{-3} cm^2/mmHg; and 0.6 to 4.4 × 10^{-3} cm^2/mmHg for abdominal aorta.

Table B6.15 lists the relative wall thickness and the retraction on excision for a variety of blood vessels. The retraction of a vessel is the amount by which a segment of vessel shortens on removal from the body, expressed as a percentage of the length of the segment in situ. The relative wall thickness is the ratio of wall thickness to mean diameter of the vessel.

B6.5.3 Tensile properties of human arteries

Table B6.16 presents typical data for the tensile properties of arterial tissues from Yamada [43]. The test specimens of tissues were strips each with a reduced middle region 10 mm length, 2–3 mm in width, and a length to width ratio of 3:1. In the tables:

1. Tensile breaking load per unit width (g/mm) = ultimate tensile strength (g/mm^2) × thickness (mm)
2. Ultimate tensile strength (g/mm^2) $= \dfrac{\text{tensile breaking load (g)}}{\text{cross-section area of the test section}}$
3. Ultimate percentage elongation (%) $= \dfrac{\text{breaking elongation (mm)}}{\text{original length of the specimen (mm)}} \times 100$

Table B6.15 Relative Wall Thickness and Retraction on Excision of Various Blood Vessels*

Vessel	*Species*	$\gamma \times$ %	*Retraction %*	*Source*
Thoracic aorta	Dog	10.5	32	[2]
Abdominal aorta	Dog	10.5	34	[2]
Femoral artery	Dog	11.5	42	[2]
Carotid artery	Dog	13.2	35	[2]
Iliac artery	Dog	—	40	[2]
Carotid artery	Dog	13.6	—	[38]
Carotid artery	Cat	14.5	—	[38]
Carotid artery	Rabbit	11.2	—	[38]
Carotid sinus	Dog	20.0	—	[38]
Carotid sinus	Cat	16.0	—	[38]
Carotid sinus	Rabbit	12.0	—	[38]
Thoracic aorta	Dog	14.0	—	[39]
Abdominal aorta	Dog	12.0	—	[39]
Femoral artery	Dog	13.0	—	[39]
Pulmonary artery	Man	2.0	—	[40]
Abdominal vena cava	Dog	2.3	30	[41]
Thoracic aorta	Man	6–9	25–15	[33]†
Abdominal aorta	Man	8–13	30–17	[33]†
Femoral artery	Man	12–19	40–25	[33]†
Carotid artery	Man	2–15	25–18	[33]†

Source: Adapted from [42].

† Measurement from [33] of young (<35) and old (>35) subjects respectively.

Table B6.16 Tensile Properties of Human Coronary Arterial Tissue* (Longitudinal Direction)

Age (yrs)	*Tensile Breaking Load/Unit width (g/mm)*	*Ultimate Tensile Strength (g/mm²)*	*Ultimate Elongation (%)*
10–19	85±3.1	140±3.0	99±2.4
20–39	82±1.8	114±9.3	78±1.6
40–59	82±1.8	104±4.7	68±3.5
60–79	79±2.9	104±4.7	4.5±3.8
Adult (average)	81	107	64

* Adapted from [43].

Table B6.16 lists the tensile data for human coronary arterial tissue in the longitudinal direction. Other arteries have similar properties [43]. Yamada [43] provides the tensile properties of animal tissues in various tables.

B6.5.4 Dynamic mechanical properties of arteries

The most direct way to study arterial viscoelasticity is to determine the response of the test tissue to oscillatory stresses. If the arterial wall is conceived to be represented by a simple Kelvin–Voigt model consisting of a spring and a dashpot in parallel, the dynamic elastic component and the viscous component of a vessel can be expressed as

$$E_D = \mathbf{E} \cos \phi$$

$$\eta\omega = \mathbf{E} \sin \phi \qquad \text{(B6.5)}$$

where **E** is the complex dynamic elastic modulus that is identical to the incremental elastic modulus under static stresses; ϕ is the phase lag of the strain behind the stress (in the case of circumferential direction, it is the phase lag of diameter behind the pressure); E_D is the dynamic elastic modulus of the vessel; and $\eta\omega$ is the viscous retarding modulus (η is the viscous constant and ω the angular frequency). For measuring the circumferential dynamic mechanical properties, the test vessel is usually subjected to an oscillatory pressure. The pressure oscillations are in a sinusoidal form. In circumferential direction, **E** can be calculated from equation (B6.2) with the recorded diameter of the blood vessel and the oscillatory pressure [44].

Table B6.17 lists the dynamic mechanical properties of different arteries at a frequency of 2.0 Hz at a mean pressure of 100 mmHg. In this table, E_p is the circumferential pressure-strain modulus defined as

$$E_p = \Delta P_i \, R_o \, / \, \Delta R_o \qquad \text{(B6.6)}$$

Table B6.17 Circumferential Dynamic Mechanical Properties of Different Human Arteries*

Vessel	*E_p (dynes-cm^{-2} × 10^{-6})*	*ϕ(radians)*	*V_p (m/s)*	*Source*
Ascending aorta	0.8	---	6.0	[29]
Carotid	6.2	---	17	[29]
Carotid	0.4	---	4.6$^+$	[45]
Thoracic aorta	0.6–1.0	0.12	6–9$^+$	[33]$^{++}$
Abdominal aorta	0.7–1.5	0.1	6–8$^+$	[33]$^{++}$
Femoral	2.5–7.0	0.15	13–18	[33]$^{++}$
Carotid	2.5–3.0	0.1	---	[33]$^{++}$
Pulmonary artery	0.1–0.16	---	2.3–2.9	[29]

* Adapted from [42].
Elastic modulus and pulse-wave velocity values collected from the literature. Those values for the PWV marked thus: $^+$ were measured, the others have been calculated from dynamic elasticity measurements; ++ measurements for young (<35) and old (>35) subjects respectively. ϕ = phase difference between wall stress and strain at 2 Hz. E_p is defined in eq (B6.6). The mean pressure was 100 mmHg.

in which ΔP_i is the pressure increment, R_o is the external diameter of the vessel and ΔR_o the external diameter change. E_p is essentially a reciprocal of the compliance of an artery and differs from elastic modulus in that it defines the stiffness of the total artery. Nevertheless, it is an indication of E_D.

Another important parameter listed in Table B6.17 is the pulse-wave velocity V_p (PWV) that can be calculated from the Moens–Korteweg equation:

$$V^2_p = Eh/2R\rho \tag{B6.7}$$

where E = elastic modulus of the wall, h = wall thickness, R = mean radius of the vessel, ρ = density of blood.

There is general understanding that the dynamic elastic modulus is not strongly frequency dependent above 2–4 Hz and that it increases from the static value at quite low frequencies. Bergel [42] provides additional values for canine vessels.

B6.5.5 Creep and stress relaxation

When a subject is suddenly strained and then the strain is maintained constant afterward, the corresponding stresses induced in the subject decrease with time, this phenomenon is called stress relaxation. If the subject is suddenly stressed and then the stress is maintained afterwards, the subject continues to deform, this phenomenon is called creep. Creep and stress relaxation are another two important phenomena in the arterial viscoelasiticity. Langewouters *et al.* [46] studied the creep responses of human thoracic and abdominal aortic segments. The pressure in the segments was changed in steps of 20 mmHg between 20 and 180 mmHg. Aortic creep curves at each pressure level were described individually by a constant plus biexponential creep model (C-model, [47])

$$A_i^c = \Delta A\left[1 - \alpha_1 \exp\left(\frac{-t_i}{\tau_1}\right) - \alpha_2 \exp\left(\frac{-t_i}{\tau_2}\right)\right] \quad (B6.8)$$

where A = aortic cross-sectional area; A_i^c = sample value of aortic creep response at time t_i; δA = change in aortic area upon a 20 mmHg pressure step; t = time; i = sample number; a_1, a_2 = creep fraction; τ_1, τ_2 = time constant. Table B6.18 lists the creep fractions and time constants for all aortic segments [46].

Stress relaxation relations for human arteries are not available; however, Tanaka and Fung [48] studied the stress relaxation spectrum of the canine aorta. They expressed the stress history with respect to a step change in strain in the form:

$$T(t, l) = G(t) \cdot T^{(e)}(l), \; G(0) = 1 \quad (B6.9)$$

where G (t) is the normalized relaxation function of time; $T^{(e)}$ (l) is a function of strain l, called elastic response. This is the tensile stress instantaneously generated in the aortic tissue when a step elongation, l, is imposed on the specimen.

If the relaxation function is written as:

$$G(t) = \frac{1}{\mathcal{A}}\left[1 + \int_0^\infty S(\tau) e^{-t/\tau} d\tau\right] \quad (B6.10)$$

in which

$$\mathcal{A} = \left[1 + \int_0^\infty S(\tau) d\tau\right]$$

is a normalized factor, then the spectrum S (t) is expected to be a continuous function of relaxation time t. A special form of S (t) is proposed

Table B6.18 Creep Constants of Human Thoracic and Abdominal Aortas*

	Thoracic aorta (n = 35)			*Abdominal aorta (n = 16)*		
Parameter	*Range*	*Mean*	*S.D.*	*Range*	*Mean*	*S.D.*
α_1	0.05–0.13	0.076	0.017	0.05–0.12	0.078	0.017
α_2	0.03–0.15	0.102	0.028	0.07–0.15	0.101	0.025
t_1 (S)	0.31–1.43	0.73	0.29	0.33–0.81	0.61	0.12
t_2 (S)	5.9–23.5	14.0	4.1	4.6–17.7	12.1	3.4
C (10^{-3} cm²/mmHg)	1.5–12.3	5.1	2.5	0.5–3.3	1.5	0.78
Age	30–78	63	14	30–78	58	15

* Adapted from [46] by permission.
α_1, α_2, creep fractions; t_1, t_2, time constants; *C*, compliance; S.D., standard deviation.

$$S(t) = c/t \text{ for } t_1 \leq t \leq t_2$$
$$= 0 \quad \text{for } t < t_1,\ t > t_2 \qquad \text{(B6.11)}$$

Values for segments of the canine aorta are given in [48].

B6.6 MECHANICAL PROPERTIES OF VEINS

B6.6.1 Static mechanical properties of veins

The structure of the venous walls is basically similar to that of the arterial walls. The main difference is that they contain less muscle and elastic tissue than the arterial walls, which raises the static elastic modulus two to fourfold [49]. Because the venous walls are much thinner than the arterial wall, they are easily collapsible when they are subject to external compressions.

Table B6.19 lists the static incremental elastic moduli of the canine jugular vein and human saphenous vein. For the purpose of comparison, the static increment elastic modulus of the canine carotid artery segments are also presented in the table. This comparison is of interest because in some arterial reconstructive surgeries, a vein is used as a substitute for an artery.

Table B6.19 Comparison of elastic Moduli between Venous and arterial Segments*

	Extension ratio		*Incremental venous elastic modulus*		*Carotid artery Incremental modulus*	
Pressure (cm H_2O)	λ_θ	λ_z	E_θ *(dynes/ cm^2 × 10^6)*	E_z *(dynes/ cm^2 × 10^6)*	E_θ *(dynes/ cm^2 × 10^6)*	E_z *(dynes/ cm^2 × 10^6)*
			Canine Jugular Vein			
10	1.457	1.481	15 ± 3*	1.2 ± 0.18†	7.62	5.16
25	1.463	1.530	47 ± 6†	4.4 ± 0.35†	8.39	7.15
50	1.472	1.597	88 ± 7†	11.8 ± 2.1	9.51	10.69
75	1.478	1.646	98 ± 7†	46 ± 13*	10.37	13.97
100	1.482	1.675	117 ± 10†	67 ± 25	10.92	16.24
125	1.484	1.686	134 ± 24†	89 ± 32	11.16	17.17
150	1.484	1.686	171 ± 9†	113 ± 13†	11.16	17.17
			Human Saphenous Vein			
10	1.357	1.169	0.27 ± 0.12†	1.61 ± 0.32*	5.30	0.017
25	1.417	1.206	0.65 ± 0.13†	2.03 ± 0.39*	5.82	0.328
50	1.500	1.266	1.89 ± 0.41†	2.75 ± 0.78	6.00	0.735
75	1.561	1.325	9.85 ± 1.6	3.18 ± 0.76	9.66	1.80
100	1.602	1.381	15.0 ± 2.6	3.56 ± 0.58	12.77	3.15
125	1.621	1.430	20.4 ± 1.6*	3.98 ± 0.96	14.79	4.59
150	1.621	1.470	25.1 ± 7.5	4.75 ± 1.2	15.51	5.93

* Adapted from [50] by permission.
* $P < 0.05$ for the comparison between the venous and carotid moduli.
† $P < 0.01$ for the comparison between the venous and carotid moduli.

Sobin [51] obtained data on the mechanical properties of human vena cava from autopsy material. The data may be expressed by the following equation:

$$T = \alpha EC\lambda\ [a(E^2 - E^{*2})] \qquad \text{(B6.12)}$$

$$E = (\lambda^2 - 1)/2$$

$$T^* = \alpha CE^*\lambda^*$$

where λ is the ratio of the changed length of the specimen divided by the reference length of the specimen, C and α are material constants, and E^* is the strain that corresponds to a selected value of stress S^*. The product of the constant αC is similar to the elastic modulus, provided that the modulus is defined as the ratio, S^*/E^*, where $S^* = T^*/\lambda^*$. Fung [1] provides typical values of these constants obtained experimentally; however, no universal constants have been discovered.

Table B6.20 Tensile Properties of Human Venous Tissue*

		Age group			
Vein	*Direction*	*20–39 yr*	*40–50 yr*	*60–69 yr*	*adult average*
		Tensile Breaking Load per Unit Width (g/mm)			
Inferior vena cava	L	102.0	87.0	68.0	89.0
	T	245.0	224.0	224.0	232.0
Femoral	L	159.0	149.0	149.0	153.0
	T	211.0	217.0	224.0	216.0
Popliteal	L	116.0	116.0	116.0	116.0
	T	180.0	197.0	158.0	182.0
		Ultimate Tensile Strength (kg/mm²)			
Inferior vena cava	L	0.15	0.11	0.08	0.12
	T	0.36	0.28	0.27	0.31
Femoral	L	0.24	0.21	0.20	0.22
	T	0.32	0.31	0.29	0.31
Popliteal	L	0.20	0.17	0.15	0.18
	T	0.31	0.29	0.20	0.27
		Ultimate Percentage Elongation			
Inferior vena cava	L	98.0	77.0	70.0	84.0
	T	58.0	47.0	44.0	51.0
Femoral	L	97.0	72.0	72.0	82.0
	T	79.0	67.0	56.0	70.0
Popliteal	L	112.0	97.0	81.0	100.0
	T	77.0	77.0	77.0	77.0

* Adapted from [43].L = longitudinal; T = transverse.

B6.6.2 Tensile properties of veins

The tensile properties of human venous tissues are presented in Table B6.20. For the testing method and definitions of the terms in the table, please refer to Section B6.5 on *Mechanical properties of arteries.*

B6.7 MECHANICAL CHARACTERISTICS OF LYMPHATIC VESSELS

The problem concerning the ontogenesis of the lymphatic vessels is still not completely solved. However, most of the evidence indicates that the large lymphatic vessels are derived from the veins [52]. Therefore, lymphatics can be considered modified veins. According to the reports by Ohhashi *et al.* [53, 54], the circumferential elastic modulus of the bovine mesenteric lymphatics ranged from 4.2×10^4 to 2.7×10^5 dynes/cm^2 at a pressure range from 0 to about 20 mmHg, and the elastic modulus of canine thoracic duct is about 2.0×10^5 dynes/cm^2. These values are less than those of veins obtained by Bergel [55]. Therefore, the lymphatics are more distensible than the veins.

B6.8 TRANSPORT PROPERTIES OF BLOOD VESSELS

Under transmural pressures, fluid or plasma will flow across the walls of blood vessels. On one hand, convective fluid motion through the blood vessel wall plays a very important role in nourishing the vessel walls, on the other hand, it is involved in atherogenesis by promoting the transport of macromolecules such as lipoproteins into the arterial wall [55–58], possibly through leaky endothelial cell junctions in regions of high endothelial cell turnover [59]. Table B6.21 lists the filtration properties of excised, presumably normal, human iliac blood vessels.

Table B6.21 Water Permeability of Iliac Vessels*

Vessel	*Pressure (mmHg)*	*Filtration rate (cm/sec × 10^6)*
Iliac artery	0–20	0
	25–80	2.58
	100	4.08
	200	6.42
Iliac vein	0–20	6.94
	21–40	9.72
	41–60	11.67
	61–80	12.22
	81–100	12.78

* Adapted from [56].

B6.9 EFFECT OF AGE, HYPERTENSION AND ATHEROSCLEROSIS ON BLOOD VESSELS

B6.9.1 Age

Two well known changes accompany aging of the cardiovascular system are dilation of thoracic aorta [60] and increased thickness of arterial wall [61]. Arterial walls become less distensible with aging [34, 62, 63]. Both dry matter and nitrogen content of artery tissue show a tendency to decrease with age in large and medium sized arteries [20]. But the relative quantity of collagen [22] and elastin [23, 24] in the arterial wall remains essentially unchanged. With aging the arterial wall becomes progressively stiffer. Bader [34] found that the circumferential elastic modulus of human thoracic aorta increased linearly with age. At 100 mmHg, the static circumferential modulus of 'young' (< 35 years) human thoracic aorta averaged 7.5×10^6 dynes/cm^2, and for the 'old' (> 35 years) the average was 16.6×10^6 dynes/cm^2 [33]. Young peripheral arteries tend to have a greater viscosity ($\eta\omega$) than the older ones [33]. Despite the overall increase in stiffness, the arterial wall itself is considerably weaker than the younger/older one [43].

B6.9.2 Hypertension

Several studies have shown that the water content of human, rat and dog arteries is increased in hypertension, and this increased water content may be associated with an increased wall thickness [64, 65]. Due to the limitations in studying samples from human subjects, animal models (mainly rats) have been employed. Mallov [66] found that the aorta from hypertensive rats had more smooth muscle than normal aorta. Greenwald and Berry [67] reported increased elastin and decreased collagen content in the aorta from spontaneous hypertensive rats when compared with the normal aorta. Wolinsky [25] observed an increase in the absolute amounts of both medial elastin and collagen contents in hypertensive rats. However, the relative percentage of these elements remained essentially constant. Experimental studies [67–69] showed an increase in vessel stiffness with the development of hypertension. This increase in vessel stiffness results in a smaller vessel diameter for a given distending pressure, i.e. a decrease in the distensibility [70].

B6.9.3 Atherosclerosis

It is generally accepted that substantial changes in the arterial wall occur with atherosclerosis in man. In human atherosclerotic arteries, it appears that there may be an absolute increase in collagen and a decrease in muscle fibers when compared with normal arteries [28]. In canine iliac artery the ratio of collagen to elastin was found to be increased, while the ratio in carotid was decreased [26]. The elastic moduli of the diseased aorta and common iliac arteries are several times higher than those reported [33] for normal arteries. The most popular model used to study the effect of atherosclerosis on arterial wall properties is the rabbit subject to a high cholesterol diet. Cox and Detweiler [26] have shown that in the iliac arteries from high cholesterol fed greyhounds, collagen and elastin contents are decreased, but the ratio of collagen to elastin is increased. In carotid arteries from the treated animals, the elastin content is increased and the collagen to elastin ratio is decreased. Their results also show that the elastic modulus of the iliacs from the cholesterol fed animals is higher than that of the normal iliacs while the treated carotids are unchanged. By using a rabbit model, Pynadath and Mukherjee [71] found that cholesterol feeding had no effect on the longitudinal dynamic elastic modulus of the aorta, but the circumferential one was affected significantly. After six weeks of feeding, the circumferential dynamic elastic modulus increased from the normal value of 2.7×10^6 dynes/cm^2 to 4.0×10^6 dynes/cm^2. This increase showed a remarkable correlation with the cholesterol content in the aortas. Although animal models shed some light on the effects of cholesterol feeding, since atherosclerotic changes in the arterial wall are so closely related to aging, it is difficult to separate the effect of atherosclerosis from those of aging. The effects of atherosclerosis on the mechanical properties of the arterial wall remain unclear. Confusion with the effects of aging and other forms of arteriosclerosis such as medial calcification make interpretation of the results difficult.

B6.10 FINAL COMMENTS

Mechanical properties of the arteries from human and various animals have been extensively studied. However, literature on lymphatic vessels is very scarce. The data on the circumferential elastic modulus of the lymphatic vessels obtained by Ohhashi *et al.* [53, 54] seem to be too low considering that the lymphatics are originating from the veins.

The overall viscoelastic properties of a large blood vessel such as the aorta are known to be nonlinear [2, 44] and anisotropic [37]. But due to the fact that the blood vessel wall is incompressible [72] and deforms orthotropically [31], the mechanical properties of blood vessels can be described mainly by six coefficients: an elastic and a viscous moduli in the longitudinal, circumferential and radial directions. Among them, only the moduli in the circumferential and longitudinal directions have been studied widely. Much fewer data in the radial direction can be found in literature. In calculation of the circumferential elastic moduli, it was usually assumed that the Poisson's ratio was 0.5 that is not strictly true when large strains are considered [36]. In fact, the measured data [37, 73] show that the Poisson's ratio is about 0.3, not 0.5 as would be predicted for an isotropic material. But the Poisson's ratio was almost constant with respect to circumferential strain and pressure in both relaxed and constricted canine carotid arteries [73].

To our best knowledge, water diffusion properties of blood vessels have been studied extensively, but their electrical and thermal properties are still unknown.

ACKNOWLEDGEMENT

This work was supported by the Medical Research Council of Canada (Grant MT-7879). The assistance of Y. Marois, M. King and Y. Douville in preparation of this material is gratefully acknowledged.

ADDITIONAL READING

Canfield, T.R. and Dorbin, P.B. (1987) Static properties of blood vessels, in *Handbook of Bioengineering* (eds R. Skalak and S. Chien), McGraw-Hill Book Company, New York, pp. 16.1–16.28.

The authors discuss the mechanical behavior of arteries and the mathematical method required for quantification of such data. The discussion is entirely concerned with the elastic or pseudoelastic behavior of blood vessels. It should be emphasized that the arterial wall also exhibits inelastic properties, such as viscosity, creep, stress & relaxation and pressure–diameter hysteresis. Very few data on mechanical properties of blood vessels are presented.

Dorbin, P.B. (1983) Vascular mechanics, in *Handbook of Physiology, Vol. 3 The Cardiovascular System*, (eds J.T. Shepherd and F. Abboud), Amer. Physiol. Soc., Washington, DC, Section 2, pp. 65–102.

This chapter reviews the essential concepts of vascular mechanics and its methods of quantification. Some of the important controversies are discussed, and further research areas are pointed out. Detailed information is provided on the structural and mechanical changes of arteries with age. The effect of vascular disorders such as arterosclerosis and hypertension on the mechanical behavior of blood vessels is discussed as well. Extensive addition literature sources are provided.

Schneck, D.J. (1995) An outline of cardiovascular structure and function, in *The Biomedical Engineering Handbook*, (ed. J.D. Bronzino), CRC Press, Boca Raton, pp. 3–14.

The cardiovascular system is described as a highway network, which includes a pumping station (the heart), a working fluid (blood), a complex branching configuration of distributing and collecting pipes and channels (the blood vessels), and a sophisticated means for both intrinsic (inherent) and extrinsic (antonomic and endocrine) control. Data on both the arterial and venous systems are tabulated. However, no detailed sources are provided for the data listed. This is a very suitable reference for biomedical engineers.

Hargen, A.R. and Villavicenco, J.L. (1995) Mechanics of tissue/lymphatic support, in *The Biomedical Engineering Handbook*, (ed J.D. Bronzino), CRC Press, Boca Raton, pp. 493–504.

From an engineering point of view, the authors discuss the lymphatic system as a drainage system for fluids and waste products from tissues. Basic concepts of lymphatic transport along with clinical disorders are discused, although briefly. Extensive additional sources are cited.

REFERENCES

1. Fung, Y.C. (1993) *Biomechanics, Mechanical Properties of Living Tissues*, 2nd edn, Springer-Verlag, New York, pp. 321–391.
2. Bergel, D.H. (1961) The static elastic properties of the arterial wall. *J. Physiol.*, **156,** 445–457.
3. Patel, D.J. and Vaishnav, R.N. (1972) The rheology of large blood vessels, *Cardiovascular Fluid Dynamics*, D.H. Bergel (ed.), Academic Press, New York, Vol. 2, pp. 1–64.
4. Fung, Y.C., Fronek, K. and Patitucci, P. (1979) Pseudoelasticity of arteries and the choice of its mathematical expression. *Am. J. Physiol.*, **237,** H620–H631.
5. Remington, J.W. (1955) Hysteresis loop behavior of the aorta and other extensible tissues. *Am. J. Physiol.*, **180,** 83–95.
6. Alexander, R.S. (1971) Contribution of plastoelasticity to the tone of the cat portal vein. *Circ. Res.*, **28,** 461–469.
7. Anitschkov, N. (1933) Experimental arteriosclerosis in animals, in *Arteriosclerosis*, E.V. Cowdry, Editor, Macmillan, New York, pp. 298–299.
8. Wilens, S.L. and McCluskey, R.T. (1954) The permeability of excised arteries and other tissues to serum lipid. *Circ. Res.*, **2,** 175–182.
9. Baldwin, A.L., Wilson, L.M. and Simon, B.R. (1992) Effect of pressure on aortic hydraulic conductance. *Arterio. Thromb.*, **12,** 163–171.
10. Fung, Y.C. (1984) *Biodynamics, Circulation*, Springer-Verlag, New York, p. 77.
11. Brecher, G.A. (1956) *Venous Return*, Grune & Stratton, New York, pp. 30–67.
12. Helps, E.P.W. and McDonald, D.A. (1954) Observation on laminar flow in veins. *J. Physiol.*, **124,** 631–639.
13. Spencer, M.P. and Denison, A.B. (1963) Pulsatile blood flow in the vascular system, in *Handbook of Physiology*, Section 2, Circulation, W.F. Hamilton and P. Dow, Editors, Am. Physiol. Soc., Washington, pp. 839–864.
14. Fry, D.L. and Greefield, J.C. Jr. (1964) The mathematical approach to hemodynamics, with particular reference to Womersley's theory, in *Pulsatile Blood Flow*, Attinger, E.O. (ed), McGraw-Hill, New York, pp. 85–99.
15. Maggio, E. (1965) *Microhemocirculation, Observable Variables and Their Biological Control*, C.C. Thomas, Springfield.
16. Whitmore, R.L. (1968) *Rheology of the Circulation*, Pergamon Press, Oxford, pp. 99–108.

17. Morse, D.E. (1979) The normal aorta: embryology, anatomy, and histology of the aorta, in *The Aorta*, J. Lindsay, Jr. and J.W. Hurst, Editors, Grune & Stratton, New York, pp. 15–37.
18. Singhal, S., Henderson, R., Horsfield, K. *et al.* (1973) Morphometry of human pulmonary arterial tree. *Circ. Res.*, **33,** 190–197.
19. Fung, Y.C. (1984) *Biodynamics, Circulation*, Springer-Verlag, New York, pp. 77–165.
20. Kirk, J.E. (1962) Arterial and arteriolar system, biochemistry, in *Blood Vessels and Lymphatics*, D.I. Abramson, Editor, Academic Press Inc., London, pp. 82–95.
21. Fischer, G.M. and Llaurado, J.G. (1966) Collagen and elastin content in canine arteries selected from functionally different vascular beds. *Circ. Res.*, **19,** 394–399.
22. Kanabrocki, E.L., Fels, I.G. and Kaplan, E. (1960) Calcium, cholesterol and collagen levels in human aorta. *J. Gerontol.*, **15,** 383–387.
23. Lansing, A., Alex, M. and Rosenthal, T.B. (1950) Calcium and elastin in human arteriosclerosis. *J. Gerontol.*, **5,** 112–119.
24. Kraemer, D.M. and Miller, H. (1953) Elastin content of the abdominal fraction of human aortae. *Arch. Pathol.*, **55,** 70–72.
25. Wolinsky, H. (1970) Response of the rat aortic media to hypertension. Morphological and chemical studies. *Circ. Res.*, **26,** 507–523.
26. Cox, R.H. and Detweiler, D.K. (1979) Arterial wall properties and dietary atherosclerosis in the racing greyhound. *Am. J. Physiol.*, **5,** H790–H797.
27. Kirk, J.E. (1962) Venous system, biochemistry, in *Blood Vessels and Lymphatics*, D.I. Abramson, Editor, Academic Press Inc., London, pp. 211–213.
28. Strandness, D.E. and Sumner, D.S. (eds) (1975) *Hemodynamics for Surgeons*, Grune & Stratton, New York, New York, pp. 161–205.
29. Patel, D.J., Greenfield, J.C. and Fry, D.L. (1964) *In vivo* pressure-length-radius relationships of certain vessels in man and dogs, in *Pulsatile Blood Flow*, E.O. Attinger, Editor, McGraw-Hill, New York, pp. 293–302.
30. Cox, R.H. (1975) Anisotropic properties of the canine carotid artery *in vitro*. *J. Biomech.*, **8,** 293–300.
31. Patel, D.J. and Fry, D.L. (1969) The elastic symmetry of arterial segments in dogs. *Circ. Res.*, **24,** 1–8.
32. Bergel, D.H. (1958) A photo-electric method for the determination of the elasto-viscous behavior of the arterial wall. *J. Physiol.*, **141,** 22–23.
33. Learoyd, B.M. and Taylor, M.G. (1966) Alteration with age in the viscoelastic properties of human arterial walls. *Circ. Res.*, **18,** 278–292.
34. Bader, H. (1967) Dependence of wall stress in the human thoracic aorta on age and pressure. *Circ. Res.*, **20,** 354–361.
35. Langewouters, G.J., Wesseling, K.H. and Goedhard, W.J.A. (1984) The static elastic properties of 45 human thoracic and 20 abdominal aortas *in vitro* and the parameters of a new model. *J. Biomech.*, **17,** 425–435.
36. Bergel, D.H. (1960) *The Visco-elastic Properties of the Arterial Wall.* PhD thesis, University of London.
37. Patel, D.J., Janicki, J.S. and Carew, T.E. (1969) Static anisotropic elastic properties of the aorta in living dogs. *Circ. Res.*, **25,** 765–779.

38. Rees, P.M. and Jepson, P. (1970) Measurement of arterial geometry and wall composition in the carotid sinus baroreceptor area. *Circ. Res.*, **26,** 461–467.
39. Gow, B.S. and Taylor, M.G. (1968) Measurement of viscoelastic properties of arteries in the living dog. *Circ. Res.*, **23,** 111–122.
40. Reid, L. (1968) Structural and functional reappraisal of the pulmonary artery system, in *Scientific Basis of Medicine, Annual Reviews*, Vol. 8, pp. 289–307.
41. Yates, W.G. (1969) Experimental studies of the variations in the mechanical properties of the canine abdominal vena cava, in SUDAAR Report 393, Stanford University, California.
42. Bergel, D.H. (1972) The properties of blood vessels, in *Biomechanics, Its Functions and Objectives*, Y.C. Fung, Editor, Prentice-Hall, Englewood Cliffs, N.J., p. 110 and p. 131.
43. Yamada, H. (1970) *Strength of Biological Materials*, F.G. Evans, Editor, Williams and Wilkins, Baltimore, pp. 106–277.
44. Bergel, D.H. (1961) The dynamic elastic properties of arterial wall. *J. Physiol.*, **156,** 458–469.
45. Arndt, J.O., Klauske, J. and Mersch, F. (1968) The diameter of the intact carotid artery in man and its change with pulse pressure. *Pfülger's Arch*,, **30,** 230–240.
46. Langewouters, G.J., Wesseling, K.H. and Goedhard, W.J.A. (1985) The pressure dependent dynamic elasticity of 35 thoracic and 16 abdominal human aortas *in vitro* described by a five component model. *J. Biomech.*, **18,** 613–620.
47. Langewouters, G.J. (1982) *Visco-Elasticity of the Human Aorta* in vitro in Relation to Pressure and Age. PhD thesis, Free University, Amsterdam, The Netherland.
48. Tanaka, T.T. and Fung, Y.C. (1974) Elastic and inelastic properties of the canine aorta and their variation along the aortic trees. *J. Biomech.*, **7,** 357–370.
49. Attinger, E.O. (1967) Modelling of pressure-flow relations in arteries and veins (Abstract). *Biorheology*, **4,** 84.
50. Wesly, R.L.R., Vaishnav, R.N., Fuchs, J.C.A. *et al.* (1975) Static linear and nonlinear elastic properties of normal and arterialized venous tissue in dog and man. *Circ. Res.*, **37,** 509–520.
51. Sobin, P. (1977) *Mechanical Properties of Human Veins*. M.S. thesis, University of California, San Diego, California.
52. Susznyák, I., Földi, M. and Szabó, G. (1967) *Lymphatics and Lymph Circulation: Physiology and Pathology*, Pergamon Press, London, pp. 33–50.
53. Ohhashi, T., Azuma, T. and Sakaguchi, M. (1980) Active and passive mechanical characteristics of bovine mesenteric lymphatics. *Am. J. Physiol.*, **239,** H88–H95.
54. Ohhashi, T. (1987) Comparison of viscoelastic properties of walls and functional characteristics of valves in lymphatic and venous vessels. *Lymphatic*, **20,** 219–223.
55. Bergel, D.H. (1964) Arterial viscoelasticity, in *Pulsatile Blood Flow*, E.O. Attinger, Editor, McGraw-Hill, New York, pp. 275–292.
56. Wilens, S.L. and McCluskey, R.T. (1952) The comparative filtration filtration properties of excised arteries and veins. *Am. J. Med. Sci.*, **224,** 540–547.
57. Tedgui, A. and Lever, M.J. (1985) The interaction of convection and diffusion in the transport of ^{131}I-albumin within the media of rabbit thoracic aorta. *Circ. Res.*, **57,** 856–863.

58. Tedgui, A. and Lever, M.J. (1987) Effect of pressure and intimal damage on ^{131}I-albumin and ^{14}C-sucrose spaces in aorta. *Am. J. Physiol.*, **253,** H1530–H1539.
59. Weinbaum, S., Tzeghai, G., Ganatos, P. *et al.* (1985) Effect of cell turnover and leaky junctions on arterial macromolecular transport. *Am. J. Physiol.*, **248,** H945–H960.
60. Bazett, H.C., Cotton, F.S., Laplace, L.B. *et al.* (1935) The calculation of cardiac output and effective peripheral resistance from blood pressure measurements with an appendix on the size of the aorta in man. *Am. J. Physiol.*, **113,** 312–334.
61. Anderson, J.R. (1980), *Muir's Textbook of Pathology*, Arnold, London, pp. 360–395.
62. Nakashima, T. and Tanikawa, J. (1971) A study of human aortic distensibility with relation to atherosclerosis and aging. *Angiology*, **22,** 477–490.
63. Mozersky, D.J., Summer, D.S., Hokanson, D.E. *et al.* (1972) Transcutaneous measurement of the elastic properties of the human femoral artery. *Circulation*, **46,** 948–955.
64. Tobian, L. (1960) Interrelationship of electrolytes, juxtaglomerular cells and hypertension. *Physiol. Rev.*, **40,** 280–312.
65. Peterson, L.H. (1963) Systems behavior, feed-back loops and high blood pressure research. *Circ. Res.*, **12,** 585–596.
66. Mallov, S. (1959) Comparative reactivities of aortic strips for hypertensive and normotensive rats to epinephrine and levarterenol. *Circ. Res.*, **7,** 196–201
67. Greenwald, S.E. and Berry, C.L. (1978) Static mechanical properties and chemical composition of the aorta of spontaneously hypertensive rats, a comparison with the effects of induced hypertension. *Cardiovas. Res.*, **12,** 364–372.
68. Feigl, E.O., Peterson, L.H. and Jones, A.W. (1963) Mechanical and chemical properties of arteries in experimental hypertension. *J. Clin. Invest.*, **42,** 1640–1647.
69. Bandick, N. and Sparks, H. (1970) Viscoelastic properties of the aortas of hypertensive rats. *Proc. Soc. Exp. Biol. Med.*, **134,** 56–60.
70. Greene, M.A., Friedlander, R., Boltax, A.J. *et al.* (1966) Distensibility of arteries in human hypertension. *Proc. Roy. Soc. Exp. Biol.*, **121,** 580–585.
71. Pynadath, T.I. and Mukherjee, D.P. (1977) Dynamic mechanical properties of atherosclerotic aorta: A correlation between the cholesterol ester content and the viscoelastic properties of atherosclerotic aorta. *Atherosclerosis*, **26,** 311–318.
72. Carew, T.E.R., Vaishnav, R.N. and Patel, D.J. (1968) Compressibility of the arterial wall. *Circ. Res.*, **23,** 61–68.
73. Dobrin, P.B. and Doyle, J.M. (1970) Vascular smooth muscle and the anisotropy of dog carotid artery. *Circ. Res.*, **27,** 105–119.

B7 The intraocular lens

T.V. Chirila

B7.1 INTRODUCTION

Although the existence of the intraocular crystalline lens, usually referred to as the lens, in the eye was recognized by the scientists of the Hellenistic period (about 2000 years ago), it was 400 years ago that the real role of the lens in vision was properly understood, and truly scientific approaches to the lens measurements and properties began to be applied only in the nineteenth century [1]. For instance, the first to weigh the human lens was Smith in 1883 [2].

The lens is positioned between the aqueous humor and vitreous body of the eye. The lens refracts the light which enters the eye through the pupil and focuses it on the retina. The lens (i) provides refractive power to the optical system of the eye; (ii) provides the accommodation necessary for normal vision; (iii) maintains its own transparency; and (iv) absorbs UV radiation and blue light, both deleterious to the subsequent ocular segments.

The lens is a biconvex body similar to a flattened globe. For descriptive purposes, it has two poles (anterior and posterior), an equator, and therefore two diameters (polar, or lens thickness, and equatorial).

The lens is composed of epithelial cells which become anuclear and elongated as they are displaced further toward the center. Because of the enormous length finally attained by these cells, they are referred to as lens fibers. The lens is surrounded by a transparent acellular capsule of variable thickness. A proper epithelium underlies the capsule along the anterior side and equator, but not under the posterior capsule. The superficial layers of cells and fibers constitute the lens cortex, and the lens

Handbook of Biomaterial Properties. Edited by J. Black and G. Hastings.
Published in 1998 by Chapman & Hall, London. ISBN 0 412 60330 6.

nucleus is situated in the center. The fibers are continuously formed throughout life and the new fibers cover the old ones which are displaced toward the nucleus.

At present, there are significantly more compositional and physical property data on animal lenses than on the human lens.

Even the determination of a straightforward property like the water content has led to variable results (Tables B7.1 and B7.2), likely due both to nonuniform distribution of the water in the lens and to the variability of methods employed for measurements. While data on the inorganic content of the human lens (Table B7.3) are generally in agreement, there was a larger variation in reporting the organic content. This is presumably due to the greater sensitivity of the organic metabolism to age and disease. The most reliable results are included in Table B7.4.

Tables B7.5–B7.7 provide some key dimensional properties of the lens while Table B7.8 focuses on perhaps the most important feature, the optical properties.

Mechanical characteristics of the lens required sophisticated procedures for measurements and the data are probably difficult to reproduce. All the available mechanical properties of the human lens are included in Tables B7.9–B7.13. Large variations in the electrical properties of animal lenses have been reported, but it seems that the only measurements performed on human lenses are those shown in Table B7.14.

B7.2 CHEMICAL COMPOSITION

Table B7.1 Water content of the normal human lens

Method	*Value (%)*	*Source*
n.a.	65[a]	[3]
Vacuum dehydration	68.6 ± 4.3[b]	[4]
	63.4 ± 2.9[c]	
Microsectioning	52.5 - 66.2[c,d]	[5]
	72.5 - 90[d,e]	
Raman microspectroscopy	69 ± 4[b]	[6]
	65 ± 4[c]	
Freeze drying	68[c]	[7]
	80[e]	
	75[f]	
Raman microspectroscopy	58.0 ± 4.7 (<70 yr)[c]	[8]
	63.0 ± 2.8 (>70 yr)[c]	
	85.3 ± 9.4[e]	
	80.9 ± 8.3[f]	

± = Standard deviation; [a] whole lens; [b] cortex; [c] nucleus; [d] age 62 years to 68 years; [e] outermost anterior cortex; [f] outermost posterior cortex.

Table B7.2 Water content of cataractous human lenses

Method	*Value (%)*	*Source*
Drying	67.6[a]	[9]
	75.4[b]	
Freeze drying	79[c,d]	[8]
	83.5[c,e]	
	78[d,f]	
	87.5[e,f]	
	68[d,e,g]	
Drying	63.8 (< 60 yr)	[10]
	67.7 (> 80 yr)	

[a] No sclerosis, average age 64.7 years;[b] advanced sclerosis, average age 70.8 years;[c] outermost anterior cortex.;[d] primary nuclear cataract;[e] subcapsular cataract;[f] outermost posterior cortex;[g] nucleus.

Table B7.3 Inorganic ions content of the normal adult human lens

Ion	*Representative value*	*Source*
Sodium	91 mg/100 g wet wt	[3]
Potassium	170 mg/100 g wet wt	[3]
Calcium	1.4 mg/100 g wet wt	[3]
Magnesium	0.29 mg/100 g wet wt	[3]
	6.2 μg/g dry wt	[11]
Zinc	21 μg/g dry wt	[3]
	25 μg/g dry wt	[11]
Copper	< 1 μg/g dry wt	[3]
	0.6 μg/g dry wt	[11]
Manganese	0.2 μg/g dry wt	[11]
Iron	0.4 μg/g dry wt	[11]
Rubidium	6.8 μg/g dry wt	[11]
Chloride	35.3 mg/100 g wet wt	[3]
Phosphate	25 mg/100 g wet wt	[12]
Sulfate	24 mg/100 g wet wt	[12]
pH	7.3 to 7.7	[13]

Table B7.4 Organic content of the human lens[a]

Component	*Representative value*	*Source*
Proteins	30% of lens (young)	[14]
	35% of lens (old)	
Ascorbic acid	30	[11]
Glutathione[b]	170 (normal lens)	[15]
	52 (cataractous lens)	
	46–150	[11]
	200–450	[12]
Taurine	10	[11]
	6.7	[12]
Alanine	11.9	[11]
Glycine	5.9	[11]
Glutamic acid	50	[11]
Serine	5.9	[11]
Urea	28.2	[11]
Inositol	462	[12]
Cholesterol	1.4 mg/lens	[11]
Phospholipids: cortex	600–725[c]	[11]
nucleus	450–650[c]	[11]

[a] Expressed as mg per 100 g wet weight of lens, unless otherwise specified; [b] there is a large variation of reported data on glutathione content; [c] variation with age.

B7.3 DIMENSIONS AND OPTICAL PROPERTIES

Table B7.5 Dimensional variation with age of the human lens [11]

Dimension	*Value(mm)*
Polar diameter (lens thickness)	3.5 to 5
Equatorial diameter	6.5 to 9
Anterior radius of curvature	8 to 14
Posterior radius of curvature	4.5 to 7.5

Table B7.6 Thickness of the human lens capsule at age 35 years [11]

Location	*Value (μm)*
Anterior pole	14
Anterior, maximum	21
Equator	17
Posterior pole	4
Posterior, maximum	23

Table B7.7 Weight, volume and density of the human lens in adult life [16]

Age range (yrs)	*Weight, mean (mg)*	*Volume, mean (mm^3)*	*Density (calc.) at beginning of decade ($g\ cm^{-3}$)*
20–30	172.0	162.9	1.034
30–40	190.3	177.3	1.048
40–50	202.4	188.1	1.061
50–60	222.3	205.4	1.072
60–70	230.1	213.0	1.082
70–80	237.1	218.3	1.091

Table B7.8 Optical refractive index and transmissivity as a function of age

Refractive index [3]: 1.420

	Transmission of radiation at wavelength (%) [17]		
	Age (years)		
	25	*54*	*82*
Wavelength (nm)			
350	1.2	1.2	1.2
400	4.8	4.8	4.8
450	38.0	30.6	21.7
500	70.0	42.7	30.0
700	75.0	51.7	37.0

Table B7.9 Variation with age of tensile modulus (Young's modulus of elasticity) of the decapsulated human lens [18][a]

	Modulus ($kN\ m^{-2}$)	
Age (years)	*Polar*	*Equatorial*
at birth	0.85	0.75
20	1.0	0.75
40	1.5	1.1
63	3.0	3.0

[a] Determined by the spinning method.

Table B7.10 Hardness of cataractous human lenses [19][a]

Age (years)	*Mean Force (N)*	*Number of lenses*
<60	0.80	13
61–70	0.87	20
71–80	1.12	31
>80	1.38	27

[a] Measured by the force necessary to cut the lens in a guillotine.

Table B7.11 Mechanical properties of the human lens capsule [20][a]

Age (years)	*Property*	*Value*
	Tensile modulus (MPa)	
20		5.6
50		4.0
80		1.5
	Ultimate tensile stress (MPa)	
< 20		2.3
> 70		0.7
b	Elongation (%)	29
b	Poisson's ratio	0.47 ± 0.5

± = Standard deviation; [a]determined from the volume–pressure relationship upon distension with isotonic saline; [b]independent of age.

Table B7.12 Force of contraction for maximum accommodation of the human lens [21][a]

Age (years)	*Force (mN)*
25	7.2
35	10.9
45	12.8
55	11.4

[a] Determined from the stress–dioptric power relationship.

Table B7.13 Spring constants of human lens and zonules[22][a]

Spring constant at 10%elongation, m N	*Age range (years)* 2–39	40–70
Lens, polar	13.5±0.80	25.4±0.24
Lens, equatorial	12.3±0.65	36.5±0.23
Zonules[b]	0.38±0.32	0.65±0.85

± = Standard deviation; [a] spring constant is defined here as $S'=F/(\Delta l/l_o)$, where F total force and $\Delta l/l_o$ is elongation; [b] determined on specimens zonule–lens–zonule, after the excision of the ciliary muscles.

Table B7.14 Translenticular electrical properties in the isolated human lens [23]

Property	*Value*
Potential difference[a]	7 mV
Short circuit current density[b]	5 uA cm^{-2}
Resistance	1.5 kΩ cm^2

[a] Anterior side positive; [b] reflects sodium transport from the posterior to the anterior lens side and is expressed as a current density; [c] calculated as a ratio between potential difference and current density.

ADDITIONAL READING

Bellows, J.G. (ed.) (1975) *Cataract and Abnormalities of the Lens*, Grune & Stratton, New York.

A valuable collection of 42 contributions on the lens, its pathology and surgery, written by known experts such as Barraquer, Bellows, Choyce, Girard, Hockwin, Kaufman, Rosen and Yanoff. The first five introductory chapters present historical aspects, development and characterization of the lens. However, most of the book is dedicated to cataract and its treatment.

Spector, A. (1982) Aging of the lens and cataract formation, in *Aging and Human Visual Function* (eds R. Sekuler, D. Kline and K. Dismukes), Alan R. Liss, Inc., New York, pp. 27–43.

A brief, but comprehensive account of the changes which take place in the composition and metabolism of the lens during aging and cataractogenesis.

Duncan, G. and Jacob, T.J.C. (1984) The lens as a physicochemical system, in *The Eye*, vol. 1b, 3rd ed. (ed. H. Davson), Academic Press, Orlando, FL, pp. 159–206.

This text develops some topics usually neglected in other books, including the structural order in the lens, optical properties of the lens, role of lens membranes, and electrolyte transport and distribution in the lens.

Cotlier, E. (1987) The lens, in *Adler's Physiology of the Eye*, 8th ed. (eds R.A. Moses and W.M. Hart), C.V. Mosby Co., St. Louis, pp. 268–290.

A systematic presentation of the anatomy, biochemistry and physiology of the lens.

Moses, R.A. (1987) Accommodation, in *Adler's Physiology of the Eye*, 8th ed., (eds R.A. Moses and W.M. Hart), C.V. Mosby Co., St. Louis, pp. 291–310.

A thorough exposition of all aspects of the mechanism of accommodation and the role of the lens in vision. A text, by now classic, on a topic much more complex than it appears.

Jones, W.L. (1991) Traumatic injury to the lens. *Optom. Clin.*, **1**, 125–42.

This review article analyzes the effects of concussive trauma to the eye, emphasizing the types of injuries to the lens. The mechanical response of the anterior and posterior segments of the eye to external forces is also described.

REFERENCES

1. Grom, E. (1975) History of the crystalline lens, in *Cataract and Abnormalities of the Lens*, (ed. J.G. Bellows), Grune & Stratton, New York, pp. 1–28.
2. Smith, P. (1883) Diseases of crystalline lens and capsule. 1. On the growth of the crystalline lens. *Trans. Ophthalmol. Soc. UK*, **3,** 79–99.
3. Kuck, J.F.R. (1970) Chemical constituents of the lens, in *Biochemistry of the Eye*, (ed. C.N. Graymore), Academic Press, London, chapter 3.
4. Fisher, R.F. and Pettet, B.E. (1973) Presbyopia and the water content of the human crystalline lens. *J. Physiol.*, **234,** 443–7.
5. Bours, J., Födisch, H.J. and Hockwin, O. (1987) Age-related changes in water and crystalline content of the fetal and adult human lens, demonstrated by a microsectioning technique. *Ophthalmic Res.*, **19,** 235–9.

6. Huizinga, A., Bot, A.C.C., de Mul, F.F.M. *et al.* (1989) Local variation in absolute water content of human and rabbit eye lenses measured by Raman microspectroscopy. *Exp. Eye Res.*, **48,** 487–96.
7. Deussen, A. and Pau, H. (1989) Regional water content of clear and cataractous human lenses. *Ophthalmic Res.*, **21,** 374–80.
8. Siebinga, I., Vrensen, G.F.J.M., de Mul, F.F.M. *et al.* (1991) Age-related changes in local water and protein content of human eye lenses measured by Raman microspectroscopy. *Exp. Eye Res.*, **53,** 233–9.
9. Salit, P.W. (1943) Mineral constituents of sclerosed human lenses. *Arch. Ophthalmol.*, **30,** 255–8.
10. Tabandeh, H., Thompson, G.M., Heyworth, P. *et al.* (1994) Water content, lens hardness and cataract appearance. *Eye*, **8,** 125–9.
11. Harding, J.J. and Crabbe, M.J.C. (1984) The lens: development, proteins, metabolism and cataract, in *The Eye*, vol. 1b, 3rd ed., (ed. H. Davson), Academic Press, Orlando, FL, pp. 207–492.
12. Paterson, C.A. (1985) Crystalline lens, in *Biomedical Foundations of Ophthalmology*, vol. 2, 2nd ed., (eds T.D. Duane and E.A. Jaeger), Harper & Row, Philadelphia, chapter 10.
13. Kuck, J.F.R. (1970) Metabolism of the lens, in *Biochemistry of the Eye*, (ed. C.N. Graymore), Academic Press, London, chapter 4.
14. Davson, H. (1990) *Physiology of the Eye*, 5th ed., Macmillan, London, Chapter 4.
15. Dische, Z. and Zil, H. (1951) Studies on the oxidation of cysteine to cystine in lens proteins during cataract formation. *Am. J. Ophthalmol.*, **34,** 104–13.
16. Scammon, R.E. and Hesdorfer, M.B. (1937) Growth in mass and volume of the human lens in postnatal life. *Arch. Ophthalmol.*, **17,** 104–112.
17. Lerman, S. (1987) Chemical and physical properties of the normal and ageing lens: spectroscopic (UV, fluorescence, phosphorescence, and NMR) analyses. *Am. J. Optom. Physiol. Optics*, **64,** 11–22.
18. Fisher, R.F. (1971) The elastic constants of the human lens. *J. Physiol.*, **212,** 147–80.
19. Heyworth, P., Thompson, G.M., Tabandeh, H. *et al.* (1993) The relationship between clinical classification of cataract and lens hardness. *Eye*, **7,** 726–30.
20. Fisher, R.F. (1969) Elastic constants of the human lens capsule. *J. Physiol.*, **201,** 1–19.
21. Fisher, R.F. (1977) The force of contraction of the human ciliary muscle during accommodation. *J. Physiol.*, **270,** 51–74.
22. van Alphen, G.W.H.M. and Graebel, W.P. (1991) Elasticity of tissues involved in accommodation. *Vision Res.*, **31,** 1417–38.
23. Platsch, K.D. and Wiederholt, M. (1981) Effect of ion substitution and ouabain on short circuit current in the isolated human and rabbit lens. *Exp. Eye Res.*, **32,** 615–25.

C1 Blood and related fluids

V. Turitto and S.M. Slack

C1.1 INTRODUCTION

This section provides data for several human biological fluids including blood, plasma or serum, cerebrospinal (CS) fluid, lymph, synovial fluid, and tear fluid. The material presented here was gleaned from a variety of sources, with emphasis placed on the most recently published work, and includes physicochemical properties (Table C1.1), cellular compositions (Table C1.2), concentrations of inorganics (Table C1.3), organics (Table C1.4), and major proteins (Table C1.5). In addition, various properties of the major proteins are presented in Table C1.7, while Tables C1.8 and C1.9 contain information regarding the components of the coagulation and complement cascades, respectively. Because of the variability in values for many properties of biological fluids, in many cases a normal singular range of such values is listed. In all cases, the data are those compiled for normal human adults and, where possible, differences with respect to gender are included. It must be stressed that fluid properties can readily change as a result of disease, aging, or drug ingestion.

Handbook of Biomaterial Properties. Edited by J. Black and G. Hastings.
Published in 1998 by Chapman & Hall, London. ISBN 0 412 60330 6.

Table C1.1 Physiochemical properties [1–3]

Property	*Whole blood*	*Plasma (serum)*
Dielectric constant	8.0–8.5	—
Freezing point Depression (°C)	0.557--0.577	0.512–0.568
Osmolality (mosm/kg)	—	276–295
pH	7.38–7.42	7.39–7.45
Refractive index	—	1.3485–1.3513
Relative viscosity	2.18–3.59	1.18–1.59
Specific gravity	1.052–1.061	1.022–1.026
Specific conductivity (S/cm)	—	0.0117–0.0123
Specific heat (cal/g/°C)	0.87	0.94
Surface tension (dyne/cm)	55.5–61.2	56.2

Property	*Synovial fluid*	*CS fluid*	*Tear fluid*
Dielectric constant	—	—	—
Freezing Point Depression (°C)	—	0.540–0.603	0.572–0.642
Osmolality (mosm/kg)	292–300	290–324	309–347
pH	7.29–7.45	7.35–7.70	7.3–7.7
Refractive index	—	1.3349–1.3351	1.3361–1.3379
Relative viscosity	> 300	1.020–1.027	1.26–1.32
Specific gravity	1.008–1.015	1.0032–1.0048	1.004–1.005
Specific conductivity (S/cm)	0.0119	—	—
Specific heat (cal/g/°C)	—	—	—
Surface tension (dyne/cm)	—	60.0–63.0	—

The refractive index, specific gravity, and surface tension were measured at 20°C, the specific conductivity at 25°C, and the relative viscosity at 37°C. The specific gravity is that relative to water. The viscosity of serum is slightly less than that of plasma due to the absence of fibrinogen. Blood viscosity depends strongly on shear rate and hematocrit and the value given in Table C1.1 is that at high shear rates (> 200 s^{-1}) and normal hematocrits (40–45%). Blood is a non-Newtonian fluid and exhibits increased viscosity with decreasing shear rate. Correlations relating blood viscosity to hematocrit, shear rate, and protein content have been described in the literature [4,5]. The reader is referred to several excellent publications for further details regarding factors affecting blood viscosity [4,6–11].

Table C1.2 Cellular composition of biological fluids [12]

A. Whole blood

Whole blood: Cell type	*Cells/μL*	*Cell size (μm)*	*Half-life in circulation*
Erythrocytes	$4.6–6.2 \times 10^6$ (M) $4.2–5.2 \times 10^6$ (F)	7–8	25 ± 2 days
Leukocytes			
Neutrophils	3000–6500	10–15	6–8 hours
Eosinophils	50–250	10–15	8–12 hours
Basophils	15–50	10–15	?
Monocytes	300–500	12–20	1–3 days
Lymphocytes	1000–3000	7–8	variable
Platelets	$1.5–3.5 \times 10^5$	2–4	3.2–5.2 days
Reticulocytes	$2.3–9.3 \times 10^4$	7–10	--
Synovial fluid:			
Cell type	*Cells/μL*		
Leukocytes	4–5		
Monocytes	35–40		
Lymphocytes	15–16		
Synovial cells	2–3		

The variability in the half-life of circulating lymphocytes is a result of the many subsets of this cell type, e.g., B-cells, helper and suppressor T-cells, etc. Cerebrospinal fluid also contains ~ 1–5 cells/μL, primarily lymphocytes.

Table C1.3 Inorganic content of various fluids [1]

Compound	*Whole blood*	*Plasma (serum)*	*Synovial fluid*
Bicarbonate	19.1–22.7	25–30	—
Bromide	0.033–0.074	0.043–0.093	—
Calcium	2.42	2.12–2.72	1.2–2.4
Chloride	77–86	100–108	87–138
Copper (μM)	11.3–19.5	13–22	—
Fluoride (μM)	5.3–23.7	—	—
Iodine (μM)	0.2–1.34	0.30–0.47	—
Iron	7.5–10.0	0.01–0.027	—
Magnesium	1.48–1.85	0.7–0.86	—
Phosphorous (total)	10.1–14.3	2.87–4.81	—
Potassium	40–60	3.5–4.7	3.5–4.5
Sodium	79–91	134–143	133–139
Zinc	0.076–0.196	0.011–0.023	—
Compound	*Cerebrospinal fluid*	*Tear fluid*	*Lymph*
Bicarbonate	18.6–25.0	20–40	—
Bromide	0.018–0.048	—	—
Calcium	1.02–1.34	0.35–0.77	1.7–2.8
Chloride	119–131	110–135	87–103
Copper (μM)	0.13–0.37	—	—
Fluoride (μM)	55	—	—
Iodine (μM)	—	—	—
Iron	0.0003–0.0015	—	—
Magnesium	0.55–1.23	—	—
Phosphorous (total)	0.442–0.694	—	2.0–3.6
Potassium	2.62–3.30	6.6–25.8	3.9–5.6
Sodium	137–153	126–166	118–132
Zinc	—	—	—

Concentrations are in mM, unless otherwise specified.

Table C1.4 Organic content of various fluids [13–15]

Species	*Whole blood*	*Plasma (serum)*	*CS fluid*
Amino acids (mg/L)	48–74	20–51	10–15
Ammonia (mg/L)	0.26–0.69	0.22–0.47	0.14–0.26
Bilirubin (mg/L)	2–14	2–8	<0.1
Cholesterol	1.15–2.25	1.7–2.1	—
Creatine (mg/L)	3–5	1.3–7.7	4.6–19
Creatinine (mg/L)	10–20	5.6–10.5	6.5–10.5
Fat, neutral	0.85–2.35	0.25–2.6	trace
Fatty acids	2.5–3.9	3.5–4.0	trace
Glucose	630–870	650–966	430–640
Hyaluronic acid	—	—	—
Lipids, total	4.45–6.1	2.85–6.75	0.01–0.02
Total nitrogen	30–41	12–14.3	0.16–0.22
Nonprotein nitrogen	0.26–0.50	0.14–0.32	0.11–0.20
Phospholipid	2.25–2.85	2.0–2.5	0.002–0.01
Urea	0.166–0.39	0.18–0.43	0.14–0.36
Uric acid (mg/L)	6–50	30.5–70.7	1.1–6.3
Water	830–865	930–955	980–990

Species	*Synovial fluid*	*Tear fluid*	*Lymph*
Amino acids (mg/L)	—	—	—
Ammonia (mg/L)	—	50	—
Bilirubin (mg/L)	—	—	8
Cholesterol	—	—	0.34–1.06
Creatine (mg/L)	—	—	—
Creatinine (mg/L)	—	—	8–89
Fat, neutral	—	—	—
Fatty acids	—	—	—
Glucose	—	0.025	1.36–1.40
Hyaluronic acid	3.32	—	—
Lipids, total	—	—	—
Total nitrogen	0.084–4.0	1.58	—
Nonprotein nitrogen	0.22–0.43	—	0.13–1.39
Phospholipid	—	—	—
Urea	0.15	0.33–1.4	—
Uric acid (mg/L)	39	—	17–108
Water	960–988	982	810–860

Concentrations are in mg/mL, unless otherwise specified.

Table C1.5 Major protein content of various fluids [12,14]

Protein	*Plasma (serum)*	*CS fluid*[1]	*Synovial fluid*
Albumin	37.6–54.9	155±39	6–10
α_1-Acid glycoprotein (orosomucoid)	0.48–1.26	1.85±0.74	—
α_1-Antitrypsin	0.98–2.45	7.0±3.0	0.78±0.017
β_2-Microglobulin	0.58–2.24	0.1–1.9	—
Haptoglobin		2.24±1.5	0.1
Type 1.1	1.45±0.34		
Type 2.1	2.06±0.67		
Type 2.2	1.74±0.70		
Ceruloplasmin	0.09–0.51	0.88±0.21	0.043±0.016
Transferrin	1.52–3.36	8.42±3.5	—
C1 Inhibitor	0.15–0.35	—	—
α_2-Macroglobulin	1.45–4.43	4.64±1.84	0.31–0.21
IgA	0.7–3.12	2.26±0.95	0.62–1.15
IgG	6.4–13.5	13.9±6.6	1.47–4.62
IgM	0.56–3.52	—	0.09–0.22
Fibrinogen	2–4	0.65	—
Lysozyme	—	—	—
Fibronectin	0.09–0.25	—	—
Hemopexin	0.53–1.21	—	—

Protein	*Synovial fluid*	*Tear fluid*
Albumin	3.94	15–26.7
α_1-Acid glycoprotein (orosomucoid)	—	—
α_1-Antitrypsin	0.015	—
β_2-Microglobulin	—	—
Haptoglobin	—	—
Ceruloplasmin	0.04	—
Transferrin	—	—
C1 Inhibitor	—	—
α_2-Macroglobulin	—	—
IgA	0.04–0.80	—
IgG	0.04–0.62	7.8
IgM	trace	—
Fibrinogen	—	—
Lysozyme	1–2.8	—
Fibronectin	—	—
Hemopexin	—	—

[1] Protein concentrations in CS fluid are given in mg/L.
All others have units of mg/mL.

Table C1.6 Fluid volumes [16]

Fluid	*Volume Male (mL)*	*Volume Female (mL)*
Whole blood	4490	3600
Erythrocytes	2030	1470
Plasma	2460	2130
Cerebrospinal fluid	100–160	100–160
Tear fluid	4–13	4–13

The following equations can be used to estimate blood volume (BV, mL), erythrocyte volume (EV, mL), and plasma volume (PV, mL) from the known body mass (b, kg) with a coefficient of variation of approximately 10%:

Males (M) $BV = 41.0 \times b + 1530$ Females (F) $BV = 47.16 \times b + 864$

$PV = 19.6 \times b + 1050$ $PV = 28.89 \times b + 455$

$EV = 21.4 \times b + 490$ $EV = 18.26 \times b + 409$

These equations, relating BV, PV, and EV to body weight, are taken from Lentner [12]. Additional correlations relating these volumes to body weight and surface area are available from the same source.

Table C1.7 Properties of major plasma proteins [16, 17]

Protein	Plasma concentration (mg/mL)	Molecular weight (Da)	p^I	S^1	D^2
Prealbumin	0.12–0.39	54 980	4.7	4.2	—
Albumin	38–52	66 500	4.9	4.6	6.1
α_1 – Acid Glycoprotein (Orosomucoid)	0.5–1.5	44 000	2.7	3.1	5.3
α_1 – Antitrypsin	2.0–4.0	54 000	4.0	3.5	5.2
α_2 – Macroglobulin	1.5–4.5	725 000	5.4	19.6	2.4
α_2 – Haptoglobin					
Type 1.1	1.0–2.2	100 000	4.1	4.4	4.7
Type 2.1	1.6–3.0	200 000	4.1	4.3–6.5	—
Type 2.2	1.2–2.6	400 000	—	7.5	—
α_2 – Ceruloplasmin	0.15–.60	160 000	4.4	7.08	3.76
Transferrin	2.0–3.2	76 500	5.9	5.5	5.0
Hemopexin	0.56–0.89	57 000	5.8	4.8	—
Lipoproteins	5.5–6	140 000–20 000 000	—	—	5.4
IgA (Monomer)	1.4–4.2	162 000	—	7	3.4
IgG	6–17	150 000	6.3–7.3	6.5–7.0	4.0
IgM	0.5–1.9	950 000	—	18–20	2.6
C1q	0.05–0.1	459 000	—	11.1	—
C3	1.5–1.7	185 000	6.1–6.8	9.5	4.5
C4	0.3–0.6	200 000	—	10.0	—
Fibrinogen	2.0–4.0	340 000	5.5	7.6	1.97

Protein	Plasma concentration (mg/mL)	$E_{280}{}^3$	$V_{20}{}^4$	CH_2O^5	Half-life (days)
Prealbumin	0.12–0.39	14.1	0.74	—	1.9
Albumin	38–52	5.8	0.733	0	17–23
α_1 – Acid glycoprotein (orosomucoid)	0.5–1.5	8.9	0.675	41.4	5.2
α_1 – Antitrypsin	2.0–4.0	5.3	0.646	12.2	3.9
α_2 – Macroglobulin	1.5–4.5	8.1	0.735	8.4	7.8
α_2 – Haptoglobin					
Type 1.1	1.0–2.2	12.0	0.766	19.3	2–4
Type 2.1	1.6–3.0	12.2	—	—	
Type 2.2	1.2–2.6	—	—	—	
α_2 – Ceruloplasmin	0.15–.60	14.9	0.713	8	4.3
Transferrin	2.0–3.2	11.2	0.758	5.9	7–10
Hemopexin	0.56–0.89	19.7	0.702	23.0	9.5
Lipoproteins	5.5–6	—	—	—	—
IgA (Monomer)	1.4–4.2	13.4	0.725	7.5	5–6.5
IgG	6–17	13.8	0.739	2.9	20–21
IgM	0.5–1.9	13.3	0.724	12	5.1
C1q	0.05–0.1	6.82	—	8	—
C3	1.5–1.7	—	0.736	—	—
C4	0.3–0.6	—	—	—	—
Fibrinogen	2.0–4.0	13.6	0.723	2.5	3.1–3.4

[1] Sedimentation constant in water at 20°C, expressed in Svedberg units.
[2] Diffusion coefficient in water at 20°C, expressed in 10^{-7} cm^2/s.
[3] Extinction coefficient for light of wavelength 280 nm traveling 1 cm through a 10 mg/ml protein solution.
[4] Partial specific volume of the protein at 20°C, expressed as ml g^{-1}.
[5] Carbohydrate content of the protein, expressed as the percentage by mass.

Table C1.8 Proteins involved in blood coagulation [19]

Protein	*Plasma concentration (μg/mL)*	*Relative molecular weight, M_r (Da)*	*Biological half-life $t_{1/2}$ (hr)*
Fibrinogen	2000–4000	340 000	72–120
Prothrombin	70–140	71 600	48–72
Factor III (tissue factor)	–	45 000	–
Factor V	4–14	330 000	12–15
Factor VII	trace	50	2–5
Factor VIII	~0.2	330 000	8–12
Factor IX	~5.0	57 000	24
Factor X	~12	58 800	24–40
Factor XI	2.0–7.0	160 000	48–84
Factor XII	15–47	80 000	50–60
Factor XIII	~10	320 000	216–240
Protein C	~4.0	62 000	10
Protein S	~22	77 000	–
Protein Z	~2.9	62 000	60
Prekallikrein	35–50	85 000	–
High molecular weight kininogen	70–90	120 000	–
α_1 Protease inhibitor	2500	55 000	–
Antithrombin III	230 ± 23	58 000	67

Table C1.9 Proteins in the compliment system

Protein	*Serum concentration (mg/L)*	*Relative molecular weight, Mr (Da)*	*Sedimentation constant $S_{20W}(10^{-13}s)$*
C1q	70 ± 14	459 000	11.1
C1r	39 ± 2	83 000	7.5
C1s	36 ± 3	83 000	4.5
C2	27 ± 5.6	108 000	4.5
C3	1612 ± 244	185 000	9.5
C4	498 ± 151	200 000	10.0
C5	153 ± 29	185 000	8.7
C6	50.9 ± 8	128 000	5.5
C7	4 – 60	121 000	6.0
C8	43.2 ± 6.5	151 000	8.0
C9	57.5 ± 12.7	71 000	4.5
Factor B	275 ± 55	92 000	5–6
Factor D	trace	24 000	3.0
Properdin	28.4 ± 5	220 000	5.4
C1 inhibitor	158 ± 14	100 000	–
Factor H	525 ± 58	150 000	6.0
Factor I	38.6 ± 5.5	88 000	5.5

ADDITIONAL READING:

Ditmer, D.S. (ed.) (1961) *Blood and Other Body Fluids*, Federation of American Societies for Experimental Biology, Washington, D.C.

This text provides a thorough compilation of the physical properties and composition of numerous biological fluids. Unlike the *Geigy Scientific Tables*, this book also reports data for many non-human species. However, citations and some measurement techniques are somewhat outdated.

Kjeldsberg C.R. and Knight J.A. (eds) (1993) *Body Fluids: Laboratory Examination of Amniotic, Cerebrospinal, Seminal, Serous & Synovial Fluids*, 3rd ed., American Society of Clinical Pathologists, Chicago.

An excellent source of information, especially for a clinician or medical technologist. Includes numerous color photographs of fluids and cells. Discusses abnormal amounts or types of specific proteins and cells in fluids as potentially diagnostic of disease states.

Lentner, C. (ed.) (1984) *Geigy Scientific Tables*, Ciba-Geigy, Basle.

This is the most comprehensive source of information available on properties and composition of body fluids. Volumes 1 and 3 provide extensive data, generally in tabular form, on fluid content (as well as measurement technique), related to gender, age and disease state.

REFERENCES

1. Ditmer, D.S. (ed.) (1961) *Blood and Other Body Fluids*, Federation of American Societies for Experimental Biology, Washington, D.C.
2. Fullard, R.J. (1988) *Current Eye Research*, **7,** 163–179.
3. Chmiel, H. and Walitza, E. (1980) *On the Rheology of Blood and Synovial Fluids*, Research Studies Press, New York.
4. Barbanel, J.C., Lowe, G.D.O. and Forbes, C.D. (1984), The viscosity of blood. in *Mathematics in Medicine and Biomechanics*, G.F. Roach (ed.), Shiva Publications, Nantwich, p. 19.
5. Begg, T.B. and Hearns, J.B. (1966) Components in blood viscosity: The relative contribution of hematocrit, plasma fibrinogen and other proteins. *Clinical Science*, **31,** 87–93.
6. Whitmore, R.L. (1968) *Rheology of The Circulation*, Pergamon Press, New York.
7. Merrill, E.W. (1969) Rheology of blood. *Physiology Reviews*, **49,** 863–867.
8. Harkness, J. (1971) The viscosity of human blood plasma: Its measurement in health and disease. *Biorheology*, **8,** 171–193.
9. Lowe, G.D.O., Barbanel, J.C. and Forbes, C.D. (eds) (1981) *Clinical Aspects of Blood Viscosity and Cell Deformability*, Springer-Verlag, New York.
10. Lowe, G.D.O and Barbanel, J.C. (1988) Plasma and blood viscosity, in *Clinical Blood Rheology*, G.D.O. Lowe (ed.), CRC Press, Boca Raton, pp. 11–44.
11. Schmidt-Schonbein, H. (1988) Fluid dynamics and hemorheology, in *Clinical Blood Rheology*, G.D.O. Lowe (ed.), CRC Press, Boca Raton, pp. 129–220.
12. Lentner, C. (ed.) (1984) *Geigy Scientific Tables*, Ciba-Geigy, Basle.

13. Bicks, R.L. (1993) *Hematology: Clinical and Laboratory Practice*, Mosby, St Louis.
14. Sokoloff, L. (ed.) (1978) *The Joints and Synovial Fluid*, Academic Press, New York.
15. Hermens, W.T., Willems, G.M. and Visser, M.P. (1982) *Quantification of Circulating Proteins: Theory and Applications Based on Analysis of Plasma Protein Levels*, Martinus Nijhoff, The Hague.
16. Colman, R.W., Hirsh, J., Marder, V.J., *et al.* (eds) (1993) *Hemostasis and Thrombosis*, Lippincott, Philadelphia.
17. Schultze, H.E. and Heremans, J.F. (1966) *Nature and Metabolism of Extracellular Proteins*, Elsevier, Amsterdam.
18. Bing, D.H. (ed.) (1978) *The Chemistry and Physiology of the Human Plasma Proteins*, Pergamon Press, Boston.
19. Stamatoyannopoulos, G., Nienhuis, A.W., Majerus, P.W., *et al.* (eds) (1994) *The Molecular Basis of Blood Diseases*, W.B. Saunders, Philadelphia.

The Vitreous Humor

C2

T.V. Chirila and Y. Hong

C2.1 INTRODUCTION

The vitreous body, also termed the vitreous humor, vitreus, or vitreous, is a clear and transparent mass (gel or liquid or a mixture of both) that fills the posterior cavity of the eye in vertebrates, between the lens and the retina. The human vitreous body is a hydrogel with a very high water content which provides an adequate support for the retina, allows the diffusion of metabolic solutes, and allows the light to reach the retina. There are currently two differing concepts on the nature of vitreous body. A significant amount of evidence supports the view that the vitreous body is basically an extracellular matrix. Another model has been developed in which the vitreous body is considered as a specialized, but simple, connective tissue. The two concepts are not yet reconciled, therefore the structure and role of the vitreous body are usually regarded from both points of view. It is accepted that the vitreous body possesses a unique macromolecular organization, a double-network system consisting of a scaffold of randomly spaced rod-like collagen fibers filled and entangled with a network of very large coiled-up macromolecules of hyaluronic acid (hyaluronan). The latter is present in the form of its sodium salt (sodium hyaluronidate). The double-network model explains satisfactorily most of the properties of the vitreous body, as well as its remarkable stability, although it probably overestimates the importance of hyaluronan. The natural vitreous body displays true viscoelastic properties which enable it to resist sudden compression shocks, offering much the best protection for the retina against contusion trauma. It is believed that the hyauronan network imparts the latter feature, while the collagen network is responsible for the plasticity and tensile strength of the vitreous body.

Handbook of Biomaterial Properties. Edited by J. Black and G. Hastings.
Published in 1998 by Chapman & Hall, London. ISBN 0 412 60330 6.

As is the case with many other structural elements of the eye, there are presently much more data on animal vitreous body than on the human counterpart. Likely, the results reviewed here cover almost everything reported so far on the human vitreous. However, in many cases it is not possible to select a most reliable single value; dependable values representing a range are thus provided in several of the following tables.

Being a very loose tissue, albeit well structured in a very specific way, the vitreous body becomes homogeneous during processing for measurements and the resulting data for its physical properties merely illustrate the behavior of a fluid consisting mainly of water and containing minute amount of inorganic and organic components. The dimensional characteristics (Tables C3.1, C3.5 and C3.6), bulk chemical composition (Tables C3.2 and C3.3) and optical properties (Table C4.7) are seemingly not affected by the morphological heterogeneity of the vitreous. However, some investigators took into account the separate existence of gel and liquid fractions in the vitreous (Tables C3.4, and C3.6).

Over the past few decades the vitreous body was perceived as a typical viscoelastic material. However, its characterization by rheometry (as shown in Table C3.8) is still in its infancy.

C2.2 GENERAL PROPERTIES

Table C3.1 Physical properties of the human vitreous body

Property	*Value*	*Source*
Volume	3.9 ml	[1]
Weight	3.9 g	[1]
Water content	99.7%	[2]
	99%	[3]
pH	7.5	[4]
	7.4–7.52	[5]
	7–7.3	[6]
Osmolality	288–323 mOsm kg^{-1}	[7]
Osmotic pressure		
(freezing point depression)	-0.554 to -0.518°C [4]	
Density	1.0053–1.0089 g cm^{-3}	[8]
Intrinsic viscosity	3–5 × 10^3 cm^3 g^{-1}	[9]
Dynamic viscosity	1.6 cP	[10]
Refractive index	1.3345	[11]
	1.3345–1.337	[1]

Table C3.2 Inorganic ions content of the human vitreous body

Ion	*Representative value*	*Source*
Sodium	2.714–3.542 mg cm^{-3}	[12]
	3.15 g/kg H_2O	[3]
	2.603–5.805 mg cm^{-3}	[6]
Potassium	130–470 μg cm^{-3}	[12]
	0.15 g/kg H_2O	[3]
	308–788 μg cm^{-3}	[6]
Calcium	56–106 μg cm^{-3}	[12]
	14–76 μg cm^{-3}	[6]
Phosphate	0.1–3.3 mEq dm^{-3}	[12]
Chloride	3.155–5.140 mg cm^{-3}	[12]
	4 g/kg H_2O	[3]
	3.477–7.621 mg cm^{-3}	[6]
Bicarbonate	1.2–3.0 g/kg H_2O	[3]

Table C3.3 Organic content of the human vitreous body (low molecular weight components)

Component	*Representative value*	*Source*
Lipids	2 μg/ml	[13]
Glucose	17–105 mg/dl	[12]
	30–70 mg/dl water	[3]
Lactic acid	70 mg/dl water	[3]
Urea	24–172 mg/dl water	[12]
Creatinine	0.3–3.0 mg/dl	[12]
Citrate	1.9 mg/dl water	[3]
Pyruvic acid	7.3 mg/dl water	[3]
Ascorbic acid	36 mg/100 g	[14]

Component	*Representative value ($\mu g\ cm^{-3}$)*	*Source*
Proteins[a]	280–1360	[13]
	450–1100	[15]
Hyaluronan	100–400	[15]
	42–399	[6]
Collagen	40–120	[15]
	30–532	[6]
Albumin	293 ± 18	[16]
Immunoglobulin (IgG)	33.5 ± 3	[16]
α_1-Antitrypsin	141 ± 2.9	[16]
α_1-Acid glycoproptein	4 ± 0.7	[16]

± = Standard deviation; [a] total protein content.

Table C3.4 Variation with age of total protein content in the liquid human vitreous [15]

Age range (years)	*Protein (mg cm^{-3})*
10–50	0.4–0.6
50–80	0.7–0.9
>80	0.9–1.0

Table C3.5 Axial length of the human vitreous body during maturation [17][a]

Age (years) and gender	*Axial length, (mm)*
<13, male	10.48
<13, female	10.22
>13, male	16.09
>13, female	15.59

[a] The axial growth of the vitreous body is essentially completed by the age of 13 years.

Table C3.6 Gel and liquid volume of the vitreous as a function of age (adapted from [18])[a]

Age (years)	*Gel volume (cm^3)*	*Liquid volume (cm^3)*
Birth	1.6	0
5	3.3	0
10	3.5	0.7
20	3.9	0.9
30	3.9	0.9
40	3.9	0.9
50	3.5	1.3
60	3.2	1.6
70	2.8	2.0
80	2.5	2.3
90	2.2	2.6

[a] The liquid vitreous appears first in childhood and by the seventh decade it occupies half of the vitreous [18, 19].

Table C3.7 Transmission of radiation through the vitreous body (adapted from [20])

Wavelength (nm)	*Transmittance (total, %)*
300	0
325	76
350	82
400	90
500	97
600	98
700	98

C2.3 MECHANICAL PROPERTIES

Table C3.8 Rheological characteristics of the human vitreous body [21]

Parameter	*Region in the vitreous*		
	Anterior	*Central*	*Posterior*
Residual viscosity η_m (Pa s)	1.4	2.2	4.9
Internal viscosity η_k (Pa s)	0.3	0.35	0.5
Relaxation time τ_m (S)	0.38	0.30	1.61
Retardation time τ_k (S)	0.27	0.41	0.46
Elastic compliance, instantaneous, Jm ($m^{-2}N^{-1}$)	0.1	0.3	0.3
Elastic modulus, internal, G_k ($N\ m^{-2}$)	2.5	1.3	1.2

ADDITIONAL READING

Balazs, E.A. (1968) The molecular biology of the vitreous, in *New and Controversial Aspects of Retinal Detachment*, (ed. A. McPherson), Harper & Row, New York, pp. 3–15.

This is a landmark paper on the nature of the vitreous body, describing the 'mechanochemical' (or 'double-network') model. This model explains satisfactorily the correlations between some properties of the vitreous (composition, rheology, volume, cell population, transparency) and the physicochemical principles governing its stability (frictional interaction, expansion/contraction, the excluded-volume concept, and the molecular-sieve effect).

Berman, E.R. and Voaden, M. (1970) The vitreous body, in *Biochemistry of the Eye*, (ed. C.N. Graymore), Academic Press, London, pp. 373–471.

A comprehensive summary of knowledge at that time on animal and human vitreous body, including development, chemical composition, metabolism, and aging effects.

Shields, J.A. (1976) Pathology of the vitreous, in *Current Concepts of the Vitreous including Vitrectomy*, (ed. K.A. Gitter), C.V. Mosby Co., St. Louis, pp. 14–42.

This book chapter presents competently the pathologic vitreous, including developmental abnormalities, inflammation, hemorrhage, effects of trauma, systemic diseases, and degenerative processes.

Gloor, B.P. (1987) The vitreous, in *Adler's Physiology of the Eye*, 8th ed., (eds R.A. Moses and W.M. Hart), C.V. Mosby Co., St. Louis, pp. 246–267.

A concise description of all aspects of the vitreous body, including properties, development, anatomy, structure, biochemistry, metabolism, and pathology.

Sebag, J. (1989) *The Vitreous. Structure, Function, and Pathology*, Springer-Verlag, New York.

This is probably only the second single-authored book in this century to be dedicated entirely to the topic of vitreous body. It is a well-structured and updated compendium. The first half of the book is dedicated to structure, properties and physiology of the vitreous. Pathology of the vitreous is analyzed in the other half from a biological angle. Although a clinician, the author manages to avoid typical clinical descriptions and to provide a text which integrates the basic scientific knowledge for both clinicians and scientists.

Williams, G.A. and Blumenkranz, M.S. (1992), Vitreous humor, in *Duane's Foundations of Clinical Ophthalmology*, vol. 2 (eds W. Tasman and E.A. Jaeger), J.B. Lippincott Co., Philadelphia, chapter 11.

This chapter (27 pages) presents the modern concepts in the pathophysiologic mechanisms of vitreous diseases, and in the clinical conditions involving the vitreous (detachment, macular holes and membranes, diabetes, proliferative vitreoretinopathy, hyalosis, amyloidosis). Aspects such as separation of the vitreous from the retina and traction of the vitreous by hypocellular gel contraction are explained according to the most recent findings.

REFERENCES

1. Redslob, E. (1932) *Le corps vitré*, Masson & Cie, Paris, pp. 299–305.
2. Duke-Elder, W.S. (1929) The physico-chemical properties of the vitreous body. *J. Physiol.*, **68,** 155–65.
3. Nordmann, J. (1968) Chimie, in *Biologie et chirurgie du corps vitré*, (eds A. Brini, A. Bronner, J.P. Gerhard *et al.*), Masson & Cie, Paris, pp. 95–167.
4. Mörner, C.T. (1894) Untersuchung der Proteïnsubstanzen in den lichtbrechenden Medien des Auges. *Z. Physiol. Chem.*, **18,** 233–56.
5. Gala, A. (1925) Observations on the hydrogen ion concentration in the vitreous body of the eye with reference to glaucoma. *Br. J. Ophthalmol.*, **9,** 516–9.
6. Lee, B. (1994) Comparative rheological studies of the vitreous body of the eye, Ph.D. Thesis, University of Pennsylvania, 1992, U.M.I./Bell & Howell Co., Ann Arbor, MI, pp. 102, 138–152.

7. Sturner, W.Q., Dowdey, A.B.C., Putnam, R.S. *et al.* (1972) Osmolality and other chemical determinations in postmortem human vitreous humor. *J. Forensic Sci.*, **17,** 387–93.
8. Visser-Heerema, J. (1936) Über das spezifische Gewicht der bei der Operation von Netzhautablösungen gewonnenen Flüssigkeit. *Arch. Augenheilkd.*, **109,** 543–61.
9. Berman, E.R. and Michaelson, I.C. (1964) The chemical composition of the human vitreous body as related to age and myopia. *Exp. Eye Res.*, **3,** 9–15.
10. Shafer, D.M. (1965) Intraocular injections as adjuncts to other retinal detachment procedures, in *Controversial Aspects of the Management of Retinal Detachment*, (eds C.L. Schepens and C.D.J. Regan), Little, Brown & Co., Boston, pp. 186–204.
11. Guggenheim, I. and Franceschetti, A. (1928) Refraktometrische Untersuchungen des Glaskörpers von Kaninchen und Mensch (unter physiologischen und pathologischen Bedingungen). *Arch. Augenheilkd.*, **98,** 448–82.
12. Naumann, H.N. (1959) Postmortem chemistry of the vitreous body in man. *Arch. Ophthalmol.*, **62,** 356–63.
13. Swann, D.A. (1980) Chemistry and biology of the vitreous body. *Int. Rev. Exp. Pathol.*, **22,** 1–64.
14. Süllmann, H. (1951) Chemie des Auges. *Tabul. Biol.*, **22,** 1–119.
15. Balazs, E.A. and Denlinger, J.L. (1984) The vitreus, in *The Eye*, vol. 1a, 3rd edn, (ed H. Davson), Academic Press, Orlando, FL, pp. 533–89.
16. Clausen, R., Weller, M., Wiedemann, P. *et al.* (1991) An immunochemical quantitative analysis of the protein pattern in physiologic and pathologic vitreous. *Graefe's Arch. Clin. Exp. Ophthalmol.*, **229,** 186–90.
17. Larsen, J.S. (1971) The sagital growth of the eye. III. Ultrasonic measurement of the posterior segment (axial length of the vitreous) from birth to puberty. *Acta Ophthalmol.*, **49,** 441–53.
18. Balazs, E.A. (1992) Functional anatomy of the vitreus, in *Duane's Foundations of Clinical Ophthalmology*, vol. 1, (eds W. Tasman and E.A. Jaeger), J.B. Lippincott Co., Philadelphia, Chapter 17.
19. Balazs, E.A. and Denlinger, J.L. (1982) Aging changes in the vitreus, in *Aging and Human Visual Function*, (eds R. Sekuler, D. Kline and K. Dismukes), Alan R. Liss, Inc., New York, pp. 45–57.
20. Boettner, E.A. and Wolter, J.R. (1962) Transmission of the ocular media. *Invest. Ophthalmol.*, **1,** 776–83.
21. Lee, B., Litt, M. and Buchsbaum, G. (1992) Rheology of the vitreous body. Part I: Viscoelasticity of human vitreous. *Biorheology*, **29,** 521–33.

PART II

Metallic Biomaterials

1

J. Breme and V. Biehl

1.1 INTRODUCTION

Compared with other biomaterials like ceramics and poylmers, the metallic biomaterials possess the outstanding property of being able to endure tensile stresses, which, in the case of alloys, may be extremely high and also of dynamic nature. This is the reason why alloys, for example those with sufficient bending fatigue strength, are widely used as structural materials for skeletal reconstructions if high acting loads are expected to occur. Typical examples for such highly loaded implants are hip and knee endoprostheses, plates, screws, nails, dental implants, etc. Nevertheless, metallic biomaterials are also used for unloaded, purely functional devices such as cages for pumps, valves and heart pacemakers, conducting wires, etc.

The main requirements which must be fulfilled by all biomaterials are corrosion resistance, biocompatibility, bioadhesion (bone ingrowth), biofunctionality (adequate mechanical properties, especially fatigue strength and a Young's modulus as close to that of the bone as possible), processability and availability. These requirements are more or less satisfactorily fulfilled by the various customary groups of biomaterials. In comparison the different materials show a different behaviour according to the demands. A corrosion resistant material may not necessarily be biocompatible and, contrarily, a more biocompatible material may be less corrosion resistant. Especially fretting corrosion may pose a problem in articulating devices like knee joints or plate/screw systems. Often unique characteristic properties of a material are responsible for its application. Typical examples are the amalgams which in spite of their reduced

Handbook of Biomaterial Properties. Edited by J. Black and G. Hastings.
Published in 1998 by Chapman & Hall, London. ISBN 0 412 60330 6.

corrosion resistance and biocompatibility were used over a long period of time for dental restoration due to their extremely good processability provided by their ability to amalgamate with mercury at room temperature within a short time, showing in this condition a high hardness.

The biocompatibility of most metallic biomaterials is based on a passive oxide layer which is always present on the metal surface and which will be restored quickly (milliseconds) after damage. These oxide layers, similar to alumina, show an inert behaviour towards the surrounding tissue. Therefore, the chemical bonding of a metallic implant with the tissue, which is observed between bioactive ceramics like hydroxyapatite and bone, seems to be improbable, and the adhesion strength between the bone and the metal will have a primarily mechanical character. With stainless steel and a cobalt–chromium base alloy ('Vitallium') metallic materials exhibiting such a passive and highly inert oxide layer have been available for about 60 years. About 25 years ago, due to the favourable properties of the special metals niobium, tantalum and titanium, their application as biomaterials became the subject of much discussion. Especially titanium and its alloys began to compete with the existing biomaterials.

Because of this competitive situation an enormous advancement of the materials was set going in different directions. Quality assurance systems for customers and surgeons were created by standardization and normalization of the existing materials. In addition, attention was devoted to the further development of the existing base materials, one example being the development of a forgeable Ni-free cobalt–chromium alloy with an extremely low carbon content, with a resulting avoidance of the precipitation of brittle carbides. Examples related to titanium materials are the development of alloys containing no toxic elements like vanadium (e.g. Ti5Al2.5Fe and Ti6Al7Nb) and the development of near β- or β-alloys. Besides a high fatigue strength these alloys have, due to a high content of the β-phase, a Young's modulus which is even lower than that of conventional titanium materials, by means of which a good load transfer is achieved. Therefore, stress shielding can be avoided and new bone formation is stimulated.

A further direction of advancement was originated by the progress being made in research and surgery and by the demand for materials with special properties for special applications. For these cases the materials, which are often composite materials, had to be tailored to the intended application. One example is the development of the alloy TiTa30 which in its thermal expansion coefficient is very similar to alumina and can therefore be crackfree bonded with the ceramic. This material is used as a dental implant. The metallic biomaterial which can resist bending stresses is inserted into the jaw. The upper part of the implant consisting of alumina, which shows a smaller deposition of plaque than the metallic materials, passes through the gingiva into the mouth cavity. Another example for the tailoring of materials is a surface treatment in order to improve the physical properties. Heart pacemaker leads, for example, which are produced by porous sintering of Ti-powder, are PVD-surface coated with Ir, TiN, TiB_2, TiC, etc. in order to increase the electrical conductivity.

In the following chapters the various groups of metallic biomaterials are characterized in terms of their composition, physical and mechanical properties and their corrosion and biological behaviour. In addition, recommendations are given for their processing (deformation, machining, welding, brazing, etc.).

1.2 GENERAL DISCUSSION

Considering the testing methods used to determine the main requirements which must be fulfilled by biomaterials, i.e. corrosion resistance, biocompatibility, bioadhesion and biofunctionality, it is obvious that only the measurement of the mechanical properties, including fatigue (biofunctionality), will supply objectively comparable results because these testing methods are standardized.

In the methods used for the investigation of corrosion resistance, biocompatibility and bioadhesion the researchers try to simulate and imitate the natural *in vivo* condition of the implant. Only in the near past have efforts been made to standardize these tests. Because of a longtime decline of standardization the tests described up until now in literature differ and the results of such diversified tests are not comparable. Corrosion measurements, for example, are performed in different solutions with changing pH values and atmospheres (aerated or de-aerated). Only if different materials have been investigated in one test and under the same conditions does a comparison of their behaviour for this test seem possible. Nevertheless, regarding the differing test results, the most corrosion resistant materials seem to be the special metals (titanium, niobium, tantalum and their alloys), followed by wrought CoCr-based, cast CoCr-based alloys and stainless steel.

The current density of various materials was determined as a function of the potential difference between the anodic and cathodic branches of the current potential curves in 0.9% NaCl with a stable redox system $Fe\ (CN)_6^{4-}/Fe\ (CN)_6^{3-}$ [1]. The saline solution containing this redox system had a resting potential closely resembling that of a tissue culture fluid which has a redox potential of 400 mV. Ti and its alloys Ta and Nb exhibit a better resistance than the stainless steel AISI 316L and a wrought CoNiCr alloy. The same ranking can be observed during the measurement of the polarization resistance of the different materials [1]. Breakdown potential measurements of various implant materials in

Hank's solution also indicated a clear order of ranking of the materials. While commercially pure titanium and Ti6Al4V had high breakdown potentials of 2.4 and 2.0 V respectively, for stainless steel and CoCr alloys (cast and wrought) this value amounted to only 0.2 and 0.42 V respectively [2]. As already described [3], Ti and its alloys with Nb and Ta belong to the group of metals which cannot undergo a breakdown of passivity in body fluids. In these fluids a breakdown at a high potential causing pitting corrosion is impossible because it is more positive than the oxygen reduction reversible potential. On the other hand, the passivation potential is less positive than the water or hydrogen-ion reduction.

In all materials the passive layer can be damaged mechanically, for example, by fretting metal on metal (plate/screw) or by the instruments used during surgery. The repassivation time of the material is therefore very important. The repassivation behaviour of different materials in a saline solution was measured using an electrode which rotates at a rate of $10\ s^{-1}$ in the solution, during which it is activated by an Al_2O_3 cutting tool. The decrease in the corrosion current is measured as a function of the time at different potentials. The repassivation is defined as being achieved when the current density amounts to 1/e (e [approximate or equal too] 2718) of the current density in the activated condition [4]. In addition, the time $t_{0.05}$ of a residual active current density of 5 % was determined. The passive oxygen surface layer (t_e) is reconstructed as a function of the material in some milliseconds, demonstrating an advantage on the part of titanium materials. The growth of the surface layer ($t_{0.05}$) of cp-titanium and the titanium alloys is accelerated as compared to that of the other materials (stainless steel, wrought and cast CoCr).

In order to avoid damaging of the surface layer, coatings of hard layers of non-abrasive materials which also show favourable fretting behaviour, are recommended, especially for the movable parts of implants. Since the highest values for the acceleration tension are achieved by ion implantation, the best reaction and binding can be expected with this procedure. By the implantation of TiN on wrought CoCr, for example, not only the fretting behaviour, but also the corrosion resistance of the material tested in 0.17 M saline solution was improved. The pitting of the surface treated material amounted to 1.16 V, while the material which had not undergone surface treatment had a potential of 0.83 V [5]. If cracks and fissures are present in the surface layer, the corrosion rate will be accelerated due to the lower pH value in these crevices. Experiments with ion implantation of nitrogen in titanium surfaces produced good results concerning the fretting behaviour. Even the fatigue strength of the alloy Ti6Al4V, which was surface treated by nitrogen ion implantation, is reported to have increased due to compression stresses generated by the high acceleration tension of the nitrogen ions [6]. Another possibility of hardening the surface of Ti and its alloys without diminishing the corrosion behaviour and fatigue properties is a short annealing in air, e.g. by induction heating and subsequent quenching. This method was applied for the improvement of the friction behaviour of hip prosthesis heads [7].

For the biocompatibility and bioadhesion tests similar restrictions as in the corrosion resistance tests must be observed. A comparison of the behaviour of the different materials is possible only if the testing conditions are identical. Results obtained in animal experiments with rats and rabbits must be treated with reservations because both animals show intense bone growth and rapid healing after the implantation.

Measurements of the concentration of various metals in different organs of a rabbit six and sixteen weeks after implantation showed after six weeks a titanium content of 45.1 ppm in the spleen and 53.4 ppm in the lung. These values correspond to the values in a normal spleen or lung. No significant changes were observed in the liver or kidneys. However, Co and Ni from cobalt-based alloys and stainless steel were found in higher concentrations in these organs [8].

Patients with total hip replacements by implants of stainless steel or of CoCr alloys who experienced difficulties after two to fifteen years due to a loosening of the prosthesis and/or allergic reactions to Cr, Co or Ni were found to have an increased content of these elements in their urine, plasma and blood. Already fifteen months after removal the contents were excessive in these fluids [9].

The level of toxicity of the various elements was determined by investigating the reaction of salts of these elements with cells of the kidneys of green African monkeys. The so-called CCR_{50} value was measured which is defined as the concentration of the studied substance which generates a reduction of survival of the renal cells of 50%. Of all the elements measured the lowest value of 3×10^{-2} μg/ml was observed for vanadium [10]. This is the reason why absolutely biocompatible biomaterials containing no toxic elements such as Ti5Al2.5Fe [11] and Ti5Al7Nb [12] were developed.

After insertion of wires of different metals into the epiphyseal region of rabbits and an exposure time of fifteen months, the histology showed different results. With materials of inert or biocompatible behaviour the cells in the vicinity of the implant were still supplied with blood, while the cells in the neighbourhood of toxic materials underwent an inflammatory reaction and died. A few elements (Cr, Co, Ni and V) have toxic effects and also have a relatively low polarization resistance. Ti and its alloys, Nb and Ta, which have a high polarization resistance, exhibit an inert behaviour. In between the materials were found which are capsulated. The results also show that not only the corrosion behaviour provided by the polarization resistance is responsible for the biocompatibility of the material exposed to the tissue. The steel 316L and the CoCr alloy, which have a polarization resistance similar to that of titanium, are encapsulated by a tissue membrane and their behaviour is not inert [13].

A sensitive and reproductive test of biocompatibility seems to be the cultivation of cells with an increasing content of fine metal powders (<20 μm). The survival rate is measured after a constant exposure time. The limit of toxicity C_{50} is defined as the value (μg/ml) of the powder concentration which produces a dying off of 50% of the cells. (The results can be found in the chapters related to biocompatibility.)

In the implant/body system there are several interactions which can generate injuries:

(a) The corrosion process produces a flow of electrons in the implant metal and a flow of ions in the surrounding tissue. The latter may disturb the physiological ion movement of the nerve cells.
(b) An inorganic reaction of the implant or of primary corrosion products is caused by the solution of metal ions in the body fluid and transport to the various organs where they are concentrated and can produce systemic or hypersensitive effects if the limit of toxicity for a certain metal is exceeded.
(c) Direct organic reaction of the implant or of primary corrosion products with proteins of the tissue takes place, causing, for example, inflammation.
(d) Generation of H_2O_2 by inflamed cells and decomposition of H_2O_2 by the formation of a hydroxyl radical, causing injury in the biological system.

Whether one of these interactions occurs or not depends on the physical and chemical properties of the various materials. Ti, Ta and Nb are reported to be biocompatible because they form protective surface layers of semi- or nonconductive oxides. These oxides are able to prevent to a great extent an exchange of electrons and therefore a flow of ions through the tissue [14] due to their isolating effect. This isolating effect may be demonstrated by the dielectric constants of the different metal oxides. There are three groups of oxides. While TiO_2 (rutile), Fe_2O_3 and Nb_2O_5 have constants even higher than that of water, Al_2O_3, Cr_2O_3 and Ta_2O_5 have a lower isolating effect and a higher conductivity. For Ni- and V-oxides dielectric constants are not available because of their high conductivity [8]. The relatively low isolating effect of Ta-oxide is indirectly proved by the cytotronic effects of Ta on the membrane properties and on the growth of spinal ganglion cells during *in vitro* tests. In contrast, Ti showed no effect on the membrane properties and on the growth of ganglion cells [15].

Concerning inorganic or organic reactions, the primary corrosion products of the metallic implants are mainly responsible for the biocompatibility of the implanted metal because they may have, due to their large surface, an interaction with the tissue or with the body fluid. The metal is transported by a solution in the body fluid to the various organs where due to an enrichment of the metal an undesirable interaction may occur.

The primary corrosion products of the most important elements in metallic implant materials vary in their thermodynamic stability. While the oxides or hydroxides of Al, Cr, Nb, Ta, Ti and V are stable due to a more negative heat of formation than that of water, the oxides and hydroxides of Co and Ni are unstable because of a less negative heat of formation than that of water [16]. The interaction between the oxide or hydroxide and the body fluid is increased if the heat of formation for the oxide or hydroxide is increased. Therefore, the thermodynamically stable corrosion products have a low solution product and a low solubility in the body fluid. This is directly demonstrated by the pk values (negative logarithm) of the solution product of the primary corrosion products [13]. While Ti, Ta-, Nb- and Cr-oxides have pk-values of >14, i.e. hydrolysis cannot play a role, Co-, Fe-, and Ni-oxides possess even negative pk values which cause a considerable solubility. In spite of a high negative heat of formation for Fe_2O_3 and Fe- and Cr-hydroxide negative pk values and a high solubility are reported [13]. A remarkable solubility of Cr in serum was observed [17], while titanium is practically insoluble due to the formation of the thermodynamically very stable oxide TiO_2.

Thermodynamically stable primary corrosion products with a low solubility in body fluid are in a stable equilibrium with only a low reactivity with the proteins of the surrounding tissue.

The hydroxyl radical is able to cause injury in biological systems, e.g. biomembranes can be deteriorated. Titanium is able to bind H_2O_2 in a Ti–H_2O_2 complex. This complex can trap the superoxide radical which is formed during the H_2O_2 decomposition. By spectrophotometric spin-trapping measurements and electron spin resonance measurements no hydroxyl radical formation rate in Ti–H_2O_2 could be detected. A similar result was observed with Zr, Au and Al [18].

The integration of metallic implants by ingrowth was studied for many different materials and implant systems. The ingrowth behaviour of miniplates of commercially pure titanium and of the stainless steel 316L was investigated by the implantation of these plates on the legs of Hanford minipigs. The miniplates were fixed to the legs of the pigs by screws. After removal following an exposure time of eight weeks a histologic examination was performed by fluorescence microscopy. In all animals where titanium plates had been used a new formation of bone could be observed in close contact to the surface of the screws and plates [19]. In contrast to this result, when stainless steel was used, there was less new bone formation and in addition granulated tissue was found between the metallic surface and surrounding bone [19]. This granulated tissue at the interface bone/implant has the disadvantage that it is not supplied with blood. Therefore, a systematic treatment of the host tissue against inflammatory reactions in the vicinity of the implant by means of injections is not successful because the antidote cannot be transported directly to the inflamed area. In addition, the granulated connective tissue is not able to transfer or sustain forces, so that a loosening of the implant will take place. Growth of the bone in close contact with the metal has already been reported in many other investigations [20–25] in which the contact area tissue/implant has been studied in detail.

Dental implants made from different materials inserted into the jaws of dogs varied in their behaviour. With titanium implants the bone grew in close contact to the metal surface. In contrast, when stainless steel was used as the implant material, a fibrous encapsulation which separated the implant from the surrounding tissue was formed. In titanium implants instead of this fibrous encapsulation an intercellular substance appeared. A similar unfavourable behaviour was found in the case of dental implants of a CoCr alloy in dogs. Histological findings showed that 28 days after the implantation newly formed bone fibrils grew into the surface of the metal. However, already after 56 days the hole of the implant was enlarged due to a decrease in the newly formed bone caused by resorption. After 112 days a vitallium implant was lost, whereas a CoCr implant which had been plasma coated with titanium again had close contact to the bone [26].

The surface roughness of metallic implants plays an important role. This influence was investigated using cylinders of titanium and titanium alloys which were implanted on the legs of rabbits. A measurable adhesion of the titanium alloys could be observed only on implants with a surface roughness of >22 μm. With increasing roughness the adhesion strength is improved.

The exposure time after the implantation also has an influence. With implants of Ti6Al4V the tensile strength required to tear the cylinders off the bone was more than doubled if the time was increased from 84 to 168 days. After the short exposure time of 84 days an implant of Ti5Al2.5Fe already had an adhesion to the bone similar to that of an implant made of bioglass.

In contrast to the titanium alloys, the adhesion of the bioglass was not dependent on the surface roughness [27]. These results show that the growth of the bone and the tissue in close contact to Ti and its alloys with formation of a strong bond must have a more biomechanical than chemical-bioactive character. Consequently, it was shown that by an increase of the surface area, e.g. by drilling holes in the contact area of the implanted cylinders to the bone, the tear-off force necessary was increased. However, if the supplementary surface was taken into consideration, the adhesion strength was not increased. A Ti5Al2.5Fe implant coated with hydroxylapatite had a maximum adhesion strength of 1.97 N/mm^2 [27] already after 84 days.

The improved fixation of the bone at a structural implant surface leads consequently to a porous implant and implant surface respectively, which allows an ingrowth of the bone. In addition to an improved fixation, the porous implant has two other advantages: its Young's modulus is decreased, which provides better transmission of the functional load and stimulation of new bone formation. In addition, the damping capacity of the implant is increased, and the shear stress generated by the functional loading is decreased because, similar to the thread of a screw, the load at this interface causes a normal stress perpendicular to the inclined area and a lower shear stress which is effective in the inclined area.

REFERENCES

1. Zitter, H. and Plenk, H. (1987) The Electrochemical Behaviour of Metallic Implant Materials as an Indicator of their Biocompatibility. *J. of Biomedical Materials Research*, **21,** 881.
2. Fraker, A.C., Ruff, A.W., Sung, P. von Orden, A.C. and Speck, K.M. (1983) Surface Preparation and Corrosion Behaviour of Titanium Alloys for Surgical Implants, in *Titanium Alloys in Surgical Implants*, (eds H.A. Cuckey and F. Kubli), ASTM STP 796, pp. 206–219.
3. Mears, D.C. (1975) The Use of Dissimilar Metals Surgery. *J. Biomed. Mat. Res.*, **6,** 133.
4. Rätzer-Scheibe, H.J. and Buhl, H. (1984) Repassivation of Titanium and Titanium Alloys, in *Proc. of the 5th World Conf. on Titanium*, Vol. 4, pp. 2641–2648.
5. Higham, P.A. (1986). Proc. Conf. Biomed Mat., Boston, Dec. 1985, 253.
6. Williams, J.M. and Buchanan, R.A. (1985) Ion Implantation of Surgical Ti-6Al-4V. *Mater. Sci. Eng.*, **69,** 237–246.
7. Zwicker, U., Etzold, U. and Moser, Th. (1984) Abrasive Properties of Oxide Layers on TiAl5Fe2.5 in Contract with High Density Polyethylene, in *Proc. of the 5th World Conf. on Titanium*, Vol. 2, pp. 1343–1350.
8. Ferguson, A.B., Akahashi, Y., Laing, P.G. and Hodge, E.S. (1962) *J. Bone and Joint Surg.*, **44,** 323.
9. Hildebrand, H.F., Mercier, J.V., Decaeslecker, A.M., Ostapzuk, P., Stoeppler, U., Roumazeille, B. and Decloulx, J., *Biomaterials.*
10. Frazier, M.E. and Andrews, T.K. (1979), in *Trace Metals in Health and Disease* (ed. N. Karash), Raven Press, NY, 71.
11. Zwicker, U., Bühler, U., Müller, R., Beck, H., Schmid, H.J. and Ferstl, J. (1980) Mechanical Properties and Tissue Reactions of a Titanium Alloy for Implant Material, in *Proc. of the 4th World Conf. on Titanium*, Vol. 1, pp. 505–514.
12. Semlitsch, M. Staub, T. and Weber, H. (1985) Titanium–Aluminium–Niobium Alloy, Development for Biocompatible, High Strength Surgical Implants. *Biomed. Tech.* **30** (12), 334–339.
13. Steinemann, S.G. and Perren, S.M. (1984) Titanium Alloys as Metallic Biomaterials, in *Proc. of the 5th World Conf. on Titanium*, Vol 2, pp. 1327–1334.

14. Zitter, K., Plenk, H. and Strassl, H. (1980) Tissue and cell reactions *in vivo* and *in vitro* to different metals for dental implant, in *Dental Implants*, (ed. G. Heimke), C. Hanser, München, p. 15.
15. Bingmann, D. and Tetsch, P. (1986) Untersuchungen zur Biokompatibilität von Implantatmaterialien. *Dt. Zeitschr. f. Zahnärztl. Implantol.*, Bd. II, 190.
16. Kubashewski, O., Evans, E.Cl. and Alcock, C.B. (1967) *Metallurgical Thermochemistry*, Pergamon Press, London.
17. Zitter, H. (1976) Schädigung des Gewebes durch metallische Implantate. *Unfallheilkunde*, **79,** 91.
18. Tengvall, P., Lundström, J., Sjoquist, L., Elwing, H. and Bjursten, L.M. (1989) Titanium–Hydrogen Peroxide Interactions. Model Studies of the Influence of the Inflammatory Response on Titanium Implants. *Biomaterials* **10** (3) 166–175.
19. Breme, J. Steinhäuser, E. and Paulus, G. (1988) Commercially Pure Titanium Steinhäuser Plate–Screw System for Maxillo facial Surgery. *Biomaterials*, **9,** 310–313.
20. Krekeler, G. and Schilli, W. (1984) Das ITI-Implantat Typ H: Technische Entwicklung, Tierexperiment und klinische Erfahrung. *Chirurgische Zahnheilkunde*, **12,** 2253–2263.
21. Kirsch, A. (1980) Titan-spritzbeschichtetes Zahnwurzel-implantat unter physiologischer Belastung beim Menschen. *Dt.Zahnärztl.Z.*, **35,** 112–114.
22. Schröder, A., van der Zypen, E. and Sutter, F. (1981) The Reaction of Bone, Connective Tissue and Epithelium to Endosteal Implants with Titanium-Sprayed Surface. *J. Max. Fac. Surg.*, **9,** 15.
23. Brånemark, P.I., Adell, R., Albrektsson, T., Lekholm, U. Lundkvist, S. and Rockler, B. (1983) Osseointegrated Titanium Fixtures in the Treatment of Edentulousness. Biomaterials, **4,** 25.
24. Schröder, A., Stich, H., Strautmann, F. and Sutter, F. (1978) über die Anlagerung von Osteozement an einem belasteten Implantatkörper. Schw. Mschr. *f. Zahnheilkunde*, **4,** 1051–1058.
25. Kydd, W.L. and Daly, C.H. (1976) Bone–Titanium Implant Response to Mechanical Stress. *J. Prosthet. Dent.*, **35,** 567–571.
26. Strassl, H. (1978) Experimentelle Studie über das Verhalten von titanbeschichteten Werkstoffen hinsichtlich der Gewebekompatibilität im Vergleich zu anderen Metallimplanteten. Teil 1, *Osterr. Z. Stomatol.*, **75** (4), 134–146.
27. Schmitz, H.J., Gross, V., Kinne, R., Fuhrmann, G. and Strunz, V., Der Einfluβ unterschiedlicher Oberflächenstrukturierung plastischer Implantate auf das histologische Zugfestigkeitsverhalten des Interface, *7. DVM-Vortragsreihe Implantate.*

Stainless Steels

1a

1A.1 COMPOSITION

Table 1a.1 Comparison of international standard stainless steels for various medical applications

Chemical composition	*Germany*[1] *Alloy No.*	*Great Britain*[2] *B.S.I. No.*	*France*[3] *AFNOR No.*	*United States*[4] *AISI/SAE No.*	*Japan*[5] *JIS No.*
X20Cr13 (cast)	1.4021	410C21	Z12Cr13	410CA-15	SUS410
X20Cr13	1.4021	420S27	Z20C13	420	SUS4020J1
X15Cr13	1.4024	420S29			
X46Cr13	1.4034	(420S45)	Z38C13M		
X20CrNi172	1.4057	431S29	Z15CN16.02	431	SUS431
X12CrMoS17	1.4104		Z10CF17	430F/J405–89	SUS430F
X5CrNi1810	1.4301	304S15	Z6CN18–09	304	SUS304
		304S16		304H	
X10CrNiS189	1.4305	303S21	Z10CNF18.9	303	SUS303
X2CrNi1911	1.4306	304S12	Z2CNF18.9	304L/	SUS19
X2CrNi189 (cast)		304S11	Z2CN19	J405–89	SUS304L
X12CrNi177	1.4310	301S21	Z12CN17.07	301	SUS301
X5CrNiMo17122	1.4401	316S16	Z6CND17.11	316	SUS316
X5CrNiMo17133	1.4436		Z6CND17.12		
X2CrNiMo17132	1.4404	315S11	Z2CND18.13	316L	SUS316L
X2CrNiMo17130		316S12	Z2CND17.12		
X2CrNiMo1810 (cast)					
X2CrNiMoN17122	1.4406	316S61	Z2CND17.12Az	316LN	SUS316L
X2CrNiMoN17133	1.4429	316S62	Z2CND17.13Az		
			Z12CN18.07		
		304C12	Z2CN18.9		
X2CrNiMo18164	1.4438	317S12	Z2CND19.15	317L	SUS17L
X5CrNiMo1713	1.4449	317S16		317	SUS317
X6CrNiTi1810	1.4541	321S12	Z6CNT18.10	321	SUS321
		321S31			
X10CrNiNb189	1.4550		Z10CNNb18–10	347	
X10CrNiMoNb1810	1.4580		Z8CNDNb18–12	318	
X2CrNiN1810				XM-21	

X = sum of alloying elements >5 wt %.
Figure after X = carbon content multiplied by 100.
L = low carbon content.
N = contains nitrogen.
1)standardized in DIN 17440 – 17443, DIN 174400 will be replaced by DIN EN 10088.
2)standardized in BS 970/1 and BS7253–1, BS7252–9: ISO 5832–1.
3)standardized in NFA 35–574, replaced by NF EN 10088–3.
4)also standardized in ASTM A276.
5)standardized in JIS Cr 4303.

Table 1a.2 Chemical composition (wt%) and application of steels for medical instruments (Ref. 2, 3, 4)

	C	*Si*	*Mn*	*P*	*S*	*V*	*Cr*	*Mo*	*Ni*	*Application*
Martensitic and austenitic free cutting steels										
X12CrMoS17	0.1–0.17	≤1.0	≤1.5	≤0.045	0.15–0.25	–	15.5 –17.5	0.1–0.3	—	handles, screws, nuts
X12CrNiS188	≤0.15	≤1.0	≤2.0	≤0.045	0.1–0.2	—	9–11.5	—	8–10	handles, screws bolts, probes
Austenitic steels										
X5CrNi1810	≤0.07	≤1.0	≤2.0	≤0.045	≤0.03	—	17–20	—	9–11.5	pincettes, scissors, forceps
X12CrNi177	≤0.15(AISI) ≤0.12	≤2.0	≤0.045	≤0.03	—	16–18	—	—	7–9	handles, drills
X5CrNiMo17122	≤0.07	≤1.0	≤2.0	≤0.045	≤0.03	—	16.5–18.5	2–2.5	10.5–13.5	pincettes, scissors, drills

Table 1a.3 Chemical composition (wt%) and application of steels for medical instruments (Ref. 3, 4, 5)

	Martensitic steels									
	C	*Si*	*Mn*	*P*	*S*	*V*	*Cr*	*Mo*	*Ni*	*Application*
X10Cr13	≤0.15	≤1.0	≤1.0	≤0.04	≤0.03	–	11.5–13.0		–	
X15Cr13	0.12–0.17	≤1.0	≤1.0	≤0.045	≤0.03	–	12–14	–	–	Pincettes, forceps probes, suture hooks
20Cr13	0.17–0.22	≤1.0	≤1.0	≤0.045	≤0.03	–	12–14	–	–	As above, curettes, drills
X40Cr13	0.4–0.5	≤1.0	≤1.0	≤0.045	≤0.03	–	12–14	–	–	Scissors, forceps, scalpels, drills
X20CrNi172	≤0.20	≤1.0	≤1.0	≤0.04	≤0.03		15.5–17.5	–	1.25–2.5	
X65CrMo17	0.60–0.75	≤1.0	≤1.0	≤0.04	≤0.03			16.0–18.0	0.75	
X38CrMoV15	0.35–0.4	0.3–0.5	0.2–0.4	≤0.045	≤0.03	0.1–1.15	14–15	0.4–0.6	–	Scissors, forceps, scalpels, curettes
X45CrMoV15	0.4–0.5	0.3–0.5	0.2–0.4	≤0.045	≤0.03	0.1–0.15	14–15	0.4–0.6	–	Scissors, forceps, scalpels, curettes
X20CrMo13 (cast)	0.18–0.15	≤1.0	≤1.0	≤0.045	≤0.03	–	12–14	0.9–1.3	≤1.0	Curettes, Sharp spoons
X35CrMo17 (cast)	0.33–0.43	≤1.0	≤1.0	≤0.045	≤0.03	–	15.5–17.5	1–1.3	≤1.0	Curettes, Sharp spoons

Table 1a.4 Chemical composition (wt%) of austenitic stainless steels (Ref. 5)

Alloy	*C*	*Si*	*Mn*	*P*	*S*	*Cr*	*Mo*	*Ni*	*Others*
X12CrNi177	≤0.15	≤1.0	≤2.0	≤0.045	≤0.03	16.0–18.0	—	6.0–8.0	—
X5CrNi1810	≤0.08	≤1.0	≤2.0	≤0.045	≤0.03	18.0–20.0	—	8.0–10.5	—
X2CrNi1911	≤0.03	≤1.0	≤2.0	≤0.045	≤0.03	18.0–20.0	—	8.0–12.0	—
X25CrNi2522	≤0.25	≤1.5	≤2.0	≤0.045	≤0.03	24.0–26.0	—	19.0–22.0	—
X25CrNi2520	≤0.25	1.5–3.0	≤2.0	≤0.045	≤0.03	23.0–26.0	—	19.0–20.0	—
X5CrNiMo17133	≤0.08	≤1.0	≤2.0	≤0.045	≤0.03	16.0–18.0	2.0–3.0	10.0–14.0	—
X2CrNiMo17133	≤0.03	≤1.0	≤2.0	≤0.045	≤0.03	16.0–18.0	2.0–3.0	10.0–14.0	—
X5CrNiMo18164	≤0.08	≤1.0	≤2.0	≤0.045	≤0.03	18.0–20.0	3.0–4.0	11.0–15.0	—
X2CrNiMo18164	≤0.03	≤1.0	≤2.0	≤0.045	≤0.03	18.0–20.0	3.0–4.0	11.0–15.0	—
X6CrNiTi1810	≤0.08	≤1.0	≤2.0	≤0.045	≤0.03	17.0–19.0	—	9.0–12.0	Ti ≥5 × wt% C

Table 1a.5 Chemical composition of steels for implant surgery (wt%) (Ref. 6)

Alloy	*C*	*Si*	*Mn*	*P*	*S*	*N*	*Cr*	*Mo*	*Ni*	*Nb*
X2CrNiMoN18133	≤0.03	≤1.0	≤2.0	≤0.025	≤0.01	0.14–0.22	17–18.5	2.7–3.2	13–14.5	—
X2CrNiMo18153	≤0.03	≤1.0	≤2.0	≤0.025	≤0.01	≤0.01	17–18.5	2.7–3.2	13.5–15.5	—
X2CrNiMoN18154	≤0.03	≤1.0	≤2.0	≤0.015	≤0.01	0.1–0.2	17–18.5	2.7–3.2	14–16	—
X2CrNiMnMoN22136	≤0.03	≤0.75	5.5–7.5	≤0.025	≤0.01	0.35–0.5	21–23	2.7–3.7	10–16	0.1–0.25

The minimum content of Cr and Mo amounts to ≥ 26 according to the sum of efficacy which is given by 3.3 × % Mo + % Cr.

1A.2 PHYSICAL PROPERTIES

Table 1a.6 Physical properties of selected steels for medical instruments (Ref. 2)

Alloy	*Magnetic Properties*	*Thermal Expansion Coefficient between 70 and 300°C ($\times 10^{-6}K^{-1}$)*	*Thermal Conductivity at 20°C (W/mK)*	*Specific Heat Capacity at 20°C (J/kgK)*	*Specific Electrical Resistivity at 20°C (μΩm)*	*Young's modulus (GPa)*	*Density (g/cm^3)*
X10Cr13		9.9	24.9		0.57	200	7.8
X15Cr13	Magnet-	11.5			0.60		
X20Cr13	izable	11.5	30	460	0.60	200	7.8
X40Cr13		11.5			0.60		
X45CrMoV15		11.0			0.65		

Table 1a.7 Physical properties of austenitic stainless steels for medical instruments (Ref. 7)

Alloy	*Magnetic Properties*	*Thermal Expansion Coefficient between 70 and 300°C ($\times 10^{-6}K^{-1}$)*	*Thermal Conductivity at 20°C (W/mK)*	*Specific Heat Capacity at 20°C (J/kgK)*	*Specific Electrical Resistivity at 20°C ($\Omega mm^2/m$)*	*Young's modulus (GPa)*	*Density (g/cm^3)*
X12CrNi177		17.	16.2	500	0.72	193	8.0
X5CrNi1810		17.8	16.2	500	0.72193	8.0	
X2CrNi1810	Para-						
	mag-						
X25CrNi2520	netic	15.1	17.5	500	0.77	200	7.8
X5CrNiMo17133							
X2CrNiMo17133		15.9	16.2	500	0.74	193	8.0
X2CrNiMoN17133							
X2CrNiMo18164		15.9	16.2	500	0.74	193	8.0
X5CrNiMo18164							
X6CrNiTi1810		16.6	16.1	500	0.72	193	8.0

Table 1a.8 Physical properties of various stainless steels (Ref. 2)

Alloy	*Magnetic Properties*	*Thermal Expansion Coefficient between 70 and 300°C ($\times 10^{-6}K^{-1}$)*	*Thermal Conductivity at 20°C (W/mK)*	*Specific Heat Capacity at 20°C (J/kgK)*	*Specific Electrical Resistivity at 20°C ($\Omega mm^2/m$)*	*Young's modulus (GPa)*	*Density (g/cm^3)*
X12CrMoS17	Ferro-	11.0	26.1	460	0.60	200	7.8
X20CrNi172	magnetic	12.1	20.2	460	0.72	200	7.8

1A.3 PROCESSING OF STAINLESS STEELS (REF. 8, 9, 10, 11, 12)

1a.3.1 Hot Working and Heat Treatment

Stainless steels are more difficult to forge than carbon or low-alloy steels because of their higher yield stress strength at elevated temperatures and the limitation of the maximum temperature at which they can be forged without microstructural damage due to the precipitation of δ-ferrite. Most austenitic stainless steels can be forged above 930°C. Above 1100°C some steels precipitate the δ-ferrite phase which decreases the forgeability. Typical forging temperatures are between 925 and 1100°C. If the precipitation of δ-ferrite does not appear, the deformation temperature can be increased to 1260°C. Nitrogen-alloyed austenitic stainless steels have a higher strength and a higher corrosion resistance than austenitic stainless steels due to the stabilization of the austenite by nitrogen. For this reason higher chromium and molybdenum contents can be used to improve the corrosion resistance.

In the forging of martensitic stainless steels, especially those with high carbon contents, precautions must be taken to avoid cracking during cooling caused by the martensitic transformation. These steels are cooled more slowly than austenitic steels to a temperature of about 590°C. Forging is recommended in the temperature range of 900–1200°C.

1a.3.2 Working of Sheet

Alloys with low carbon contents (ferritic or austenitic stainless steels) are suitable for cold deformation such as bending, folding or deep-drawing. In general, austenitic stainless steels show better cold work properties than ferritic stainless steels.

In the deformation of ferritic stainless steels a temperature of 100–300°C should be used to achieve a better workability. If higher deformation rates are required, an intermediate annealing at 750–800°C should be performed.

Deformation of austenitic stainless steels results in a much higher work hardening than in ferritic stainless steels. Therefore, higher deformation forces, harder and more wear-resistant tools are required.

In drawing, excessively high speeds must be avoided. Best results are obtained with a speed of 6–8 m/min.

In deep drawing a high holding-down force prevents the formation of folds, but results in a higher danger of cracks due to the higher stresses. Deformation should be carried out in one step because of the high rate of work hardening. Oil with graphite or MoS_2 is used as a lubricant. Before the subsequent heat treatment the lubricant must be removed carefully in order to avoid a reaction with the steel.

1a.3.3 Descaling

Descaling of hot worked stainless steels can be accomplished by mechanical or by chemical cleaning, or by a combination of both methods. The surface can be cleaned by sand blasting, but unless it is machined after blasting, only nonmetallic blast material should be used in order to avoid contamination and a reduction of the corrosion resistance. Following blast cleaning stainless steels are usually acid pickled and washed with water. Common etching acids are:

(a) 1.5–2.0% NaOH
(b) 10% H_2SO_4
(c) 10% HNO_3 / 2% HF

1a.3.4 Machining of Stainless Steels

Stainless steels are generally more difficult to machine than low-carbon steels due to their high work hardenability. The non-free machining steels have a tendency to develop long, stringy chips, which reduce the life of the tool. The cutting speed is lower and a higher power is necessary than with low-carbon steels. Because of the low thermal conductivity good lubrication and cooling are important requirements.

The machinability of martensitic stainless steels decreases with in creasing carbon content because of the higher amount of chromium carbides. Austenitic stainless steels have a high work-hardenability which causes a cold deformation of the surface during machining, which decreases the machinability.

By additions of manganese and copper the work hardenability is reduced and machinability improved. Strength and hardness are increased by carbon and nitrogen, which however causes a poorer machinability. Machining parameters of stainless steels are given in Table 1a.9.

The turning of stainless steels requires tools with top rake angles on the high side of the 5–10° range in order to control the formation of chips. Carbide-tipped tools can be used and allow higher speeds than high-speed tools. An interruption of the cuts should be avoided. Blade-type and circular cutoff tools can also be employed.

The drilling of stainless steels should be carried out with a sharp three-cornered punch in order to avoid work hardening.

Thread rolling is possible with automatic screw machines of sufficient power and rigidity.

Milling can be accomplished with high-speed cutters and tools with carbide inserts, particularly in the case of alloys which are difficult to machine. The best surface quality is obtained by using helical or spiral cutters at high speeds.

Table 1a.9 Nominal machining parameters for stainless steels (Ref. 10)

Alloy	*Type of Machining*	*Tool Material*	*Depth of Cut (mm)*	*Speed (m/min)*	*Feed (mm/rev)*
Martensitic	Turning	HSS	0.75–3.8	20–38	0.18–0.38
		carbide	0.75–3.8	80–180	0.18–0.38
Austenitic	Turning	HSS	0.75–3.8	23–30	0.18–0.38
		carbide	0.75–3.8	100–160	0.18–0.38
Martensitic	Drilling	M1, M7, M10	—	12–18	0.025–0.46*
Austenitic				12–18	0.025–0.46*
Martensitic	Tapping	M1, M7, M10	—	3–12	—
Austenitic				4–8	
Martensitic	Milling	M2, M7	—	27–34	0.025–0.15 mm/tooth
		C6	—	82–107	0.025–0.15 mm/tooth
Austenitic		M2, M7	—	23–24	0.05–0.15 mm/tooth
		C6	—	79–82	0.025–0.15 mm/tooth
Martensitic Austenitic	Power hardening		—	50–90 strokes/min	0.1 mm/stroke

* Depending on hole diameter

Band sawing and power hacksawing are possible with high-speed steel blades.

The grinding of stainless steels can be performed with alumina and silicon carbide wheels, but the latter will have a reduced wheel life.

1a.3.5 Brazing

The chromium oxide film on the surfaces prevents wetting of the base metal by the molten filler and must therefore be removed by a suitable flux. Stainless steels can easily be joined together with other metallic materials or stainless steels of other composition. All conventional brazing processes, such as furnace, torch, induction and resistance brazing, can be employed. The most commonly used process is furnace brazing.

The filler metals used in brazing stainless steels can be alloys of silver, nickel, copper and gold, with the silver alloys being those most frequently employed. The chemical composition and the properties of the standard brazing filler metals used for joining stainless steels are listed in Table 1a.10. Furnace brazing in a reducing or inert atmosphere (argon, vacuum) requires no fluxes, but for torch brazing (reducing flame) they are always necessary. The commercially available fluxes contain boric acid, borates, fluorides, fluoborates and a wetting agent. They are available as powders, pastes and liquids.

Table 1a.10 Chemical composition and brazing temperature range of filler metals for brazing stainless steels (Ref. 13, 14)

	Chemical Composition (wt%)									*Brazing*
Filler Metal	*Ag*	*Cu*	*Zn*	*Cd*	*Ni*	*Sn*	*Li*	*Mn*	*In*	*Temperature Range (°C)*
AgCu	53–93	balance	—	—	—	—	≤0.5	—	—	765–980
Ag55Sn	54–57	20–23	balance	—	—	2–5	—	—	—	650
Ag56InNi	55–57	balance	—	—	3.5–4.5	—	—	—	13–15	730
AgCuZn	20–70	20–40	14–40	—	≤3.5	≤5.5	—	—	—	650–870
AgCuZnCD	30–50	14–35	13–25	12–25	—	—	—	—	—	620–840
AgCuZnMn	20–50	15–40	21–37	—	≤2.5	—	—	1.5–8	—	700–870

1a.3.6 Welding

Stainless steels can be welded by fusion (e.g. arc welding) or pressure welding (e.g. resistance welding) techniques. Steels which do not contain more than 0.03% sulphur, phosphorous or and selenium can be fusion welded by most welding techniques, such as shielded metal arc welding, submerged arc welding, inert gas metal welding, gas tungsten inert gas welding, plasma arc welding and flux cored arc welding.

Because of their low thermal conductivity and higher electrical resistance stainless steels require 20–30% less heat input than carbon steels during resistance welding. The resulting slow cooling rate may lead to a lower corrosion resistance because of the precipitation of chromium carbides.

Free-machining stainless steels are unweldable because of their high sulphur content.

To avoid contamination, especially by carbon, the stainless steel parts should be cleaned to remove organic substances.

Extra low carbon stainless steels, such as X2CrNiMo17133 do not tend to precipitate carbide and can therefore be welded without the danger of a diminished corrosion resistance.

Table 1a.11 lists electrodes and welding rods suitable as filler metals for the arc welding of stainless steels.

Table 1a.11 Filler metals for arc welding of stainless steels (Ref. 11, 15)

Steel	*Condition of Weld for Service*	*Electrode or Welding Rod*
X12CrNi177 X5CrNi1810	As welded or annealed	X8CrNi2011
X2CrNi1911	As welded or stress relieved	X8CrNi1811
X25CrNi2520	As welded	X25CrNi2520
X5CrNiMo17133*	As welded or annealed	X5CrNiMo17133
X2CrNiMo17133*	As welded or stress relieved	X2CrNiMo17133
X5CrNiMo18164*	As welded or annealed	X5CrNiMo18164
X2CrNiMo18164*	As welded or stress relieved	X2CrNiMo18164
X6CrNiTi1810	As welded or stabilized and stress relieved	X8CrNi1811
X20Cr13**	Annealed or hardened and stress relieved	X20Cr13
X20CrNi1810***	As welded	X25CrNi2520 X8CrNi2011

* Welds may have poor corrosion resistance in as welded condition.
Restoration by subsequent heat treatment possible:
X5CrNiMo17133, X5CrNiMo18164: full annealing at 1065–1120°C;
X2CrNiMo17133, X2CrNiMo18164: stress relieving at 870°C.
** Careful preheating and postweld heat treatment are required to avoid cracking.
*** Careful preheating required.

Preheating of austenitic stainless steels usually has no beneficial effect on the welding results.

Thermal stress relief can be carried out in wide temperature and time ranges, depending on the amount of relaxation required. Table 1a.12 gives two examples of the temperature and time required to achieve different stress relief.

In general, ferritic stainless steeels are less weldable than austenitic steels because of a grain coarsening during the welding operation and the risk of the formation of both austenite and martensite during cooling. This may reduce the toughness and ductility of the steel. Martensite can be eliminated by annealing, but this is not the case with coarsened ferrite.

Martensitic stainless steels are very difficult to weld because, during the welding operation, they become harder and less ductile, whereby cracking may occur. Whether preheating and postweld annealing are necessary in the case of the martensitic stainless steels depends on the carbon content. Table 1a.13 shows the recommended preheating temperatures, depending on the carbon content for martensitic stainless steels.

As compared to carbon steels, a resistance welding of austenitic stainless steels is possible with shorter welding times and lower welding currents than in the case of carbon steels because of their higher electrical resistivity. By comparison, the welding pressure must be higher for stainless steels.

Martensitic and ferritic stainless steels can also be resistance welded, but the welded seam shows a brittle behaviour in the as-welded condition. Therefore a postweld thermal treatment is required.

Table 1a.12 Examples of the temperature and time required to achieve various degrees of stress relief in austenitic steels (Ref. 11)

Temperature (°C)	*Time (min/cm section thickness)*	*Stress Relief (%)*
840–900	25	85
540–650	95	35

Table 1a.13 Dependence of the preheating temperature on the carbon content for martensitic stainless steels (Ref. 11)

Carbon Content (wt%)	*Preheating Treatment*
0<0.1*	No preheating or postweld treatment
0.1–0.2	Preheating to 260°C, welding at 260°C, slow cooling
0.2–0.5	Preheating to 260°C, welding at 260°C, annealing

* Not a standard carbon content.

1a.3.7 Heat Treatment

Table 1a.14 summarizes the various recommended heat treatments for martensitic, precipitation hardened, austenitic and ferritic austenitic steels.

Table 1a.14 Recommended heat treatments for various stainless steels (Ref. 1, 2, 8, 16)

Alloy	*Hot Deformation (°C)*	*Soft Annealing (°C)*	*Hardening (°C)*	*Hardening Medium*	*Annealing (°C)*
X20C13	750–1150	750–780	950–1000	Oil	650–700
X12CrMoS17	750–1100	800–850	1020–1050	Oil	550–600
X5CrNiMo17133	800–1150		1050–1100	Water, air	
X2CrNiMo17133	800–1150		1000–1100	Water, air	
X5CrNi1810	800–1150		1000–1050	Water, air	
X2CrNi1810	800–1150		1000–1050	Water, air	
X6CrNiTi1810	800–1150		1020–1070	Water, air	

1A.4 MECHANICAL PROPERTIES

Table 1a.15 Mechanical properties of steels for medical instruments (Ref. 2, 3)

Steel	*Condition*	*Young's Modulus *10³ (MPa)*	*Tensile Yeild Strength * (0.2 %) (MPa)*	*Ultimate Tensile Strength (MPa)*	*Ratio Yield /Tensile Strength*	*Elongation at Fracture* (%)*	*Reduction of Area (%)*
			Martensitic steels				
X15Cr13	As forged	216	—	≤720	—	—	—
X20Cr13	+ Annealed	216	—	≤740	—	—	—
X45CrMoV15		220	—	≤900	—	—	—
X20CrMo13	As cast	—	—	≤800	—	—	—
X35CrMo17	+ Annealed	—	—	≤950	—	—	—
			Martensitic and austenitic free cutting steels				
X12CrMoS17	As forged + Annealed	216	—	540–740	—	16	—
X12CrNiS188	As forged + Quenched	200	195	500–700	—	35	—
			Austenitic steels				
X5CrNi1810	As forged* + Quenched	200	220–235	550–750	0.3–0.4	43–45	—
X5CrNiMo17122	As forged* + Quenched	200	240–255	550–700	0.36–0.44	43–45	—
X12CrNi177	Wire, cold deformed	185–195	—	1250–2450**	—	—	>40

* Longitudinal/transversal.
** Depends on the degree of cold deformation.

Table 1a.16 Mechanical properties of austenitic stainless steels (minimum values at room temperature) (Ref. 5, 9, 17)

Alloy (bar)	*Condition*	*Tensile Yield Strength (MPa)*	*Ultimate Tensile Strength (MPa)*	*Ratio Yield/ Tensile Strength*	*Elongation at Fracture (%)*	*Reduction of Area (%)*
X12CrNi177	Annealed	205	515	0.40	40	
	Full hard	965	1280	0.75	9	
X5CrNi1810	Hot finished + annealed	205	515	0.40	40	50
	Cold finished	310	620	0.50	30	40
X2CrNi1911	Hot finished + annealed	170	480	0.35	40	50
	Cold finished + annealed	310	620*	0.50	30	40
X25CrNi2520	Hot finished + annealed	205	215	0.95	40	50
	Cold finished + annealed	310	620	0.50	30	40
X5CrNiMo17133	Hot finished + annealed	205	515	0.40	40	50
	Cold finished + annealed	310	620	0.50	30	40
X2CrNiMo17133	Hot finished + annealed	170	515	0.33	40	50
	Cold finished + annealed	310	620	0.50	30	40
X5CrNiMo1713	Hot finished + annealed	205	515	0.40	40	50
	Cold finished + annealed	310	620	0.50	30	40
X2CrNiMo18164	Annealed	240	585	0.41	55	65

* Typical values.

Table 1a.17 Mechanical properties of martensitic stainless steels (minimum values at room temperature) (Ref. 2, 5)

Alloy (bar)	*Condition*	*Tensile Yield Strength (MPa)*	*Ultimate Tensile Strength (MPa)*	*Ratio Yield/ Tensile Strength*	*Elongation at Fracture (%)*	*Reduction of Area (%)*
X10Cr13	Hot finished + annealed	275	485	0.57	20	45
	Cold finished + annealed	275	485		16	45
X20Cr13	Hardened + tempered 204°C	1480	1720	0.86	8	25
X20CrNi172	Hardened + tempered 260°C	1070	1370	0.78	16	55
	Hardened + tempered 593°C	795	965	0.82	19	57
X65CrMo17	Hardened + annealed	415	725	0.57	20	--
	Hardened + tempered 316°C	1650	1790	0.92	5	20

Table 1a.18 Mechanical properties of steels for implant surgery (Ref. 6)

Alloy	*Condition*	*Tensile Yield Strength* (0.2%) (MPa)*	*Ultimate Tensile Strength (MPa)*	*Ratio Yield/ Tensile Strength*	*Elongation at Fracture* (%)*
X2CrNiMoN18133	Solution Treated	300	600–800	0.38–0.5	40
X2CrNiMo18153		190	490–690	0.28–0.39	40
X2CrNiMoN18154		285	590–800	0.36–0.48	40
X2CrNiMnMoN22136		500	850–1050	0.48–0.59	35

* Minimum values.

Special requirements:

1. Allowed melting procedures: vacuum arc furnace or electroslag remelting.
2. After the solution heat treatment the material has to be free of delta-ferrite.
3. Grain size of at least ASTM4.
4. Resistance to intercrystalline corrosion determined according to Table 1a.5.
5. Microscopic purity concerning inclusions of oxides and sulfides determined according to Table 1a.5.

Table 1a.19 Mechanical properties of wire for implant surgery (Ref. 6)

Alloy	*Condition*	*Ultimate Tensile Strength (MPa)*	*Elongation at Fracture* (%)*
X2CrNiMoN18133	Solution	800–1000	30
X2CrNiMoN18154	treated	800–1000	40
X2CrNiMoN18133	Cold	1350–1850	—
X2CrNiMoN18154	worked	1350–1850	—

*Minimum values.
The values depend on the diameter of the wire (solution heat treated) and on the degree of deformation (decrease of diameter and increase of degree of deformation = increase of value).

Table 1a.20 Mechanical properties of X2CrNiMo17133 stainless steel as a function of cold working (Ref. 18)

Degree of Cold Working (%)	*Tensile Yield Strength (MPa)*	*Ultimate Tensile Strength (MPa)*
0	255	584
31	831	912
50	1036	1138
63	1169	1255
70	1204	1344
76	1252	1421

Table 1a.21 Influence of heat treatment on the mechanical properties of steels for medical instruments (Ref. 2)

	Condition	*Tensile Yield Strength* (0.2%) (MPa)*	*Ultimate Tensile Strength (MPa)*	*Ratio Yield/ Tensile Strength*	*Elongation at Fracture* (%)*	*Reduction of Area (%)*
		Martensitic steels				
X15Cr13	Quenched	450	650–800	0.56–0.69	10–15	25–30
X20Cr13	+ tempered	550	750–950	0.58–0.73	8–14	20–30
		Martensitic and austenitic free cutting steels				
X12CrMo5	Quenched + tempered	450	640–840	0.54–0.70		11

* Minimum values.
The values of the elongation at fracture and of the impact strength depend on the direction of sampling (longitudinal = higher values; transversal = lower values) and on the thickness of the sheet or rod (increase of thickness = decrease of value).

Table 1a.22 Influence of a cold deformation on the mechanical properties of steels for implant surgery (standard qualities, other qualities – for all steels – as agreed upon) (Ref. 6)

Alloy	*Condition*	*Tensile Yield Strength* (0.2%) (MPa)*	*Ultimate Tensile Strength (MPa)*	*Ratio Yield/ Tensile Strength*	*Elongation at Fracture* (%)*
X2CrNiMoN22136	As cold worked,	690	860–1100	0.63–0.8	12
X2CrNiMo18154	dia.≤19 mm	650	860–1100	0.63–0.8	12

* Minimum values.

Table 1a.23 Influence of heat treatment on the hardness of various stainless steels (Ref. 1)

Alloy	*Heat Treatment*	*VHN*
X20Cr13	Hardened and annealed I	190–235
	Hardened and annealed II	230–275
X12CrMoS17	Soft annealed (800–850°C)	160–210
	Soft annealed + drawn	160–210
	Hardened + annealed (1020–1050°C/oil/550–600 °C/air)	190–235
X5CrNiMo17133 X2CrNiMo17133	1050–1100°C/water quenched	130–180
X5CrNi1810 X2CrNi1810	1000–1050°C/water quenched	130–180
X6CrNiTi1810	1020–1070°C/water quenched	130–190

1A.5 FATIGUE

Table 1a.24 Fatigue limit (2×10^6 cycles) by the staircase method* of X2CrNiMo17133 stainless steel (Ref. 18)

Tensile Strength (MPa)	*Degree of Cold Work (%)*	*Stress Ratio, R*	*Fatigue Limit (MPa)*
658	7	0	283
1211	57	0	362
1211	57	-1	505

*Explanation:
(1) Starting with a stress S_o.
(2) if specimen fails before $2\times10^{+6}$ cycles → new specimen with a stress $S - \Delta S_o$
if specimen does not fail before $2\times10^{+6}$ cycles → new specimen with a stress $S_o + \Delta S$.
(3) Do (2) for 15–20 samples and evaluate with standard statistical methods.

Table 1a.25 High cycle fatigue strength of hip endoprostheses of stainless steel, measured in 0.9% NaCl solution at 37°C. Testing conditions according to DIN 58840 (simulation of a loosened shaft) (Ref. 19)

Alloy	*Maximum load in 2×10^7 cycles (kN)* *0.9% NaCl (f = 2 Hz)*
hot wrought X2CrNiMo17133	2
hot wrought X3CrNiMoNbN2317	5.5–7.5

Table 1a.26 High cycle fatigue strength σ_D of various stainless steels (Wöhler curves) and rotating fatigue strength σ_R(Ref. 20, 21, 22)

Alloy	*σ_D (MPa)*	*σ_R (MPa)*	*R*
X2CrNiMo17133	250–320	250	
X2CrNiMo18153	Annealed	250–320	–1
	Cold worked	350–415	
X2CrNiMnMoN22136	Hot forged	500–650	

Table 1a.27 Fatigue properties of various stainless steels (Ref. 23)

Alloy	*Heat treatment*	*Testing condition* *Type*	*R*	*α_k*	*Medium*	*Fatigue limit at NB=10^7 (MPa)*
X20Cr13	30 min/1020°C/oil	RB*	-1	1	Air	481
	+ 2 h/550°C/air			1	30% NaCl	69
				3.6	Air	206
				3.6	30% NaCl	49
X20Cr13	30 min/1020°C/oil	RB	-1	1	Air	412
	+ 2 h/625°C/air			1	30% NaCl	78
				3.6	Air	177
				3.6	30% NaCl	29
X5CrNi1810	30 min/1050°C/ water	RB	-1	1	Air	220–250
X5CrNiMo17133	15 min/1050°C/ water	RB	-1	1	Air	265
					30% NaCl	216

* RB = rotating bending.

1A.6 CORROSION AND WEAR

Table 1a.28 Sum of efficacy and breakdown potential of various stainless steels in 1 M NaCl at room temperature (Ref. 21)

Alloy	*Sum of Efficacy*	*Breakdown Potential (V)*
X5CrNi1810	19	0.25
X5CrNiMo17133	25	0.25
X2CrNiMo17132	26.5	0.5
X2CrNiMoN18164	29.5	0.7
X2CrNiMoV1813	25	0.65

Table 1a.29 Rate of formation of corrosion products for the stainless steel X2CrNiMo17133 in Hank's solution during current-time-tests (Ref. 24)

Alloy	*Metal Converted into Compound (ng/cm^2h)*
X2CrNiMo17133	
Mechanically polished	7.8
Chemically polished	230

Table 1a.30 Corrosion properties of the stainless steel X2CrNiMo17133 in 0.9% NaCl. Potential referred to standard calomel electrode (SCE) (Ref. 18)

Testing Method	*Result*
ASTM F746–81 test (mV)	300 ±25
Scratch test (mV)	530 ±20
Potentiodynamic test	
Current 10 $\mu A/cm^2$ (mV)	560 ±25
Repassivation (mV)	90 ±25
Critical pitting temperature test	
Potentiostatic 200 mV (°C)	95 ±5
Potentiostatic 350 mV (°C)	65 ±5
Critical crevice temperature test	
Potentiostatic 200 mV (°C)	25 ±5
Potentiostatic 350 mV (°C)	<25

Table 1a.31 Polarization current (i) and polarization resistance (R_c) of the stainless steel X2CrNiMo17133 in 0.9% NaCl and in 0.9% NaCl with a stable redox system [$Fe(CN)_6^{4-}$ / $Fe(CN)_6^{3-}$] at 37°C corresponding to a potential of the body fluid of 400 mV (Ref. 25, 26)

		R_c ($k\Omega cm^2$)	
Alloy	*i ($\mu A/cm^2$)*	*0.9% NaCl*	*0.9% NaCl + redox*
X2CrNiMo17133	0.006	1670	4.38

Table 1a.32 Repassivation time of the stainless steel X2CrNiMo17133 in 0.9% NaCl and breakdown potential in Hank's solution (Ref. 21)

Alloy	*Breakdown Potential (mV) vs. Standard Calomel Electrode*	*Repassivation Time (ms)*	
		-500 mV	*+500 mV*
X2CrNiMo17133	200–300	72 000	35

Table 1a.33 Electrochemical data for the stainless steel X5CrNi1810 in 0.1 M NaCl; influence of the pH-value (Ref. 27)

Alloy	*Corrosion Potential E_{corr} (mV)*	*Passive Current Density I_p (μA/cm²)*	*Breakdown Potential E_b (mV)*
X5CrNi1810			
pH 7	-395	0.56	770
pH 2	-661		-270

Table 1a.34 Coefficients of friction of sliding materials (Ref. 20, 24)

Material	*Lubricant*	*Coefficient of friction*
X2CrNiMo17133 vs.		
High density polyethelyne	Synovial fluid:	
	in vitro	0.10
	in vivo	0.02
Cartilage vs.		
cartilage	in vivo	0.008

Table 1a.35 Influence of the N^+ -implantation* on weight loss during wear testing** of the stainless steel X5CrNi1810 (Ref.29)

Alloy	*Weight loss (μg) after*		
	1000 cycles	*3000 cycles*	*5000 cycles*
X5CrNi1810	200	780	1000
N^+-implanted X5CrNi1810	320	460	440

* Implantation parameters: 100 keV nitrogen ions

$$3 \times 10^{17} \frac{N^+}{cm^2} \text{ nominal dose}$$

** Testing conditions: dry; load: 5 N; speed 150 cycles/min; wear against high speed steel (66 HRC); wear distance: 23 mm/cycle.

1A.7 BIOLOGICAL PROPERTIES

Table 1a.36 Influence of heat treatment (oxidation) on shear strength between X2CrNiMo17133 screw implants and bone (rat femur after various times of insertion (Ref. 28)

Time after insertion (days)	*Shear strength (MPa)*	
	Control	*Heat treated**
4	0.01 ± 0.001	0.03 ± 0.01
5	0.04 ± 0.01	0.21 ± 0.07
6	0.28 ± 0.06	0.68 ± 0.07
10	0.58 ± 0.09	1.23 ± 0.19
35	1.58 ± 0.18	2.61 ± 0.21

* Heat treatment: 200 min/280°C/air.

REFERENCES

1. Product information, Röchling Werke, Germany.
2. DIN 17440 (1985), Beuth.
3. DIN 17441 (1985), Beuth.
4. DIN 17442 (1977), Beuth.
5. *ASM Metals Handbook*, Vol. 3: Properties and Selection: Stainless Steels, Tool Materials and Special-Purpose Metals.
6. DIN 17443 (1986), Beuth.
7. *ASM Metals Handbook*, Vol. 3: Properties and Selection: Stainless Steels, Tool Materials and Special-Purpose Materials.
8. Heimann, W. Oppenheim, R. and Weizling, W. (1985) Nichtrostende Stähle, in *Werkstoffkunde Stahl*, Bd. 2: Anwendungen, Springer-Verlag.
9. Harris, T. and Priebe E. Forging of Stainless Steels, in *ASM Metals Handbook*, Vol. 14: Forming and Forging.
10. Kosa, T. and Ney, R.P. Machining of Stainless Steels, in *ASM Metals Handbook*, Vol. 16: Machining.
11. Arc Welding of Stainless Steels, in *ASM Metals Handbook*, Vol. 6: Welding Brazing, Soldering.
12. Resistance Welding of Stainless Steels, in *ASM Metals Handbook*, Vol. 6: Welding Brazing, Soldering.
13. Brazing of Stainless Steels, in *ASM Metals Handbook*, Vol. 6: Welding Brazing, Soldering.
14. DIN 8513 (1979), Beuth.
15. DIN 8856 (1986), Beuth.
16. Bergman, W. (1991) *Werkstofftechnik, Teil 2: Anwendungen*, Hanser Verlag, München.
17. American Standard ASTM F138.
18. Cigada, A., De Soutis, G., Gratti, A.M., Roos, A. and Zaffe, D. (1993): In vivo Behaviour of a High Performance Duplex Stainless Steel, *J. of Appl. Biomaterials*, **4**, 39–46.

19. Kunze, E. (1988) Vergleichende Untersuchungen zum Langzeit-Ermüdungsverhalten von Hüftgelenkprothesen an Luft und in NaCl-Lösung. *Metall*, **2**, 140–145.
20. Thull, R. (1979) Eigenschaften von Metallen, für orthopädische Implantate und deren Prüfung. *Orthopädie*, **7**, 29.
21. Breme, J. and Schmidt, H.-J. (1990) Criteria for the Bioinertness of Metals for Osseo-Integrated Implants, in *Osseo-Integrated Implants*, Vol. 1, (ed. G. Heimke), pp. 31–80.
22. Webster, J.G. (ed) (1988) *Encyclopedia of Medical Devices and Instrumentation*, Vol. 1, Wiley-Interscience Publication.
23. Schmidt, W. (1981) Werkstoffverhalten bei schwingender Beanspruchung. Thyssen Edelst. Techn. Ber., **7** (1), 55–71.
24. Mears, D.C. (1977) Metals in Medicine and Surger. *International Metals Review*, Review 218, June, 119–155.
25. Breme, J. (1988) Titanium and Titanium Alloys, Biomaterials of Preference, in *Proc. of the 6th World Conf. on Ti*, Vol. 1, pp. 57–68.
26. Zitter, H. and Plenk, H. (1987) The Electrochemical Behaviour of Metallic Implant Materials as an Indicator of their Biocompatibility. *J. of Biomedical Materials Research*, **21**, 881.
27. Geis-Gerstorfer, J., Weber, H. and Breme, J. (1988) Electroche mische Untersuchung auf die Korrosionsbeständigkeit von Implantatlegierungen. *Z. f. Zahnärztl. Implantologie* **4**, (1), 31–36.
28. Hazan, R., Brener, R. and Oron, V. (1993) Bone growth to metal implants is regulated by their surface properties. *Biomaterials* **14** (8), 570–574.
29. Cavalleri, A. Gzuman L., Ossi, P.M. and Rossi, I. (1986) On the Wear Behaviour of Nitrogen Implanted 304 Stainless Steel, *Scripta Metallurgica* **20**, 37–42.

CoCr-based alloys

1b

1B.1 COMPOSITION

Table 1b.1 Comparison of international standards for Co-based alloys

Chemical composition	*Germany DIN*	*Great Britain BSI*	*France AFNOR*	*International Organization for Standardization ISO*	*United States ASTM*	*Japan JIS*
Co29Cr5Mo (cast)	5832–4 13912–1	7252- Part 4	Project S 94–054	5832/IV	F75	T6115
Co29Cr5Mo (wrought/PM)	5832–12	7252- Part 12	Project S 94–053	5832/XII	F799	T6104
Co20Cr15W10Ni	5832–5	7252- Part 5	Project S 90–406	5832/V	F90	
Co20Cr35Ni10Mo	5832–6	7252- Part 6	NFISO5832–6	5832/VI	F562	
Co20Cr16Ni16Fe7Mo (wrought/cast)	5832–7	7252- Part 7	Project S 94–057	5832/VII	F1058	
Co20Cr20Ni5Fe3Mo3W	5832–8	7252- Part 8	Project S 94–058	5832/VIII	F563	

Table 1b.2 Chemical composition of cast Co alloys (wt%) (Ref. 1, 2, 8)

Alloy	*Cr*	*Mo*	*Ni*	*Fe*	*C*	*Si*	*Mn*	*Ti*	*Co*
CrCo29Cr5Mo	26.5–30.0	4.5–7.0	≤2.5	≤1.0	≤0.35	≤1.0	≤1.0	--	balance
CoCrMo*	15.0–32.5	4.0–7.5	≤2.0	<1.5	≤0.05	≤1.0	≤1.0	≤5	33.0–75.0

* Alloys used for dental restoration (according to standards sum of Co + Cr ≥ 85%, Cr + Mo + Ti ≥25%, Be ≤ 0.01%).

Table 1b.3 Chemical composition of wrought Co alloys (wt%) (Ref. 3, 4, 5, 6, 7, 9)

Alloy	*Cr*	*Mo*	*Ni*	*Fe*	*C*	*Si*	*Mn*	*P*	*S*	*W*	*Ti*	*Co*
Co20Cr15W10Ni	19.0–21.0	---	9.0–11.0	≤3.0	≤0.15	≤1.0	≤2.5	≤0.04	≤0.03	14.0–16.0	---	Balance
Co20Cr35Ni10Mo*	19.0–21.0	9.0–10.5	33.0–37.0	≤1.0	≤0.15	≤0.15	≤0.15	≤0.015	≤0.010	---	≤1.0	Balance
Co20Cr16Ni16Fe7Mo	18.5–21.5	6.5–8.0	14.0 18.0	balance	≤0.15	---	1.0–2.5	≤0.015	≤0.015	---	---	39.0–42.0
Co20Cr20Ni5Fe3Mo3W	18.0–22.0	3.0–4.0	15.0–25.0	4.0–6.0	≤0.05	≤0.05	≤1.00	---	≤0.010	3.0–4.0	0.5 3.5	Balance

* Other elements: single ≤0.1, sum: ≤0.4.
Be ≤0.001.

1B.2 PHYSICAL PROPERTIES

Table 1b.4 Physical properties of CoCr-alloys (Ref. 1, 8, 10)

Alloy	*Density* (g/cm^3)	*Melting Point (interval)* (°C)	*Transformation Temperature hcp→fcc* (°C)	*Young's Modulus* (GPa)	*Thermal Conductivity at 20°C* (W/mK)	*Electrical Restistivity at 20°C* (μΩm)
G-Co29Cr5Mo	8.2–8.4	1235 (eutectic) 1300–1400	890	210–330		
Co20Cr15W10Ni			650			
Co20Cr3Ni10Mo	8.43	1315–1427	650	235		1.03

1B.3 PROCESSING OF CoCr-ALLOYS (REF. 11, 12, 13, 14)

CoCr-alloys can be classified in two different groups:

(a) cast CoCr-alloys
(b) wrought CoCr-alloys

As a result there are two different methods for producing biomedical devices. Both groups of alloys contain more than 20 wt% chromium, thus providing a good resistance due to a passive oxide layer on the surface.

The cast alloys (e.g. G–Co29Cr5Mo) contain up to 0.5 wt% carbon to improve the castability by lowering the melting temperature to ~1350°C compared to 1450–1500°C for binary CoCr-alloys. Normally these alloys are investment cast (lost wax process). An improved casting quality can be achieved by a vacuum melting and casting process, whereby an oxidation is avoided. The lower melting temperature due to the alloying elements (e.g. carbon) results in a fine grain size and allows a decrease in the mould temperature from 1000°C to 900°C. The casting temperature ranges from 1350 to 1450°C depending on the alloy composition. The cast microstructure consists of a dendritic matrix with dispersed carbides ($M_{23}C_6$, M_7C_3, M_6C, where M = Co, Cr or Mo) and of other intermetallic compounds. In the as cast condition the alloys have reduced strength and ductility. Therefore, a heat treatment must follow the casting procedure. A solution heat treatment is performed at 1210–1250°C leading to a complete solution of the carbides in the matrix. The carbide forming elements increase the strength by a solid-solution hardening. In order to avoid an excessive grain growth, the carbides are not completely dissolved. This measure results in a planing of the grain boundaries.

As an alternative to the near net shape casting the devices are sometimes produced by the powder metallurgical route. The compacting of the material is performed by HIP (~10000 MPa, 1100° C). Because of the relatively high costs this method is used only for highly loaded implants like femoral stems of total hip prostheses. Hipping of cast CoCr-alloys is recommended for a decrease of defects like gas or shrinkage pores, whereby an improvement of the mechanical properties is achieved.

Wrought CoCr-alloys have a lower Cr content (19–21 wt%) than cast alloys. Cr is substituted by Mo or W. In order to stabilize the fcc phase a certain content of Ni, Fe or Mn is necessary. Because of the high strength of the alloys at elevated temperatures higher forces must be applied for forging these alloys. For a plastic deformation the alloys must be annealed in order to produce the fcc structure which can be retained to room temperature. The hcp transformation, which causes an improvement of the mechanical properties, is induced by the mechanical deformation. After hot working the microstructure consists of a fcc matrix with fine hcp platelets. A hardening process may be achieved by cold working followed by aging between 500 and 600°C for 1–4 h, resulting in precipitation of Co_3Mo, which increases the hardness. Table 1b.10 shows the influence of hot working and heat treatment. Table 1b.11 summarizes the influence of cold working on the mechanical properties of the CoCr-alloys.

The alloy Co20Cr35Ni10Mo is hot forged or rolled at temperatures between 870 and 1125°C. This multiphase alloy with a high strength and ductility is aged between 540 and 590°C after the hot working process. Table 1b.11 shows the influence of a deformation and of a heat treatment on the mechanical properties of the alloy.

1b.3.1 Machining of CoCr-Alloys

Since CoCr-alloys have a low thermal conductivity, a high shear strength and a high work hardening rate and since they contain hard intemetallic compounds, they are expensive to machine because high cutting forces must be applied.

For turning CoCr alloys, tungsten carbide tools are usually applied. Ceramic coated carbide, boron nitride and high speed steels can also be used. Water soluble oils are applied as cutting fluids. Table 1b.5 gives the turning parameters for CoCr-alloys.

Drilling of CoCr-alloys is accomplished by similar methods. The speeds and feeds must be reduced because of the slower cooling rate and lubriant efficiency.

Milling of CoCr-alloys requires, like turning, higher forces and climb milling is preferred. Cuts deeper than 1.5 mm are not possible. Besides high-speed cutters carbide tools can also be used. Table 1b.7 gives the milling parameters for CoCr-alloys.

All types of sawing, such as band sawing, circular sawing and hack-sawing, can be applied. A good supply of cutting fluid during the sawing operation is important.

Table 1b.5 Turning parameters of cast and wrought CoCr-alloys (Ref. 11)

Alloy	*Condition*	*Roughing Speed (m/min)*	*Finishing Speed (m/min)*	*Depth of Cut (mm)*	*Feed Rate (mm/rev)*
Cast CoCr	As cast or as cast and aged	3–15	3–18	Rough: 2.5–5 Finish: 0.8	Rough: 0.13–0.18 Finish: 0.13
Wrought CoCr	Solution treated or solution treated and aged	5–17	6–27	Rough: 5 Finish: 0.8	Rough: 0.25 Finish: 0.13

Table 1b.6 Drilling parameters of cast and wrought CoCr-alloys (Ref. 11)

Alloy	*Condition*	*Speed (m/min)*	*Feed Rate (mm/rev)*
Cast CoCr	As cast or as cast and annealed	2–4.5	0.025–0.15
Wrought CoCr	Solution treated	6	0.05–0.1
	Solution treated and aged	4.5	0.05–0.1

Table 1b.7 Milling parameters of cast and wrought CoCr-alloys (Ref. 11)

Alloy	*Type of Milling*	*Depth of Cut (mm)*	*Speed (m/min)*	*Feed Rate (mm/rev)*
Cast CoCr	Face	1	3.6–4.5	0.05
	with HSS tools	8	1.5–2.0	0.075
Wrought CoCr	Face	1	4.5–9.0	0.05
	with HSS tools	8	2.0–6.0	0.1
Cast CoCr	Face	1	9–15	0.13
	with carbide tools	4	6–14	0.15
Wrought CoCr	Face	1	18–21	0.13
	with carbide tools	4	17–20	0.13–0.15
Cast CoCr	Finish with HSS tools	0.5	3.0–3.6	0.025–0.05
Wrought CoCr	Finish with HSS tools	0.5	3.6–4.5	0.025–0.05
Cast CoCr	Finish with Carbide tools	0.5	12–18	0.025–0.05
Wrought CoCr	Finish with carbide tools	0.5	18–21	0.025–0.05

Grinding of CoCr-alloys requires good control of the parameters because of the sensitivity of the alloys to microcracks and because of alterations in the microstructure.

Brazing of CoCr-alloys can be performed either in a hydrogen atmosphere or in vacuum. As filler metals Ni- or Co-base alloys or Au–Pd-alloys can be used. In order to achieve a better wetting by the filler metals an electroplating or flashing with Ni is performed. Copper filler metals should be avoided because of the danger of an embrittlement of the seam. Table 1b.8 shows the compositions of a typical Co-base filler metal.

Table 1b.8 Chemical composition (wt%) of a Co-based filler metal (Ref. 12)

Cr	*Ni*	*Si*	*W*	*Fe*	*B*	*C*	*P*	*S*	*Al*	*Ti*	*Zr*	*Co*
18–20	16–18	7.5–8.5	3.5–4.5	1.0	0.7–0.9	0.35–0.45	0.02	0.02	0.05	0.05	0.05	Balance

1b.3.2 Arc Welding of CoCr-Alloys

CoCr-alloys can be welded by tungsten inert gas welding (TIG), metal inert gas welding (MIG) and shielded metal arc welding (SMAW). Before welding the parts must be carefully cleaned by grinding, machining or washing with a solvent. Sand-blasting should be avoided because of the danger of contamination of the surface. TIG is accomplished with a thoriated tungsten electrode (W + 2% ThO_2). Automatic MIG is possible with argon or helium as shielding gases and with an electrode material corresponding to the base metal. The heat input provided by the current and voltage respectively and by the welding speed (Table 1b.9) should be low in order to produce a high cooling rate providing a favourable microstructure (for grains and fine precipitations of carbides). Therefore SMAW is performed in a flat position with a rapid welding speed and with little weaving.

Table 1b.9 Recommended parameters for the welding of CoCr-alloys by different processes (Ref. 12)

Parameter	*TIG*	*MIG*
Power supply	DC transformer	DC transformer
Electrode diameter (mm)	1.1–1.6	0.9
Filler metal	—	According to base metal
Shielding gas	Ar	Ar
Welding position	flat	flat
Current (A)	12–70	130–160
Voltage (V)	10–20	22–25
Arc starting	High frequency	—
Welding speed (m/min)	0.4–2.3	0.75

CoCr-alloys are welded in the solution-treated condition with electrodes of a similar composition to the base metal. CoCr-alloys are more difficult to weld than wrought CoCr-alloys. Table 1b.9 gives recommended parameters for the welding of CoCr-alloys by different processes.

1B.4 MECHANICAL PROPERTIES

Table 1b.10a Mechanical Properties of cast CoCr and powder metallurgically produced (pm) alloys (Ref. 1, 2, 8, 15, 16)

Alloy	*Condition*	*Young's Modulus × 10^3 (MPa)*	*Tensile Yield Strength* (0.2%) (MPa)*	*Ultimate Tensile Strength (MPa)*	*Ration Yield/ Tensile Strength*	*Elongation at Fracture* (%)*	*Reduction of Area (%)*	*Hardness HV*
Co29Cr5Mo	As cast		≥450	≥665	≥0.69	≥8	≥8	
CoCrMo*	As cast	210–	500–650	1277		4–10		300–400
	HIP	330	841			14		

* Alloys used for dental restoration.

Table 1b.11 Influence of the hot working procedure and of the heat treatment on the mechanical properties of cast CoCrMo (Ref. 16)

Treatment	*Tensile Yield Strength (MPa)*	*Ultimate Tensile Strength (MPa)*	*Ratio Yield/ Tensile Strength*	*Elongation at Fracture (%)*
As cast	430–490	716–890	0.55–0.60	5–8
Solution annealed 1230°C/1 h/water quenched	450–492	731–889	0.55–0.62	11–17
Solution annealed + aged 650°C/20 h	444–509	747–952	0.47–0.68	10–13.5
Cast and extruded 1200°C + annealed 1100°C/2 h	731	945	0.77	17
Cast and hot forged and rolled 1175°C + cold rolled 10% + 1050°C/40 min air cooled	876	1360	0.64	19

Table 1b.12 Influence of the cold working procedure on the mechanical properties of the alloy Co20Cr15W10Ni (Ref. 16)

Treatment	*Tensile Yield Strength (MPa)*	*Ultimate Tensile Strength (MPa)*	*Ratio Yield/ Tensile Strength*	*Elongation at Fracture (%)*
Annealed	450–650	950–1200	0.47–0.54	37–60
Cold worked (17.5%)	1180	1350	0.87	22
Cold worked (4%)	1610	1900	0.85	10
Cold worked	1300	1520	0.85	—

Table 1b.13 Influence of deformation and heat treatment on the mechanical properties of the alloy Co20Cr35Ni10Mo (Ref. 16)

Treatment	*Tensile Yield Strength (MPa)*	*Ultimate Tensile Strength (MPa)*	*Ratio Yield/ Tensile Strength*	*Elongation at Fracture (%)*
Wrought, annealed >1050°C	300	800	0.37	40
Cold worked (50%)	650	1000	0.65	20
Cold worked (55%)	1413	1827	0.77	12
Cold worked (55%) + aged + 538°C/4 h	1999	2068	0.97	10
Hot forged >650°C below the recrystallization temperature (950°C)	—	1300	—	—

1B.5 FATIGUE

Table 1b.14 High cycle fatigue strength of various CoCr alloys (Ref. 16, 17)

Alloy	*Condition*	*R*	*Fatigue Reversed-Stress (MPa)*	*R*	*Rotating Bending Fatigue Strength (MPa)*
G-Co29Cr5Mo	As cast	-1	200–300	-1	300
Co20Cr35Ni10Mo	As cast		200–300		—
Co20Cr15W10Ni	Wrought		540–600		500
pm-Co29Cr5Mo	HIP		370–430		725

Table 1b.15 Influence of the heat treatment on the fatigue strength (10^7 cycles) of CoCr-alloys (Ref. 16, 18)

Alloy	*Treatment*	*R*	*Tensile Fatigue Strength (MPa)*
G-Co29Cr5Mo	As cast		300
	As cast + polished		>200
	As cast + shot peened		>260
	Solution annealed (1230°C/1 h/water quenched		220–280
	Annealed 1170°C	-1	280–350
Co20Cr15W10Ni	Cold worked (17.5%)		490
	Cold worked (44%)		587
Co20Cr35Ni10Mo	Annealed >1050°C		340
	Cold worked (50%)		435
	Cold worked (50%)		405
	Hot forged + annealed		400–450
	Hot forged > 650°C		520

Table 1b.16 High cycle fatigue strength of hip endoprostheses of CoCr alloys, measured in 0.9% NaCl solution at 37°C. Testing conditions similar to DIN 58840 (simulation of a loosened shaft, 50 mm free length) (Ref. 19)

Alloy	*Maximum load in 2 × 10^7 cycles (kN)* Air (f = 25 Hz)	0.9% NaCl (f = 2 Hz)
Cast Co29CrMo	7	5.5–6.5
Wrought CoNiCrMo	5.5	4.5

1B.6 CORROSION AND WEAR

Table 1b.17 Influence of the pH value on the electrochemical data of the alloy Co29Cr5Mo in 0.1 M NaCl (Ref. 20)

Metal/Alloy	*Corrosion Potential E_{corr} (mV)*	*Passive Current Density I_p (μA/cm²)*	*Breakdown Potential E_b (mV)*
Co29Cr5Mo			
pH 7	-391	1.36	340
pH 2	-465	0.54	476

Table 1b.18 Repassivation time in 0.9% NaCl and breakdown potential in Hank's solution of CoCr alloys (Ref. 21)

Alloy	*Breakdown Potential (mV) vs Calomel Electrode*	*Repassivation Time (ms)*	
		-500 mV	*+500 mV*
G-Co29Cr5Mo	+420	44.4	36
Co20Cr35Ni10Mo	+420	35.5	41

Table 1b.19 Polarization current (i) and polarization resistance (R_c) of CoCr alloys in 0.9% NaCl and in 0.9% NaCl with a stable redox system at 37°C [$Fe(CN)_6^{4-}/Fe(CN)_6^{3-}$], corresponding to a potential of the body fluid of 400 mV (Ref. 22, 23)

Material	*i (μA/cm²)*	*R_c (kΩ cm²)*	
		0.9% NaCl	*0.9% NaCl + redox*
Co20Cr15W10Ni	0.004	2500	3.32

Table 1b.20 Rate of formation of corrosion products for the alloys Co29Cr5Mo in Hank's solution under constant natural potential (Ref. 24)

Alloy	*Metal (Converted into Compound) (ng/cm² h)*
Co29Cr5Mo	
Mechanically polished	150
Chemically polished	20

Table 1b.21 Coefficients of friction of sliding materials (Ref. 17, 24)

Material	*Lubricant*	*Coefficient of Friction*
G-Co29Cr5Mo/ G-Co29Cr5Mo	Dry	0.80
	Distilled H_2O	0.38
	Synovial fluid	0.16
	Globulin solution	0.16
	Albumin solution	0.18
	in vivo	0.04
G-Co29Cr5Mo/HDPe	Synovial fluid	
	in vitro	0.04
	in vivo	0.02
Co20Cr35Ni10Mo/ Co20Cr35Ni10Mo	H_20	0.58
Cartilage/Cartilage	*in vivo*	0.008

Table 1b.22 Influence of nitrogen ion implantation on the mean wear rate and the coefficient of friction of the cast alloy Co29Cr5Mo (Ref. 25, 26)

Alloy	*Testing Load (N)*	*Mean Wear Rate ($mm^3/10^6$)*	*Coefficient of Friction*
Co29Cr5Mo	132	3.22	
Co29Cr5Mo nitrogen implanted	132	5.93	
Co29Cr5Mo	10	0.260	0.131
Co29Cr5Mo nitrogen implanted	10	0.185	0.89

Testing conditions: Co29Cr5Mo – pin on UHMWPE disk; lubricant: bovine serum; testing speed: 85 mm/s.

1B.7 BIOLOGICAL PROPERTIES

Table 1b.23 Biocompatibility of cp-Co, cp-Cr, cp-Ni and NiCrCo alloys; survival rate of L-32 cells incubated with powders (Ref. 27, 28)

Metal/Alloy	*Powder Concentration (mg/l)*	*Survival Rate (%)*
Co	25	45
	50	18
Cr	200	65
	400	62
Ni	200	0.9
	400	0.1
Co20Cr15W10Ni	200	33
	400	23
Co20Cr35Ni10Mo	200	25
	400	14

Table 1b.24 50% lethal concentration (LC50) of powders from Table 1b.23 (Ref. 27)

Metal/Alloy	*LC50 (mg/l)*
Co	30
Cr	>400
Ni	25
Co20Cr15W10Ni	80
Co20Cr35Ni10Mo	100

REFERENCES

1. DIN/ISO 5832–4 (draft) (1980), Beuth.
2. American Standard ASTM F75 (1982) (ASTM F75–67).
3. DIN/ISO 5832–5 (draft) (1992), Beuth.
4. DIN/ISO 5832–6 (draft) (1980), Beuth.
5. DIN/ISO 5832–7 (draft) (1992), Beuth.
6. American Standard ASTM F75 (1990) (ASTM F90–68).
7. American Standard ASTM F562 (1984) (ASTM 578A).
8. CoCr-alloy producing industries.
9. DIN/ISO 5832–8 (draft) (1992), Beuth.
10. MP35N Alloys, Latrobe Steel Company, Pennsylvania.
11. *ASM Metals Handbook*, Vol. 16: Machining.
12. Brazing of Heat-Resisting Alloys, in *ASM Metals Handbook*, Vol. **6**. Welding, Brazing Soldering.
13. *ASM Metals Handbook*, Vol. **14**: Turning and Forging.
14. *Encyclopedia of Mat. Sci. Eng.* (1986), Pergamon Press.
15. DIN 13912 (1982), Beuth.
16. Pilliar, R.M., Manufacturing Processes of Metals: The Processing and Properties of Metal Implants, in *Metal and Ceramic Biomaterials*, Vol. **1**.
17. Thull, R. (1979) Eigenschaften von Metallen, für orthopädische Implantate und deren Prüfung. *Orthopädie*, **7,** 29.
18. Lorenz, M. Semlitsch, M., Panic, B., Weber, H. and Willhert, H.G. (1978) Fatigue Strength of Cobalt-Base Alloys with High Corrosion Resistance for Artificial Hip Joints. *Engineering in Medicine*, **7** (4), 241.
19. Kunze, E. (1988) Vergleichende Untersuchungen zum Langzeit-Ermüdungsverhalten von Hüftgelenkprothesen an Luft und in NaCl-Lösung. *Metall*, **2,** 140–145.
20. Geis-Gerstorfer, J., Weber, H. and Breme, J. (1988) Electrochemische Untersuchung auf die Korrosionsbeständigkeit von Implantatlegierungen. *Z. f. Zahnärztl. Implantologie* **4,** (1), 31–36.
21. Breme, J. and Schmidt, H.-J. (1990) Criteria for the Bioinertness of Metals for Osseo-Integrated Implants, in *Osseo-Integrated Implants*, Vol. 1, (ed. G. Heimke), pp. 31–80.
22. Zitter, H. and Plenk, H. (1987) The Electrochemical Behaviour of Metallic Implant Materials as an Indicator of their Biocompatibility. *J. of Biomedical Materials Research*, **21,** 881.
23. Breme, J. (1988) Titanium and Titanium Alloys, Biomaterials of Preference, in *Proc. of the 6th World Conf. on Ti*, Vol. 1, pp. 57–68.
24. Mears, D.C. (1977) Metals in Medicine and Surgery. *International Metals Reviews*, Review 218, June, 119–155.
25. Greer, K.W. and Jones, D.E. (1994) The importance of standardization of wear test parameters in the simulation of three wear mechanisms, *Proc. of the 20th Annual Meeting of the Society for Biomaterials*, p. 408.
26. Taylor, S.K. Serekian, P. and Manley, M. (1992) Effect of nitrogen ion implantation on CoCr wear performance against UHMWPE, *Proc. of the 4th World Biomaterials Congress*, p. 275.
27. Hildebrand, H.F. (1993) *Biologische Aspekte beim Einsatz von Implantatwerkstoffen*, DGM Hochschulseminar, Saarbrücken, Germany.
28. Breme, J. (1993) *Metalle als Biomaterialien*, DGM Hochschulseminar, Saarbrücken, Germany.

Titanium and titanium alloys 1c

1C.1 COMPOSITION

Table 1c.1 Comparison of international standards for titanium and titanium alloys

*Chemical Composition**	*Germany DIN***	*Great Britain BSI*	*France AFNOR*	*International Organization for Standardization ISO*	*United States ASTM*	*Japan JIS*
Ti-1 Ti-2 Ti-3 Ti-4	5832–2 and 17850 respectively	2TA1 2TA2 2TA6 BS7252–2	NFISO5832–2 and S 90–404 respectively	5832/II	F67/Grade 1 F67/Grade 2 F67/Grade 3 F67/Grade 4	H4600
Ti6Al4V	5832–3 and 17851 respectively	2TA10, 2TA13 BS7252–3	NFISO5832 and S94–080 respectively	5832/III	F136	H4607
Ti5Al2.5Fe	5832–10 and 17851 respectively	BS7252–10	–	5832/X	–	–
Ti6Al7Nb	5832–11 and 17851 respectively		S94–081	5832/XI	F1295	–

* Ti-1–Ti-4 = commercially pure titanium; others: direct chemical composition, e.g. Ti6Al4V: 6 wt%, Al, 4 wt% V, balance Ti.
** terms of delivery: DIN 17860, DIN 17862.

Table 1c.2 Chemical composition of cp-titanium (wt%) (Ref. 1, 2)

cp-Titanium	*Fe max.*	*O approx.*	*N max.*	*C max.*	*H max.*	*Ti*
Grade I	0.2	0.1	0.05	0.08	0.013	
Grade II	0.25	0.2	0.06	0.08	0.013	Balance
Grade III	0.3	0.25	0.06	0.1	0.013	
Grade IV	0.35	0.3	0.07	0.1	0.013	

Table 1c.3 Chemical composition of (α+β)-titanium alloys (wt%) (Ref. 1, 3, 4)

Alloy	*Al*	*V*	*Fe*	*Nb*	*Ta*	*O*	*N*	*C*	*H*	*Others Single*	*Others Sum*	*Ti*
Ti6Al4V	5.5–6.75	3.5–4.5	0.3	---	---	0.2	0.05	0.08	0.015	0.1	0.4	Balance
Ti5Al2.5Fe	4.5–5.5	---	2.0–3.0	---	---	0.2	0.05	0.08	0.015	0.1	0.4	Balance
Ti6Al7Nb	5.5–6.5	---	0.25	6.5–7.5	0.5	0.2	0.05	0.08	0.009	---	---	Balance

Table 1c.4 Chemical composition-(wt%) of β and near β titanium alloys (experimental alloys) (Ref. 5, 6)

Alloy	*Al*	*Mo*	*Zr*	*Ta*	*Nb*	*Sn*	*Ti*
Ti15Mo5Zr3Al	3,8	15	5				
Ti12Mo5Zr5Sn		11.5	5			4.5	Balance
Ti30Nb					30		
Ti30Ta				30			

1C.2 PHYSICAL PROPERTIES

Table 1c.5 Physical properties of commercially pure titanium (Ref. 1, 7, 9

Young's modulus	(GPa)	105–110
Density	(g/cm^3)	4.5
Melting point	(°C)	1700
Boiling point	(°C)	3600
Transformation temperature α--β	(°C)	885
Crystal structure		>850°C β bcc <850°C α hex
Magnetic properties		paramagnetic
Heat of transformation	(kJ/kg)	67
Thermal neutron-capture cross section	(cm^2)	5.8×10^{-22}
Specific heat at 15°C	(kJ/kg K)	0.52
Heat fusion	(kJ/kg)	419
Thermal conductivity at room temperature	(W/mK)	17
Thermal expansion coefficient between 20 and 200°C	(K^{-1})	9×10^{-6}
Specific heat resistivity at 20°C	(μΩm)	0.5

Table 1c.6 Physical properties of (α+β)-titanium alloys (Ref. 1, 7, 8, 9)

Property	*Ti6Al4V*	*Ti5Al2.5Fe*	*Ti6Al7Nb*
Young's modulus (GPa)	100–110	110–116	110
Density (g/cm^3)	4.43	4.45	4.52
Type of phase at room temperature (°C)	α+β	α+β	α+β
Microstructure	Al–A9	Al–A9	Al–A9
Transformation temperature (°C)	990±15	950±15	1010±15
Thermal conductivity at room temperature (W/mK)	6.5	—	—
Coefficient of thermal expansion between 30–200°C (×10^{-6}K^{-1})	8.6	9.3	—
Specific heat at 20°C (kJ/kg K)	0.56	—	—
Specific electrical resistivity at 20°C (52 mm^2/m)	1.66	—	—

Table 1c.7 Influence of alloying elements and heat treatment on Young's modulus (Ref. 10, 11)

Alloy	*Heat Treatment*	*Young's Modulus (GPa)*
Ti30Ta	As rolled	80
	1 h/1000°C/H_2O	63
Ti30Nb	As rolled	70
Til5Mo5Zr3Alell	Solution heat treated at 840°C	75
	Solution heat treated at 740°C	88
	Solution heat treated at 740°C + aged at 600°C	113

1C.3 PROCESSING OF cp-Ti AND Ti ALLOYS [1]

Provided that the following characteristics of titanium are taken into consideration, almost all processing procedures are possible:

1. high affinity to the gases oxygen, nitrogen and hydrogen
2. high reactivity to all metals producing intermetallic compounds
3. relatively low Young's modulus and therefore backspringing
4. relatively low thermal conductivity
5. tendency to stick to the tools

1c.3.1 Hot working and heat treatment

Titanium and titanium alloys are fabricated into semi-finished products by conventional methods such as forging, rolling, pressing, drawing etc.

When Ti materials are heated, care must be taken to avoid an excessive pickup of oxygen, nitrogen and hydrogen. Heating and annealing should therefore take place in a neutral or slightly oxidizing atmosphere. During heating in a gas-fired furnace direct contact with the flame must be avoided because of the risk of hydrogen pickup and of local overheating. During a short heating period oxygen pickup is restricted to the surface area. This surface zone must be removed by chemical or mechanical methods. Because hydrogen is able to penetrate the matrix rapidly, a reducing atmosphere must be avoided. The hot working temperature depends on the alloy composition and should be selected to obtain the best mechanical properties and grain structure (A1–A9 according to ETTC2, Ref. 11). Table 1c.8 summarizes the deformation temperatures for the various Ti materials. Table 1c.9 gives the temperature ranges and recommended annealing times for stress relieving, soft annealing and solution treating + age hardening. Where the cross-section is very small, annealing is favourably carried out in a high vacuum furnace. Prior to this annealing treatment the oxide film must be removed from the surface in order to avoid diffusion of oxygen into the material.

Table 1c.8 Deformation temperatures for various titanium materials (Ref. 1.13)

Alloy	*Deformation temperature (°C)*
cp-Ti Grade 1	650–870
Grade 2	650–870
Grade 3	700–900
Grade 4	700–930
Ti6Al4V	760–1040

Table 1c.9 Recommendation for the heat treatment of cp-Ti and Ti alloys (Ref. 1, 7)

Alloy	*Stress Relief*	*Soft Annealing*	*Solution Annealing + Age Hardening*
Ti grade I Ti grade II Ti grade III Ti grade IV	15 min–2 h at 450°C/air	15 min–8 h at 650–750°C	—
Ti6Al4V	3 min/mm min. 30 min max. 4 h at 500–600°C/air	min. 15 min max. 4 h at 700–850°C/air slow cooling rate to 550 °C	15–60 min at 820–950°C/H_2O + 2 h at 480–600°C/air
Ti5Al2.5Fe			15–60 min at 800–920°C/H_2O + 2–4 h at 480–600°C/air

1c.3.2 Working of sheet

At room temperature cp-Ti, grades I and II, can be worked very well, grades III and IV only moderately well. The Ti alloys, because of their high yield/tensile strength ratio, can be worked only under certain conditions.

For deep drawing special coatings in the form of polymer foils have proved to be effective. At high temperatures colloidal graphite and common hot press greases with graphite or molybdenum disulphide additives have been successful. The Fe-, Ni- and Cr-contents should be limited to 0.05, 0.1 and 0.33 wt%, respectively, in order to allow during a short annealing treatment (1–5 min at 750–850°C) a grain growth producing an average grain size of 50–70 μm. Due to this grain growth a deformation by twinning, with a resulting increased deep drawability, occurs (Ref. 14).

Superplastic forming is a material-saving and cost-reducing processs for manufacturing parts of complicated shape because it can be carried out together with diffusion welding in a single operation. Especially fine grained alloys like Ti6Al4V and Ti5Al2.5Fe can be used for a superplastic deformation. Other special deformation processes such as stretch forming, spinning or explosion forming are also possible.

1c.3.3 Descaling

With thick-walled parts the oxide layer on the surface generated during deformation and/or heat treatment is removed by sand-blasting and/or pickling. The workpiece is treated in an aqueous solution of 20 Wt. %. HNO_3 and 2% Wt. % HF.

Thin walled pieces are only pickled in an electrolytic or salt bath. It is important that not only the surface layer of oxide, but also the underlying oxygen enriched diffusion zone is removed. Otherwise, the machinability and the service life of turning and milling tools would be negatively affected.

1c.3.4 Machining

The machining of titanium materials presents no difficulties provided the following characteristic properties are taken into account:

1. relatively low thermal conductivity which may cause high thermal stresses at the cutting edge of the tool
2. low Young's modulus which yields to the pressure of the tool
3. tendency to stick to the tool

The titanium materials must therefore be machined at low cutting speeds, at a relatively high feed rate with an ample supply of coolant (sulphur containing oil; mixture of tetrachloride carbon, molybdenum sulphide and graphite; 5% aqueous solution of sodium nitrite, 5–10% aqueous solution of water-soluble oil or sulphurized chlorinated oil). The cutting tools should be sharp and mounted as rigidly as possible. Recommended parameters for turning and milling are given in Table 1c.10.

Since titanium dust and chips can easily catch fire, safety precautions must be taken.

Threads should be cut on a lathe, as thread-cutting discs are subject to seizure.

Sawing causes no difficulties if a high blade pressure is used and the coolant supply is ample. Coarse toothed blades (4 teeth per inch) are recommended.

For grinding, aluminium oxide (5–10 m/sec) and silicon carbide (20–30 m/sec) can be used.

Table 1c.10 Recommendations for the cutting and milling of cp-Ti and Ti alloys (Ref. 7)

Alloy	*Cutting Speed (m/min)*	*Feed (mm/rev)*	*Depth of Cut (mm)*	*Cutting Angle*	*Relief Angle*
		Rough cutting			
cp-Ti TC	30–75	0.2–0.4		0–6°	6–8°
HSS	7.5–4.0	0.1–1.25		6–15°	5–7°
			>2.5		
Ti alloys TC	15–25	0.2–0.4		0–6°	6–8°
HSS	3–15	0.1–0.4		6–15°	5–7°
		Forecutting			
cp-Ti TC	60–100	0.1–0.4		6–6°	6–8°
HSS	18–50	0.075–0.2		6–15°	5–7°
			0.75–2.5		
Ti alloys TC	20–50	0.1–0.4		6–6°	6–8°
HSS	5–15	0.075–0.2		6–15°	5–7°
		Finish cutting			
cp-Ti TC	60–100	0.075–0.3		0–15°	6–8°
HSS	20–50	0.05–0.1		5–6°	5–7°
			0.1–0.75		
Ti alloys TC	20–70	0.075–0.3		0–15°	6–8°
HSS	9–15	0.05–0.1		5–6°	5–7°
		Milling			
cp-Ti TC	25–30	0.07–0.15			
HSS	50–60	0.1–0.2	>1.25 face cutter	–	–
Ti alloys TC	7.5–20	0.07–0.2	>2.5 gear cutter		
HSS	15–30	0.1–0.2			

TC = hard metal (tungsten carbide).
HSS = high speed steel.

1c.3.5 Soldering and brazing

Immediately before soldering and brazing the oxide layer which is always present on the surface of titanium materials must be removed. For direct applications using a torch, aluminium–zinc and tin–zinc solders are suitable. The higher temperatures required for brazing present the difficulty of avoiding the formation of intermetallic phases. With almost all metals titanium forms brittle intermetallic phases in the fusion zone. The only exception is Ag, so that this metal forms one of the main constituents of brazers. The sources of heat used for brazing and soldering are the acetylene torch, high frequency induction coils, infrared radiation, an inert-gas-shielded arc with graphite or tungsten electrodes, furnaces with an argon atmosphere (min. 99.99% and/or a dew point below -50°C) and high vacuum furnaces. If brazing is not performed under vacuum or in a controlled atmosphere, fluxes are necessary to dissolve the oxide layers and prevent a pickup of gases.

1c.3.6 Welding

The inert-gas-shielded arc processes (TIG and MIG) are mainly used for fusion welding. In special cases resistance, ultrasonic, electron beam, diffusion and laser welding are applied. With the cp-Ti grades the weld attains mechanical properties approximating those of the base metal. A slight decrease in ductility may occur with high tensile grades. Under passivating conditions, titanium welds have the same corrosion resistance as the base metal. On the contrary, in reducing media the weld may be subjected to a more severe corrosive attack than the base metal. During the welding operation, the weld, the heat affected zone and the underside of the weld are shielded from the atmosphere. The filler rod used is an uncoated wire of the same grade or of a grade with a lower hardness than the base metal. Careful preparation of the joint is necessary, i.e. surface impurities must be removed by grinding or pickling in order to avoid porosity. Even fingermarks can produce a hardening of the weld. Sheet up to 2.5 mm thickness can be welded by a single layer. In order to avoid local oxygen concentrations oxidation products, such as those found at the tip of the electrode, must be cut off. The effectiveness of the inert gas is responsible for the welding rate. The optimum argon flow rate has proved to be about 6–8 l/mm. After welding the appearance of a dark blue or gray oxide layer indicates an insufficient inert gas shielding and an embrittlement of the weld due to oxygen and/or nitrogen pickup. The hardness of a good weld may exceed that of the fully recrystallized base metal by a maximum of 50 VHN. If, after a slight grinding of the surface, a hardness test should give a higher value, the weld must be completely removed because of embrittelement.

Electron beam welding is particularly suitable for titanium materials. It offers many advantages such as very narrow seams and small heat affected zones, weldability of thick diameters, high welding speed and reproducibility of even complex welds.

Titanium materials can be spot welded without any particular preparation under similar conditions to those of stainless steel. Using flat-tipped electrodes, spot welding can be performed without inert gas. A hardening of the zone by up to 50 VHN compared with the base metal is regarded as normal and does not diminish the strength of the joint. Seam and flash-butt welding are also possible if an argon atmosphere is used.

Diffusion welding is of particular importance for titanium materials because these materials are more amenable to a homogeneous band in the solid state state than other metals. After welding, the joint zone shows a higher temperature under high vacuum or, in an inert atmosphere, a microstructure very similar to that of the base metal.

1C.4 MECHANICAL PROPERTIES

Table 1c.11 Mechanical properties of commercially pure titanium (Ref. 1, 14)

cp-Titanium	*Condition*	*Tensile yield strength (0.2 %) (MPa)*	*Ultimate tensile strength (MPa)*	*Ratio yield/ tensile strength*	*Elongation at fracture* (%)*	*Reduction of area* (%)*	*Hardness*	*Bend radius (105°) for sheet thickness t <2 mm*	*>2 mm <5 mm*
Ti grade I		200	290–410	0.49–0.69	30	35	120	2 t	3 t
Ti grade II	sheet,	250	390–540	0.46–0.64	22	30	150	3 t	4 t
Ti grade III	as	320	460–590	0.54–0.7	18	30	170	4 t	5 t
Ti grade IV	rolled	390	540–740	0.53–0.72	16	30	200	5 t	6 t

* Minimum values.

Table 1c.12 Influence of a cold deformation on the mechanical properties of commercially pure titanium (Ref. 15)

cp-Titanium	*Condition (%)*	*Tensile Yield Strength (0.2%) (MPa)*	*Ultimate Tensile Strength (MPa)*	*Ratio Yield/ Tensile Strength*	*Elongation at Fracture (%)*
Ti grade I	30	555	635	0.87	18
	40	560	645	0.87	16
	55	605	710	0.85	15
	60	620	725	0.86	14
	65	640	730	0.88	14.5
Ti grade II	30	605	680	0.89	18
	40	645	740	0.87	17
	50	680	780	0.87	16
	60	685	795	0.86	16
	65	692	810	0.85	16.5

Table 1c.13 Mechanical properties of β and near β-titanium alloys (experimental alloys) (Ref. 5, 10, 16)

Alloy	*Tensile Yield Strength (0.2%) (MPa)*	*Ultimate Tensile Strength (MPa)*	*Ratio Yield/ Tensile Strength*	*Elongation at Fracture (%)*	*Reduction of Area (%)*
Ti15Mo5Zr3Al	870–1173	882–1177	1.0	15–20	43–80
Ti12Mo5Zr5Sn	1002	1010	0.99	17.8	56
Ti30Nb	500	700	0.71	20	60
Ti30Ta	590	740	0.80	28	58

Remarks: The alloys Ti15Mo5Zr3Al and Ti12Mo5Zr5Sn were investigated in the as forged and aged (600°C) condition. The alloys Ti30Nb and Ti30Ta, which can be used due to their thermal expansion coefficient adapted to that of alumina for a direct bonding to the ceramic for the production of dental implants, were tested in the as rolled condition.

Table 1c.14 Influence of heat treatment on the mechanical properties of β- and near β-titanium alloys (Ref. 5,10)

Alloy	*Condition*	*Tensile yield strength (0.2 %) (MPa)*	*Ultimate tensile strength (MPa)*	*Ratio yield/ tensile strength*	*Elongation at fracture (%)*	*Reduction of area (%)*
Ti15Mo5Zr3Al	SHT at 840°C	870	882	0.99	20	83.2
	SHT at 740°C	968	975	0.99	16.9	64.5
	SHT at 740°C aged at 600°C	1087	1099	0.99	15.3	57.5
Ti30Ta	Annealed at 1100°C	650	800	0.81	8	42
	Annealed at 1200°C	660	800	0.83	8	38
	Annealed at 1300°C	665	800	0.83	8	30
	Annealed at 1400°C	680	800	0.83	6	18

SHT = solution heat treatment.

Table 1c.15 Influence of a cold deformation on the mechanical properties of β-titanium alloys (Ref. 5)

Alloy	*Condition*	*Tensile yield strength (0.2 %) (MPa)*	*Ultimate tensile strength (MPa)*	*Ratio yield/ tensile strength*	*Elongation at fracture (%)*	*Reduction of area (%)*
Ti15Mo5Zr3Al	45% CW + aged at 600°C	1284	1312	0.98	11.3	43.8

CW = cold worked.

Table 1c.16 Mechanical properties of (α+β)-titanium alloys (Ref. 1, 3, 17, 18)

Alloy	*Condition* *Sheet as rolled thickness (mm)*	*Tensile yield strength (0.2 %) (MPa)*	*Ultimate tensile strength (MPa)*	*Ratio yield/ tensile strength*	*Elongation at fracture* (%)*	*Reduction of area* (%)*	*Hardness*	*Bend radius (105°) for sheet thickness t <2 mm*	*>2 mm <5 mm*
Ti6Al4V	-6	870	950	0.92	8	25	310	9 t	10 t
	6–100	830	920	0.90	8	25	310		
Ti5Al2.5Fe	-6	780	860	0.91	8	25	310	9 t	10 t
Ti6Al7Nb	Extruded	811–952	869–1008	0.93–0.94	7–13	24–44			
	hot rolled + hot forged	943–1008	1016–1086	0.93	11–16	40–55			
Ti6Mn	-6	1058	1095	0.97	11.5	26	360	--	--

Ti6Mn was developed for a coating with hydroxyapatite. Due to a thermal expansion coefficient of this alloy, which is near to that of the ceramic, an extremely high shear strength of the surface layer has been achieved.

Table 1c.17 Influence of a solution treating and ageing on the mechanical properties of Ti6Al4V (Ref. 1)

Condition	*Tensile Yield Strength (0.2%) (MPa)*	*Ultimate Tensile Strength (MPa)*	*Ratio Yield/ Tensile Strength*	*Elongation at Fracture (%)*	*Reduction of Area (%)*
Sheet ≤ 12.5 mm 15–60 min at 800–920°C/H_2O + 2–4 h 480–600°C/air	1070	1140	0.94	8	20

Table 1c.18 Fracture toughness of Ti-alloys (Ref. 5,19).

Alloy	*Condition*	*Fracture Toughness K_{IC} ($N/mm^{3/2}$)*
Ti6Al4V	Annealed	1740
	Solution treated + annealed	2020
Ti5A12.5Fe	Annealed (2 h/700°C/air)	1225
	Solution treated + annealed (1 h/900°C/water//2 h/700°C/air)	1785
Ti15Mo5Zr3A1	Solution treated at 740°C	4580
	Solution treated at 740°C + annealed at 600°C	2430
	40% cold worked + annealed at 600°C	980

Table 1c.19 Influence of a plasma nitriding (PVD) on the mechanical properties of commercially Ti6Al4V (Ref. 20)

Treatment	*Tensile Yield Strength (0.2%) (MPa)*	*Ultimate Tensile Strength (MPa)*	*Ratio Yield/ Tensile Strength*	*Elongation at Fracture (%)*
Untreated	809	894	0.90	20
Vacuum annealed 20 h/850°C	815	924	0.88	21
Plasma nitrided* 20 h/850°C/N_2	805	914	0.88	20
Plasma nitrided* 20 h/850°C/NH_3	880	984	0.89	20

* Plasma nitriding at 20–40 kW.

1C.5 FATIGUE

Table 1c.20 High cycle fatigure strength σ_B and rotating fatigue strength σ_R of titanium and titanium alloys (Wöhler curves) (Ref. 10, 21, 22, 23, 24)

Alloy	*R*	*σ_B (MPa)*	*R*	*σ_R (MPa)*
cp-Ti	–1	230–280	–1	200
Ti6Al4V	–1	400–450	–1	500–660
Ti5A12.5Fe	–1		–1	450–550
Ti6Al7Nb	–1	—	–1	450–600
cp-Nb	–1	—	–1	150
cp-Ta	–1	—	–1	200
Ti30Ta	–1	—	–1	400

Table 1c.21 Rotating bending fatigue tests of unnotched and notched titanium alloys (Ref. 19)

Alloy	*R*	*Condition*	*Stress Concentration Factor*	*Fatigue Strength for Alternating Tensile Stresses (>10^7 cycles) (MPa)*
Ti6Al4V	–1		1.0	725
Ti5AL12.5Fe	–1	Wrought + annealed	1.0	725
	–1	Wrought + solution		
	–1	treated + annealed	3.6	300
	–1	Cast + HIP	3.6	300
	–1	Cast + HIP	1.0	450

Table 1c.22 High cycle fatigue strength of hip endoprostheses of titanium alloys, measured in 0.9% NaCl solution at 37°C. Testing conditions similar to DIN 58840 (simulated loosened shaft, 50 mm) (Ref. 23, 25)

Alloy	*Maximum load in 2×10^7 cycles (kN) 0.9% NaCl (f = 2 Hz)*
Hot wrought Ti6Al4V	6.5–8.0
Wrought Ti5A12.5F	8
Ti6ALI7Nb	3.5–6.0

Table 1c.23 Influence of the mean stress S_m on the fatigue strength of Ti6Al4V (Ref. 26)

S_m (MPa)	*R*	*Notch Factor K_f*	*Fatigue Strength (MPa) at 10^7 cycles*
0	-1	1	400
		2.82	250
250	-0.1	1	300
	0.33	2.82	125
500	0.33	1	250
	0.66	2.82	100
750	0.7	1	125
	0.81	2.82	80

Table 1c.24 Influence of the notch factor on the fatigue strength of Ti6Al4V (Ref. 27, 28, 29, 30)

Notch Factor K_f	*Stress Ratio R*	*Fatigue Strength (MPa)*
1	–1	400
1.7	–1	300
3.7	–1	150
6.0	–1	100

Table 1c.25 Influence of interstitial elements on the rotating bending strength of Ti6Al4V (Ref. 31)

Chemical composition of the base alloy (wt%)							
Al	V	Fe	C	N	O	H	Ti
6.03	3.96	0.10	0.02	0.009	0.1	0.005	balance

Composition	*Heat Treatment*	*Notch Factor* K_f	*R*	*Fatigue Strength (MPa)*
Base alloy	1 h 815°C/furnace →	1	–1	610
	600°C air	3	–1	210
Base alloy	1 h 855°C/furnace →	1	–1	510
+ 0.07% N	600°C air	3	–1	180
Base alloy	1 h 870°C/furnace →	1	–1	550
+ 0.2% O	600°C air	3	–1	210
Base alloy	1 h 840°C/furnace →	1	–1	560
+ 9.2% C	600°C air	3	–1	230
Base alloy	1 h 930°C/furnace →	1	–1	580
+ 0.07% N	600°C air	3	–1	240
+ 0.2% O				
+ 0.2% C				

Table 1c.26 Influence of texture and test directions on the rotating bending fatigue strength of Ti6Al4V (fine equiaxed microstructure in rolled plates) (Ref. 32)

Type of Texture and Method of Production	*R*	*Test Direction*	*Fatigue Strength (MPa) at 10^7 cycles*
Basal (0002 tilted out of the rolling plane by about 30°) cross rolling in lower (α+β)-field	–1	Rolling direction	625
Transverse (0002 aligned parallel to the rolling direction) uni-directional in the higher (α+β)-field, 950°C	–1	Rolling direction	630
		Transverse direction	590
Basal/transverse (both are present), unidirectional roll-at about 930°C	–1	Rolling direction	720
		Transverse direction	690

Table 1c.27 Influence of heat treatment (annealing and precipitation hardening respectively) on the fatigue strength of Ti6Al4V (Ref. 30, 33)

Condition	*Yield Strength (MPa)*	*Tensile Strength (MPa)*
As annealed	900	955
As hardened	1100	1195

Condition	S_m	K_f	*R*	*Fatigue Strength (MPa) at 10^7 cycles*
As annealed	0	1	–1	510
	0	3.3	–1	300
As hardened	0	1	–1	600
	0	3.3	–1	280
As annealed	200	1	–0.3	425
	200	3.3	–0.01	200
As hardened	200	1	–0.5	600
	200	3.3	0	200
As annealed	300	1	0.14	400
	300	3.3	0.23	165
As hardened	300	1	–0.22	550
	300	3.3	–0.2	190

Table 1c.28 Influence of the beta field heat treatment on the fatigue strength of Ti6Al4V (Ref. 34)

Heat Treatment	*R*	*Fatigue Strength (MPa) at 10^7 cycles*
0.5 h 1010°C/AC + 2 h 700°C/AC	0	525
5 h 1000°C/AC + 2 h 700°C/AC	0	620
0.5 h 1010°C/H_20 + 2 h 700°C/AC	0	750
5 h 1010°C/H_20 + 2 h 700°C/AC_2	0	650

Table 1c.29 Influence of the surface treatment on the rotating bending fatigue (fine lamellar microstructure, produced by annealing in 15 min/1050°C/H_20 + 1 h/800°C/H_20) (Ref. 35)

Surface Treatment	*R*	*Fatigue strength (MPa) at 10^7 cycles*
Electrically polished	–1	680
Mechanically polished (7 μm)	–1	750
Mechanically polished (80 μm)	–1	605
Mechanically polished (80 μm) + 1 h 500 °C	–1	550
Mechanically polished (180 μm)	–1	600
Mechanically polished (80 μm)+ 1 h 800 °C	–1	450

Table 1c.30 Influence of the surface treatment on the rotating bending fatigue of Ti6Al4V (fine equiaxed microstructure produced by rolling at 800°C/H_2O + 1 h/800°C(H_2O) (Ref. 35)

Surface Treatment	*R*	*Fatigue Strength (MPa)*
Electrically polished	–1	610
Shot peened	–1	710
Shot peened + 1 h 500 °C	–1	390
Shot peened + 1 h 500 °C 20 μm surface removed	–1	800
Shot peened + 20 μm surface removed	–1	820

Table 1c.31 Influence of surface working on the rotating bending of Ti6Al4V (Ref. 27, 36)

Surface Working	*Notch Factor (K_f)*	*R*	*Fatigue Strength (MPa)*
Mechanically polished	1	–1	620
Mechanically polished and cold roll bent	1	–1	660
Ground	1	–1	540
Mechanically polished	2.02	–1	330

Table 1c.32 Influence of plasma nitriding (PVD) on the rotating bending fatigue of Ti6Al4V (Ref. 20)

Treatment	*R*	*Maximum Bending Stress at 10^7 cycles (MPa)*
Untreated	–1	600
Vacuum annealed 20 h/850 °C	–1	370
Plasma nitrided* 20 h/850 °C/N_2	–1	470
Plasma nitrided*20 h/700 °C/NH_3	–1	550
Solution treated 1 h/940 °C/vac. + Ar cooled	–1	530
Solution treated 1 h/940 °C/vac. + Ar cooled + plasma nitrided* 20 h/770 °C/N_2	–1	500

* Plasma nitriding at 20–40 kW.

1C.6 CORROSION AND WEAR

Table 1c.33 Electrochemical data for titanium and titanium alloys in 0.1 M NaCl under different conditions (Ref. 16, 37, 38).

Metal/Alloy	*Corrosion Potential* E_{corr}*(mV)*	*Passive Current Density* I_p *(μA/cm²)*	*Breakdown Potential* E_b *(mV)*
cp-Ti			
pH 7	-628	0.72	
pH 2	-459	113	>1500
Ti5Al2.5Fe			
pH 7	-529	0.68	
pH 2	-567	0.71	>1500
Ti6Al4V			
pH 7	-510	0.92	
pH 2	-699	0.69	>1500
Ti6Al7Nb			
pH 7		0.45	>1000
Ti30Ta			
pH 7		0.3	>1500
Ti40Nb			
pH 7		0.2	>1500

Table 1c.34 Polarization current (i) and polarization resistance (R_c) of titanium and titanium alloys in pure saline at 37°C (Ref. H37) and in 0.9% NaCl with a stable redox system [$Fe(CN)_6^{4-}/Fe(CN)_6^{3-}$] (Ref. 39)

Material	*i (μA/cm²)*	R_c *(kΩcm²)* *Pure saline*	*Saline + redox*
cp-Ti	0.010	1000	714
cp-Ta	0.003	3000	1430
cp-Nb	0.004	2500	455
Ti6Al4V	0.008	1250	455

Table 1c.35 Repassivation time in 0.9% NaCl and breakdown potential in Hank's solution of titanium and titanium alloys (Ref. 16, 22, 40, 41)

Metal/Alloy	*Breakdown Potential (mV) vs. calomel electrode*	*Repassivation Time (ms)* *-500 mV*	*+500 mV*
cp-Ti	2400	43	44.4
cp-Ta	2250	—	—
Ti30Ta	>1500	41.7	47.5
Ti40Nb	>1500	44.6	43.4
Ti6Al4V	>2000	37	41
Ti5Al2.5Fe		110–130	120–160
Ti4.5Al5Mo1.5Cr	2400		
Ni45Ti	1140		

Table 1c.36 Electrochemical data for anodic titanium and titanium alloys at 37°C in different solutions (de-aired) versus standard calomel electrode (SCE) (Ref. 42)

Metal/Alloy	*Corrosion Potential vs. SCE E_p (mV)*	*Passive Current Density I_b (μAcm^{-2})*	*Breakdown Potential E (mV)*	*Solution**
cp-Ti	-440 – -490	1.0–3.0	1300	1
	-94–-140	0–1.0	1750	2
	-94	5.0–9.0	1950	3
Ti6Al4V	-200–-250	0.9–1.0	1155–1240	1
	-240–-300	0.8–1.5	1900	2
	-180–-250	0.9–2.0	1550	3
Ti15V3Cr3Sn3A1 mill	-480–-495	3.0–5.0	1900	1
	-480–-500	4.0–5.0	1700	2
	-490–-520	3.0	>2000	3
annealed 6h/510°C/air	-800–-840	3.0–4.0	1000	1
	-650–-740	1.0–2.0	1300	2
	-590–-600	3.0–4.0	1800	3

* Key: 1 = Ringer's solution; 2 = Hank's solution; 3 = 0.17 M NaCl solution.

Table 1c.37 Repassivation rates in artificial saliva versus standard calomel electrode (Ref. 43)

Material	*Corrosion Potential (mV)*	*Potential (mV) after 1 h*	*2 h*	*36 h*
Titanium	-355	-308	-260	-160

Table 1c.38 Galvanic corrosion between titanium and other alloys in artificial saliva (Ref. 43)

Couples	*Potential difference (mV)*	*I_{galv} after 20 h (nA cm^{-2})*	*Titanium position*
Ti–HGC	-134	4	Anode
Ti–non gamma 2 amalgam	130	10	Cathode
Ti–CoCrMo cast alloy	90–117	2	Cathode
Ti–HGC–CoCrMo	-22	3	Anode
HGC–CoCrMo	225	500	—

HGC = high gold containing alloy.

Table 1c.39 Repassivation time of titanium and titanium alloys in contact with different metallic materials (Ref. 44)

NaCl, pH = 7.4 (shortcut alloy)	*HCl, pH = 3 (activated alloy)*	*Repassivation Time t_e (ms)*
cp-Ti	cp-Ti	—
	Ti30Ta	37.7
	Ti6Al4V	41.8
	cp-Nb	480.0
	Co30Cr6.5Mo	38.7
	Co28Cr5Mo	38.4
	X3CrNiMo1812	1000.0
Ti30Ta	cp-Ti	43.0
	Ti30Ta	48.6
	Ti6Al4V	39.0
	cp-Nb	1080.0
	Co30Cr6.5Mo	44.1
	Co28Cr5Mo	(4200)
	X3CrNiMo1812	1000.0
Ti6Al4V	cp-Ti	44.0
	Ti30Ta	34.2

Table 1c.40 Influence of the surface treatment on the fretting corrosion behaviour of Ti6Al4V (Ref. 45)

Material Combination	*Total Weight loss (μg)*	*Ti (μg)*	*V (μg)*
Untreated–untreated	2423	3925	78.5
Untreated–nitrogen ion implanted	1295	1260	31.2
Untreated–PVD coated with TiN	1002	902	15.0
Untreated–plasma ion nitrided	807	716	6.4
PVD- PVD	713	470	8.5
Plasma ion nitrided–plasma ion nitrided	273	87	0.5

Testing conditions:
- plate screw system with a micromotion of 100 μm.
- 14 days at 1 Hz for 1 200 000 cycles.
- testing medium was calf serum solution.

Table 1c.41 Influence of the surface treatment on the wear behaviour of Ti6Al7Nb as a result of a pin-on-disk test (Ref. 46)

Property	*PVD coated with 3 μm TiN layer*	*Oxygen diffusion hardened (ODH) (30 μm hardened surface)*
Wear factor ($10^{-7}mm^3/Nm$)	2.111	1.353
Coefficient of friction	0.078	0.051
Surface roughness R_z (μm)	0.159	0.330
Wetting angle (°)	47	49

Table 1c.42 Influence of ion implantation of nitrogen on the wear properties of commercially pure Ti and Ti6Al4V (Ref. 47)

Material	*Friction Couple*	*Total Wear (mg)*	*Friction Coefficient*
cp-Ti*	Untreated–untreated	632.3	0.48
	Nitrided–nitrided 4 h/940°C/N_2:H_2=2:1	54.3	0.10
Ti6Al4V**	Untreated–untreated	600.0	0.46
	Nitrided–nitrided 4 h/940°C/N_2:H_2=2:1	40.1	0.10
	Nitrided–nitrided 6 h/800°C/N_2:H_2=1:1	92.3	0.12

* Friction distance = 1257 m.
** Friction distance = 1885 m.

Table 1c.43 Rate of formation of corrosion products for titanium and titanium alloys in Hank's solution during current-time-tests (Ref. 48)

Alloy	*Metal converted into compound (ng/cm²h)*
cp-Ti	
Mechanically polished	4.1
Chemically polished	3.5
Ti16Mo	1.5
Ti5Ta	0.26

1C.7 BIOLOGICAL PROPERTIES

Table 1c.44 Biocompatibility of cp-Ti and Ti alloys, survival rate of L132 cells incubated with powders (Ref. 49)

Metal	*Powder Concentration (mg/1)*	*Survival Rate of Cells*
cp-Ti	>400	
Ti6Al4V	>400	
Ti5Al2.5Fe	>400	>80%
Ti30Ta	>400	
Ti30Nb	>400	

Table 1c.45 Influence of the implantation time (in vivo) on the surface roughness and peak-to-valley (P–V) height of Ti6Al4V femoral heads (Ref. 50)

			Implantation Time					
	Before Implantation		*85 months*		*110 months*		*124 months*	
Position	*R_a (nm)*	*P–V*	*R_a (nm)*	*P–V*	*R_a (nm)*	*P–V*	*R_a (nm)*	*P–V*
Anterior	43±10	370±72	58±50	746±509	250±147	2044±1178	86±81	812±763
Posterior	41±6	591±333	150±125	2281±1842	114±96	1175±778	142±131	1045±890
Medial	51±14	411±159	44±29	649±259	118±69	1224±731	412±11	401±125
Lateral	52±9	364±68	71±55	722±474	117±106	1195±1009	40±16	527±156

1C.8 TiNi – SHAPE MEMORY

Table 1c.46 Properties of the alloy Ni45Ti (Ref. 37, 51, 52)

	Above (= austenitic)	*Transition temperature (55°C)*	*Below (= martensitic)*
Density (g/cm^3)		6.4–6.5	
Melting point (°C)		1310	
Young's modulus (GPa)	83–110		21–69
Tensile yield strength (0.2%) (MPa)	621–793		34–138
Ultimate tensile strength (MPa)	827–1172		103–862
Ratio yield/tensile strength	0.75–0.68		0.33–0.16
Elongation at fracture (%)	1–15		up to 60
Electrical conductivity (S/m)		1–1.5	
Corrosion potential (mV)			
in 0.1 M NaCl pH 7		-431	
pH 2		-518	
Passive current density ($\mu A/cm^2$)			
in 0.1 M NaCl pH 7		0.44	
pH 2		0.61	
Breakdown potential (mV)			
in 0.1 M NaCl pH 7		890	
pH 2		960	

REFERENCES

1. DTG Product Information, Germany
2. DIN 17850 (1990), Beuth.
3. Semlitsch, M., Staub, F. and Weber, H. (1985) Development of a Vital, High-Strength Titanium Aluminium-Niobium Alloy for Surgical Implants: Proc. 5th European Conf. on Biomaterials, Paris, Sept. 4–6, 1985.
4. DIN 17851 (1990), Beuth.
5. Steinemann, S.G., Mäusli, P.-A., Szmukler-Moncler, S., Semlitsch, M., Pohler, O., Hintermann, H.-E. and Perren, S.M. (1993) Beta-Titanium Alloy for Surgical Implants, Proc. of the 7th World Conf. on Titanium, pp. 2689–2696.
6. Mäusli, P.-A., Steinemann, S.G. and Simpson, J.P. (1984) Properties of surface oxides on titanium and some titanium alloys, in *Proc. of the 6th World Conference on Titanium*, Vol. 3, pp. 1759–1764.
7. DIN 17869 (draft), (1990), Beuth.
8. Specification Properties, IMI 367-alloy.
9. Microstructure Standard for titanium Alloy Bars, Technical Committee of European Titanium Producers, Publication ETTC2.
10. Breme, J. Wadewitz, V. and Burger, K. (1988) Verbund Titanlegierungen/Al_2O_3-Keramik für dentale Implantate – Entwicklung geeigneter Legierungen, in *Verbundwerkstoffe – Stoffverbunde* (ed. G. Ondracek), DGM 1988, pp. 123–130.
11. Breme, J., Biehl, V., Schulte, W., d'Hoedt, B. and Donath, K. (1993) Development and functionality of isoelastic Dental Implants of Titanium Alloys. *Biomaterials*, **14** (12), 887–892.

12. Hülse, K., Kramer, K.-H. and Breme, J. (1989) Influence of Small Additions of Fe, Cr and Ni on the Recrystallisation Behaviour of cp-Ti. *Proc. of the 6th Intern. Conf. on Ti*, Soc. Franc. de Métallurgie, 1675–1683.
13. Zwicker, U. (1974) *Titan und Titanlegierungen*, Springer-Verlag.
14. DIN 17864 (draft), (1990), Beuth.
15. Ramsdell, J.D. and Hull, E.D. (1960) Characterstics of cold-rolled and annealed Ti, Bureau of Mines Rep. of Inv. 5656.
16. Breme, J. and Wadewitz, V. (1989) Comparison of Ti–Ta, Ti-Nb Alloys, *J. of Oral & Max. Implants*, **4** (2), 113–118.
17. Breme, J., Zhou, Y. and Groh, L. (1995) Development of a titanium alloy suitable for an optimized coating with hydroxyapatite, *Biomaterials*, **16,** 239–244.
18. DIN 17860 (1990), Beuth.
19. Borowy, K.H. and Kramer, K.H. (1984) On the Properties of a New Titanium Alloy (TiAl5Fe2.5) as Implant Material, in *Proc. of the 5th World Conf. on Ti*, Vol. 2, 1381–1386.
20. Lanagan, J. (1988) Properties of plasma nitrided titanium alloys, *Proc. of the 6th World Conf. on Titanium*, Vol. 4, pp. 1957–1962.
21. Thull, R. (1979) Eigenschaften von Metallen, für orthopädische Implantate und deren Prüfung. *Orthopädie,* **7,** 29.
22. Breme, J. and Schmidt, H.-J. (1990) Criteria for the Bioinertness of Metals for Osseo-Integrated Implants, in *Osseo-Integrated Implants*, Vol. 1 (ed. G. Heimke), pp. 31–80.
23. Semlitsch, M. and Weber, H. (1992) Titanlegierungen für zementlose Hüftprothesen, in *Die zementlose Hüftprothese* (E. Hipp, R. Gradinger and R. Asherl), Demeter Verlag, pp. 18–26.
24. Semlitsch, M. and Panic, B. (1994) 15 years of experience with test criteria for fracture-proof anchorage stems of artificial hip joints, in *Technical Principles, Design and Safety of Joint Implants* (eds G.H. Buchhorn and H.-G. Willert), Hogrefe & Huber Publishers, pp. 23–36.
25. Kunze, E. (1988) Vergleichende Untersuchungen zum Langzeit-Ermüdungsverhalten von Hüftgelenkprothesen an Luft und in NaCl-Lösung. *Metall,* **2,** 140–145.
26. Reactive Metals Inc. Niles, Ohio, RMI-Titanium 1969.
27. Weinberg, I.G. and Hanna, I.E. (1957) an evaluation of the fatigue properties of Ti and Ti-alloys, TML Rep. 77.
28. Mote, W.M. and Frost, R.B. (1958) The engineering properties of commercial Ti-alloys, TML Rep. 92.
29. Weltzin, R.B. and Koves, G. (1968) Impact fatigue testing of Ti alloys. *J. of Materials*, **3,** 469–480.
30. *ASM Metals Handbook* (1961), Vol. 1: Properties and Selection of Metals.
31. Dittmar, C.B., Bauer, G.W. and Evers, D (1957) The effect of microstructural variables and interstitial elements on the fatigue behavior of Ti and commercial Ti alloys, Mallory, Sharen Titanium Corp. AD-110726WADC-TR 56–304, 95.
32. Lütjering, G. and Gysler, A. (1984) Fatigue, in *Proc. of the 5th Conf. on Ti*, pp. 2065–2083.
33. Hempel, M. and Hillnhagen, E. (1966) Dauerschwingfestigkeit der technischen Titanlegierungen TiAl5Sn2.5 und TiAl6V4, *Arch. f. Eisenhüttenwesen*, **37,** 263–277.

34. Rüdinger, K. and Fischer, D. (1984) Relationship between primary alpha content, tensile properties and high cycle fatigue behaviour of Ti6Al4V, in *Proc. of the 5th Conf on Ti*, pp. 2123–2130.
35. Wagner, L. Gerdes, C. and Lütjering, G. (1984) Influence of surface treatment on fatigue strength of Ti6Al4V, in Proc. of the 5th Conf. on Ti, Vol. 4, 2147–2154.
36. Liu, H.W. (1956) Effect of surface finish on the fatigue strength of TiAl6V4-alloy, Dept. of Theoretical and Applied Mechanics, University of Illinois, T.U.A.M. Rep. 533.
37. Geis-Gerstorfer, J., Weber, H. and Breme, J. (1988) Electrochemische Untersuchung auf die Korrosionsbeständigkeit von Implantatlegierungen. *Z. f. Zahnärztl. Implantologie* **4,** (1), 31–36.
38. DIN 17851 (1990), Beuth.
39. Breme, J. (1988) Titanium and Titanium Alloys, Biomaterials of Preference, in *Proc. of the 6th World Conf. on Ti*, Vol. 1, pp. 57–68.
40. Fraker, A.C, Ruff, A.W. *et al.* (1983) Surface Preparation and Corrosion. Behaviour of Titanium Alloys for Surgical Implants, in *Titanium Alloys in Surgical Implants*, ASTM STP796, (eds H.A. Luckey and F.Kubli), pp. 206–19.
41. Breme, J., Wadewitz, V. and Ecker, D. (1986) Untersuchungen zum Einfluβ des Gefügezustandes auf das Korrosionverhalten der Implantatlegierung TiAl5Fe2, 5. Z. *f Zahnärztl. Implantologie*, Bd. II 32–37.
42. Gagg, C., Corrosion Characteristics of Ti15V3Cr3Sn3Al (Ti15–3) Alloy in a Physiological Environment.
43. Elagli, K., Traisnel, M. and Hildebrand, H.F. (1993) Electrochemical Behaviour of Titanium and Dental Alloys in Artificial Saliva. *Electrochimica Acta*, **38** (14), 1769–1774.
44. Wadewitz, V. and Breme, J. (1989) Titan-Legierungen für dentale Implantate. *Z. Zahnärztl. Implantol. V*, 116–120.
45. Maurer, A., Brown, S.A. and Merrit, K. (1992) Effects of Surface Treatments on Fretting Corrosion of Ti6A14V, *Proc. of the 4th World Biomaterials Congress*, pp. 200.
46. Streicher, R.M., Weber, H., Schön, R. and Semlitsch, M. (1991) Wet behaviour of different ceramic surfaces in comparison to TiN and OHD treated Ti6Al4V alloy paired with polyethylene, in *Ceramics in Substitutive and Reconstructive Surgery (ed. P Vincenzini)*, Elsevier, pp. 197–205.
47. Hu, Y.-S.. Dai, D.-H. and Dong, Y.-L. (1988) The ion nitriding of titanium materials and its applications, *Proc. of the 6th World Confer. on Titanium*, Vol. 4, pp. 1801–1804.
48. Mears, D.C. (1977) Metals in Medicine and Surgery. *International Metals Reviews*, Review 218, June, 119–155.
49. Hildebrand, H.F. (1993) Biologische Aspekte beim Einsatz von Implantatwerkstoffen, DGM Hochschulseminar, Saarbrücken, Germany.
50. Easter, T.L., Graham, R.M., Jacobs, J.J., Black, J. and LaBerge, M. (*1994*) Clinical Performance of Ti6Al4V Femoral Components: Wear Mechanisms vs. Surface Profile, *Proc. of the 20th Annual Meeting of the Society for Biomaterials*, pp. 185.
51. Ebel, B. (1990) Zur Biokompatibilität von Implantatwerkstoffen, KfK 4476.
52. Tautzenberger, P. and Stöckel, D. (1987) Vergleich der Eigenschaften von Thermobimetallen und Memory-Elementen, **1,** 26–32.

Dental Restoration Materials 1d

1D.1 AMALGAMS

1d.1.1 Composition of alloys

Table 1d.1 Chemical composition of dental amalgams (wt%) (Ref. 1, 2)

*Alloy powder**	*Ag*	*Sn*	*Cu*	*Zn*	*Hg*
LCS	66–73	25–29	<6	<2	0–3
HCB	69	17	13	1	—
HCSS, HCSL	40–60	25–30	15–30	—	—

The mercury concentration after amalgamization is <50 %.
* LCS = low-copper spherical.
HCB = high-copper blended.
HCSS = high-copper single-composition spherical.
HCSL = high-copper single-composition lathe-cut.

1d.1.2 Physical properties

Table 1d.2 Physical and mechanical properties of amalgams (Ref. 2)

Thermal expansion coefficient	25×10^{-6}/K
Thermal conductivity	23 W/mK
Ultimate tensile strength	≥60 MPa
Ultimate compression strength	≥300 MPa
Fracture toughness K_{IC}	<1 MPa $m^{1/2}$

1d.1.3 General properties and processing

General properties of dental amalgams (Ref. 1, 2)

By definition amalgam is an alloy of mercury with one or more other metals. Dental amalgams are produced by mixing an alloy powder with mercury. Usually the alloy powder is called 'amalgam' and the composition of amalgam denotes the composition of the powder. The two basic physical shapes of the alloy powder are:

1. irregular shaped particles (length 20–120 μm, width 10–70 μm, thickness 10–35 μm) produced by lathe cutting.
2. spherical particles (diameter < 30 μm) produced by atomization.

Amalgams for dental restorations are classified by their copper content in two basic types:

1. low-copper type, < 6 wt% Cu, used since the late 19th century.
2. high-copper type (non-gamma-2 amalgam), >6 wt% Cu, used since 1960.

The high-copper type is available in two alloy groups, classified by the mixture of different powder shapes:

2.1 mixed alloys consisting of
2.1.1 2/3 conventional lathe cutting + 1/3 spherical powder of Ag–Cu eutecticum (total composition see Table 1d.1 composition of eutecticum: Ag30Cu)
2.1.2 1/3 conventional lathe cutting powder + 2/3 spherical powder (Ag25Sn15Cu)
2.2 one-component amalgams consisting of
2.2.1 ternary alloys, spherical shape
2.2.2 ternary alloys, irregular shape
2.2.3 quaternary alloys, non-spherical shape

During amalgamization the powder reacts with the mercury, producing different phases, depending on the amalgam powder:

1. low copper type: $\underset{\gamma\ \text{phase}}{Ag_3Sn} + Hg \rightarrow \underset{\gamma_1\ \text{phase}}{Ag_2Hg_3} + \underset{\gamma_2\ \text{phase}}{Sn_{7-8}Hg} + \underset{\gamma_3\ \text{phase}}{Ag_3Sn}$

2. high copper type, mixed alloy (a(i)), reacts in two steps:

step one: $\underset{\gamma\ \text{phase}}{Ag_3Sn} + Hg \rightarrow \underset{\gamma_1\ \text{phase}}{Ag_2Hg_3} + \underset{\gamma_2\ \text{phase}}{Sn_{7-8}Hg} + \underset{\text{unreacted}}{Ag_3Sn}$

step two: $\underset{\gamma_2\ \text{phase}}{Sn_{7-8}Hg} - \underset{\text{eutetic beads}}{Ag\text{–}Cu} \rightarrow Cu_6Sn_5 + Ag_2Hg_3$

The result of the amalgamization is a microstructure consisting of unreacted Ag_3Sn and Ag–Cu surrounded by a layer of Cu_6Sn_5 and the γ_1 matrix. The microstructure of the one-component non-gamma-2 amalgams is similar to that of the mixed alloy except that the Cu_6Sn_5 particles are decomposed in the γ_1 phase and form no layer.

Processing of dental amalgams

For dental restoration (fillings) the mercury is mixed with the (amalgam) alloy immediately before application. The alloy is delivered in powder or pellet form. The amount of mercury after amalgamization must be below 50 wt%. Trituration is accomplished manually in a mortar with a pestle or more often automatically using a capsule of mercury with a given weight and an alloy pellet. The amalgam is placed in the cavity of the tooth in small portions which are pressed with a force of 40–50 N. On the surface of the filling a mercury-rich phase should appear, allowing a good bonding to the following portion. When the cavity is completely filled, the mercury-rich phase must be removed, and the filling can be modelled to the desired shape. 24 hours after the amalgamization the filling must be polished in order to achieve a smooth surface, resulting in a low corrosion rate.

1d.1.4 Mechanical properties

Table 1d.3 Mechanical properties of dental amalgams (Ref. 2)

*Amalgam**	*Ultimate compression strength (MPa)* After 1 h	*Ultimate compression strength (MPa)* After setting	*Creep (%) (7 days after amalgamization, pressure 38 MPa)*
LCL	120–170	380–450	2.5–3.5
LCS	140–180	380–450	0.3–1.5
HCB	120–330	410–460	0.2–1.7
HCSS, HCSL ternary alloy	230–320	460–540	0.002–0.3
HCSS, HCSL quaternary alloy with indium	210–410	430–480	0.06–0.1

* LCL = low-copper lathe-cut. LCS = low-copper spherical. HCB = high-copper blended. HCSS = high-copper single-composition spherical. HCSL = high-copper single-composition lathe-cut.

1d.1.5 Corrosion and wear

Table 1d.4 Average passive current density, range of passivity, corrosion and breakdown potential of a non-gamma-2 amalgam in artificial saliva (Ref. 3)

Alloy	*Passive Current Density ($\mu A\ cm^{-2}$)*	*Range of Passivity (mV vs. SCE)*	*Corrosion Potential (mV vs. SCE)*	*Breakdown Potential (mV vs. SCE)*
Non-gamma-2 amalgam	1.5	-300 – +300	-400	300

Table 1d.5 Repassivation rates in artificial saliva versus standard calomel electrode (Ref. 3)

Material	*Corrosion Potential (mV)*	*Potential (mV) after* 1 h	2 h	36 h
Non-gamma-2 amalgam	-400	-408	-382	-290

Corrosion of amalgams

1. Corrosion of conventional amalgams
The heterogeneous structure of conventional amalgams is responsible for high corrosion. The γ_2 phase is the most active phase in electrochemical corrosion because it is less noble than γ and γ_1. Therefore an anodic dissolution occurs. The corrosion products of the γ_2 phase are

1.1 Sn^{2+} ions, in the presence of saliva SnO_2 and $Sn(OH)_6Cl$
2.2 the released Hg reacts with particles of the γ phase.

2. Corrosion of the high copper type amalgams
Because of the absence of the γ_2 phase, the Cu_6Sn_5 phase is the electrochemically based phase. However, the total corrosion current in the non-gamma-2 amalgams is much lower than in the conventional types. Therefore, the amount of corrosion products is much lower than in gamma-2 alloys. An additional advantage of these amalgams is the lack of mercury during corrosion.

Generally, to achieve a low corrosion in amalgams certain requirements must be fulfilled:

- a polished surface
- no contact with gold (this would lead to a high corrosion of the amalgams, setting mercury free and resulting in a reaction between gold and mercury).

Table 1d.6 Rate of release of mercury vapour per unit area of different types of almagam dipped in an isotonic NaCl solution (pH = 6) (Ref. 4)

*Alloy**		*Rate of Hg Release (ng/min mm²)*
LCL	New	0.011
	Old	0.011
HCB	New	0.133
	Old	0.017
HCSS,	New	0.022
HCSL	Old	0.022
In-containing	New	0.222
one component	Old	0.350

LCL = low-copper lathe-cut. HCB = high-copper blended. HCSS = high-copper single-composition spherical. HCSL = high-copper single-composition lathe-cut. New = tested within 2 months after amalgamization. Old = tester after 1.5 years after amalgamization.

1D.2 NOBLE METALS

1d.2.1 Composition of alloys

Table 1d.7 Chemical composition of high gold-containing dental cast alloys (wt%) (Ref. 5, 6, 8)

*Type**	*Au + Pt Metals*	*Au*	*Pt*	*Pd*	*Ir*	*Rh*	*Ag*	*Cu*	*Zn*	*Ta*	*In*	*Re*	*Fe*	*Sn*
HGC-1	88.6	87.5		1.0	0.1		11.5							
HGC-2	80.5–81.2	75.7–79.3	0.3–1.4	1.6–3.3			12.3–15.0	4.1–5.5	0.4–1.0	0–0.1				
HGC-3	78.0–78.5	74.0–74.4	0–2.4	2.0–3.5	0.1		9.6–13.5	7.0–11.5	0.9–1.0					
HGC-4	75.5–80.0	65.5–71.0	4.4–12.9	0.0–2.0	0.1	0–1.1	10.0–14.0	8.2–10.0	0.5–4.0					
HGC-1-C	95.0–97.0	80.0–85.0	5.0–11.0	3.3–4.4	0.2	1.6	3.0–5.0							
HGC-2-C	95.0	70.0	7.5	15.0	0.5	2.0	5.0							
HGC-3-C	98.0–99.0	82.6–86.0	9.7–10.4	0–2.2	0.1–0.3	0–1.6					1.0–2.0			
HGC-4-C	82.9–97.4	73.8–84.4	8.0–9.0	5.0–8.9	0.1		1.2–9.2	0.3–4.4	0–2.0	0–0.2	1.5–2.5	0–0.2	0–0.2	0.5 0.8

HGC = high gold-containing (Au + Pt metals > 75 wt%, Pt metals = Pt, Pd, Ir, Rh, Re, Os).
1 = soft, 2 = medium hard, 3 = hard, 4 = extra hard.
c = ceramic alloy (bonding with ceramic is possible).

Table 1d.8 Chemical composition of low gold-containing dental cast alloys (wt%) (Type 4: extra hard) (Ref. 5, 7, 8)

*Type**	*Au + Pt metals*	*Au*	*Pt*	*Pd*	*Ir*	*Ag*	*Cu*	*Sn*	*Zn*	*In*	*Ga*	*Re*	*Ta*	*Fe*	*Co*
LGC-4	48.0–66.7	40.0–62.2	0–4.4	0 9.9	0.1	23.3–35.0	7.0–12.0	0–1.5	0.4–3.5	0–5.0					
LGC-4-C	74.8–89.8	43.0–55.1		29.0–38.5	0.1–0.2	0–19.5	0–0.3	0–0.5		0–9.0	0–1.5	0–0.2	0–0.1	0–0.2	0–2.8

* LGC-4 = low gold-containing, extra hard (60 wt% ≤ Au + Pt metals ≤ 75 wt%).
LGC-4-C = low gold-containing, extra hard, fusible (C = ceramic alloy (a bonding with ceramic is possible).

Table 1d.9 Chemical composition of AgPd and Pd-alloys (wt%) (Ref. 5, 8)

Type	*Au + Pt metals*	*Au*	*Pt*	*Pd*	*Ir*	*Ag*	*Cu*	*Sn*	*Zn*	*In*	*Ru*	*Ga*	*Ge*
AgPd-1	29.5	2.0		27.5		70.0		0.2	0.3				
AgPd-4	29.5–40.0	≤2.0		27.4–39.9	0.1	52.0–58.5	0–10.5	≤2.0	1.5–4.0	≤2.0			
Pd-4-C	52–88	0–17	≤1.0	25–70		7.2–38.0	0–11.6	1.9–7.5	≤2.0	0–4.0	≤0.8	0–7.2	≤0.5

Key: see Table 1d.7.

1d.2.2 Physical properties

Table 1d.10 Physical Properties of precious dental alloys (Ref. 5, 8)

Alloy	*Density (g/cm^3)*	*Melting Temperature (interval) (°C)*	*Mean Coefficient of Expansion ($10^{-6}/K$) 25–600°C*	*Young's Modulus (GPa)*
HGC-1	17.2	1030–1080		
HGC-2	16.1–16.4	900–1040		92–95
HGC-3	15.6–15.8	900–975		
HGC-4	15.6–16.8	900–1000		98–109
HGC-1-C	18.3–18.6	1090–1370	14.1–14.8	
HGC-2-C	17.3	1285–1370	13.6	
HGC-3-C	18.4–19.5	1045–1220	14.2–14.7	100–105
HGC-4-C	16.7–18.1	900–1260	14.0–16.8	102–113
LGC-4	12.1–14.1	770–1065		94–106
LGC-4-C	14.0–14.8	1150–1315	13.8–14.8	
AgPd-1	11.1			
AgPd-4	10.6–11.1	950–1150		
Pd-4-C	11.2–12.2	1100–1290	14.0–15.4	122–126

Key: see Table 1d.7.

1d.2.3 Processing of Precious Metal Alloys (Ref. 2, 5, 8)

Casting

Precious metal alloys are normally cast by means of the lost wax process. The well-known method of wax modelling is applied. For the commonly used casting procedure, centrifugal and vacuum pressure casting, the alloys can be heated by the following methods:

- resistence
- propane/oxygen torch (reducing flame zone)
- HF induction
- electrical arc

The alloys are melted in graphite or ceramic crucibles. After removal of the crucible the alloys can if required be hardened. After casting or brazing the alloys are descaled. Mechanical cleaning can be carried out with rotating tools, ceramic grinding wheels or rubber polishers.

Heat Treatment

Depending on the type of alloy and its application, the dental alloys are heat treated. After the casting the alloys are quenched. A homogenization at 700°C followed by rapid cooling should be carried out in order to decompose grain segregations, especially in alloys containing platinum. After a cold deformation the alloys should be stress-relieved. Precipitation hardening is performed by:

- slow cooling from 700°C to room temperature
- cooling from 450 to 250°C in 30 minutes, followed by quenching
- heating between 350 and 450°C for 15 minutes, followed by quenching

Table 1d.12 gives the recommended heat treatments for various noble metal alloys used in dental restoration.

Brazing

Brazing can be carried out with a torch or in a furnace. For larger surfaces furnace brazing is preferable. The best strength properties are obtained with a solder gap of 0.05 to 0.2 mm between the surfaces. Table 1d.11 shows the chemical composition and the brazing temperatures of various filler metals.

Bonding with Ceramics

Precious metal alloys are cast by the lost wax process. After removal of the crucible with carbide tools the castings are sand-blasted with alumina (100–150 μm, pressure 2 bar) to roughen the surfaces and to provide by increasing the surface an improvement in the adhesion strength. After cleaning with water and hot steam an additional cleaning of the alloys is performed by annealing for 10 minutes at 980°C. The bonding procedure takes place in the temperature range of 800–900°C. After bonding the surface must be carefully cleaned in order to provide good corrosion resistance. The final step of the process is a polishing operation with rotating cotton or wool buffers and a small amount of polishing paste.

Table 1d.11 Chemical composition (wt%) and brazing temperatures of various filler metals (Ref. 5, 8)

Filler Metals for Brazing	*Brazing Temp.(°C)*	*Au*	*Pt*	*Pd*	*Ir*	*Ag*	*Cu*	*Zn*	*In*	*Re*
HGC, LGC	700–840	50–73	≤19	≤1.0	≤0.1	8.0–28	0–9.0	6.0–14	≤2.0	≤0.1
AgPd	760–820	73	0.9	1.0	0.1	13.0		12.0		
HGC-C, LGC-C	700–1120	50–73	≤1.9	≤1.0	≤0.1	10.0–28.0	0–5.0	12.0–14.0	≤2.0	≤0.1
Pd-4-C	1030–1120	50–73	≤1.9	≤1.0		10.0–28.0	3.0–5.0	12.0–14.0	≤2.0	

Key: see Table 1d.7.

Table 1d.12 Recommended heat treatments for various noble metal alloys (Ref. 5, 8)

	Precipitation Hardening		*Soft Annealing*		*Oxidizing without Vacuum*	
Alloy	*Time (min)*	*Temperature (°C)*	*Time (min)*	*Temperature (°C)*	*Time (min)*	*Temperature (°C)*
HGC	15	400	15	700–800		
HGC-C	15	500–600	15	950	10	960–980
LGC	15	400–500	15	700–800		
LGC-C	15	600	15	950	10	980
AgPd	15	550				
Pd-4-C	15	600	15	950	10	980

Key: see Table 1d.7.

1d.2.4 Mechanical properties

Table 1d.13 Mechanical properties of high gold-containing dental cast alloys (Ref.5, 8)

Type		*Tensile Yield Strength (0.2 %) (MPa)*	*Ultimate Tensile Strength (MPa)*	*Ratio Yield/ Tensile Strength*	*Elongation at Fracture (%)*	*Hardness HVHN*
HGC-1		80	170	0.47	45	55
HGC-2		180–240	370–390	0.49–0.61	35–45	95–110
HGC-3	s	330–350	460	0.72–0.76	35–40	145
	h	350–390	550–590	0.64–0.66	20–23	170–190
HGC-4	s	300–420	500–580	0.60–0.72	15–37	155–195
	h	540–780	710–870	0.76–0.90	5–18	225–295
HGC-1-C	s	90–130	220–280	0.41–0.46	29–38	60–75
	h	105–140	230–300	0.46–0.47	27–38	70–90
HGC-2-C	s	230	400	0.58	20	105
	h	240	410	0.59	18	125
HGC-3-C	s	370–420	460–515	0.80–0.82	8–15	150–160
	h	470–490	530–590	0.83–0.89	6–9	185–200
HGC-4-C	s	380–480	530–580	0.72–0.83	7–14	150–200
	h	470–600	550–650	0.85–0.92	3–6	220–230

Key: see Table 1d.7.
s = soft, h = hardened.

Table 1d.14 Mechanical properties of low gold-containing dental cast alloys (Ref.: 5, 8)

Type		*Tensile Yield Strength (0.2 %) (MPa)*	*Ultimate Tensile Strength (MPa)*	*Ratio Yield/ Tensile Strength*	*Elongation at Fracture (%)*	*Hardness VHN5*
LGC-4	s	310–400	480–510	0.65–0.78	18–43	155–170
	h	555–830	640–890	0.87–0.93	3–13	220–275
LGC-4C	s	310–590	570–790	0.54–0.75	11–26	180–250
	h	550–700	710–900	0.77–0.78	6–18	235–285

Key: see Table 1d.7.
s = soft, h = hardened

Table 1d.15 Mechanical properties of AgPd and Pd-alloys (Ref.: 5, 8)

Type	*Tensile Yield Strength (0.2 %) (MPa)*	*Ultimate Tensile Strength (MPa)*	*Ratio Yield/ Tensile Strength*	*Elongation at Fracture (%)*	*Hardness VHN5*
AgPd-1	80	230	0.35	33	55
AgPd-4	285–595	510–950	0.56–0.63	3–31	140–310
Pd-4-C	340–630	630–900	0.54–0.70	8–30	180–285

Key: see Table 1d.7.

1d.2.5. Corrosion and wear

Table 1d.16 Polarization current (i) and polarization resistance (R_c) of gold in 0.9% NaCl and in 0.9% NaCl with a stable redox system [$Fe(CN)_6^{4-}$ / $Fe(CN6^{3-}]$ at 37 °C corresponding to the potential of the body fluid of 400 mV (Ref. 7, 12)

Material	*i (μA/cm²)*	*R_c (kΩcm²)*	
		0.9% NaCl	*saline + redox*
Au	0.009	1100	0.28

Table 1d.17 Average passive current density, range of passivity, corrosion and breakdown potential of a high gold containing alloy (HGC) in artificial saliva (Ref. 3)

Alloy	*Passive Current Density (μA cm⁻²)*	*Range of Passivity (mV vs. SCE)*	*Corrosion Potential (mVvs. SCE)*	*Breakdown Potential (mVvs. SCE)*
HGC	1.5	-100 – +400	-137	400

Table 1d.18 Repassivation rates in artifical saliva versus standard calomel electrode (Ref. 3)

Material	*Corrosion Potential (mV)*	*Potential (mV) after*		
		1 h	*2 h*	*36 h*
HGC	-137	-48	-26	-26

1D.3 CoCr-ALLOYS

See Chapter 1b, CoCr-alloys.

1D.4 NiCr-ALLOYS (REF. 9, 10, 11)

NiCr-alloys are difficult to classify because of the wide range of the chemical composition, as shown in Table 1d.19. The NiCr-alloys in dentistry are generally used for porcelain veneered and unveneered crowns, fixed and removable partial dentures and bridgework. As the processing is similar to that of the CoCr-alloys, it is not described here (see Chapter 1b.3). The requirements for these specific applications determine the chemical composition. The corrosion resistance of the NiCr-alloys is provided by the chromium content which produces a passive oxide layer on the surface. Beryllium is added as a solid solution strengthener and supports the self-fluxing at the porcelain veneering temperature. It is also responsible for the good chemical bonding to the porcelain. As it lowers the melting temperature, beryllium also improves the stability.

Aluminium also produces a passive oxide layer, aids in the bonding to the porcelain and strengthens the alloy due to the precipitation of $AlNi_3$. Silicon lowers the melting temperature and, like manganese, acts as a deoxidizer. Molybdenum and niobium are added to improve corrosion resistance and, like iron, are used to adapt the thermal expansion coefficient to the coefficient of the porcelain.

The wide composition range results in an equally wide range of physical (Table 1d.20) and mechanical properties (Table 1d.21). The high rigidity and strength of these alloys as compared to that of the precious metal alloys make them suitable for the production of small prosthetic devices.

Table 1d.19 Chemical composition (wt%) of the NiCr-alloys used in dentistry Ref. 11)

Ni	*Co*	*Fe*	*Cr*	*Mo*	*Nb*	*Ti*	*W*	*Be*	*Ga*	*Si*	*C*	*Others*
58	0	0	12	0.5	0	0	0	0	0	0	≤0.5	Al, Ce, B,
—	—	—	—	—	—	—	—	—	—	—		Mn, Sn, Y, V,
82	2	9	26	16	7	3	4	1.5	7.5	3		Ta, La, Cu

Table 1d.20 Physical and mechanical properties of NiCr-alloys used in dentistry (Ref. 11)

Melting interval	940–1430 °C
Young's modulus	170–220 GPa
Density	7.8–8.6 g/cm^3
Mean coefficient of linear thermal expansion between 25–600 °C	13.9–15.5 10^{-6}/K

Table 1d.21 Mechanical properties of NiCr-alloys used in dentistry (Ref. 12)

Tensile Yield Strength (0.2%) (MPa)	*Elongation at Fracture (%)*	*Hardness (VHN5)*
255–800	3–25	160–395

REFERENCES

1. Cahn, R.W., Haasen, P. and Kramer, E.J. (eds) (1992) *Materials Science and Technology*, Vol. **14,** VCH.
2. Combe, E. (1984) *Zahnärztliche Werkstoffe*, Hanser.
3. Elagli, K., Traisnel, M. and Hildebrand, H.F. (1993) Electrochemical Behaviour of Titanium and Dental Alloys in Artificial Saliva. *Electrochimica Acta*, **38**(14), 1769–1774. 881.
4. Berglund, A. (1993) An in *vitro* and in *vivo* study of the release of mercury vapor for different types of amalgam alloys. *J. Dent. Res.* **72** (5), 939–945.
5. Product information, Degussa, Germany.
6. DIN 13906–1 (=EN 21562, ISO 1562) (1990). Beuth.
7. DIN 13906–2 (invalid, replaced by DIN 28891) (1990). Beuth.
8. Product information, Wieland Edelmetalle, Germany.
9. Fraker, A.C., Corrosion of Metallic Implants and Prosthetic Devices, in *Metals Handbook*, 9th Ed., Vol. **13**: Corrosion, p. 1351.
10. *Encyclopedia of Materials Science and Engineering*, Vol. **2,** (1986) Pergamon Press, pp. 1057–1058.
11. NiCo-alloy producing industries.
12. Zitter, H. and Plenk, H. (1987) The Electrochemical Behaviour of Metallic Implant Materials as an Indicator of their Biocompatibility. *J. of Biomedical Materials Research*, **21,** 881.

2 Composite materials

L. Ambrosio, G. Carotenuto and L. Nicolais

2.1 TYPES OF COMPOSITES AND COMPONENT MATERIALS

Composites are combined materials created by the synthetic assembly of two or more components – a selected reinforcing agent and a compatible matrix binder – in order to obtain specific and advanced characteristics and properties. The components of composite do not dissolve or otherwise merge completely into each other, but nevertheless do act in concert. The components as well as the interface between them can usually be physically identified, and it is the behavior and properties of the interface that generally control the properties of the composite. The properties of a composite cannot be achieved by any of the components acting alone.

The composites can be classified on the basis of the form of their structural components: fibrous (composed of fibers in a matrix), laminar (composed of layers of materials), and particulate (composed of particles in a matrix). The particulate class can be further subdivided into flake (flat flakes in a matrix) or skeletal (composed of a continuous skeletal matrix filled by a second material). In general, the reinforcing agent can be either fibrous, powdered, spherical, crystalline, or whiskered and either an organic, inorganic, metallic, or ceramic material.

2.2 FIBRE TYPES AND PROPERTIES

A summary of the most important reinforcing filaments and their properties is presented in Tables 2.1–2.7.

Handbook of Biomaterial Properties. Edited by J. Black and G. Hastings.
Published in 1998 by Chapman & Hall, London. ISBN 0 412 60330 6.

2.2.1 Glass fibers

Glass fibers are the most common of all reinforcing fibers for polymeric matrix composites. Their main advantages are low cost, high tensile strength, high chemical resistance and good insulating properties. On the other hand they display a low tensile modulus, a relatively high density comparated to the other fibers, a high sensitivity to wearing and a low fatigue resistance. Depending on the chemical composition of the glass they are commercially available in different grade: A, C, E, R, S. At one time 'A' or alkali glass was quite common as the basic material for glass fibre production. Today this has been virtually completely superseded by 'E' or electrical grade glass. E-glass is a very low alkali content borosilicate glass which provides good electrical and mechanical properties, coupled with good chemical resistance. Another glass produced in commercial quantities for fibers production is the C-glass, a special chemical resistant glass. This is used in the manufacture of surfacing tissues to provide additional chemical resistance over E-glass. For specific application 'R' and 'S' glasses are available as fibers. These are high strength glasses used mostly for aerospace applications.

Table 2.1 Compositions and properties of various glasses (4)

Compound	*A*	*C*	*E*	*R*	*S*
SiO_2	72.0	64.6	52.4	60.0	64.4
Al_2O_3, Fe_2O_3	1.5	4.1	14.4	25.0	25.0
CaO	10.0	13.4	17.2	9.0	—
MgO	2.5	3.3	4.6	6.0	10.3
Na_2O, K_2O	14.2	9.6	0.8	—	0.3
B_2O_3	—	4.7	10.6	—	—
BaO	—	0.9	—	—	—

Table 2.2 Properties of fiberglass (2)

Property	Grade of class A	B	E	S
Physical properties				
Specific gravity	2.50	2.49	2.54	2.48
Mohs gravity	—	6.5	6.5	6.5
Mechanical properties				
Tensile strength, psi×10^6 (MPa)				
At 72 °F (22 °C)	440 (3033)	440 (3033)	500 (3448)	665 (4585)
At 700 °F (371 °C)	—	—	380 (2620)	545 (3758)
At 1000 °F (538 °C)	—	—	250 (1724)	350 (2413)
Tensile modulus elasticity at 72 °F (22 °C), psi×10^6 (GPa)	—	10.0 (69.0)	10.5 (72.4)	12.4 (85.5)
Yield elongation, %	—	4.8	4.8	5.7
Elastic recovery, %	—	100	100	100
Thermal properties				
Coefficient of thermal linear expansion, in./in./°F×10^{-6} (m/m/°C)	4.8 (8.6)	4.0 (7.2)	2.8 (5.0)	3.1 (5.6)
Coefficient of thermal conductivity, Btu-in./hr/sq ft/°F (watt/motor K)	—	—	72 (10.4)	—
Specific heat at 72 °F (22 °C)	—	0.212	0.197	0.176
Softening point, °F(°C)	1340	1380	1545	
Electrical properties				
Dielectric strength, V/mil	—	—	498	—
Dielectric constant at 72 °F (22 °C)				
At 60 Hz	—	—	5.9–6.4	5.0–6.4
At 10^6 Hz	6.9	7.0	6.3	5.1
Dissipation (power) factor at 72 °F (22 °C)				
At 60 Hz	—	—	0.005	0.003
At 10^6 Hz	—	—	0.002	0.003
Volume resistivity at 72 °F (22 °C) and 500 V DC, ½-cm	—	—	10^{15}	10^{16}
Optical properties				
Index of refraction	—	—	10^{13}	10^4
Acoustic Properties				
Velocity of sound, ft/sec (m/sec)	—	—	17,500 (5330)	19,200 (5850)

2.2.2 Aramid fibers

The most common aramid fiber available is the Kevlar 49. These fibers are composed of a highly oriented crystalline polymer and present the highest tensile strength/weight ratio. On the other hand the disadvantages that they present are the low compressive strength, difficulty of manufacturing and a sensitivity to ultraviolet light and water. However, Kevlar fibers find applications in sporting goods.

Table 2.3 Thermal Properties of Kevlar 49 (8)

Property	*Value*
Long-term use at elevated temperature in air, °C (°F)	160 (320)
Decomposition temperature, °C (°F)	500 (932)
Tensile strength, MPa (Ksi)	
At room temperature for 16 months	No strength loss
At 50°C (122 °F) in air for 2 months	No strength loss
At 100°C (212 °F) in air	3170
At 200 °C (392 °F) in air	2720
Tensile modulus, GPa (10^3 Ksi)	
At room temperature for 16 months	No modulus loss
At 50 °C (122 °F) in air for 2 months	No modulus loss
At 100 °C (212 °F) in air	113.8 (16.5)
At 200 °C (392 °F) in air	110.3 (16.0)
Shrinkage, %/°C (%°F)	4×10^{-4} (2.2×10^{-4})
Thermal coefficient of expansion, 10^{-6} cm/cm °C	
Longitudinal, 0–100 °C (32–212 °F)	-2
Radial, 0–100 °C (32–212 °F)	+59
Specific heat at room temperature, J/g°C (Btu/lb°F)	1.42 (0.34)
Thermal conductivity at room temperature, J cm/sec m^2°C (Btuin/hr ft^2 °F)	
Heat flow perpendicular to fibers	4.110 (0.285)
Heat flow parallel to fibers	4.816 (0.334)
Heat of combustion, kJ/g (Btu/lb)	34.8 (15,000)

Table 2.4 Properties of Kevlar 29 (2)

Specific gravity	1.44
Tensile strength (GPa)	2.76
Tensile modulus (GPa)	58
Elongation (%)	4.0
Filament diameter (μm)	12.1

2.2.3 Boron fibers

These fibers are characterized by an extremely high tensile modulus coupled with a large diameter, offering an excellent resistance to buckling that contributes to a high compressive strength of the composites. Their high cost is due to the processing operations. For this reason boron fibers find application only in aerospace and military contexts.

Table 2.5 Typical Properties of Boron fibers and of other Commercially Available Reinforcement Filaments (1)

Filament material	*Diameter (μm)*	*Manufacturing technique*	*Average strength N/m^2 (Ksi)*	*Density (g/cm^3)*	*Modulus (GN/m^2)*
Boron	100–150	CVD	34 (500)	2.6	400
SiC-coated boron	100–150	CVD	31 (450)	2.7	400
SiC	100	CVD	27 (400)	3.5	400
B_4C	70–100	CVD	24 (350)	2.7	400
Boron on carbon	100	CVD	24 (350)	2.2	—
Al_2O_3	250	Melt withdrawal	24 (350)	4.0	250
Beryllium	100–250	Wire drawing	13 (200)	1.8	250
Tungsten	150–250	Wire drawing	27 (400)	19.2	400
'Rocket Wire' AFC-77	50–100	Wire drawing	41(600)	7.9	180

2.2.4 Graphite fibers

Carbon fibers owe their success in high performance composites to their extremely high tensile modulus/weight and tensile strength/weight ratios, high fatigue strength and low coefficient of thermal expansion, coupled with a low ratio of cost to performance. Carbon fibers are commercially available with a variety of moduli ranging from 270 GPa to 600 GPa. They are produced following two different processes, depending on the type of precursors.

Table 2.6 Carbon fibre precursors (2)

Precursor material	*Carbon content (%wt)*	*Carbonization yield (%wt)*
Cellulose fibre	45	10–15
Polyacrylonitrile	68	40
Lignin	70	50
Hydrocarbon pitch	95	85–90

Table 2.7 Properties of some carbon fibers (2)

Fibre precursor	*Fibre type*	*Trade name*	*Diameter (μm)*	*Specific gravity*	*Tensile strength (GPa)*	*Tensile modulus (GPa)*	*Elongation (%)*	*Carbon content (%wt)*
Hydrocaron pitch	Carbon	Kureha	10.5	1.6	1.03	—	2.5	99.5
Lignin	Carbon		10–15	1.5	0.6	—	1.5	90
Cellulose	Graphite	Thornel	6.6	1.67	2.0	390	0.6	99.9
Polyacrylonitrile	Carbon	Graphil HT	8	1.76	3.2	230	—	—
Polyacrylonitrile	Graphite	Graphil HM	8	1.87	2.4	330	—	—

2.3 MATRIX MATERIALS

Polymer matrix resins bind the reinforcing fibers and fabrics together in composite structures. Resins also act as sizing, load distributors, and vibration dampeners in the composite structure. A wide variety of thermoset and thermoplastic resins are used in polymer composites. A summary of the most important materials used as composite matrix and their properties is presented.

2.4 THERMOPLASTIC MATRIX

Although many commercial applications for filled thermoplastics exist, use of thermoplastics in advanced composites is still in the developmental stage. In fact, the industry is still split on the use of thermoplastics for advanced composites. According to some, it is difficult to improve the rigidity, stability and thermal and chemical resistance of the thermoset resins currently available. Others believe that the majority of the thermoplastic resins available today not only possess the high-service temperature characteristics required, but also hold the potential of quicker and more economical processing once the existing problems are resolved. The various thermoplastics and their characteristics are described in the following paragraphs:

Polyamides, commonly referred to as nylons, are produced by condensation between diamines and diacids or by self-condensation of an amino acid. Like many other resins, the exact chemistry of polyamides can vary and, therefore, so can the final properties. However, all polyamides have low-service temperatures and low melting points.

Polyamideimides are marketed by Amoco Chemicals under the trade name Torlon. A polyamideimide is also a good candidate for the production of thermoplastic prepregs.

Polycarbonates are noted for an extremely high-impact strength in an unreinforced state. However, compared to such other crystalline polymers as PEEK, a polycarbonate does not bond well to reinforcing fibers. It also has poor chemical resistance, which can be greatly improved by alloying it with thermoplastic polyesters. Although only a small quantity of polycarbonate with carbon fiber reinforcement is used today, primarily for interior aircraft structures, polycarbonate is potentially one of the more promising matrix resins for advanced composites, especially in alloyed versions such as General Electric's Xenoy and Bayer's Makroblend.

Polyetheretherketones (PEEK) have excellent properties for use in advanced polymer composites, including low flammability, low smoke and toxic gas emission, and broad chemical and solvent resistance. PEEK possesses a continuous service temperature of 200°C to 240°C (392°F to 464°F) and has a very high melting point of 334°C (633°F). PEEK also provides excellent abrasion resistance at its service temperature, radiation resistance, excellent fatigue and wear resistance and a relatively low specific gravity of 1.32. It is possible to process PEEK on conventional extrusion and molding equipment, and its highly crystalline nature responds well to fiber reinforcement.

Polyetherimides (PEI) have been commercially introduced by General Electric as ULTEM, and the company states that it could be a possible matrix for carbon fiber.

Polyether sulfones (PES) are also amorphous in structure. Although PES has poor resistance to solvents, it possesses several valuable properties. The resin is capable of providing thousands of hours of service at temperatures up to 180°C (356°F) and has very good load-bearing properties. It is dimensionally stable up to 200°C (392°F) and, like PEEK, possesses excellent flame resistance and favorable processing characteristics. In addition to thermoset polyimides, several thermoplastic polyimides are offered for high-temperature applications. Although difficult to process, these resins maintain favorable performance characteristics up to a higher temperature, 371°C (700°F), than their thermoset counterparts.

Polyphenylene sulfides (PPS), partially crystalline polymers, are produced by the reaction of p-dichlorobenzene and sodium sulfide. This polymer has metallic-like properties and responds well to reinforcement. PPS possesses good creep and good moisture resistance and a low coefficient of thermal expansion.

2.5 THERMOSETS MATRIX

The basic difference between thermoset and thermoplastic resins is the reaction heat. A thermoset resin is cured by the application of heat and often by the addition chemicals called curing agents. Once cured, the material is infusible, unsoluble and can softened or reworked with the addition of heat.

A thermoplastic, on the other hand, is capable of being repeatedly softened by addition of heat and hardened by decreasing temperature. The change occurring thermoplastic resin with the addition of heat is primarily physical, not chemical. This different provides one major advantage for thermoplastics: any scrap from fabrication can be reused.

Thermoset resins can vary greatly with respect to service temperature, solvent resist and other important characteristics. A description follows of the various thermoset resin their basic characteristics.

2.6 VINYL ESTER RESINS

Vinyl ester resins are thermosetting resins that consist of a polymer backbone with acrylate or methacrylate termination. The backbone component of vinyl ester resins can derived from an epoxide resins, polyester resins, urethane resin, and so on, but those base epoxide resins are of particular commercial significance.

Vinyl ester resins are produced by the addition of ethylenically unsaturated carbo acids (methacrylic or acrylic acid) to an epoxide resin (usually of the bisphenol epichlorohydrin type). The reaction of acid addition to the epoxide ring (esterification exothermic and produces a hydroxyl group without the formation of by-products. Appropriate diluents and polymerization inhibitors are added during or after esterification.

Epoxide resins that have been used to produce vinyl ester resins include:

- bisphenol A types (general-purpose and heat-resistant vinyl esters)
- phenolic-novolac types (heat-resistant vinyl esters)
- tetrabromo bisphenol A types (fire-retardant vinyl esters)

Vinyl ester resins contain double bonds that react and crosslink in the presence of free radicals produced by chemical, thermal or radiation sources.

2.7 EPOXIDE RESINS

Epoxide are materials which contain two or more glycidyl groups per molecule. The uncured resins range from free flowing liquids to high melting solids, which can be cross-linked by reaction with an appropriate curing agent.

Typical curing agents include primary and secondary amines, polyamides and organic anhydrides. Other curing agents used are the catalytic curing agents, such as the boron trifluoride complexes. No by-products are evolved during cure. The resultant cured resins are generally hard thermoset materials with excellent mechanical, chemical and electrical properties.

These materials can be conveniently divided into six classes of resins:

- bisphenol A based (e.g. diglycidyl ether of bisphenol-A (DGEBA))
- glycidyl esters
- glycidyl amines (e.g. tetraglycidyl amine of 4,4-diamino-diphenylmethane)
- novolacs brominated resins (e.g. diglycidyl ether of tetrabromobisphenol A)
- cycloaliphatic resins (e.g. Tetraglycidyl ether of tetraphenylene ethane)

2.8 DILUENTS

Diluents are added to epoxide resins primarily to lower viscosity and thus to improve handling characteristics. They also modify the cured properties of the resin. Diluents can be divided into two classes: (a) the reactive diluents and (b) the non-reactive diluents.

2.8.1 Reactive diluents

- Butane-1,4-diol diglycidyl ether
- n-Butyl glycidyl ether (nBGE)
- Glycidyl methacrylate
- Phenyl glycidyl ether (PGE)
- 2-Ethylhexyl glycidyl ether (2EHGE)
- Iso-octyl glycidyl ether (IOGE)
- Diethylene glycol monobutyl glycidyl ether
- Cresyl glycidyl ether (CGE)
- p-t-Butylphenil glicidyl ether
- Epoxide 7 (C8–C10 glycidyl ether)
- Epoxide 8 (C12–C14 glycidyl ether)
- Dibromocresyl glycidyl ether (BROC)
- Dibromophenyl glycidyl ether (DER 599)

2.8.2 Non reactive diluents

- Benzyl alcohol
- Furfuryl alcohol
- Dibutyl phthalate (DBP)

2.9 CURING AGENTS FOR EPOXIDE RESINS

These are known variously as curing agents, hardeners, activators or catalysts. They are required to convert liquid and solid epoxide resins into tough infusible thermoset polymers. The curing agents promote this curing reaction by opening the epoxide ring and become chemically bound into the resin in the process. Each of the curing agents for epoxide resins will now be discussed in turn.

2.9.1 Amine curing agents

Amine curing agents may be primary or secondary amines, aliphatic, alicyclic or aromatic. The reaction with an epoxide resin is an addition reaction where the amine links directly with an epoxide group to form a combined polymer, with hydroxyl groups formed during the reaction. The amines commonly used are the following:

- Ethylenediamine (EDA)
- Trimethylhexamethylenediamine (TMD)
- Diethylenetriamine (DTA)
- 2-Hydroxyethyldiethylenetriamine (T)
- Dipropylenetriamine (DPTA)
- Triethylenetetramine (TETA)
- Tetraethylenepentamine (TEPA)
- Diethylaminopropylamine (DEAPA)
- Dimethylaminpropylamine (DMAPA)
- m-Xylylenediamine (mXDA)
- N-Aminoethylpiperazine (AEP)

2.9.2 Anhydride curing agent

These consist of organic anhydrides and are used in roughly stoichiometric proportions with epoxide resins. The anhydride commonly used are the following:

- Phthalic anhydride (EPA)
- Tetrahydrophthalic anhydride (THPA)
- Methyltetrahydrophthalic anhydride (MTHPA)
- Endomethylenetetrahydrophthalic anhydride (NA)
- Hexahydrophthalic anhydride (HHPA)
- Methylhexahydrophthalic anhydride (MHPA)
- Trimellitic anhydride (TMA)
- Pyromellitic dianhydride (PDMA)
- Dodecenylsuccinic anhydride (DDSA)

2.9.3 Accelerators for anhydride cured systems

Various accelerators can be used with epoxy/anhydride systems to promote cure. Some accelerators in use are:

- Benzyldimethylamine (BDMA)
- Tris(dimethylaminomethyl)phenol
- 1-Methylimidazole (DY 070 from Ciba-Geigy)
- N-Butylimidazole
- 2-Ethyl-4-mathylimidazole
- Triamylammonium phenate (DY 063 from Ciba-Geigy)

2.9.4 Polyamide curing agents

The polyamides used to cure epoxide resins are all reactive compounds with free amine groups. They may be amidopolyamines, aminopolyamides or imidazolines. They are mostly used in coating systems and in adhesive formulations. Some suppliers of polyamide curing agents are listed below:

- Ancamide (Anchor Chemical Co, Ltd)
- Araldite (Ciba-Geigy Plastics & Additives Co.)
- Versamid, Genamid, Synolide (Cray Valley Products Ltd)
- Plastamid (Croda Resin Ltd)
- Grilonit (Grilon (UK) Ltd)
- Beckopox (Hoechst AG(Reichhold Albert Chemie AG))
- Euredur (Schering Chemicals Ltd)
- Epikure (Shell Chemicals UK Ltd)
- Casamid (Thomas Swan & Co. Ltd)
- Uracure (Synthetic Resins Ltd)
- Thiokol (Thiokol Chemicals Ltd)
- Wolfamid (Victor Wolf Ltd)

2.9.5 Other curing agents

Several other types of curing agent are used with epoxide resins for laminating applications or in moulding compounds. Examples of these curing agents are:

- Dicyandiamide (Dicy)
- Boron trifluoride complexes
- Boron trifluoride monoethylamine
- 2-Ethyl-4-methylimidazole
- N-n-Butylimidazole

2.10 POLYESTER RESINS

The basic materials used to make a polyester resin are a dibasic organic acid or anhydride and a dihydric alcohol.

2.10.1 Catalysts or initiators

Catalyst or initiators for unsaturated polyester resin system consist of organic peroxides. Some commercially available catalysts are:

- Diacyl peroxides (benzoyl peroxide, 2,4-dichlorobenzoyl peroxide, dilauroyl peroxide, diacetyl peroxide).
- Ketone peroxides (methyl ethyl ketone peroxide, cyclohexanone peroxide, acetylacetone peroxide, methyl isobutyl ketone peroxide).
- Hydroperoxides (t-butyl hydroperoxide, cumene hydroperoxide).
- Dialkyl and diaralkyl peroxides (dicumyl peroxide, di-t-butyl peroxide, t-butyl cumyl peroxide, 2,5-dimethyl-2,5-bis(t-butylperoxy)hexane).

- Peroxyesters (t-butyl peroxybenzoate, t-butyl peroxydiethylacetate, t-butyl peroxyester, t-butyl peroxyisononanoate, t-butyl peroctoate, di-t-butyl diperoxyphthalate, t-buthyl peroxypivalate).
- Perketals (2,2-bis(t-butylperoxy)butane, 1,1-bis(t-butylperoxy)cyclohexane, 1,1-bis(t-butylperoxy)-3,3,5-trimethylcyclohexane).

2.10.2 Accelerators or promotors

These are materials which when used in conjunction with an organic peroxide catalyst increase the rate at which that peroxide breaks down into free radicals. Some of the commercially available accelerators are:

- Cobalt accelerators: cobalt siccatolate, naphthenate or octoate
- Manganese accelerators: manganese salts
- Vanadium accelerators
- Tertiary amine accelerators:
  dimethylaniline (used to accelerate diacyl peroxide catalysed system);
  diethylaniline (used to accelerate benzoyl peroxide catalysed system);
  dimethyl-p-toluidine (used to accelerate benzoyl peroxide catalysed system).

2.11 LAMINATE PROPERTIES

Current attitudes regarding composite materials emphasize the relationship of structural performance to the properties of a ply. A 'ply' is a thin sheet of material consisting of an oriented array of fibers, embedded in a continuous matrix material. These plies are stacked one upon other, in a definite sequence and orientation, and bonded together yielding a laminate with tailored properties. The properties of the laminate are related to the properties of the ply by the specification of the ply thickness, stacking sequence, and the orientation of each ply. The properties of the ply are, in turn, specified by the properties of the fibers and the matrix, their volumetric concentration, and geometric packing in the ply. Generally, the material is preformed and can be purchased in a continuous compliant tape or sheet form which is in a chemically semicured condition. Fabrication of structural items involves using this 'prepreg' material, either winding it on to a mandrel or cutting and stacking it on to a mold, after which heat and pressure or tension is applied to complete the chemical hardening process.

The basis for engineering design of a such material is then the properties of a cured ply or lamina as it exists in a laminate. This ply is treated as a thin two-dimensional item and is mechanically characterized by its stress–strain response to: (i) loading in the direction of the filaments, which exhibits a nearly linear response up to a large fracture stress; (ii) loading in the direction transverse to the filament orientation, which exhibits a significantly decreased moduli and strength, and (iii) the response of the material to an in-plane shear load.

By the contrast with isotropic metallic materials, an oriented ply, in the form of a thin sheet, is anisotropic and requires four elastic (plane stress) constants to specify its stiffness properties in its natural orientation

$$\sigma_1 = Q_{11}\epsilon_1 + Q_{12}\epsilon_1$$
$$\sigma_2 = Q_{12}\epsilon_1 + Q_{22}\epsilon_2$$
$$\sigma_6 = Q_{66}\epsilon_6 \tag{2.1}$$

where $\sigma_6 = \tau_{12}$ and $\epsilon_6 = \tau_{12}$ or in matrix form

$$\begin{vmatrix}\sigma_1\\ \sigma_2\\ \sigma_3\end{vmatrix} = \begin{vmatrix}Q_{11} & Q_{11} & 0\\ Q_{11} & Q_{11} & 0\\ 0 & 0 & Q_{11} & \end{vmatrix} \cdot \begin{vmatrix}\epsilon_1\\ \epsilon_2\\ \epsilon_3\end{vmatrix} \tag{2.2}$$

where the plane stress stiffness moduli are

$$Q_{11} = E_{11}/(1 - \nu_{12}\,\nu_{21})$$
$$Q_{22} = E_{22}/(1 - \nu_{12}\,\nu_{21})$$
$$Q_{12} = \nu_{21}E_{11}/(1 - \nu_{12}\,\nu_{21})$$
$$Q_6 = G_{12} \tag{2.3}$$

where ν_{ij} is the Poisson ratio, defined as $-\epsilon_i/\epsilon_j$.

If, however, the ply is rotated with respect to the applied stress or strain direction additional moduli appear, which results in the direction-indicated shear coupling rotation simple extension

$$\begin{vmatrix}\sigma_1\\ \sigma_2\\ \sigma_3\end{vmatrix} = \begin{vmatrix}Q^*_{11} & Q^*_{12} & Q^*_{16}\\ Q^*_{12} & Q^*_{22} & Q^*_{26}\\ Q^*_{16} & Q^*_{26} & Q^*_{66}\end{vmatrix} \cdot \begin{vmatrix}\epsilon_1\\ \epsilon_2\\ \epsilon_3\end{vmatrix} \tag{2.4}$$

where

$$Q_{11}^* = U_{11} + U_2\cos(2\theta) + U_3\cos(4\theta)$$
$$Q_{22}^* = U_1 - U_2\cos(2\theta) + U_3\cos(4\theta)$$
$$Q_{12}^* = U_4 - U_3\cos(4\theta)$$
$$Q_{66}^* = U_5 - U_3\cos(4\theta)$$
$$Q_{16}^* = -½\, U_2\sin(2\theta) - U_3\sin(4\theta)$$
$$Q_{26}^* = -½\, U_2\sin(2\theta) + U_3\sin(4\theta) \tag{2.5}$$

The invariants U_i to the rotation are

$$U_1 = \tfrac{1}{8}\,(3Q_{11} + 3Q_{22} + 2Q_{12} + 4Q_{66})$$
$$U_2 = \tfrac{1}{2}\,(Q_{11} - Q_{22})$$
$$U_3 = \tfrac{1}{8}\,(Q_{11} + Q_{22} - 2Q_{12} - 4Q_{66})$$
$$U_4 = \tfrac{1}{8}\,(Q_{11} + Q_{22} + 6Q_{12} - 4Q_{66})$$
$$U_5 = \tfrac{1}{8}\,(Q_{11} + Q_{22} - 2Q_{12} + 4Q_{66}) \qquad (2.6)$$

In addition, lamination can result in up to 18 elastic coefficients and increased deformational complexities, but the additional coefficients can all be derived from the four primary coefficients using the concept of rotation and ply-stacking sequence. These complications are the result of geometric variables. If the laminate is properly constructed, the in-plane stretching or stiffness properties can still be specified by four elastic coefficients. We shall consider laminates of this nature.

Note that both short and continuous fibers are handled in the same manner. These calculations, while tedious, are analytically simple. The 'plane stress', the Q_{ij} terms, are employed because lamination neglects the mechanical properties through the ply thickness. These stiffnesses are sometimes regrouped into new constants called 'invariants', the U_i terms, for analytical simplicity. To compute the properties of the laminate one then sums the ply (h_k) properties through the thickness of the laminate, weighted by the thickness (h_k) of each oriented ply

$$A_{ij} = \sum_{k=1}^{N} (Q_{ij})_k\, h_k$$

For a balanced (same number of $\pm\theta$) and symmetrical system ($+\theta$ or $-\theta$ at same distance above and below the midplane) the laminate solution is

$$A_{11} = U_1 + U_2 \cos(2\theta) + U_3 \cos(4\theta)$$
$$A_{22} = U_1 - U_2 \cos(2\theta) + U_3 \cos(4\theta)$$
$$A_{12} = U_4 - U_3 \cos(4\theta)$$
$$A_{66} = U_5 - U_3 \cos(4\theta) \qquad (2.7)$$

Note the inverted terms A_{jj} yield the required elastic properties of the laminate in terms of the individual ply properties E_{11}, E_{12} and G_{12}.

$$E_{11} = (A_{11}A_{22} - A^2_{12})/A_{22}$$
$$E_{22} = (A_{11}A_{22} - A^2_{12})/A_{11}$$
$$\nu_{12}/E_{11} = A_{12}/(A_{11}A_{22} - A^2_{12}) \quad G_{12} = A_{66} \qquad (2.8)$$

These calculations have been thoroughly tested and agree closely with experiment. The circles and squares are the experimental points and the lines are the theoretical predictions for a nylon fiber reinforced rubber. The angle ply laminate is predicted from the ply properties. The ply properties are in turn correlated with the transformation equations and the micromechanics. The micromechanics employed in this demonstration are based upon the 'self-consistent method' developed by Hill (8). Hill rigorously modeled the composite as a single fiber, encased in a cylinder of matrix, with both embedded in an unbounded homogeneous medium which is macroscopically indistinguishable from the composite. Hermann (9) employed this model to obtain solution in terms of Hill's 'reduced moduli'. Halpin and Tsai (10) reduced Hermann's solution to simpler analytical form and extended its use for a variety of filament geometries

$$E_{11} = E_f V_f + E_m V_m$$

$$\nu_{12} = \nu_f V_f + \nu_m V_m$$

$$p/p_m = (1 + \eta\xi V_f)/(1 - \eta V_f) \tag{2.9}$$

where

$$\eta = (t_f/t_m - 1)/(p_f/p_m + \zeta)$$

$$\xi = (e/d);\ \zeta_{G12} = 1\ \zeta_{G23} = 1/(3 - 4\nu_m)$$

$$p = E_{22}, G_{12}, G_{23};\ p_f = E_f, G_f;\ p_m = E_m, G_m \tag{2.10}$$

These equations are suitable for single calculation and were employed previously for the single ply and angle ply properties. The short fiber composite properties are also given by the Halpin–Tsai equations where the moduli in the fiber orientation direction is a sensitive function of aspect ratio (l/d) at small aspect ratios and has the same properties of a continuous fiber composite at large but finite aspect ratios.

If the ply is used in the construction of a balanced and symmetrical 0/90 laminate and is mechanically tested, bilinear stress/strain curve is obtained, and the stiffness is the sum, through the thickness of the plane stress stiffness of each layer. As the laminate is deformed each ply possesses the same in-plane strain, and when the strain on the 90 layers in the laminate prevents the 90° layer from carrying its share of the load, $Q_{ij}(90°)=0$. This load is transferred to the unbroken layers, the 0° layers for our illustration, and results in a loss of laminate stiffness or modulus. Continual loading will ultimately produce a catastrophic failure of the laminate when the strain capability of the unbroken, 0°, layers is exceeded. For a 0/90 construction, employing glass/epoxy material, the ratio of the ultimate failure stress to the crazing stress is 6.1. Note a change in stiffness as the 90° and then the 45° layers fail, and the correspondence of the theoretical ultimate strength of 356 MPa with the experimental results of 346 MPa. While the strain for transverse ply failure is constant from laminate to laminate, the stress required to craze the system as well as cause final failure is a function of laminate geometry, because the construction of the laminate specifies the stiffness properties (crazing stress = stiffness × allowable transverse ply strain). It must be noticed that the area under the stress/strain curve is proportional to the impact energy. Therefore, lamination permits the engineer to tailor a fixed prepreg system to meet the conflicting stress/strain demands at different points in a structure. A further point, the crazing stress threshold is generally at or below the creep fracture or fatigue limit for all classes of composites (for glass/epoxy the fatigue limit lies between 0.25 and 0.30 of static ultimate strength). Boron and graphite are fatigue insensitive filaments, thus no fatigue damage is realized below first ply failure.

Thus, the material properties of a laminate are specified in terms of the ply engineering moduli, E_{11}, E_{22}, ν_{12} and G_{12}; the engineering strains to failure, ϵ_1, ϵ_2 and ϵ_6; and the thermal expansion coefficients, ϵ_1 and ϵ_2.

2.12 COMPOSITE FABRICATION

Various fabrications used in the reinforced plastics industry are discussed below:

2.12.1 Hand lay-up and spray-up procedures

In one of the simplest and labor intensive procedures, pigmented, catalysed resin is applied to the surface of the mold. This gel coat in room temperature lay-up techniques will end up on the surface of the finished composite (FRP). Catalysed resin-impregnated mat is then applied over the gel coat and this and subsequent layers are brushed or rolled to assure good contact between layers and to remove any entrapped air. This procedure is continued until the desired thickness of the composite is attained.

The assembled composite may be cured at room temperature or at elevated temperatures for faster cycles. This procedure, which was originally called contact molding, may be upgraded by the application of a vacuum or pressure bag placed over a Cellophane film on the final layer to reduce void formation in the composite. The laminate may also be built up by a spray-up process in which a mixture of chopped glass strands and catalysed resin is sprayed on the gel coat instead of resin-impregnated mat. In any case, the inner surface will be less smooth than the first layer formed by the gel coat. Tanks, boats and pipe may be fabricated by this technique.

2.12.2 Centrifugal casting

Fiber-reinforced plastic pipe (FRP) can be produced by rotating a mixture of chopped strand and catalysed resin inside a hollow mandrel. Because of differences in specific gravity, there is a tendency for these composites to be less homogeneous than those produced by other techniques.

In addition to being available as continuous filaments and staple fibers in mats, fiberglass textiles are also available as biaxial, triaxial, knitted and three dimensional braided patterns. Many different resin matrices are in use but the emphasis in this chapter will be on unsaturated polyester and epoxy resins. While the strength and stiffness are controlled primarily by the reinforcements, the resinous matrix contributes to thermal conductivity and flexibility. The ultimate properties of these composites are based on a harmonious contribution of both the continuous and discontinuous phases.

2.12.3 Matched die molding

Matched die molding of a premix of chopped glass, roving, and catalyzed resin is used for relatively large scale production of reinforced articles. Uncured dough-like compositions are called bulk molding compounds (BMC). Uncured resin-impregnated sheets are called sheet molding compound (SMC). These compounds are supplemented by thick molding compounds (TMC) and XMC. TMC is produced continuously on a machine that resembles a 2 roll mill. XMC, in which the continuous impregnated fiber are arranged in an X-pattern, is produced on a filament winding machine.

Autoclave molding

Autoclave molding, the process of curing thermoset resins at elevated temperature and pressure in an inert environment, has an important role in the fabrication of continuous fiber reinforced thermoplastics. While most companies view thermoplastics as an alternative to traditional autoclave long-cycle processing, they have come to accept the following reasons for the autoclave processing of thermoplastic matrices:

- Availability
- High temperature and pressure capability
- Reduced tooling requirements
- Uniform pressure distribution.

The dominant reason for the autoclaves' role in thermoplastics production is its availability. Aerospace first- and second-tier contractors, who conducted much of the developmental work in parts fabrication, all have autoclaves on hand.

While it may seem defeatist to use the autoclave for thermoplastic resins which undergo no chemical reaction and lend themselves to rapid fabrication, autoclave use offers other advantages.

In the industry, many fabricators own autoclaves capable of processing high temperature thermosets (e.g. polyimides) at operating temperatures up to 800 °F and pressures of 150 to 200 psi; which can also accommodate high temperature thermoplastics such as PEEK, which is normally processed in the 700 to 750 °F range. One disadvantage, particularly for production-sized autoclaves, is the inability to finely control cool-down rate – a critical process step for the semicrystalline thermoplastics. This situation can be improved by implementing integrally cooled tooling.

Where high consolidation pressures are required, the autoclave can reduce tooling costs by eliminating the need for matched metal tooling, when compared to a molding process (e.g. compression molding or thermoforming). Less expensive tooling aids can be used for consolidation via the autoclave's pressurized environment. The autoclave also provides uniform pressure over the part's area and eliminates pressure distribution concerns associated with a matched tool in a press.

Thermoforming

Thermoforming offers vast potential for high volume thermoplastic composite parts fabrication. There are many thermoforming variations; but by basic definition, thermoforming is the heating of a reinforced thermoplastic matrix sheet or kit above the softening temperature, followed by forcing the material against a contour by mechanical (e.g. matched tooling, plug) or pneumatic (e.g. differential air or hydraulic) means. The material is then held and cooled sufficiently for shape retention, and removed from the mold. Thermoforming implies only those processes applicable to thermoplastic resins, and is often used in the same context as the term 'compression molding' which also applies to thermosets. In this section, the process is defined as the preheating of the lay-up or reconsolidated sheet, followed forming via a matched mold.

Phillips Petroleum has applied this technology to fabric reinforced Ryton (PPS) materials. A conveyorized infrared oven is used to rapidly preheat the lay-up to 600 °F in two to three minutes. The charge is quickly transferred to a preheated mold in a fast closing press for part forming. Total cycle times of one to three minutes are feasible with this automated approach.

High production rates can be achieved using thermoforming technology. However, it is difficult to form high quality continuous fiber reinforced thermoplastic parts with demanding geometries, due to the restricted movement of the fiber.

Du Pont's long discontinuous fiber sheet products with PEEK and J-2 resins provide easier fabrication of complex shapes. This product form is particularly attractive to helicopter manufacturers for the press forming of highly contoured secondary structure parts.

Transfer molding

Transfer molding is used for the manufacture of small components and is particularly useful with multi-cavity tools and where small inserts are to be moulded in. Materials used are polyester and epoxide dough moulding compounds, although a new liquid resin injection technique is reported.

Heated steel molds, preferably hard chrome plated, are used, which may be of multicavity design. Tooling costs are higher than for compression moulding since appropriate gates and runners must be included in the mould.

A pre-weighed quantity of DMC is placed in a heated transfer pot by hand. A punch or ram compresses the material and causes it to flow into the heated tool cavity where it cures. The tool is mounted between the platens of a press.

Factors to be considered with transfer molding are transfer and tool clamping pressures and transfer time. To reduce transfer time and increase overall efficiency the molding compound may be pre-heated in an oven or high frequency pre-heater such as a micro-wave oven.

Mold temperatures range from 155 to 170°C both for polyester and epoxide resin compounds, with molding pressures ranging from 5 to 100 MPa depending on the type of compound to be processed, mold design and temperature. Cure time in the mold (excluding pre-heat time) is usually of the order of 10–30 s per millimetre of wall thickness for both types of compound.

Injection molding

Injection molding, a technique used extensively for the processing of thermoplastic materials, has also been developed to process thermosetting resin systems. Due to high mould costs it is generally only suitable for the large scale production of small-to-medium sized components. Materials processed in this way are polyester and epoxy DMC and also phenolics, ureas, melamines and diallyl phthalate moulding compounds. These latter materials are generally more difficult to process than either polyester or epoxy DMC.

Thermoset moldings produced by injection moulding are used widely in the electrical and automotive fields, thus large production runs are common.

Injection molding has advantages over both compression and transfer molding in that the process is more automated and far higher production rates can be achieved. Although mould costs are higher than for compression molding, overall finished component costs are generally lower. With small weight components, scrap from runners can be high compared with compression molding but for large mouldings this becomes relatively insignificant. Injection molding is also better for thick parts since, with the pre-heating of the DMC before injection into the mold, shorter molding cycles are possible.

While injection molding machines designed specifically for processing thermoset materials are available, a number of manufacturers offer replacement screw and barrel assemblies and stuffer hoppers to convert conventional thermoplastic injection moulding machines to process thermosets.

Molding compound is transferred in the cold state by pressure from the material hopper into the main injection chamber. Here it can be pre-heated before injection into the heated mould tool. Injection, through a special nozzle, can be either by ram or screw pressure. If screw feed is used, the screw must be of the type designed to process thermosets as opposed to thermoplastics.

Early machines were designed with vertical clamping pressure on the mold but today horizontal machines are mostly used. Since thermosetting materials are liquid until gelation occurs, clamping pressure has to be maintained on the mould until the resin has cured. Unless this is done, excessive flash will form. Heated matched metal molds are used, which may be of multi-cavity design. These molds must be designed for use with thermosetting resins, taking into account the fact that thermoset moldings are harder, more rigid and less easily deformed than thermoplastics.

A typical temperature sequence for injection molding DMC would be: feed hopper and feed zone – ambient temperature; metering section 50–60°C; nozzle 80–90°C; mould temperature 135–185°C for polyester DMC or 160–22°C for epoxy DMC; injection pressure 80–160 MPa. Cure time is generally of the order of 10–20 s per millimetre of wall thickness. Very little finishing of moldings is necessary.

Where fully automatic molding machines are used, hydraulic ejection with perhaps a 'joggle' facility is necessary, since thermosets have a tendency to stick in the mold.

2.12.4 Filament winding

Filament winding is a technique used for the manufacture of pipes, tubes, cylinders and spheres and is frequently used for the construction of large tanks and pipework for the chemical industry. By suitable design, filament wound structures can be fabricated to withstand very high pressures in service. In general, products fabricated by filament winding have the highest strength to weight ratios and can have glass contents of up to 80% by weight.

The process is suitable for use both with polyester and epoxide resin systems and a variety of fibres including glass, carbon, aramid and metals, providing that these materials are available in continuous filament lengths. Glass fibre is by far the most common reinforcement used and will be used as the example in the description of the process.

Filament winding is basically a simple process, although numerous modifications have been developed to improve product quality. Moldings can be produced by either a wet lay-up process or from prepreg.

In recent years filament winding has been extended to the continuous production of pipe using a continuous steel band mandrel. In this way continuous lengths of pipe can be produced, with diameters ranging from about 0.3 to 3.5 m.

2.12.5 Wet lay-up

With the wet lay-up process glass rovings are drawn through a resin bath to impregnate them with resin. The impregnated rovings are then wound under tension round a rotating mandrel. Generally the feed head supplying the rovings to the mandrel traverses backwards and forwards along the mandrel.

The mandrel, which may be segmented for large diameter pipes, is generally wrapped with a release film, such as Cellophane, prior to wrapping with glass and resin. The mandrel may incorporate some means of heating the resin system, such as embedded electric heaters, or provision for steam heating. Alternatively, the fully wrapped mandrel and laminate may be transferred to a curing oven to effect cure.

In order to provide a resin-rich, corrosion resistant inner lining to the pipe, the mandrel may be wrapped with a surfacing tissue followed by one or two layers of chopped strand mat or woven tape prior to filament winding. This first layer is usually allowed to cure partially before winding commences to prevent the resin from being squeezed out into the main laminate.

The winding angle used during construction of pipes or tanks depends on the strength/performance requirements and may vary from longitudinal through helical to circumferential. Often a combination of different winding patterns is used to give optimum performance. Accurate fibre alignment is possible.

For pipe construction, steel mandrels are generally used. However, where cylinders or spheres are to be made, an alternative material has to be used so that it can be removed once the resin system has cured. In these cases the mandrel can be made from wax, a low melting metal alloy, or an inert plaster held together with a water soluble binder. Clearly, in these cases the mandrel can only be used once. Material choice for the mandrel will depend on the cure cycle needed for the resin system.

In addition to winding with continuous filament rovings, machines have been developed which permit winding with tapes or slit-width chopped strand mat and woven rovings. These reinforcements may be used alone or combined with continuous filament rovings. Thus considerable design flexibility exists for the production of large simple shapes.

Improved chemical resistance can be achieved by the use of a thermoplastic or synthetic rubber liner. If the liner is sufficiently rigid it can be supported on a light frame and used as the mandrel, if not then it can be wrapped round the mandrel first. A grade of polypropylene is available which has a woven glass cloth partially rolled into one side to improve adhesion of the resin system (Celmar).

Dunlop has recently developed a new process for pipe production to produce pipes in the range 200–2000 mm diameter. Essentially the process is similar to conventional filament winding. A mandrel, suitably coated with release agent, is wrapped with an epoxide resin impregnated glass tape over this is wound a 150 mm high-strength steel strip angled to give 50% overlap. Epoxide resin system is applied to the steel strip to ensure that each layer is fully encapsulated. From three to 13 layers of steel may be applied to satisfy different pressure ratings. The pipe is finished by wrapping with further resin impregnated glass tape and the resin system cured. Pipe produced in this way has excellent corrosion resistance coupled with a high strength/weight ratio. It is said to provide up to 50% weight saving over conventional steel pipe.

Various processes are available for the 'on-site' construction of large filament wound storage tanks. By manufacturing these on site, transport problems are overcome and integral structures can be produced. With the various processes either horizontal or vertical mandrels are first constructed from preformed GRP sheets. These are then wrapped with resin impregnated glass rovings.

Filament wound vessels can be produced from prepreg tapes and rovings. This technique is often used with carbon fibre to reduce fibre damage during the winding operation and to permit the use of resin systems which cannot be handled by wet lay-up techniques. Here, it is essential to use a heated mandrel to melt the resin and hence displace air and consolidate and cure the laminate. Resin content of the laminate can be controlled more accurately with prepreg since the prepreg can be made with exactly the right resin content. The use of prepregs also makes for cleaner operation.

Filament winding has been used to provide a protective laminate on the outside of steel pressure pipes where external corrosion can take place. An example of this use is in the protection of the splash zone of steel riser pipes used on sea based oil and gas production platforms. Here, care has to be taken in the design of such a composite structure since the coefficient of expansion of the filament wound glass wrap can be lower than that of the steel core. If such a composite structure is produced using a heat cured resin system (say 120°C cure) and then subjected to subzero temperatures in use, the steel pipe can shrink away from the laminate and permit entry of water by capillary action. Thus the object of wrapping the pipe to prevent corrosion can be defeated, since corrosion can then still take place under the laminate. once the bond has broken it can never be remade.

2.12.6 Centrifugal moulding

Centrifugal moulding or casting is a method used for making cylindrical objects with uniform wall thickness. It is mainly used for the production of large diameter pipes, up to 5 m in diameter, from either polyester or vinyl ester resin systems, although epoxide resin systems may also be used. Pipes produced in this way are void-free and smooth on both the inner and outer surfaces. Threaded sections can be molded into the external wall if required. More recently, a system has been developed for producing tapered and curved poles by centrifugal casting.

Molds need to be bored and polished to a mirror finish and of sufficient strength to withstand, without distortion, the high G-force exerted during spinning. A steam jacket or other means of heating may be built into the mould to cure the resin system, or alternatively hot air may be blown through the mold.

Release agents used include silicones, bake-on PTFE types or PVA, although silicones are generally preferred. If the exterior of the finished pipe is to be painted then a silicone release agent should not be used. Choice of resin system must depend on application and a heat cured resin may be used, particularly where chemical resistance is required. In addition, the process lends itself to the use of several different resin systems incorporated in the one pipe, such as an abrasion resistant outer skin, a general purpose centre and a chemically resistant inner skin. The resin system used should have some degree of flexibility to give good impact resistance to the pipe, coupled with good chemical resistance. To achieve both of these requirements in the one resin system may require a compromise in properties.

Various methods of fabrication can be used. With large diameter moulds, glass and resin can be applied by the hand lay-up technique using a slow gel resin system so that the whole mold can be coated and the mould spun before gelation of the resin takes place. Here, it is necessary to tailor the reinforcement to shape to avoid overlaps.

Alternatively, the reinforcement may be wrapped round a mandrel, inserted into the mould and then unwound onto the mould surface. The mandrel is removed before resin is injected into the mold. With this technique a faster gelling resin system may be used. Woven fabrics and chopped strand mat are suitable reinforcements.

A third method, capable of being fully automated, is generally preferred. Here, resin and glass are applied to the mold surface utilizing a travelling feeder arm fitted with a chopper and spray gun, which passes slowly backwards and forwards through the mold while the mold is rotated. The laminate can be built up in layers of 0.5–1 mm thickness per pass once the reinforcement and resin system have been placed in the mold it is rotated at up to 2500 revolutions per minute (rpm) depending on mold diameter, the larger the mould diameter the slower the speed. For example, with a 2 m diameter mould a rotation speed of about 180 rpm is used. At this speed the mould surface is rotating at about 68 km/h (42.4 mph).

After the main resin system has gelled, a chemically resistant topcoat may be applied while the mold is still rotating. Mold rotation is continued until all the resin has cured.

In all of the above techniques, a relatively flexible glass reinforced resin pipe is produced, with properties similar to some of those made by filament winding. To produce stiffer pipes a modification to the spray technique has been developed and is in use commercially. Stiffer pipes, particularly in the larger diameter range, offer considerable advantages in handling and installation and maintain their shape during installation.

With this modified process, which is fully automatic, the mold is coated with release agent and rotated at a suitable speed. The feeder arm is designed in such a way that it can deliver programmed amounts of resin, chopped glass and a filler such as sand, to the mold surface as it moves in and out of the mold. In this way a layer of abrasion resistant sand filled resin system can be applied to the mold surface over this is applied a layer of glass reinforced resin. By suitable design of the chopper unit, fibre orientation can be controlled. Next a layer of sand filled resin is applied followed by a further layer of glass reinforced resin. Depending on the type and size of pipe to be produced, several more layers of GRP alternated with filled resin may be added. Finally, the inner surface is coated with a suitable chemically resistant layer of resin, which may be lightly filled or reinforced, to give a smooth corrosion resistant lining.

The equipment used can be programmed to feed materials to the mould to build up the pipe wall thickness at a rate of between 0.5 and 1 mm per pass and to compact the materials by centrifugal force throughout the whole production cycle once the final layer of resin has been applied, hot air is passed through the mold to assist curing of the resin system. The mould is cooled to ambient temperature to assist removal of the finished pipe, which is pushed out using a hydraulically operated ram. Using this technique, rigid hard wearing pipes can be produced, tailored to meet end user requirements. This is a simplified version of the pipes produced commercially, to illustrate pipe construction. In practice several more layers of glass and sand filled system may be incorporated in the pipe wall. A range of bends and joints is also available to meet most needs.

In the Usui process for producing tapered pipes, the glass fibre reinforcement is wound round a tapered mandrel to make a preform. This is inserted into the mould in the centrifugal machine and the mandrel removed. Resin is poured in and the mold tilted to a pre-determined angle and then rotated until the resin has cured.

To produce a curved tapered pipe, a flexible mold is used. This is bent to the required shape once the preform has been placed in position. It is also claimed that base plates can be simultaneously molded on by this method. These base plates are first preformed and then inserted into the mold where they become firmly bonded into the pole. Typical applications include poles for street lighting, flag poles and aerials.

2.12.7 Continuous sheet manufacture

For the purposes of this book, only those processes for which polyester resins and, to a limited extent, epoxide resins are used will be described. It should be noted, however, that the decorative laminates used in building and transport applications are in the main manufactured from melamine faced phenolic resin/paper laminates.

Several patented processes exist for continuous sheet production, all of which are similar in broad principle.

Resin and glass reinforcement are sandwiched between two sheets of release film, such as Melinex, Mylar or Cellophane and passed through rollers to consolidate the laminate before curing in an oven. Resin is applied to the release film either by spray or trickle process, care being taken to ensure that application is uniform. Glass reinforcement is laid in the resin and a second layer of release film applied. This sandwich is passed through a series of rollers to expel all air bubbles and consolidate the laminate to the correct thickness. During the next stage the laminate sandwich is either passed directly through an oven to produce flat sheet or through rollers or dies and then an oven to produce corrugated sheet. Once cured the sheet is trimmed to the required width and cut into suitable lengths. Depending on the process, corrugations may run longitudinally or transversely. Production speeds of up to 12 m/min are possible.

To produce clear sheeting the refractive index of the resin system must match that of the glass reinforcement. For this reason special resins have been developed which match the refractive index of E-glass. For translucent sheeting A-glass may be used but, due to its low refractive index, it is unsuitable for use in transparent sheeting. In any case today A-glass is rarely found.

Generally the glass reinforcement used consists of chopped strand mat with a soluble polyester powder binder or chopped rovings deposited directly into the resin film. However, for certain applications woven fabrics may be used. With the latter and to a much lesser extent with chopped strand mat, the glass cloth may be drawn through a resin bath and excess resin removed between doctor blades or rollers, before placing between two layers of release film and processing as before.

With high quality sheeting a surfacing tissue may be used to ensure a resin-rich finish. Such sheeting must be installed with the resin-rich surface exposed to the weather.

Resin systems are generally specifically formulated for each machine, since gel time and viscosity must suit the particular operating conditions of the machine. Resin systems used include those suitable for producing clear fire retardant sheeting.

By the correct choice of resin system, sheeting can be manufactured which will not yellow to any extent after exposure to tropical weather conditions for several years. However, to ensure that this is the case the resin system must be chosen with care and must be fully cured. Also the release film must be removed before installation and the laminate should contain not less than 75% by weight of resin. In other cases the resin content of the laminate may fall between 65 and 75% by weight.

2.12.8 Pultrusion

Pultrusion is a technique used for producing continuous fibre reinforced sections in which the orientation of the fibres is kept constant during cure. The process is suitable for use with both polyester and epoxide resin systems, reinforced with glass, carbon or synthetic fibres. An infinite number of profiles can be produced using appropriate dies and includes rods, tubes and flat and angled sections. All profiles have high strength and stiffness in the lengthwise direction, with fibre content generally around 60–65% by volume.

The reinforcements used consist of continuous fibres such as glass rovings or continuous carbon fibre tows, woven rovings or chopped strand mat or a combination of the two, depending on the strength and rigidity required in the molded profile.

Two processes are available which use liquid resin systems. In the first the reinforcement is drawn through an impregnating bath containing catalysed resin. For this process, a resin system with a long pot-life at room temperature is necessary. The reinforcement is then drawn through a heated die which removes excess resin, determines the cross-sectional shape and cures the resin system.

In the second process the reinforcement, accurately positioned and under tension, is drawn through a heated metal die where impregnation of the fibres and cure of the resin system takes place. Here, by the use of appropriate resin injection equipment, a short pot-life system can be used. Typical resin injection pressures are between 0.1 and 0.5 MPa. To speed up cure, the reinforcement may be pre-heated to about 100°C before passing through the die. Production rates of I m/min can be achieved. By careful design of the pulling mechanism, consistent profiles can be produced with no bending or twisting of the fibres. With some resin systems a tunnel oven may be required after the die to give a suitable post cure.

Apart from the wet processes it is also possible to make pultruded sections from prepregs. The forming procedure is the same as that used with wet resin systems. The prepreg is drawn through a heated die which melts the resin, compresses the prepreg into the required shape and cures the resin. This is a somewhat cleaner process than that using a resin bath.

It is reported that sandwich panels are being produced in the USA by pultrusion. In this process a plywood core is completely encased in a 3 mm thick glass polyester skin, resin penetrating the plywood during production to give increased bond strength and moisture resistance.

2.13 MECHANICAL PROPERTIES

A summary of the mechanical properties of the most important matrix materials and their composites with different reinforcing fibers are presented in Tables 2.8–2.39.

Table 2.8 Properties of a Typical Filled and Unfilled Polypropylene (1)

Properties	*PP*	*PP 40% Talc*	*PP 40% $CaCO_3$*	*PP 40% Glass*	*PP 30% Graphite*
T_g °C	170	168	168	163	168
Heat deflection temperature, 1.82 MPa °C	55	100	80	160	120
Maximum resistance to continuous heat °C	100	120	110	135	125
Coefficient of linear expansion cm/cm×10^{-5} °C	9	6	4	3	3
Tensile strength, MPa	35	32	26	82	47
% Elongation	150	5	15	2	0.5
Flexural strength MPa	48	60	45	100	62
Compressive strength, MPa	45	52	35	64	55
Notched Izod impact J/m	42	27	42	90	56
Hardness Rockwell	R90	R100	R88	R105	R100
Specific gravity	0.90	1.25	1.23	1.22	1.04

Table 2.9 Properties of a Typical PEEK Resin (1)

Properties	*PEEK*	*PEEK 30% Glass*	*PEEK 30% Graphite*
T_g°C	334	334	334
Heat deflection temperature, 1.82 MPa °C	165	282	282
Maximum resistance to continous heat °C	150	270	270
Coefficient of linear expansion cm/cm×10^{-5} °C	5.5	2.1	1.5
Tensile strength MPa	100	162	173
% Elongation	40	2	2
Flexural strength MPa	110	255	313
Notched Izod impact J/m	150	110	70
Hardness Rockwell	R123	R123	R123
Specific gravity	1.32	1.44	1.32

Table 2.10 Properties of a Typical Polyetherimide Resins (1)

Properties	*PEI*	*PEI 10% Glass*	*PEI 20% Glass*	*PEI 30% Glass*	*PEI 30% Graphite*
T_g °C	216	216	216	216	216
Heat deflection temperature, 1.82 MPa °C	195	200	205	210	210
Maximum resistance to continuous heat °C	165	170	175	180	180
Coefficient of linear expansion cm/cm×10^{-5} °C	5	4	3	2	2
Tensile strength MPa	105	114	138	169	216
% Elongation	7	5	4	3	2
Flexural strength MPa	144	193	205	225	283
Compressive strength MPa	140	155	162	175	220
Notched Izod impact J/m	55	60	85	110	75
Hardness Rochvell	M110	M116	M120	M125	M127
Specific gravity	1.3	1.35	1.45	1.5	1.4

Table 2.11 Properties of Typical Polycarbonate Sheets (1)

Properties	*PC*	*PC 10% Glass*	*PC 30% Glass*	*PC 40% Glass*	*PC 40% Graphite*	*Polyester carbon-ate*
T_g °C	150	150	150	150	150	160
Heat deflection temperature, 1.82 MPa °C	139	142	144	144	146	150
Maximum resistance to continuous heat °C	125	130	130	130	130	135
Coefficient of linear expansion cm/cmx10^{-5} °C	7	2	1	1	1	8
Tensile strength MPa	65	65	135	165	165	73
% Elongation	110	6	3	3	2	90
Flexural strength MPa	93	105	155	93	240	240
Notched Izod impact J/m	130	110	90	100	90	300
Hardness Rockwell	M70	M75	M92	R118	R119	M85
Specific gravity	1.2	1.28	1.4	1.35	1.35	1.2

Table 2.12 Properties of Polyphenylene Sulfide Resins (1)

Properties	*PPS*	*PPS 40% Glass*	*PPS 40% Graphite*
T_g °C	290	290	280
Heat deflection temperature, 1.82 MPa °C	133	260	260
Maximum resistance to continuous heat °C	120	240	240
Coefficient of linear expansion cm/cm×10^{-5} °C	5	2	1
Tensile strength MPa	65	135	160
% Elongation	2	2	1.5
Flexural strength MPa	95	185	210
Compressive strength MPa	95	160	180
Notched Izod impact J/m	25	80	55
Hardness Rockwell	R123	R123	R123
Specific gravity	1.3	1.65	1.45

Table 2.13 Properties of a Typical Polyarylate (1)

Heat deflection temperature, 1.82 MPa °C	174
Maximum resistance to continuous heat °C	150
Coefficient of linear expansion cm/cm×10^{-5} °C	6.5
Tensile strength MPa	68
% Elongation	50
Flexural strength MPa	74
Compressive strength MPa	93
Notched Izod impact J/m	210
Hardness Rockwell	R125
Specific gravity	1.2

Table 2.14 Properties of Typical Polyamide-Imide Plastics (1)

Properties	*PAI*	*PAI 30% Glass*	*PAI 30% Graphite*
T_g °C	275	275	275
Heat deflection temperature, 1.82 MPa °C	275	275	275
Maximum resistance to continuous heat °C	260	260	260
Coefficient of linear expansion cm/cm×10^{-5} °C	3.6	1.8	2.0
Tensile strength MPa	150	195	205
% Elongation	13	6	6
Flexural strength MPa	200	315	315
Compressive strength MPa	258	300	300
Notched Izod impact J/m	135	105	45
Hardness Rockwell	E78	E94	E94
Specific gravity	1.39	1.57	1.41

Table 2.15 Properties of Typical Polysulfones (1)

Properties	*Polysulfone (Udel) Glass*	*Polysulfone 30% Graphite*	*Polysulfone 30%*	*Polyether sulfone (Victrex)*	*PES 20% Glass*	*PES 30% Graphite*	*Modified Polysulfone*	*Modified Polysulfone 30% Glass*
Heat deflection temperature, 1.82 MPa °C	190	198	190	200	210	210	150	150
Maximum resistance to continuous heat °C	170	175	175	185	200	200	150	150
Coefficient of linear expansion cm/cm×10^{-5} °C	6	2.5	2.5	5.5	2	1	4	5
Tensile strength MPa	70	100	100	138	127	190	43	115
% Elongation	5	115	115	85	2	115	50	2
Flexural strength MPa	106	200	215	120	175	250	85	175
Compressive strength MPa	176	95	175	95	150	150	125	150
Notched Izod impact J/m	64	58	64	110	75	75	150	75
Hardness Rockwell	M69	M95	M80	M88	M98	R123	R117	M80
Specific gravity	1.25	1.5	1.36	1.4	1.5	1.5	1.35	1.5

Table 2.16 Properties of typical Nylons (1)

Properties	*Nylon 6*	*Nylon-6 30% glass*	*Nylon-6 30% graphite*	*Nylon-66*	*Nylon 66 30% glass*	*Nylon 66 30% graphite*	*Nylon 66 40% clay*	*Nylon 66 50% mica*
T_g °C	226	215	215	265	265	265	265	215
Heat deflection temperature, 1.82 MPa °C	78	210	215	75	250	260	190	230
Maximum resistance to continuous heat °C	65	190	205	100	225	240	150	170
Coefficient of linear expansion cm/cm × 10^{-5} °C	8	4	5	8	2	2	3	3
Tensile strength MPa	62	138	205	82	180	227	75	90
% Elongation	30	5	3	60	4	3	9	9
Flexural strength MPa	96	150	135	103	180	170	160	150
Compressive strength MPa	55	130	155	55	110	88	50	85
Notched Izod impact J/m	R119	M85	M80	M85	M85	R120	M80	M80
Hardness Rockwell	1.13	1.38	1.28	1.14	1.37	1.35	1.4	1.4
Specific gravity	96	275	315	103	275	330	205	400

Table 2.17 Properties of typical Nylons (1)

Properties	*Nylon 69*	*Nylon 6–10*	*Nylon 6–12*	*Nylon 6–12 35% Glass*	*Nylon 11*	*Nylon 12*	*Aramid*
T_g °C	205	220	210	210	192	177	275
Heat deflection temperature, 1.82 MPa °C	55	60	69	216	150	146	260
Maximum resistance to continuous heat °C	60	70	75	200	140	135	150
Coefficient of linear expansion cm/cm×10^{-5} °C	8	8	8	6	10	8	3
Tensile strength MPa	58	60	50	145	55	55	120
% Elongation	80	125	200	4	200	225	5
Flexural strength MPa	40	40	44	80	40	42	172
Compressive strength MPa	100	90	90	150	80	80	207
Notched Izod impact J/m	60	60	60	96	96	110	75
Hardness Rockwell	R111	R105	M78	M93	R108	R105	E90
Specific gravity	1.09	1.08	1.08	1.35	1.04	1.01	1.2

Table 2.18 Typical properties of Discontinuous Graphite-Fiber-Reinforced Thermoplastic Composites (8)

Property	*Nylon 66 30% C*	*Polysulfone 30%*	*Polyester 30%*	*Polyphenilene sulfide 30%C*	*ETFE 30%C*
Specific gravity	1.28	1.32	1.47	1.45	1.73
Water absorption (24hr), %	0.5	0.15	0.04	0.004	0.015
Equilibrium, %	2.4	0.38	0.23	0.1	0.24
Mold shrinkage, %	1.5–2.5	2–3	1–2	1	1.5–2.5
Tensile strength, ksi (MPa)	35 (241)	19 (131)	20 (138)	27 (186)	15 (103)
Tensile elongation, %	3–4	2–3	2–3	2–3	2–3
Flexural strength, ksi (MPa)	51 (351)	25.5 (176)	29 (200)	34 (234)	20 (138)
Flexural modulus of elasticity, Msi (GPa)	2.9 (20)	2.05 (14.1)	2.0 (13.8)	2.45 (16.9)	1.65 (11.4)
Shear strength ft-lb/in (J/m)	13 (89.6)	7 (48.1)	–	–	7 (48.2)
Izod impact strength ft-lb/in (J/m)	1.5 (80.1)	1.1 (58.7)	1.2 (64.1)	1.1 (58.7)	4–5 213–267)
Thermal deflection temperature at 264 psi (1.82 MPa), °F	495 (257)	365 (185)	430 (221)	500 (260)	465 (241)
Coefficient of linear thermal expansion, in/in., °F×10^{-5} (m/m/°C×10^{-5})	1.05 (1.89)	0.7 (1.26)	0.5 (0.9)	0.6 (1.08)	0.8 (1.44)
Thermal conductivity, BTU-in/hr ft² °F (W/m°C)	7.0 (12.1)	5.5 (9.5)	6.5 (11.2)	5.2 (9.0)	5.6 (9.7)
Surface resistivity, Ω/m²	3–5	1–3	2–4	1–3	3–5

Table 2.19 Typical properties of Discontinuous Graphite-Fiber-Reinforced Thermoplastic Composites (8)

Property	*Polypropilene 30%C*	*Polycarbonate 30% C*	*VF2-TFE 20%C*
Specific gravity	1.06	1.36	1.77
Water absorption (24hr), %	—	—	0.03
Equilibrium, %	—	—	—
Mold shrinkage, %	5	2	2.5–3.5
Tensile strength, ksi (MPa)	5.4 (37.2)	11.5 (79.2)	12.3 (84.7)
Tensile elongation, %	2.2	2.1	3–4
Flexural strength, ksi (MPa)	6.7 (46.2)	17.1 (118)	17.2 (119)
Flexural modulus of elasticity, Msi (GPa)	0.60 (4.1)	1.08 (7.44)	1.10 (7.58)
Shear strength ft-lb/in (J/m)	—	—	7.5 (51.7)
Izod impact strength ft-lb/in (J/m)	0.7 (37.4)	3.0 (160.2)	2.6 (138.8)
Thermal deflection temperature at 264 psi 1.82 MPa), °F	295 (146)	293 (145)	248 (120)
Coefficient of linear thermal expansion, in./in., °F×10^{-5} (m/m/°C×10^{-5}	3.0 (5.4)	1.6 (2.8)	1.6 (2.8)
Thermal conductivity, BTU-in/hr ft^2 °F (W/m°C)	3.0 (5.7)	—	—
Surface resistivity, Ω/m^2	3–5	—	—

Table 2.20 Properties of a Typical Styrene Polymer (1)

Properties	*PS*	*PS 30% Glass*
Heat deflection temperature, 1.82 MPa °C	90	105
Maximum resistance to continuous heat °C	75	95
Coefficient of linear expansion cm/cm×10^{-5} °C	7.5	4.0
Tensile strength MPa	41	82
% Elongation	1.5	1.0
Flexural strength MPa	83	117
Compressive strength MPa	90	103
Notched Izod impact J/m	21	20
Hardness Rockwell	M65	M70
Specific gravity	1.04	1.2

Table 2.21 Properties of Typical Polyester Resins (1)

Properties	*PET*	*PET 30% glass*	*PET 45% glass*	*PET 30% glass*	*PBT*	*PBT 30% glass*	*PBT 45% glass*	*PBT 30% glass*
T_g °C	255		255	255	245	245	245	245
Heat deflection temperature, 1.82 MPa °C	220		225	225	85	210	210	215
Maximum resistance to continuous heat °C	200		210	210	80	200	200	205
Coefficient of linear expansion cm/cm×10^{-5} °C	6.5		2	3	6	2.5	2	3
Tensile strength MPa	58		165	175	50	220	90	155
% Elongation	100		3	115	100	3	3	2
Flexural strength MPa	110		175	260	100	175	140	215
Compressive strength MPa	90		155	105	98	145	105	100
Notched Izod impact J/m	35		75	75	40	50	50	70
Hardness Rockwell	M97		R118	R125	M72	M90	M80	R120
Specific gravity	1.35		1.6	1.4	1.34	1.5	1.7	1.41

Table 2.22 Properties of Typical Polyimides (1)

Properties	*PI*	*PI 40% graphite*
T_g °C	330	365
Heat deflection temperature, 1.82 MPa °C	315	360
Maximum resistance to continuous heat °C	290	810
Coefficient of linear expansion cm/cm×10^{-5} °C	5	4
Tensile strength MPa	96	44
% Elongation	9	3
Flexural strength MPa	165	145
Compressive strength MPa	240	125
Notched Izod impact J/m	83	38
Hardness Rockwell	E70	E27
Specific gravity	1.4	1.65

Table 2.23 Properties of DAP (1)

Properties	*DAP*	*Fiber glass filled*	*Mineral filled*
Heat deflection temperature, 1.82 MPa °C	155	225	200
Maximum resistance to continuous heat °C	100	210	200
Coefficient of linear expansion cm/cm×10^{-5} °C	—	3	3.5
Tensile strength MPa	27.6	50	45
% Elongation	4.6	4	4
Flexural strength MPa	62.0	90	65
Compressive strength MPa	150	205	170
Notched Izod impact J/m	14	50	16
Hardness Rockwell	E115	E84	E61
Specific gravity	11.3	1.80	1.75

Table 2.24 Properties Of Typical Amino Plastics (1)

Properties	*Cellulose-filled UF*	*Fberglass-filled MF*
Heat deflection temperature, 1.82 MPa °C	175	200
Maximum resistance to continuous heat °C	100	175
Coefficient of linear expansion cm/cm×10^{-5} °C	4.0	1.6
Tensile strength MPa	65	50
% Elongation	0.7	0.7
Flexural strength MPa	90	130
Compressive strength MPa	275	310
Notched Izod impact J/m	16	100
Hardness Rockwell	M120	M120
Specific gravity	1.50	1.9

Table 2.25 Properties of fiberglass Composites with Different Thermosets (1)

Properties	*Diallyl phthalate*	*Epoxy*	*Phenolic*	*Polyester*	*Polyamide*
Heat deflection temperature 1.8 MPa °C	225	150	200	200	350
Maximum continuous use temperature °C	210	140	175	160	310
Coefficient of linear expansion cm/cm×10^{-5} °C	3	2	2	2.5	1.3
Tensile strength, MPa	50	83	41	70	44
% Elongation	4	4	1.5	1	1
Flexural strength, MPa	90	103	172	172	145
Compressive strength, MPa	205	100	200	200	300
Notched Izod impact J/m	50	25	175	200	300
Hardness Rockwell	E84	M105	M110	M50	M118
Specific gravity	1.8	1.9	1.5	2	1.6

Table 2.26 Properties of the Most Common Resin for High Performance Composites

Materials	*Tensile strength (MPa)*	*Flexural modulus (MPa)*	*Density (gcm^{-3})*	*Max service temperature (°C)*	*Coefficient of thermal expansion (10^{-50}°C^{-1})*	*Water absorption (24 h%)*
Epoxy	35–85	15–35	1.38	25–85	8–12	0.1
Polyimide	120	35	1.46	380	9	0.3
PEEK	92	40	1.30	140	6–9	0.1
Polyamide/imide	95	50	1.38	200	6.3	0.3
Polyether/imide	105	35	1.27	200	5.6	0.25
Polyphenylene/sulfide	70	40	1.32	75	9.9	0.2
Phenolics	50–55	10–24	1.30	50–175	4.5–11	0.1–0.2

Table 2.27 Properties of Polyester Composites Reinforced by Continuous and Chopped Fiberglass

Continuous Filament (%)	*Chopped Glass (%)*	*Tensile Strength MPa*	*Flexural Strength MPa*	*Transverse Tensile Strength MPa*	*Transverse Flexural Strength MPa*
75	0	690	1200	24	35
65	10	660	1135	27	90
45	20	570	980	60	155
25	50	500	810	95	200
15	60	410	680	125	260

Table 2.28 Typical properties of cured polyester resins

	Cast resin properties				*Laminate properties*				
Resin	*Flexural strength (MPa)*	*Tensile strength (GPa)*	*Tensile Modulus (GPa)*	*% Elongation*	*HDT (°C)*	*% glass*	*Flexural strength (MPa)*	*Tensile strength (MPa)*	*Tensile modulus (GPa)*
Orthophthalic	100	65–75	3.2	2.0–4.0	55–110	30	150	90	7
Isophthalic	140	70–75	3.5	3.5	75–130	30	230	120	8
Neo-pentylglycol	130	70	3.4	2.4	110	30	170	90	7
Isophthalic/ neopentylglycol	130	60	3.4	2.5	90–115	30	160	90	7
HET acid	80	40–50	3.2	1.3–4.0	55–80	30	150	85	7
Isophthalic/ HET acid	85	55	3.2	2.9	70	30	150	90	7
Bisphenol A	130	60–75	3.2	2.5–4.0	120–136	30	170	90	7
Chlorinated paraffin	110	50–60	3.4	1.2–4.8	55–80	30	140	90	7
Isophthalic/ chlorinated paraffin	90	60	2.0	4.8	50	30	140	100	7

Table 2.29 Characteristics of Epoxy resins (8)

Resin	*Description*	*Characteristics and end uses*
Epocryl® Resin 12	A neat dimethacrylate ester of a low-molecular-weight bisphenol A epoxy resin	Nominal 1 000 000 cp (1 kPa sec) viscosity designed for molding, adhesives, and electrical prepreg
Epocryl® Resin 370	A neat diacrylate ester of a low-molecular-weight bisphenol A expoxy resin	Base resin for formulation of UV-cure inks and coating
CoRezyn VE-8100 Derakane® 411-C-50 Epocryl® Resin 321	A dimethacrylate ester of an intermediate-molecular-weight bisphenol A epoxy resin containing 50 wt% styrene	Nominal 100 cP (5 dPa sec) viscosity designed for chemical-resistant FRP applications: hand lay-up and filament winding
Corrolite 31–345 CoRezyn VE-8300 Derakane® 411–45 Epocryl® Resin	A dimethacrylate ester of a high-molecular-weight bisphenol A epoxy resin containing 45 wt% styrene	Nominal 500 cP (5 dPa sec) viscosity designed for Chemical-resistant FRP applications: hand lay-up and filament winding
Derakane® 470–36	A methacrylate ester of a phenolicnovolac epoxy resin containing 36 wt% styrene	Nominal 200 cP (2 dPa sec) viscosity designed for solvent resistance and high-service-temperature FRP applications
Epocryl® Resin	A methacrylate ester of a low-molecular-weight bisphenol A epoxy resin containing 40 wt % styrene	Nominal 500 cP (5 dPa sec) viscosity designed for solvent resistance and high-service-temperature FRP applications. Exhibits high tensile strengths and elongation with high modulus. Designed for filament winding and hand lay-up applications
Derakane® 510A40	A dimethacrylate ester of a brominated bisphenol A epoxy resin containing 40 wt% styrene	Nominal 350 cP (3.5 dPa sec) viscosity designed to impart fire retardancy for chemical-resistant FRP applications

Table 2.30 Shear Properties of Composites of Kevlar 49 Fiber in Epoxy Resins (8)

Epoxy System (weight ratio)	*Cure Cycle hours/°C (hours/°F)*	*Shear Failure Stress MPa (CV)*	*Shear Strain at Failure Stress % (CV)*	*Secant Shear Modulus at 0.5% Shear Strain MPa (CV)*
XD 7818/ERL 4206/Tonox 60–40	2.5/80 + 2/160 (2.5/176 + 2/320)	21.4 (2.6)	1.35 (2.2)	1884 (3.9)
DER 332/ Jeffamine T-403 (100/39)	24/60 (24/140)	29.4 (2.0)	173 (2.3)	1923 (4.7)
ERL 2256/Tonox 60–40 (100/25/28.3)	16/50 + 2/120 (16/122 + 2/248)	23.0 (8.6)	1.49 (2.2)	1775 (0.9)
Epon 826/RD2/ Tonox 60–40 (100/25/28.3)	3/60 + 2/120 (3/140 + 2/248)	23.4 (6.3)	1.91 (6.5)	1520 (3.9)
XB 2793/Tonox 60–40 (100/25.6)	2/90 + 2/160 (2/194 + 2.320)	21.9 (0.3)	1.69 (2.9)	1600
XD 7818/XD 7575.02/XD 7114/Tonox 60/DAP (50/50/45/14.1/14.1)	5/80 + 3/120 (5/176 + 3/248)	39.7 (0.9)	2.43 (2.5)	1852 (1.7)
XD 7818/XD 7114/Tonox LC (100/45/50.3)	5/60 + 3/120	31.9 (3.4)	1.91 (4.5)	1850 (1.5)

Table 2.31 Properties of a typical PMMA Sheet* (1)

Heat deflection temperature at 1.8 MPa (°C)	96
Maximum resistance to continuous heat (°C)	90
Coefficient of linear expansion cm/cm/°C×10^{-5}	7.6
Tensile strength (MPa)	72
Percent elongation	5
Flexural strength (MPa)	110
Compressive strength (MPa)	124
Notched Izod impact (J/m)	74
Hardness Rockwell	M93
Specific gravity	1.19

*Polymethyl methocrylate (PMMA) is largely used for biomedical applications, optical fibers and cultured marble.

Table 2.32 Properties of Typical Polyfluorocarbons (1)

Properties	*PFTE*	*PCTFE*	*PVDF*	*PVF*
Heat deflection temperature 1.8 MPa (°C)	100	100	80	90
Maximum resistance to continuous heat (°C)	250	200	150	125
Coefficient of linear expansion cm/cm °C × 10^{-5}	10	14	8.5	10
Tensile strength, MPa	24	34	55	65
Flexural strength MPa	50	60	75	90
Notched Izod impact J/m	160	100	150	100
% Elongation	200	100	200	200
Hardness, Rockwell	D52	R80	R110	R83
Specific gravity	2.16	2.1	1.76	1.4

Table 2.33 Properties of typical Filled PTFE (1)

Properties	*Unfilled PTFE*	*15% Glass*	*25% Glass*	*15% Graphite*	*60% Bronze*
Thermal conductivity mW/MK	0.244	0.37	0.45	0.45	0.46
Tensile strength MPa	28	25	17.5	21	14
% Elongation	350	300	250	250	150
Notched Izod impact J/m	152	146	119	100	75
Coefficient of friction, 3.4 MPa load	0.08	0.13	0.13	0.10	0.10
Wear factor 1/pPa	5013	280	26	102	12
Shore durometer hardness	51D	54D	57D	61D	70D
Specific gravity	2.18	2.21	2.24	2.16	3.74

Table 2.34 Properties of Typical LDPE Plastics (1)

Glass transition temperature (°C)	-25
Coefficient of linear expansion cm/cm °C$\times 10^{-5}$	15
Tensile strength MPa	20
%Elongation	350
Shore hardness	47D
Specific gravity	0.925

Table 2.35 Properties of a typical Filled and Unfilled HDPE (1)

Properties	*HDPE*	*30% Glass-Filled HDPE*
Melting point (°C)	130	140
Heat deflection temp. at 1.82 MPa (°C)	40	120
Maximum resistance to continuous heat (°C)	40	110
Coefficient of linear expansion cm/cm°C$\times 10^{-5}$	10	5
Tensile strength MPa	27	62
% Elongation	100	1.5
Flexural strength MPa	—	76
Compressive strength MPa	21	43
Notched Izod impact J/m	133	64
Hardness Rockwell	D40	R75
Specific gravity	0.95	1.3

Table 2.36 Thermal and Electrical Properties of Kevlar 49 Fabric/Epoxy Composites (8)

Property	*Value*
Thermal conductivity (46 volume % fiber)	
Across fabric layers, W/m °K	0.22
Parallel to warp, W/m °K	0.91
Thermal coefficient of expansion (20–100°C)	0
Dielectric constant (58 volume % fiber)	
Perpendicular at 9.3×10^9 Hz (room temperature)	3.3
Parallel at 9.3×10^9 Hz (room temperature)	3.7
Perpendicular (48 volume % fiber) at 10^6 Hz	4.1
Dielectric strength (48 volume % fiber), V/mm (V/mil)	24.4
Volume resistivity (48 volume % fiber), ½-cm	5×10^{15}
Surface resistivity (48 volume % fiber), ½ cm	5×10^{15}
Arc resistance (48 volume % fiber), seconds	125

Table 2.37 Property of Unidirectional Thornel 300-Kevlar 49/Epoxy Hybrid Composites (8)

		Tension				Compression				Flexure					
Ratio Thornel to Kevlar	*Specific gravity*	*Modulus GPa*	*Modulus (Msi)*	*Ultimate stress MPa*	*Ultimate stress (ksi)*	*Stress at 0.02% offset (ksi)*	*Stress at 0.02% offset (ksi)*	*Ultimate stress MPa*	*Ultimate stress (ksi)*	*Stress at 0.02% offset MPa*	*Stress at 0.02% offset (ksi)*	*Ultimate stress sMPa*	*Ultimate stress (ksi)*	*Short-beam-shear stress*	*Short-beam shear stress*
100/0	1.60	145	(21.1)	1565	(227)	678	(98.4)	1007	(146)	1605	(223)	1606	(233)	91	(13.2)*
75/25	1.56	120	(17.4)	1281	(186)	469	(68.8)	938	(136)	1248	(181)	1358	(197)	76	(11.0)
50/50	1.51	108	(15.7)	1213	(176)	413	(59.9)	688	(99.8)	827	(120)	1103	(160)	56	(8.1)
0/100	1.35	77	(11.2)	1262	(183)	182	(26.4)	286	(41.5)	339	(49.2)	634	(91.9)	49	(7.1)

Table 2.38 Properties of Epoxy Resin Composites with Different Reinforcing Fibers

Properties	*E-Glass*	*S-Glass*	*Aramid Kevlar 49*	*Graphite*	*Boron*
Thermal conductivity W/mK	0.9	1.1	0.9	5	1
Linear expansion cm/cm°C×10^{-5}	1.2	1.1	1	2	1
Tensile strength MPa	450	700	800	700	1600
Elastic modulus MPa	24 000	30 000	33 000	60 000	207 000
Fracture toughness MPa $m^{1/2}$	22	25	34	18	35
Specific gravity	2.1	2.0	1.4	1.6	2.1

Table 2.39 Properties of Fiberglass-reinforced Polyester Composites with Different Fabrication Techniqes (1)

Properties	*SMC*	*BMC*	*Preform mat*	*Cold-molding*	*Spray-press up*	*Filament wound (epoxy)*	*Pultruded*
Glass content %	22	25	30	25	40	55	60
Heat deflection temp.	225	225	205	190	190	190	175
Maximum resistance to continuous heat °C	180	175	185	180	185	150	200
Coefficient of linear expansion °C×10^{-5}	1.0	1.0	1.4	1.4	1.6	4	5
Tensile strength KPa	90	48	110	110	95	120	80
% Elongation	1	0.5	1.5	1.5	1.0	2.0	2.0
Flexural strength KPa	165	100	220	190	150	1250	1000
Compressive strength MPa	80	30	150	125	135	400	340
Notched Izod impact J/m	640	240	800	560	425	2660	2750
Hardness Rockwell	H75	H95	H70	H70	H70	M110	H96
Specific gravity	1.9	1.9	1.9	1.6	1.5	1.9	1.8

2.14 ANTIOXIDANTS AND EFFECT OF ENVIRONMENTAL EXPOSURE

Many of the polymeric matrices will require some type of antioxidants to improve aging properties. The most common primary antioxidants are hindered phenols such as butylated hydroxytoluene (BHT). Typical low toxic antioxidants are reported in Tables 2.40–2.42.

Table 2.40 Typical antioxidants of low toxicity (3)

Primary antioxidants (usually hindered phenols)	Butylated hydroxytoluene (BHT)
Thioester antioxidants (usually derivates of thiodipropionic acid)	Dilaryl thiodipropionate (DLTDP) Distearyl thiodipropionate (DSTDP)
Phosphite antioxidants (usually derivates of aromatic phosphites)	Distearyl pentaerythritol diphosphite Tris (nonylphenyl) phosphite

The toxicity of commonly used polymer stabilizers and additives are classified in the following table.

Table 2.41 Toxicity of commonly used polymer stabilizers and additives (3)

Stabilizer	*Toxicity*
Fatty acid derivates of calcium, zinc and magnesium	Low toxicity. Used in non-toxic medical applications
Barium fatty acid compounds	Moderately toxic
Lead & cadmium derivates	Highly toxic. Not recommended in the US for use in medical applications (cadmium pigments considered of low toxicity in England)
Amines (antioxidants)	Generally toxic, with aromatic amines showing carcinogenic tendencies. Newer types less toxic
Butylated hydroxytoluene (BHT) (antioxidant)	Considered non-toxic as also used in foods. Recently investigated and found non-carcinogenic
Octyl tin compounds	Only class of tin compound classified as of low toxicity and used in medical applications e.g. di-(n-octyl)tin maleate polymer

Table 2.42 Toxicity data on some common plasticizers used in plastic manufacture (3)

Plasticizer	Toxicity
Adipates	To date animal experiments indicate possible carcinogenicity
Glycolates	Generally of low toxicity levels. However studies underway as commercial form are phthalyl derivates
Phosphates	Generally cause irritation to skin and mucous membranes
Phthalates	Although commercially used in medical devices, environmental effects and toxicological properties continually under investigation
Epoxidized soya bean oil	Chelating type of plasticizer with low toxicity

2.15 THE RADIATION STABILITY OF COMMERCIAL MATERIALS

The radiation resistance of common polymeric materials used as matrix for composite are shown in Tables 2.43–2.52. Generally, polystyrene and urethane rubber have the most resistance.

Table 2.43 The radiation resistance of common materials used as matrix of polymeric composites (3)

Material	*Stability effect*
ABS	Stable for single dose of 2.5 Mrad
Polyamides	Suitable for single doses of 2.5 Mrad level
Polyethylene	Stable under ordinary conditions at 2.5 Mrad
Polypropylene	Embrittles – newer variations more resistant
Poly(vinyl chloride)	Withstands single dose radiation cycle – but discolors – some HCl liberated
Polystyrene	Most radiation – stable of common polymers
Poly(tetrafluoroethylene)	Poor resistance to radiation – copolymers less affected
Polysulfone	Stable under ordinary conditions at 2.5 Mrad
Polyacetals	Embrittles – discolors
Polyurethane	Stable under ordinary conditions at 2.5 Mrad
Polymethylmethacrylate	Embrittles – discolors
Rubber natural	Stable under ordinary conditions when properly compounded
Rubber butyl	Poor stability at low radiation levels
Rubber silicones	Stable under ordinary conditions at 2.5 Mrad
Urethanes	Excellent radiation resistance

Table 2.44 The radiation resistance of common materials used as matris of polymeric composites (3)

Material Thermoplastics	*Stability*	
Acrylonitrile/Butadiene/Styrene (ABS)	Good	
Cellulosics	Fair	Undergoes chain scission,
esters more stable		
Fluoinated ethylene propylene (FEP)	Fair	Copolymers more resistant than Homopolymer
Polyacetal	Poor	Embrittles
Polyamides aromatic	Excellent	
Polyamides aliphatic	Fair	Hardens as levels increased
Polycarbonates	Good	Yellow – mechanical properties unchanged
Polyesters (aromatic)	Good	
Polyethylene	Good	lowers melt flow
Polymethylmethacrylate	Poor	Degrades-turns brown
Polyphenylene sulfide	Good	
Polyproplyene	Fair	Improved stability if properly stabilized
Polysulfone	Excellent	Yellow natural color
Polystyrene	Excellent	
Polytetrafluoroethylene	Poor	Acid evolved
Polyvinylchloride homopolymer	Good	If properly stabilized
Polyvinylchloride Copolymer	Fair	HCl evolved – turns brown
Styrene/Acrylonitrile (SAN)	Good	More resistant than ABS

Table 2.45 The radiation resistance of common materials used as matrix of polymeric composites (3)

Material Thermosetting resin	*Stability*	
Epoxies	Excellent	Very stable with the use of aromatic curing agen
Phenol or urea formaldehyde	Good	
Polyimides	Excellent	
Polyesters	Good	
Polyurethanes	Excellent	

Table 2.46 The radiation resistance of common materials used as matrix of polymeric composites (3)

Material elastomers	*Stability*
Polyisobutylene (butyl)	Poor
Natural	Good
Urethanes	Excellent
Nitrile	Good
Polyacrylic	Poor
Styrene-butadiene	Good
EPDM	Good
Silicones	Good

Table 2.47 The radiation resistance of polymers (3)

Textiles	*Stability*
Polyesters	Excellent
Cellulosics	Poor
Nylon	Fair

Table 2.48 Synergism between a UV absorber and a thermal antioxidant (6)

Additive (0.4 pph) UV stabilizer	*Antioxidant*	*Time to embrittlement of low-density polyethylene (in hours)*
None	None	400
Octylphenyl salicylate	None	1600
None	Tri (nonylphenyl) phosphite	1800
Octylphenyl salicylate	Tri (nonylphenyl) phosphite	7000
2-Hydroxy-4-n-octoxybenzophenone	None	2000
None	Tri (nonylphenyl) phosphite	1000
2-Hydroxy-4-n-octoxybenzophenone	Tri(nonylphenyl) phosphite	8500

Table 2.49 Stability of hydrocarbon polymers with bound phenolic antioxidants (6)

Material	*Hours to react with 10 cc of O_2 at 140°C*
Low-density polyethylene:	
Uninhibited	3
Reacted with diazooxide	14
High-density Polyethylene:	
Commercially stabilized	175
Reacted with diazooxide	411
Polypropylene	
Uninhibited	<1
Reacted with diazooxide	31

Table 2.50 Additives incorporated into natural rubber and as bound antioxidants (6)

Additive	*Hours to absorb 1% by wt. of O_2*	
	Before extraction	*After extraction*
N,N′-Diethyl-p-nitrosoaniline	39	30
p-Nitrosodiphenylaniline	60	53
p-Nitrosophenol	31	30
2,6-Diter-butyl-p-cresol	47	4

2.16 POLYMERS AGING

Table 2.51 Summary of effects of moisture and ambient aging on epoxy composites (7)

		Flexural strength, MN/m^2 (ksi)								
Orient	*Temperature K(°F)*	*Control*	*24-h H_2O boil*	*Retention %*	*6-week humidity*	*Retention*	*20-week ambient*	*Retention %*	*52-week ambient*	*Retention %*
				B/5505 boron/epoxy						
[0]	297 (75)	2070 (300)	1950 (283)	94	2120 (308)	103	2180 (316)	105	2280 (330)	110
[0]	450 (350)	1730 (251)	393 (57)	23	683 (99)	39	1030 (149)	59	910 (132)	53
[0±45]	450 (350)	862 (125)	545 (79)	63	641 (93)	74	882 (128)	102	807 (117)	94
				A-S/3501 graphite/epoxy						
[0]	297 (75)	1680 (244)	1680 (244)	100	1680 (244)	100	1850 (268)	110	1620 (235)	96
[0]	450 (350)	1300 (188)	434 (244)	34	386 (56)	30	703 (102)	54	593 (86)	46
[0±45]	450 (350)	676 (98)	365 (53)	54	276 (40)	41	545 (79)	81	386 (56)	57

Table 2.52 Summary of thermal aging of epoxy and polyimide system (7)

Material system	*Orientation*	*Aging temperature K(°F)*	*Test temperature K(°F)*	*Aging time, h*	*Retention of tensile strength, %*
B/E	[O]	394 (250)	450 (350)	1000	99
	[CP]				94
	[O]	450 (350)	450 (350)	1000	100
	[CP]				100
G/E	[O]	394 (250)	450 (350)	1000	94
	[CP]				100
	[0]	450 (350)	450 (350)	1000	100
	[CP]				100
G/PI	[O]	505 (450)	505 (450)	1000	98
	[CP]				92
	[O]	561 (550)	561 (550)	1000	87
	[CP]				100

2.17 COMPOSITE MATERIALS IN MEDICINE

In recent years, carbon fiber has been recognized as a material with many exciting applications in medicine. Several commercial products utilize carbon fiber as a reinforcing material which serves to enhance the mechanical properties of the polymeric resin systems in which it is included. The attractive feature of carbon reinforced polymer for this application is that the orientation and fiber content can be varied in the implant to provide the mechanical property orientation necessary for good function. The carbon fiber can be distributed in matrix material to provide strength in only those locations and directions where it is needed. The implant must be designed in a way that fatigue failure does not occur and the matrix material is not attacked by the physiological environment. The matrix materials used are listed in Table 2.53.

Table 2.53 Polymeric materials used as matrix for carbon fibers composites (3)

Polymer	*Polymer type*	*Commercial name and manufacturer*
Polysulfone	Thermoplastic	UDEL MG-11, Union Carbide, Dallas, TX
Poly-methyl methacrylate	Thermoplastic	PMMA I.V. 0.4, Rohm & Haas, Philadelphia, PA
Epoxy (low viscosity)	Thermoset	Stycast 1267
Epoxy (high viscosity)	Thermoset	C-8W795 & H.R. 795, Hysol Corp., Los Angeles, CA

Table 2.54 Mechanical properties of carbon fibers used in carbon prosthesis

Fibre-type	*Density (g/cm^3)*	*Diameter (μm)*	*Tensile strength (MPa)*	*Elastic modulus (GPa)*	*Strain to failure (%)*	α *(/10^{-6}K)*
T300	1.75	7	3430	230	1.5	-1.5
HM 35	1.79	6.7	2350	358	0.6	-0.5

These polymers were combined with unsized carbon fiber, into ±15° laminated, test specimens approximately 2.5 cm×7.5 cm×0.3 cm. Testing was performed in three point bending giving the results in Table 2.55.

Table 2.55 Typical Mechanical Properties of Polymer-Carbon Composites (3)

Polymer	*Ultimate strength (MPa)*	*Modulus (GPa)*
PMMA	772	55
Polysulfone	938	76
Epoxy Stycast	535	30
Epoxy Hysol	207	24

Because a composite hip will be subjected to the physiological environment in use, an accelerated test was performed to evaluate changes in properties. In this test, the samples were immersed in 0.9% saline solution maintained at 90°C for one week; the results are shown in Table 2.56.

Table 2.56 Accelerated Test Data (3)

	Strength (MPa)		*Modulus (GPa)*	
Matrix	*Before*	*After*	*Before*	*After*
Polysulfone	807	723	77	67
PMMA	687	594	76	73
Epoxy (Stycast)	535	323	30	21

Blood compatible materials are essential to circulatory support devices. Numerous materials have been considered for use in prosthetic devices.

2.17.1 Carbons in heart valve prostheses

Carbons are widely used in prosthetic heart valves, as a result of their favorable mechanical and biological properties. Pyrolytic carbons, deposited in a fluidized bed, have high strength, and high fatigue and wear resistance. Compatibility with blood and soft tissue is good.

Table 2.57 Representative Mechanical Properties of LTI, Glassy, and Vapor-Deposited Carbons (3)

Property	*Glassy carbon*	*Vapor-deposited carbon*	*LTI carbon*	*LTI carbon with silicon (5–12%)*
Density, g/cm^3	1.5	1.9	1.9	2.1
Crystallite size, Å	30	10	35	35
Flexural strength 1000 psi	20	80	70	85
Young's modulus, 10^6 psi	4.0	2.5	3.0	4.0
Strain to fracture, %	1.0	5.0	2.0	2.0
Fatigue limit/fracture strength	1.0	1.0	1.0	1.0
Strain energy to fracture, 100 psi	1	12	7	9

2.17.2 Wound closure biomaterials

Virtually every operation requires the use of materials to close the wound for subsequent successful healing. The material must retain adequate strength during the critical period of healing; it should also induce minimal tissue reaction that might interfere with the healing process. The complexity involved in wound healing calls for different types of wound closure materials.

Table 2.58 Mechanical Properties of Suture Materials (3)

Suture	*Yield stress (GPD)*	*Breaking stress (GPD)*	*Yield strain (%)*	*Breaking strain (%)*	*Modulus of elasticity*	*Specific work of rupture (N/Tex)×10^{-2}*
Dexon	0.80	6.30	1.9	22.6	55	6.63
Vicryl	0.97	6.55	1.8	18.4	67.5	5.46
Mersilene	1.20	4.20	2.7	8	53	1.32
Silk	1.33	3.43	1.9	11.5	79.0	2.36
Nurolon	0.34	3.80	1.6	18.2	21.0	2.80
Ethilon	0.41	6.25	2.2	33	20.0	8.96
Prolene	0.52	5.14	1.2	42	58.5	14.69

2.18 METAL MATRIX COMPOSITES

The metal matrix composites can be described as materials whose microstructure comprises a continuous metallic phase into which a second phase (ceramic materials) has been artificially introduced during processing, as reinforcement.

2.18.1 Matrix materials

The most common matrices are the low-density metals, such as aluminum and aluminum alloys, and magnesium and its alloys. Some work has been carried out on lead alloys, mainly for bearing applications, and there is interest in the reinforcement, for example, of titanium-, nickel- and iron-base alloys for higher-temperature performance. However, the problems encountered in achieving the thermodynamic stability of fibers in intimate contact with metals become more severe as the potential service temperature is raised, and the bulk of development work at present rests with the light alloys.

2.18.2 Reinforcements

The principal reinforcements for metal matrices include continuous fibers of carbon, boron, aluminum oxide, silica, aluminosilicate compositions and silicon carbide. Some ceramic fibers are also available in short staple form, and whiskers of carbon, silicon carbide and silicon nitride can be obtained commercially in limited quantities. There is also interest in the use of refractory particles to modify alloy properties such as wear and abrasion resistance. In this case, particle sizes and volume fractions are greater than those developed metallurgically in conventional alloys, and incorporation of the particles into the metal is achieved mechanically rather than by precipitation as a consequence of heat treatment. Most metal–matrix composites consist of a dispersed reinforcing phase of fibers, whiskers or particles, with each reinforcing element ideally separated from the next by a region of metal. A summary of properties of the most important metal matrix composites is presented in Tables 2.59–2.69.

Table 2.59 Summary of Mechanical Properties of A13 Aluminum-28 v/o Thornel-50 Composite (5)

Property	*Value*
Ultimate tensile strength	730 MN/m² (106 000 psi) at 20 °C 660 MN/m² (95 000 psi) at 500 °C
Rule-of-mixtures strength	700 MN/m² (101 000 psi) at 20 °C 550 MN/m² (80 000 psi) at 500 °C
Transverse tensile strength	~83 MN/m² (~12 000 psi)
Tensile elastic modulus, E	145 GN/m² (21.0×10⁶ psi)
Shear modulus, G (calculated)	55 GN/m² (7.9×10⁶ psi)
Density	2.4 g/cm³ (0.0805 lb/in.³)
Strength-to-density ratio	2.4×10⁶ cm (1.25×10⁶ in.)
Modulus-to-density ratio	620×10⁶ cm (248×10⁶ in.)
Poisson's ratio, m (calculated)	0.306

Table 2.60 Summary of Transverse Tensile Strengths of Various Aluminum–Graphite Composite Systems (5)

Composite		*Average*				
Fiber	*Matrix*	*(MN/m²)*	*(psi)*	*High (psi)*	*Low (psi)*	*Number of tests*
Thornel-50	Al-12Si	26	3777	6500	433	9
Courtaulds	220 Al	42	6117	8690	3760	20
Courtaulds	356 Al	70	10,008	14,600	5500	26
Courtaulds HM	Al-10Mg	29.5	4280	4500	3600	5
Whittaker–Morgan	356 Al	50	7300	11,300	4100	5
Whittaker–Morgan	7075 Al	21	3040	5100	400	5

Table 2.61 Uniaxial Tensile Data for Aluminum–Silicon Alloy–Thornel-50 Composite Thermally Cycled 20 Times from -193 to +500°C (5)

Sample number	*Ultimate tensile strength (psi)*	*Rule-of-mixture strength (%)*
C7	103 000	103
C8	100 000	99
C9	100 000	99
C10	99 000	99
Average	101 000	100

Table 2.62 Transverse Tensile Strengths for 356 Aluminum–Courtaulds HM Graphite Composite (5)

	Transverse strength	
Sample number	*(MN/m²)*	*(psi)*
808A	91	13 100
808A	88	12 700
808A	74	10 700
808A	68	9900
808B	79	11 500
837A	67	9700
837A	67.5	9800
837A	76	11 100
837B	67	9700
837B	72	10 400

Table 2.63 Corrosion Behavior of Aluminum–Graphite Composite for 1000hr (5)

	356 aluminum		*356 aluminum–25 v/o Thornel-50*	
Environment	(23°C)	(50°C)	(23°C)	(50°C)
Distilled water	Nil	Nil	1.2	1.2
3.5% NaCl solution	1.1	4.9	4.7	9.8

Table 2.64 Tensile Properties of Al_2O_3-Whisker-Nickel Composites at 25 and 1000 °C(5)

Type of composite	*Test temperature (°C)*	*Whisker volume fraction (v/o)*	*Composite strength (MN/m²*	*Strength-to-density ratio (10⁶ cm)*
Continuous	25	22	1230	1.63
	25	51	1050	1.68
	25	39	1350	2.0
	1000	16	282	0.114
	1000	21	495	0.665
	1000	21	495	0.67
	1000	29	759	1.08
Discontinuous	25	28	621	0.845
	25	19	1180	1.52
	25	11	938	1.14
	1000	17	451	0.542
	1000	28	106	0.144
	1000	10	269	0.33
	1000	20	618	0.80

Table 2.65 Off-Axis Tensile Properties of Ti-6Al-4V-28 v/o SiC (5)

	Average Strength (ksi)			
Filament orientation (degrees)	*Ultimate tensile strength*	*Proportional limit*	*Elastic modulus (10⁶ psi)*	*Poisson's ratio*
0	142	117	36	0.275
15	135	117	35	0.277
30	113	104	32	0.346
45	107	75	31	0.346
90	95	53	28	0.250

Table 2.66 Properties of Ti-6Al-4V-50 v/o Borsic Composites (5)

Temperature (°F)	*Orientation (degrees)*	*Tensile strength (ksi)*	*Failure strain (min./in.)*	*Elastic modulus (10⁶ psi) Tensile*	*Elastic modulus (10⁶ psi) Flexure*	*Coefficient of expansion (10⁻⁶/°F)*
70	0	140	3340	41.5	34.4	2.50
70	15	100	3220	36.8	33.3	—
70	45	66	4220	31.2	31.8	—
70	90	42	3130	29.8	31.2	3.17
500	0	119	—	—	33.2	2.80
700	0	107	—	—	32.4	—
850	0	109	—	—	31.5	3.17
850	15	86	—	—	29.9	—
850	45	53	—	—	27.6	—
850	90	35	—	—	24.4	3.64

Table 2.67 Summary of Mechanical Properties of Magnesium-Graphite Composites (5)

Composite	*Strength (psi)*	*Strength (MN/m2)*	*E (10^{-6}psi)*	*E (GN/m^2)*	*Density (gm/cm^3)*	*Strength/ density (10^{-6}cm)*	*Modulus/ density (10^{-6}cm)*
Mg-42v/o Thornel-75	65 000	450	26.6	184	1.77	2.5	1000
Mg-ZK60A	50 000	345	6.5	45	1.80	1.9	250

Table 2.68 Room-Temperature Properties of Lead–Graphite Composites (5)

Composite	*Strength lb/in.^{2}*	*Modulus of elasticity 10^{-6}lb/in.^{2}*	*Density lb/in.^{3}*	*Strength/ density 10^{-6} in.*	*Modulus/ density 10^{-6} in.*
Pure lead	2 000	2.0	0.41	0.005	4.9
Lead-base bearing (75Pb–15Sb–10Sn)	10 500	4.2	0.35	0.03	12.0
Lead-graphite 41 vol% Thornel-75 Fibers	104 000	29.0	0.270	0.385	107.0
Lead-graphite 35 vol% Courtaulds HM	72 000	17.4	0.28	0.26	62.3

Table 2.69 Summary of Mechanical Properties of Zinc and Zinc–Graphite Composite (5)

System	*Strength (psi)*	*Modulus of elasticity (10^{-6} psi)*	*Density lb/in.^{3}*	*Strength/ density (10^{-6} in.)*	*Modulus/ density (10^{-6} in.)*
Z-35 v/o Thornel/75	110 900	16.9	0.191	0.58	88.5
Alloy AG40A	41 000	10.0	0.240	0.17	41.7

2.19 CERAMIC MATRIX COMPOSITES

Composite structures in ceramics have been developed for two major reasons. First, they provide a means to enhance dramatically the performance of the so-called functional ceramics; these are systems where electrical, dielectrical, piezoelectric or sensitizing properties are greatly amplified by appropriate composite design. Secondly, they are used to avoid or diminish the brittle behaviour of structural ceramic systems.

A summary of properties of the most important ceramic matrix composites is presented in Tables 2.70–2.74.

Table 2.70 Glass and Glass ceramics suitable as matrices (4)

Matrix type	*Major constituent*	*Minor constituent*	*Maximum use temperature*
	Glass		
7740 Boro-silicate	B_2O_3, SiO_2	Na_2O, Al_2O_3	600°C
1723 Alumino-silicate	Al_2O_3, MgO, CaO, SiO_2	B_2O_3, BaO	700°C
7930 High silica	SiO_2	B_2O_3	1150°C
	Glass ceramics		
LAS I	Li_2O, Al_2O_3, MgO, SiO_2	ZnO, ZrO, BaO	1000°C
LAS II	Li_2O, Al_2O_3, MgO, SiO_2, Nb_2O_5	ZnO, ZrO_2, BaO	1100°C
LAS III	Li_2O, Al_2O_3, MgO, SiO_2, Nb_2O_3	ZrO_2	1200°C
MAS	MgO, Al_2O_3, SiO_2	BaO	1200°C
BMAS	BaO, MgO, Al_2O_3, SiO_2	—	1250°C

Table 2.71 Properties of silicon nitride and carbon/silicon nitride (4)

Property	Si_3N_4	C/Si_3N_4
Bulk density (g/cm^3)	3.44	2.7
Fibre content (vol.%)	—	30
Bending strength (MPa)	473±30	454±42
Young's modulus (GPa)	247±16	188±18
Fracture toughness (MPa $m^{1/2}$)	3.7±0.7	15.6±1.2
Work of fracture (J/m^2)	19.3±	4770±770

Table 2.72 Room temperature strengths of RBSN* and SiC/RBSN (4)

Test	*Axial strength (MPa)* 0% Fiber	23% Fiber	40% Fiber
Four point bend	107±26	539±48	616±36
Three point bend	—	717±80	958±45
Tensile	—	352±73	536±20

* RBSN – Reaction bonded silicon nitride.

Table 2.73 Properties of brittle fibre/SiC matrix composites (4)

Reinforcement	*Matrix*	*Vol %*	*Comp. density % Th.*	*Fracture toughness (MPa $m^{1/2}$)*	*4 Point bending strength, MPa*
SiC Fibers	SiC	45	70–77	—	213–230
		39.5	68–75	—	224–410
SiC Cloth	SiC	41.6	75–90	—	419–437
		37.9	73–89	—	187–217
SiC chopped	SiC	25.4	51–81	—	90–177
fibers		21.9	71–77	—	50–94
SiC cloth plain	SiC	35.5	62–83	1.8–3.6	72–107
weave satin		46.3	65–85	—	71–196
weave		50.2	68–84	—	44–97
SiC chopped	SiC	16.8	69–82	—	61–106
fibers		24.3	68–76	—	74–98
		25.4	51–81	—	90–177
SiC cloth	SiC	41–45	64–90	—	107–476
SiC fibers	SiC	39–57	68–77	—	38–410
SiC fibers	SiC	—	>90	>25	320
C fibers	SiC	—	>90	>25	530

Table 2.74 Room temperature of some unreinforced ceramics and ceramic matrix composite (4)

Material	*Flexural strength MPa*	*Fracture toughness MPa $m^{1/2}$*
Al_2O_3	550	4–5.0
SiC whiskers/Al_2O_3	800	8.7
SiC	500	4.0
SiC fibers/SiC	750	25.0
ZrO_2	200	5.0
SiC/ZrO_2	450	22.0
Borosilicate glass	60	0.6
SiC fibers/borosilicate glass	830	18.9
Glass ceramic	200	2.0
SiC fibers/glass ceramics	830	17.0
Reaction bonded Si_3N_4	260	2–3.0
SiC whiskers/reaction bonded Si_3N_4	900	20
Hot pressed Si_3N_4	470	3.7–4.5
SiC whiskers/hot pressed Si_3N_4	800	56

REFERENCES

1. Seymour, R.B. (1990) *Polymer Composites*, VSP, Utrecht, The Netherlands.
2. Weatherhead, R.G. (1980) *FRP Technology*, Applied Science Publishers, London.
3. *Biocompatible Polymers, Metals, and Composites*, edited by M. Szycher, Technomic Publishing Co. Inc.
4. Islam, M.U., Wallance, W. and Kandeil, A.Y. (1985) *Artificial Composites for High Temperature Applications*, Noyes Data Corporation, Park Ridge, New Jersey, USA.
5. Kreider, Kenneth G. (1974) *Metallic Matrix Composites*, Vol. 4, Academic Press, New York and London.
6. Hawkins, W.L. (1984) *Polymer Degradation and Stabilization*, Springer-Verlag.
7. Environmental Effects on Advanced Composite Materials, symposium presented at the seventy-eighth Annual Meeting ASTM, Philadelphia, 1975.
8. Hill, R. (1964) *J. Mech. Phys. Solids*, **12,** 199.
9. Hermann, J.J. (1970) *Proc. Konigl. Nederl. Akad. Weteschappen Amsterdam*, **B70,** 1.
10. Halpin, J.C. and Pagano, N.J. (1964) *J. Compos. Mater.*, **3,** 720.

3 Thermoplastic Polymers In Biomedical Applications: Structures, Properties and Processing

S.H. Teoh, Z.G. Tang and G.W. Hastings

3.1 INTRODUCTION

In general thermoplastic polymers are made up of long linear chain molecules which exhibit large scale chain mobility and deformation under shear forces above their softening temperature. This change is reversible. Above this temperature the thermal motions of the chain segments are sufficient to overcome inter- and intra-molecular forces. At room temperature the material is a viscoelastic solid. Their behaviour is dependent on chain morphology, structure, crystallinity and the types of additives added (often to aid processing). The materials can easily be processed into different type of products and are considered to be the most important class of plastic materials commercially available. The processability of this class of plastics is a key characteristic for developing biomedical applications.

Nine potential biomedical applications areas have been identified (Jones and Denning, 1988):

1. Membranes in extracorporeal applications such as oxygenators;
2. Bioactive membranes e.g., controlled release delivery systems and artificial cells;

Handbook of Biomaterial Properties. Edited by J. Black and G. Hastings.
Published in 1998 by Chapman & Hall, London. ISBN 0 412 60330 6.

3. Disposable equipment e.g., blood bags and disposable syringes;
4. Sutures and adhesives including biodegradable and non-biodegradable materials;
5. Cardiovascular devices such as vascular grafts;
6. Reconstructive and orthopaedic implants;
7. Ophthalmic devices such as corneas and contact lens;
8. Dental restorative materials including dentures;
9. Degradable plastic commodity products.

This section focuses on 12 thermoplastic polymers which have found wide application in the above. Each part deals with one polymer or one group of polymers of structural similarity. The content includes the chemical structure, structure-property relationships, tables of physical, mechanical and thermal properties, and processing conditions of each candidate thermoplastic. Some properties can be predicted from the structural characteristics of the polymers.

In general, for a given polymer, higher molecular weight tends to improve mechanical properties, but the increase in the resistance to flow in the fluid state makes processing more difficult and costly. A wide range of molecular weight is generally more appropriate for processing of each polymer. The effect of branching in otherwise linear molecules is significant. Short but numerous branches irregularly spaced may reduce considerably the ability of portions of linear chains to form crystal-like domains, and the corresponding polymer will display a lower stiffness, a good example being the highly branched low-density polyethylene of lower degree of crystallinity than the less branched high density product. Tacticity of polymer molecules greatly affects crystallinity and stiffness. For example, commercial polypropylene is usually about 90~95% isotactic, and is stiff, highly crystalline and with a high melting point, whereas the atactic polypropylene is an amorphous somewhat rubbery material of little value. Within the range of commercial polymers, the greater the amount of isotactic material the greater the crystallinity and hence the greater the softening point, stiffness, tensile strength, modulus and hardness. The inter-molecular and intra-molecular forces also influence the properties of polymers. The hydrogen bonds or van der Waal's and other dispersion forces between adjacent molecules produce a large increase in melting temperature. A high energy barrier to molecular rotations hinders the ability of molecules to take up the required conformations to form crystals. Polymethylmethacrylate (PMMA), and polycarbonate exist in an amorphous state and are completely transparent. The crystallinity is controlled by both structural factors and processing conditions. From the processing standpoint, the higher the crystallinity, the bigger the shrinkage observed after product processing. Thermoplastic polymers exist in semi-crystalline and amorphous states. The ratio of these two states affects material properties strongly and can be characterized using X-ray analysis and by observing the thermal behaviour of the polymers. Amorphous thermoplastics are normally transparent and do not have a fixed melting temperature like that of the semi-crystalline thermoplastics. They are also less resistant to solvent attack. Semi-crystalline thermoplastics, because of the presence of crystallites, are more fatigue and wear resistant. A typical case is polyacetal which has more than 20 years of *in vivo* experience as an occluder in the Björk–Shiley tilting disc mechanical heart valves.

A main requirement for a polymeric candidate is its biocompatibility with biological tissues and fluids. Biocompatibility will depend on the polymer intrinsic chemical nature and the additives present. It is a complex issue not dealt with here. It is not always possible to distinguish the medical-grade polymers from the conventional polymers. They may come from a batch intended for general purposes, but are selected on the basis of clean condition or trace element analysis or mechanical properties. Subsequent processing requires clean room conditions and care to avoid any contamination. There is still some inherent uncertainty about constituents unless there has been complete disclosure and/or only a 'pure' polymer is used. With new developments in polymeric biomaterials, the situation should improve.

It is hoped that the following sections will be of value to researchers in science and engineering and to clinical practitioners who are engaged in the development and material selection of new thermoplastic polymers for biomedical applications.

3.2 POLYETHYLENE

Commercially, polyethylene is produced from ethylene in various densities (from linear low to ultra high). There are four quite distinct processes to the preparation of commercial polymers of ethylene: (a) high pressure processes, (b) Ziegler processes, (c) the Phillips process, (d) the Standard Oil (Indiana) process. High pressure polymers (British patent 471590, 1930) are of the lower density range for polyethylene (0.915–0.94 g/cm^3) and usually also of the lower range of molecular weights. Until the mid-1950s, all commercial polyethylenes were produced by high pressure processes. These materials were branched materials and of moderate number average molecular weight, generally less than 50 000. Ziegler polymers (Ziegler, 1955) are intermediate in density (ca. 0.945 g/cm^3) between the high pressure polyethylenes and those produced by the Phillips and Standard Oil processes. Phillips polymers have the highest density of any commercial polythylenes (ca. 0.96 g/cm^3) Ziegler and Phillips processes produce polymers at lower temperature and pressures with a modified structure giving a higher density, greater hardness higher softening points. The Standard Oil process gives a density of about 0.96 g/cm^3) similar to the Phillips materials. Processes, such as a gas phase process developed by Union Carbide for making linear low density polyethylene (LLDPE), were aimed to produce polyethylenes with short chain branch but no long chain branch. High pressure polymers have more branching and even with side chains as long as the main chain. In contrast, the high density polyethylene (HDPE) produced by the Ziegler or Phillips methods has only 3 to 5 branches per 1000 C-atoms and the linear low density PE has very few branches. The weak point in the chain which is sensitive to degradative environmental effects is located at the branching site. The amount of branches in polyethylene also influences the crystallinity of polyethylene. A higher degree of crystallinity and associated denser packing leads to higher density and larger crystals (LDPE< 1 μm; LLDPE, 2–4 μm; HDPE, 2–8 μm). The crystallinity is increased with slower cooling rate. Only the HDPE and the ultra high molecular weight polyethylene (UHMWPE) find extensive medical applications.

Chemically, polyethylene is inert and there are no effective solvents at room temperature. However, polyethylene is subject to oxidation and halogenation. Chemicals like nitric acid produce oxidative deterioration and affect mechanical properties of polyethylene. The environmental oxidation of polyethylene happens at high temperature, under ultra-violet light and/or high energy irradiation, e.g., gamma irradiation. Polyethylene should be kept from contact with halogenating agents and environments. The lower molecular weight polyethylene may be dissolved at high temperature and swollen by chemicals such as benzene and xylene. The resistance to environmental stress cracking (ESC) increases with molecular weight, (copolymers being more resistant than homopolymers).

3.3 POLYPROPYLENE

Polypropylene is an addition polymer of propylene. The chemical structure of polypropylene is often described as the repeating unit of 2-methyl ethylene. During polymerization, the CH_3 groups characteristic of this olefin can be incorporated spatially into the macromolecule in different ways. The resulting products have different properties and are classified as a. isotactic polypropylene, where the CH_3 groups are on the same side of the main chain; b. syndiotactic polypropylene, where the CH_3 groups are symmetrically arranged on the two sides of the main chain; c. atactic polypropylene, where the CH_3 groups are randomly distributed in the spatial relationship to the main chain.

The atactic polymer is an amorphous somewhat rubbery material of little value, whereas the isotactic polymer stiff, highly crystalline and with high melting point. Commercial polymers are usually about 90–95% isotactic. Within the range of commercial polymers, the greater the amount of isotactic material, the greater the crystallinity, and hence the greater the softening point, stiffness, tensile strength, modulus, and hardness. The properties of the polymer will depend on the size and type of crystal structure formed in its construction.

Molecular weights of polypropylenes are in the range M_n = 38 000–60 000 and M_w = 220 000–700 000 with the values of M_w/M_n = 5.6–11.9, higher than those encountered normally in polyethylene. The high molecular weight polymer from propylene was introduced in 1954 by G. Natta using a modified Ziegler process, and commercialized in 1957 by Montecatini under a trade name Moplen. This was followed in 1983 by the Spheripol process; in 1988, the Valtec process; and in 1990, Himont process. The greatest influence of molecular weight and molecular weight distribution is on the rheological properties. Rheological investigations show that polypropylene deviates more strongly from Newtonian behaviour than does polyethylene. The effect of shear rate on the apparent melt viscosity is greater for polypropylene

Although polypropylene and polyethylene are similar structurally,. polypropylene has a lower density around 0.90 g/cm^3 and a higher T_g and T_m. The higher melting point of polypropylene gives the option for autoclave sterilization. The chemical resistance of polypropylene is similar to high density polyethylene, but it is more susceptible to oxidation, chemical degradation and crosslinking (irradiation, violet light and other physical means) than polyethylene. Polypropylene is better in creep resistance and in resisting environmental stress cracking than polyethylene.

3.4 POLYURETHANE

Polyurethanes are block copolymers containing blocks of low molecular weight polyethers or polyesters linked together by a urethane group. The variety of linkages in polymers results from the further reaction of urethane groups with isocyanates and of isocyanates with amines, water, or carboxylic acids.

Attention in this section will be focussed on the thermoplastic polyurethane elastomers. These polymers are based on three monomers: (1) an isocyanate source, (2) a macroglycol or carbonate, and (3) a chain extender, or curing agent. The isocyanates can be either aromatic or aliphatic. Although the aliphatic based polyurethanes are more expensive, and inferior in physical properties they do not show the embrittlement, weakening, and progressive darkening of the aromatic equivalents.

The final physical and biological properties of the polyurethanes depend principally on the type of macroglycol used in the synthesis. The polyether-based polyurethanes are less sensitive to hydrolysis, and are thus more stable *in vivo*. The polycaprolactone-based polyurethanes, due to their quick crystallization, can be used as solvent-activated, pressure-sensitive adhesives. For medical applications, the polyether-based polyurethanes, particularly those based on polytetramethylene ether glycol (PTMEG) have been used. Among chain extenders, there are two choices: either difunctional or multifunctional monomers. For the production of linear elastomers, only difunctional chain extenders are used, of these, diols and diamines are by far the most important. The chain extenders for the thermoplastic polyurethanes must be linear diols, among which, 1,4-butane diol has been chosen for medical applications. This chain extender produces thermoplastic polyurethanes with high physical properties, excellent processing conditions and clear polymers.

Polyurethane elastomers are a mixture of crystalline (hard segment) and amorphous domains(soft segment), and the hard segments are considered to result from contributions of the diisocyanate and chain extender components. They significantly affect mechanical properties, particularly modulus, hardness and tear strength. Soft segments therefore affect the tensile strength and elongation at yield and break.

Polyurethanes are sensitive to strong acids, strong alkalis, aromatics, alcohols, hot water, hot moist air and saturated steam. The hydrolytic stability of polyurethanes in applications must be considered carefully. However, polyurethanes are resistant to weak acids, weak alkalis, ozone, oxygen, mineral grease, oils and petroleum. There are doubts for the oxidation stability of polytetramethylene ether glycol based polyurethanes. Polycarbonate urethane is a promising substitute with good oxidation stability.

The thermoplastic polyurethanes are characterized by the following properties: a. high elongation at break and high flexibility (also at low temperature), b. low permanent deformation on static and dynamic loading, c. favourable friction and abrasion performance, d. high damping power, e. high resistance to high energy and UV radiation, and f. plasticizer free,

3.5 POLYTETRAFLUOROETHYLENE

Polytetrafluoroethylene, PTFE, is the polymerization product of tetrafluoroethylene discovered in 1938 by R.J. Plunkett of Du Pont. The polymer is linear and free from any significant amount of branching. The highly compact structure leads to a molecule of great stiffness and results in a high crystalline melting point and thermal stability of the polymer.

The weight average molecular weights of commercial PTFE are in the range 400 000 to 9 000 000. The degree of crystallinity of the polymer reaches 94%. The properties of PTFE moldings are considerably influenced by the processing conditions and polymer grades. After processing, cooling conditions determine the crystallinity of the molding. Slow cooling leads to higher crystallinity which affects the physical properties as well as mechanical and thermal properties.

PTFE is a tough, flexible material of moderate tensile strength with excellent resistance to heat, chemicals and to the passage of an electric current. The polymer is not wetted by water and absorption is not detectable. The permeability to gases is low, the water vapour transmission rate being approximately half that of low density polyethylene and polyethylene terephthalate. It has the lowest coefficient of friction of all solids and the dynamic and static coefficients of friction are equal, i.e. stick-slip does not occur. Abrasion resistance is low. The thermal stability of PTFE is excellent up to 300 °C but it is degraded by high energy radiation.

Phase transition behaviour precludes the use of the conventional molding methods, and PTFE can be processed by employing a process similar to that of metallurgical sintering. In 1963, Shinsaburo Oslinge of Sumitomo Industries in Japan discovered a process for expanding PTFE during extrusion. The e-PTFE has been considered for fabrication of vascular grafts.

Apart from its good slip and wear characteristics the advantages of PTFE are: a. almost universal chemical resistance, b. insolubility in all known solvents below 300 °C, c. high thermal stability, d. continuous service temperature range -270 to 260 °C, e. low adhesion, f. low coefficient of friction, g. outstanding electrical and dielectric properties, h. resistant to stress cracking and weathering, but limited use in structural components because of the low modulus of elasticity.

3.6 POLYVINYLCHLORIDE

Commercial PVC polymers are largely amorphous, slightly branched molecules with the monomer residues arranged in a head-to-tail sequence. The molecular weights for most commercial polymers are in the range of M_w = 100 000–200 000, M_n = 45 000–64 000 although values may be as low as 40 000 and as high as 480 000 for the weight average molecular weight. The ratio of M_n/M_w is usually about 2 for the commercial material although it may increase with the higher molecular weight grades.

The polarity and strong inter-chain attraction gives a higher hardness and stiffness than polyethylene. Thus PVC has a higher dielectric constant and power factor than polyethylene, although at temperatures below the glass transition temperature the power factor is still comparatively low (0.01–0.05 at 60 Hz) because of the immobility of the dipole. PVC is mainly used in a plasticized form. There are many materials that are suitable plasticisers for PVC. They have similar solubility parameters to PVC, i.e., about 19.4 $MPa^{1/2}$ and are also weak proton acceptors and may be incorporated by mixing at elevated temperatures to give mixtures stable at room temperature.

The release of low molecular weight plasticizer has resulted in polymeric plasticisers being developed, but esters are still widely used and are effective in plasticisation. (Black, 1992; Brydson, 1982, and Park and Lakes, 1992).

Characteristic properties are:

3.6.1 Unplasticized PVC

a. high mechanical strength, rigidity and hardness, b. low impact strength in unmodified form, c. translucent to transparent (depending on method of manufacture), d. good electrical properties in the low voltage and low frequency range, and e. high chemical resistance.

3.6.2 Plasticized PVC

a. flexibility adjustable over a wide range, b. depending on type of plasticiser, toughness very temperature dependent, c. translucent to transparent, d. good electrical properties in the low voltage and low frequency range, e. chemical resistance is dependent on the formulation and very dependent on temperature, and f. the polymers contain less than 1 ppm vinyl chloride monomer.

3.7 POLYAMIDES

Chemically, the polyamides may be divided into two types: a. those based on diamines and dibasic acids, and b. those based on amino acids or lactams (Chapman and Chruma, 1985). Commercial use of nylons is dominated by two products, one from each type, nylon 66 and nylon 6 from ϵ-caprolactam.

Aliphatic polyamide is linear and easy to crystallize but crystallinity varies widely with conditions. Crystàlline content may be 50–60% by slow cooling and 10% by fast cooling. High interchain attraction in the crystalline zones and flexibility in the amorphous zones leads to polymers which are tough above their apparent glass transition temperatures (Brydson, 1982).

Polyamides have excellent fibre-forming capability due to interchain H-bonding and a high degree of crystallinity which increases strength in the fibre direction (Park and Lakes, 1992). Polyamides are hygroscopic and lose strength *in vivo*. The amorphous region of polyamide chains is sensitive to the attack of water. The greater the degree of crystallinity, the less the water absorption and hence the less the effect of humidity on the properties of the polymer. The reversible absorption of water is associated with a change in volume and thus of dimensions.

The mechanical properties of moulded polyamide materials depend on molecular weight, crystallinity and moisture content. In the dry, freshly molded state, all polyamide grades are hard and brittle. When conditioned they are tough and wear resistant. High melting points result in good mechanical properties up to temperatures in the region of 120–150 °C.

They are only soluble in a few solvents (formic acid, glacial acetic acid, phenols and cresols), of similar high solubility parameter. Nylons are of exceptionally good resistance to hydrocarbons. Esters, alkyl halides, and glycols have little effect on them. Alcohols can swell the polymers and sometime dissolve some copolymers. Mineral acids attack the nylons but the rate of attack depends on the type of nylon and the nature and concentration of the acid. Nitric acid is generally active at all concentrations. The nylons have very good resistance to alkalis at room temperature. Resistance to all chemicals is more limited at elevated temperature (Brydson, 1989).

Generally, polyamides are characterized by: a. high strength, stiffness and hardness, b. high heat distortion temperature, c. high wear resistance, good slip and dry-running properties, d. good damping capacity, e. good resistance to solvents, fuels and lubricants, f. non-toxicity, g. good processability, h. aliphatic polyamides are partially crystalline and thus opaque, and i. moisture content impairs mechanical properties and affects dimensions of moldings.

3.8 POLYACRYLATES

Polyacrylates are based on acrylic acid, methacrylic acid, and their esters. Among them, polymethylmethacrylate (PMMA) and polyhydroxy ethylmethacrylate (PHEMA) have found wide applications as biomedical materials. The clinical history of polyacrylates began when it was unexpectedly discovered that the fragments of PMMA plastic aircraft canopies stayed in the body of the wounded without any adverse chronic reactions (Jones and Denning, 1988; Park and Lakes, 1992).

In normal conditions, PMMA is a hard transparent material. Molecular weight is the main property determinant. High molecular weight PMMA can be manufactured by free radical polymerization (bulk, emulsion, and suspension polymerisation). Bulk polymerization is used for cast semifinish products (sheet, profiles and even tubes), and the cast polymer is distinguished by superior mechanical properties and high surface finish

(Brydson, 1982 and Domininghaus, 1993). Cast material has a number average molecular weight of about 10^6 whilst the T_g is about 106°C. The extensive molecular entanglement prevents melting below its decomposition temperature (approx. 170°C).

An amorphous polymer, PMMA has a solubility parameter of about 18.8 $MPa^{1/2}$ and is soluble in a number of solvents with similar solubility parameters. Solvents include ethyl acetate (δ: 18.6 $MPa^{1/2}$), ethylene dichloride (δ: 20.0 $MPa^{1/2}$), trichloroethylene (δ: 19 $MPa^{1/2}$), chloroform (δ: 19 $MPa^{1/2}$), and toluene (δ: 20 $MPa^{1/2}$). The polymer is attacked by mineral acids but is resistant to alkalis, water and most aqueous inorganic salt solutions. A number of organic materials although not solvents may cause crazing and cracking (e.g. aliphatic alcohols).

The characteristic properties of PMMA are, a. high hardness, stiffness and strength, b. homopolymers are brittle, copolymers are tough, c. scratch-resistant, high gloss surface capable of being polished, d. water-white transparency, copolymers exhibit inherent yellowish color, e. high heat distortion temperature, f. good electrical and dielectric properties, g. resistant to weak acids and alkaline solution as well as to non-polar solvents, grease, oils and water, h. susceptible to stress cracking, i. flammable, j. good processability and machinability, k. rather low resistance to creep at temperature only slightly above room temperature, and l. high melt viscosity due to the high chain stiffness caused by restricted rotations about the C-bonds in the backbone chains

3.9 POLYACETAL

Polyacetal can be divided into two basic types, acetal homoploymer and acetal copolymer. Both homopolymer and copolymer are available in a range of molecular weights (M_n = 20 000–100 000). The homopolymer is a polymer of formaldehyde with a molecular structure of repeated oxymethylene units (Staudinger, 1932). Large-scale production of polyformaldehyde, i.e. polyacetal, commenced in 1958 in the USA (US Patent 2 768 994, 1956) (British patent 770 717, 1957). Delrin (1959) was the first trade mark for this polymer by Du Pont Company. The copolymers were introduced by the Celanese Corporation of America, and the first commercial product named Celcon (1960). One of the major advantages of copolymerization is to stabilize polyacetal because the homopolymer tends to depolymerize and eliminate formaldehyde. The most important stabilization method is structural modification of the polymer by, for example, copolymerization with cyclic ether.

As can been seen polyacetal has a very simple structure of a polyether. Unlike polyethylene, polyacetal has no branching, and its molecules can pack more closely together than those of polyethylene. The resultant polymer is thus harder and has a higher melting point than polyethylene (175°C for homopolymer), exhibiting a high crystallinity (77–85%).

No effective solvents have been found for temperatures below 70°C. Swelling occurs with solvents of similar solubility parameter (δ: 22.4 $MPa^{1/2}$). However, polyacetal should be kept away from strong acids, strong alkalis, and oxidizing agents. Water can not degrade it but may swell it or permeate through it and affect the dimensions of its products. Prolonged exposure to ultra-violet light will induce surface chalking and reduce the molecular weight of the polymers. Polyacetals, both homopolymer and copolymer are also radiation sensitive. The radiation damage threshold is estimated at 0.5 Mrad with 25% damage at 1.1 Mrad (Szycher, 1991).

Generally, the polyacetals have the following characteristics, a. high tensile strength, shear strength, stiffness, and toughness, b. predictable stress/ strain relationships, c. predictable dimensional behavior, d. chemical and corrosion resistance, e. abrasion resistance, f. light weight and good appearance, g. acceptability for food contact application (most grades), h. ease of processing, and i. competitive costs.

The enormous commercial success of the polyacetals is owed to their very high resistance to creep and fatigue. The acetal resins show superior creep resistance to the nylons.

3.10 POLYCARBONATE

Polycarbonate, PC, is a linear thermoplastic based on the bis-phenol A dihydroxy compound. In 1898 Einhorn reacted dihydroxybenzenes with phosgene in solution in pyridine (Brydson, 1982), and production began in both Germany and USA in 1958. General purpose polycarbonate is a linear polyester of carbonic acid in which dihydric phenols are linked through carbonate groups, while standard grades are made from bisphenol A and phosgene (Carhart, 1985).

The rigid molecular back bone of bis-phenol A PC leads to high melting temperature (T_m = 225–250°C) and high glass transition temperature (T_g = 145°C). The polymer does not show any crystallinity. After annealing polymer between 80 and 130°C there is a small increase in density and hence there must be a decrease in free volume, and a large drop in impact strength; impact strength may be reduced by annealing crystallization and aging (Brydson, 1982).

The limited crystallinity contributes to the toughness of PC. Highly crystalline samples prepared by heating for prolonged periods above their T_g or by precipitation from solution are quite brittle. Although of good impact strength and creep resistance tensile strain of 0.75% or more produces cracking or crazing. The refractive index of PC lies in the range of 1.56 to 1.65 (higher than PMMA and silicone rubber) and the transparency of 85 to 90% is reached in the region of visible light (Domininghaus, 1993).

The chemical resistance of PC is poor and hydrolysis of aliphatic PC s is more prominent than that of bis-phenol A PC s. There is resistance to dilute (25%) mineral acids and dilute alkaline solutions other than caustic soda and caustic potash. Where the resin comes into contact with organophilic hydrolysing agents such as ammonia and the amines, the benzene rings give little protection and reaction is quite rapid. The absence of both secondary and tertiary C-H bonds leads to a high measure of oxidative stability. Oxidation takes place only when thin films are heated in air to temperatures above 300°C.

Typical properties include: a. low density, b. high strength, stiffness, hardness and toughness over the range from -150 to + 135°C unreinforced and from -150 to +145°C when reinforced, c. crystal clear transparency, high refractive index, high surface gloss, d. can be colored in all important shades, transparent, translucent or opaque with great depth of color, e. good electrical insulation properties which are not impaired by moisture, f. high resistance to weathering for wall thicknesses greater than 0.75 mm, g. high resistance to high energy radiation, and h. self-extinguishing after removal of the ignition source.

The main disadvantages are: a. processing requires care, b. limited chemical resistance, c. notch sensitivity and susceptibility to stress cracking.

3.11 POLYETHYLENE TEREPHTHALATE

Polyethylene terephthalate, PET, is a thermoplastic polyester made by condensation reaction of ethylene glycol with either terephthalic acid or dimethyl terephthalate (Margolis, 1985). By the end of the 1920s J.R. Whinfield and J.T. Dickson discovered PET (BP 578079). It was first commercialized by Du Pont in 1930 (Brydson, 1982) as Dacron®, followed by ICI with Terylene® Films and blow-molded articles have become very important commercially.

The average molecular weights are distributed from 15 000 to 20 000. The physical properties of PET are largely determined by the degree of crystallinity, which varies between 30 and 40% depending on the processing conditions. The rate of crystallization of PET is considerably less than that of polyacetal (POM) and HDPE. The growth rate of the spherulites is only 10 μm/mm for PET compared with 400 μm/mm for POM and 5000 μm/mm for HDPE (Domininghaus, 1993). To achieve better crystallinity, the mould temperature should be equivalent to that for maximum growth. This point is about 175°C, higher than for POM and HDPE. Rapid-crystallization agents, nucleating agents, reduce the process cycle time and permit lower mould temperatures below 100°C, leading to very fine spherulites and hard stiff mouldings. Extrusion and rapid quenching below the temperature at which most crystallization occurs (between 120 and 200°C), produces amorphous materials and this may be followed with uniaxial orientation for fibres and biaxial orientation for films. The orientation is carried out at 100–120°C, the glass transition temperature, T_g being 86°C.

The permeability of water vapor through PET is higher than that of polyolefins but lower than that of polycarbonate, polyamide, and polyacetal. Antioxidants are necessary to prevent to the oxidation of polyether segments in thermoplastic polyester elastomer. Chemical resistance of PET is generally good to acids, alkalis, and organic solvents.

Typical properties for partially crystalline PET include, a. high strength and stiffness, b. favorable creep characteristics in comparison with POM, c. hard surface capable of being polished, d. high dimensional stability, e. good electrical, mediocre dielectric properties, and f. high chemical resistance except to strong acid and alkaline solution.

3.12 POLYETHERETHERKETONE

Polyetheretherketone, PEEK, is a polymer combining stiff conjugated aromatic groups and flexible ether segments. It was first prepared in the laboratory in 1977 and then marketed in 1978 by ICI, under the trade name of Victrex (Brydson, 1982).

The distribution of aromatic rings and polar flexible groups in the chain affects the glass transition temperature, such that PEEK has a T_g around 145°C and T_m ca. 335°C, PEK (polyether ketone) T_g ca. 165°C and T_m ca. 342°C. Normally the chain stiffness and bulkiness of aromatic rings make it difficult for these polymers to crystallize and although they invariably remain mainly amorphous (Mascia, 1989), PEEK is a partially crystalline thermoplastic. The maximum crystallinity of 48% is achieved from the melt at 256°C and by subsequent conditioning of moldings at 185°C (Domininghaus, 1993). PEEK polymers are capable of melt processing (Brydson, 1982). Other specific features are excellent gamma radiation resistance, and good resistance to environmental stress cracking. PEEK shows excellent chemical resistance and can be used in aggressive environments.

Generally, the main characteristics of this material include, a. high tensile and flexural strength, b. high impact strength, c. high fatigue limit, d. high heat distortion temperature (315°C for 30 glass reinforced), e. good electrical properties over a wide range of temperature, f. favourable slip and wear properties, g. high chemical resistance, h. high resistance to hydrolysis, j. high resistance to radiation, k. low flammability, very low gas and smoke emission, and l. easy processing, no thermal after-treatment of injection moldings.

3.13 POLYSULFONE

Polysulfone is a polymer which has properties matching those of light metals (Park and Lakes, 1992). The first commercial polysulfone was introduced in 1965 by Union Carbide as Bakelite Polysulfone, now called Udel®. In 1967 3M offered Astrel 360 referred to as a polyarylsulfone. In 1972 ICI introduced a polyethersulfone Victrex®. A high toughness polysulfone was released in the late 1970s by Union Carbide. Although the commercial polymers are linear and most have regular structures they are all principally amorphous. The backbone aromatic structure leads to high values of the glass transition temperature between 190 and 230°C. The Union Carbide materials have a secondary transition at -100°C and the ICI polymer at -70°C. Typical M_n values are ca. 23 000. Commercial materials are described variously as polysulfones (Udel), polyarylsulfones (Astrel), polyether sulfones or polyarylethersulfones (Victrex) (Brydson, 1982).

The polymer is manufactured from bisphenol A and 4, 4-dichlorosulphonyl sulfone by multi-step condensation. The most distinctive feature of the backbone chain of those polymers is the diphenylene sulfone group. The sulphur atom in each group is in its highest state of oxidation and tends to draw electrons from the adjacent benzene rings, hence resisting any tendency to lose electrons to an oxidizing agent. Polysulfones thus show outstanding oxidation resistance. The aromatic nature of the diphenylene sulphone can absorb considerable energy applied as heat or radiation and so resists thermal degradation. The diphenylene sulfone group thus confers on the entire polymer molecule the inherent characteristics of thermal stability, oxidation resistance, and rigidity at elevated temperatures.

The potential for energy dissipation confers good impact strength and ductility down to -100°C with high elongation to break and tensile strength. Under most conditions, impact properties rival those of bisphenol A polycarbonate. Unlike polycarbonate, however, polysulfone can exhibit excellent resistance to hydrolysis or reduction of molecular weight even at elevated temperatures. Tests on the hydrolysis stability of polysulfones have been carried out up to 10 000 hours without observed loss of molecular weight.

The polymers are stable in aqueous inorganic acids, alkalis, salt solutions, aliphatic hydrocarbons, and paraffin oils, are transparent, capable of steam sterilization, and free from taste and smell. They should not come in contact with ketones, aromatic solvents, chlorinated hydrocarbons, and polar organic solvents. They may show stress crazing on exposure to steam or water. A polyethersulfone, however, exhibited no crazing even after 300 hours and retained 90% of initial tensile impact strength. For a thermoplastic material, creep is low at moderate temperatures but is significant at temperatures approaching the glass transition. However, the wear properties of this material are not as good as PE and POM (Teoh *et al.*, 1994).

Generally polysulfone has the following characteristic properties, a. high strength, stiffness and hardness between -100 and +150°C short-term to 180°C, b. high thermal stability and heat distortion temperature, c. crystal clear (slightly yellowish) transparency, d. high processing temperature, e. high melt viscosity, f. high chemical resistance, g. susceptibility to stress cracking with certain solvents, h. high resistance to β-, γ-, X- and IR-radiation, i. high transmittance for microwaves, and j. high flame resistance and low smoke development.

Table 3.1 Chemical structures of thermoplastic polymers in biomedical applications

1. Polyethylene (PE)	$—[—(CH_2—CHR)_m—(CH_2—CH_2)_n—]—$ R = H, Me, Et, . . . m = 1, 2, . . . n = 1, 2, . . . if R = H, linear and high density if R ≠ H, branched and lower density
2. Polypropylene (PP)	$—[CH_2–CH\ (CH_3)]—$
isotactic	(structure below)
syndiotactic	(structure below)
atactic	(structure below)
3. Polyurethane (PU)	$—\{O–[(CH_2)_xO]_n–CONH–R–NHCO–O(CH_2)_y–OCONH–R–NHCO\}—$ $—\{O–[(CH_2)_xO]_n–CONH–R–NHCO–NH(CH_2)_y–NHCONH–R–NHCO\}—$ R = aliphatic or aromatic groups x and n for soft segment, y for extender in rigid segment
4. Polytetrafluoroethylene (PTFE)	(structure below)

Polypropylene, isotactic:

```
   H         H         H
   |    H    |    H    |
  /C\   |   /C\   |   /C\
   |   \C/   |   \C/   |
   H    |    H    |    H
       CH3       CH3
```

Polypropylene, syndiotactic:

```
   H         H         H
   |    H    |   CH3   |
  /C\   |   /C\   |   /C\
   |   \C/   |   \C/   |
   H    |    H    |    H
       CH3        H
```

Polypropylene, atactic:

```
   H         H         H
   |    H    |   CH3   |
  /C\   |   /C\   |   /C\
   |   \C/   |   \C/   |
   H    |    H    |   CH3
       CH3        H
```

Polytetrafluoroethylene (PTFE):

```
      F   F
      |   |
 —[—C—C—]—
      |   |
      F   F
```

Table 3.1 *Continued*

5. Polyvinylchloride (PVC)	$—[—CH_2—CHCl—]—$ (structure: —[—C—C—]— with H, H above and H, Cl below)
6. Polyamide (PA)	$—[NH–(CH_2)_x–NHCO—(CH_2)_y–CO]—$ $nylon_{x+1,y+1}$ and $—[NH-(CH_2)_x–CO]—$ $nylon_{x+1}$
7. Polyacrylate (PMMA)	$—(CH_2—C(R)(COOR')—)—$
8. Polyacetal (POM)	$—\{(CH_2 — O)_n —[CH_2—CH_2—(R)_x—O]_m\}—$ $R = CH_2$ $x = 0, 1, 2$ $m = 0, 1, 2$ $n = 1, 2, 3$ if $x = m = 0$, homopolymer if $x \neq m \neq 0$ copolymer
9. Polycarbonate (PC)	$—[—O—C_6H_4—C(CH_3)_2—C_6H_4—O—C(=O)—]—$

Table 3.1 *Continued*

10. Polyethylene terephthalate (PET)	$-[CH_2-CH_2-O-C(=O)-C_6H_4-C(=O)-O]-$
11. Polyetheretherketone (PEEK)	$-[-C_6H_4-C(=O)-C_6H_4-O-C_6H_4-O-]-$
12. Polysulfone (PS)	$-[-C_6H_4-C(CH_3)_2-C_6H_4-O-C_6H_4-S(=O)_2-C_6H_4-O-]-$
	$-[-C_6H_4-S(=O)_2-C_6H_4-O-]-$
	$-[-C_6H_4-O-C_6H_4-S(=O)_2-C_6H_4-C_6H_4-S(=O)_2-]-$

Table 3.2 Properties of thermoplastic polymers in biomedical applications

a. Physical properties

Physical properties	*Unit*	*PE*	*PP*	*PU*	*PTFE*	*PVC*	*PA*
Density	g/cm^3	0.954–0.965	0.90–0.915	1.02–1.28	2.10–2.20	1.16–1.70	1.02–1.15
Water absorption	%	0.001–0.02	0.01–0.035	0.1–0.9	0.01–0.05	0.04–0.75	0.25–3.5
Solubility parameter	MPa$^{1/2}$	16.4–16.6	16.3	16.4–19.5	12.6	19.4–21.5	23.02
Refractive index, n_D^{20}		1.52–1.54	1.47–1.51	1.5–1.65	1.35–1.38	1.52–1.57	1.52–1.57

Physical properties	*Unit*	*PMMA*	*POM*	*PC*	*PET*	*PEEK*	*PS*
Density	g/cm^3	1.12–1.2	1.40–1.42	1.2–1.26	1.31–1.38	1.29–1.49	1.13–1.60
Water absorption	%	0.1–0.4	0.2–0.4	0.15–0.7	0.06–0.3	0.15–0.51	0.14–0.43
Solubility parameter	MPa$^{1/2}$	18.58	22.4	19.4–19.8	21.54	20.2	20.26–22.47
Refractive index, n_D^{20}		1.49–1.51	1.48	1.56–1.60	1.51		1.56–1.67

b. Mechanical properties

Mechanical property	*Unit*	*PE*	*PP*	*PU*	*PTFE*	*PVC*	*PA*
Bulk modulus	GPa	0.8–2.2	1.6–2.5	1.5–2	1–2	3–4	2.4–3.3
Tensile strength	MPa	30–40	21–40	28–40	15–40	10–75	44–90
Elongation at break	%	130–500	100–300	600–720	250–550	10–400	40–250
Young's modulus	GPa	0.45–1.3	1–1.6	0.0018–0.009	0.3–0.7	1.0–3.8	1.4–2.8
Elastic limit	MPa	20–30	20–33	28–40	15–30	23–52	40–58
Endurance limit	MPa	13–19.6	11–18.2	21–30	9–18	13.8–31.2	22–31.9
Fracture toughness	MPa m$^{1/2}$	2.2–4	1.7–2.1	0.1–0.4	2.5–3	1–4	1.8–2.6
Hardness	MPa	60–90	60–100	50–120	27–90	70–155	100–160
Compressive strength	MPa	30–40	30–45	33–50	30–60	32–80	60–100
Poisson's ratio		0.4–0.42	0.4–0.45	0.47–0.49	0.44–0.47	0.37–0.43	0.38–0.42
Shear modulus	GPa	0.18–0.46	0.4–0.6	0.0008^{-4}–0.003	0.11–0.24	0.7–1.1	0.52–0.9

Table 3.2 *Continued*

b. Mechanical properties

Mechanical property	*Unit*	*PMMA*	*POM*	*PC*	*PET*	*PEEK*	*PS*
Bulk modulus	GPa	3–4.8	4–5.6	2.8–4.6	3–4.9	4–4.5	3.8–4.6
Tensile strength	MPa	38–80	70–75	56–75	42–80	70–208	50–100
Elongation at break	%	2.5–6	15–80	80–130	50–300	1.3–50	25–80
Young's modulus	CPa	1.8–3.3	2.55–3.5	2–2.9	2.2–3.5	3.6–13	2.4–2.9
Elastic limit	MPa	35–70	65–72	53–75	50–72	12–60	58–70
Endurance limit	MPa	19.3–38.5	28–42	29.2–41.3	30–43.2	33–36	34.8–42
Fracture toughness	MPa $m^{1//2}$	0.8–1.3	1–1.5	2.5–3.2	1.2–2	2.3–2.5	1.3–2
Hardness	MPa	100–220	110–220	110–180	97–210	100–120	180–240
Compressive strength	MPa	45–107	70–80	100–120	65–90	80–120	72–100
Poisson's ratio		0.4–0.43	0.38–0.43	0.39–0.44	0.38–0.43	0.38–0.43	0.38–0.42
Shear modulus	GPa	0.6–1.2	0.79–1	0.95–1.05	0.83–1.1	1.2–1.4	0.8–1

c. Thermal properties

Thermal property	*Unit*	*PE*	*PP*	*PU*	*PTFE*	*PVC*	*PA*
Service temperature in air without mechanical loading (short-term)	°C	90–130	140	80–130	300	55–100	130–200
Service temperature in air without mechanical loading (long-term)	°C	70–100	100	60–80	250	50–85	70–120
Minimum service temperature	°C	–63 to –53	–123 to –23	–123 to –23	–263 to –253	–43 to –28	–60 to –50
Melting(T_m)/decomposing (T_d*) ranges	°C	125–135	160–180	180–250*	322–327	150*	220–267
Glass transition temperature T_g	°C	–113 to –103	–30 to –3	–73 to –23	20 to 22	–23 to 90	20 to 92

Table 3.2 *Continued*

c. Thermal properties

Thermal property	*Unit*	*PE*	*PP*	*PU*	*PTFE*	*PVC*	*PA*
Softening temperature	°C	40–50	70–100	100		40–110	80–200
Specific heat	J/g.K	1.95–2.20	1.70–2.35	0.4–1.76	1.00–1.01	0.85–1.80	1.26–1.8
Thermal expansion	10^6/K	100–200	80–200	150–210	100–150	60–210	80–150
Thermal conductivity	W/m K	0.42–0.52	0.12–0.24	0.29–1.80	0.19–0.25	0.13–0.26	0.23–0.29
Thermal property	*Unit*	*PMMA*	*POM*	*PC*	*PET*	*PEEK*	*PS*
Service temperature in air without mechanical loading (short-term)	°C	76–108	110–140	160	180–200	300	160–260
Service temperature in air without mechanical loading (long-term)	°C	65–98	90–110	135	100	250	150–200
Minimum service temperature	°C	–123 to –73	–123 to –73	–133 to –123	–133 to –38	–123 to –103	–123 to –73
Melting(T_m)/decomposing (T_d*) ranges	°C	~170*	164–175	225–250	245–255	335	>500*
Glass transition temperature T_g	°C	106–115	-13–-75	145	67–127	144	167–230
Softening temperature	°C	70–115	110–163	138–148	70–185	140–315	150–216
Specific heat	J/g K	1.28–1.5	1.40–1.46	1.17–130	1.05–1.60	1.5–1.6	1.1–1.30
Thermal expansion	10^6/K	62–105	90–125	40–75	50–120	15–47	53–58
Thermal conductivity	W/mK	0.10–0.19	0.22–1.1	0.14–0.22	0.15–0.34	0.25–0.92	0.13–0.28

Table 3.3 Processing conditions for thermoplastc polymers in biomedical applications

Thermoplastics	*Process*	*Special process*	*Pre-treatment*	*Remarks*
1. Polyethylene	Injection moulding Extrusion Blow film extrusion Flat film extrusion Blow moulding Thermoforming Compression moulding	Film processing for PE-LD Rotational moulding for PE-powders Block, sheet, tube, profile, and film processings for PE-HD and PE-HD-UHMW Powder sintering technology for PE-UHMW	No pre-drying treatment except hygroscopic additives are added. Stabilizers and antioxidants are needed for specific processing.	PE-UHMW in solid or porous form has been used in biomedical study and application. Its most outstanding properties are wear or abrasion resistance, excellent impact resistance, and fatigue resistance. PE-UHMW has been used in fabrication of acetabular cup for hip joint prostheses.
2. Polypropylene	Injection moulding Extrusion Blow moulding Compression moulding Thermoforming	Extrusion: blown film, flat film, sheet, tube, monofilaments Injection: Long-lasting integral hinges Biaxially oriented packaging film Tapes	No pre-drying treatment except hygroscopic additives are added. Stabilizers and antioxidants are needed for specific processing.	Polypropylene has exceptionally high flex life, excellent environmental stress cracking resistance, excellent wear resistance, higher temperature resistance (withstanding steam sterilization), and low cost. Fiber applications such as suture, sewing ring, braided ligament, skin and abdominal patches. Promising applications in thin-wall packaging competing with polystyrene. Polypropylene has lower specific heat and the flow properties are more sensitive to temperature and shear rate. The mold shrinkage is lower than polyethylene but higher than with polystyrene. It has higher melt strength is important for extrusion blow molding of hollow objects. Lower molecular weight grades are suited for extrusion of monofilaments and injection molding of thin-walled articles. Cold forming may be done at room temperature (rolling), and forging, pressure forming, rolling and stamping at temperatures below the crystallite melting region (150 to 160°C). Film processing especially in oriented form competing with polyethylene.

Table 3.3 *Continued*

Thermoplastics	*Process*	*Special process*	*Pre-treatment*	*Remarks*
3. Polyurethane	Injection moulding Extrusion	Sheet extrusion Shape extrusion Cast or blow film extrusion Fiber processing	Polyurethane, especially aliphatic type is hygroscopic; the pellets must be dried before extrusion.	Characteristics high flexibility and high impact resistance, and excellent biocompatibility. Film forms of polyurethane have been used in fabrication of vascular graft and patches, heart valve leaflets, blood pumps, diaphragms for implantable artificial heart, and carriers for drug delivery. Elastomeric fibers (Spandex) made from polyurethane copolymer have been used in surgical hoses. Unfavorable processing conditions will induce residual stresses in the products which impair the biostability of polyurethane-based prostheses. To avoid residual stresses in polyurethane tubes, an upper limit of drawn down ratio of 1.5:1.0 are recommended for the appropriate stretching during extrusion. If water bath for tube processing is too cold, residual stresses are also induced. A recommended temperature for the water bath is between 21–27°C.
4. Polytetra-fluorethylene	Sintering Ram extrusion Paste extrusion Coating followed by sintering Impregnation	High temperature sintering process for parts, sheets, plates Ram extrusion for rods, tubes, profiles, wire coatings, and fibers Insulating films, crucibles Expanded tubular form	PTFE is a hydrophobic polymer and pre-drying is not necessary.	Exceptional chemical resistance, temperature resistance, and radiation and weathering resistance. Outstanding electrical properties as insulator or dielectric material. Low adhesion and low coefficient of friction. Exceptional flame resistance. Expanded PTFE (Gortex) has been used in fabrication of blood vessel prostheses.

Table 3.3 *Continued*

Thermoplastics	*Process*	*Special process*	*Pre-treatment*	*Remarks*
5. Polyvinylchloride	Extrusion Calendering Injection molding Extrusion blow molding Stretch blow molding Compression molding Sintering	Blown film Flat film Sheets Tubes and profiles Cable sheathing Bristles and mono filaments	Proper stored polyvinylchlorde can be used without pre-drying. Premixing of ingredients will be considered for plasticized PVC.	Plasticized PVC favours calendering, while unplasticized PVC prefers extrusion. Injection moulding is difficult for both plasticized and unplasticized PVCs except careful control of processing conditions or special design of machine. Characteristic flame resistance. Decomposition happens at high temperature. Overheat in processing should be avoided. Tubular, sheet, plate, and film forms of PVC have been used in medical devices such as blood bags and catheters. Implants of PVC are not encouraged.
6. Polyamides	Injection molding Extrusion Extrusion blow molding	Injection: thin-wall articles, engineering components Extrusion: bristles, packaging, tapes, fiber, wire, film, sheet, tubes, profiles, sheathing	Polyamides, especially aliphatic types are hygroscopic. Pre-drying is needed before processing, and also precaution will be considered during and after process.	Excellent friction properties and good wear and abrasion resistance. Excellent hydrocarbon resistance. Films are used for packaging. Fiber form is employed as suture materials.
7. Polyacrylates	Injection molding Extrusion Compression molding Thermoforming	Primary forms: sheet, rod, and tube Casting from monomer for optical properties Extrusion from thermoplastic resins to produce sheet. Injection moulding for small complex parts	Polyacrylates can easily pick up moisture from environment. Pre-drying is necessary.	Excellent transparency, good scratch resistance. Good processability and machinability. Monomer and polymer powder casting to produce bone cement. Hydrogel has been used to fabricate contact lens. Monomer–polymer doughs is used for processing dentures.

Table 3.3 *Continued*

Thermoplastics	*Process*	*Special process*	*Pre-treatment*	*Remarks*
8. Polyacetal	Injection molding Extrusion Blow molding Compression molding	Injection moulding Extrusion	Polyacetal is less hygroscopic than nylon. However, acetal polymer must be stored in dry place.	Oustanding creep and fatigue resistance. Good toughness and impact resistance. Excellent strength for engineering application. Processing temperature must be carefully controlled. Fiber and film forms of polyacetal are not available. Polyacetal, Delrin, has been used in disc of mechanical heart valves.
9. Polycarbonate	Injection molding Extrusion Blow moldings Thermoforming Hot bending	Injection and extrusion Films: extruded and solvent cast, uniaxially oriented amorphous and partially, crystalline Tube, rod, profile, sheet: extrusion	Polycarbonate can pick up enough moisture to deteriorate quality of products. Pre-drying is necessary.	Applications have been found in consideration of toughness, rigidity, transparency, self-extinguishing characteristics, good electrical insulation and heat resistance. Polycarbonate has been used in the manufacture of contact lenses.
10. Polyethylene-terephthalate	Injection moulding Extrusion Blow molding	Fiber process Uniaxially oriented tapes Films, packaging film, sheet, articles Biaxially oriented film and sheet	Polyethyleneterephthalate is hygroscopic. Pre-drying is necessary.	Characteristic crystallization. Both amorphous and crystallized products can be made through control of crystallization. The benefits from PET products are their stiffness, warp resistance, and dimension stability. Fiber form of PET has been used to fabricate blood vessels and by-pass prostheses. Suture made from PET. Dacron® sewing ring and medical fabrics.

Table 3.3 *Continued*

Thermoplastics	*Process*	*Special process*	*Pre-treatment*	*Remarks*
11. Polyetheretherketone	Injection molding Compression molding Extrusion Composite	Injection molding for articles Extrusion: film/cast and oriented monofilament wire covering Composite: carbon fiber/PEEK composite	PEEK is hydrophobic polymer but pre-drying is necessary for quality control.	Characteristic high strength at high temperature. Excellent resistance to hydrolysis and environmental stress cracking. Carbon fiber/PEEK composite investigated in bone fracture fixation.
12. Polysulphone	Injection molding Extrusion Blow molding Thermoforming	Injection molding for articles Extrusion: film and sheet which can be thermoformed	Polysulphone is hygroscopic and pre-drying is required to avoid vapor formation during processing.	Good rigidity, creep resistance, and toughness. Hydrolysis resistance and can undergo repeated steam sterilization. Transparent products can be made and used in medical field. Hollow fiber and membrane devices have been used in hemodialysis. Carbon fiber/polysulphone composite has been used for bone fracture fixation.

Table 3.4 Trade names of thermoplastic polymers in biomedical applications

1. Polyethylene (PE)		
	PE-LD and PE-HD	
Eltex(Solvay, BE)	Fertene Maplen (Himmont, IT)	Ladene (SABIC, Saudi Arabia)
Finathene (Fina, BE)	Rumiten (Rumianca, IT)	Escorene (Exxon Chem, US)
Alathon, Sclair (Du Pont Canada Inc., CA)	NeoZex (Mitsui, JP)	Fortiflex (Soltex Polymer, US)
Boalen (Petrimex, CS)	Nipolon (Toyo Soda, JP)	Norchem (USI, US)
Hostalen (Hoechst, DE)	Novatec (Mitsubishi, JP)	Paxon (Allied Signal Corp., US)
Lupolen (BASF, DE)	Hi Zex (Mitsol, JP)	Microthene, Petrothene (USI Chem., US)
Vestolen (Huls, DE)	Mirason (Mitsui Polychem., JP)	HiFax (Himont, US)
Ertileno (Union ERT, ES)	Sholex (Showa Denko, JP)	Marlex (Phillips Petrol., US)
Natene (Rhone-Poulenc, FR)	Sumikathene (Sumitomo Chem., JP)	Super Dylan (Arco Chem., US)
Lacqtene (Atochem, FR)	Suntec (Asahi Chem., JP)	Tenite (Easrman Chem., US)
Carlona (Shell, GB)	Staflene (Nisseki Plastic Chem., JP)	Hipten (Hemijska Ind., YU)
Rigidex, Novex (BP Chemicals, GB)	Yukalon (Mitsubishi Petroleum, JP)	Okiten (INAOKI, YU)
Tipolen (Tiszai Vegyi Kombinat, HU)	Stamylan (DSM, NL)	
Eraclene (EniChem Base, IT)	Ropol (Chem. Komb. Borcesti; RO)	
	PE-HD-UHMW	
Hostalen GUR (Hoechst AG, DE)	Lupolen UHM (BASF AG, DE)	
	PE-LLD	
Eltex (Solvay, BE)	Rumiten (Rumianca, IT)	Escorene (Exxon Chem., US)
Alathon, Sclair (Du pont Canada, CA)	Mirason (Mitsui Polychem., JP)	Marlex TR130 (Phillips Petroleum, US)
Novapol LL (Novacor Chem., CA)	Novatex (Mitsubishi Chem., JP)	Microthene, Petrothene (USI Chem., US)
Lupolen (BASF, DE)	Sumikathene (Sumitomo Chem., JP)	Norchem (USI/Exxon Chem., US)
Lotrex (Orkem Norsolor SA, FR)	Ultzex (Mitsui Petrochemical, JP)	Rexene (EI Paso Chem., US)
News (Neste Oy Chem., FI)	Stamylex (DSM, NL)	Tenite (Eastman Chem., US)
Visqueen (ICI, GB)	Ladene (SABIC, Saudi Arabia)	
Eraclear (EniChem., IT)	Dowlex (Dow Chemical, US)	
2. Polypropylene (PP)		
Asota, Ecofelt (Chemic Linz, AT)	Eltex (Solvay, FR)	Stamylan (DSM, NL)
Marlex (Phillips Petroleum Co., BE)	Carlona (Shell, GB)	Bicor (Mobil Chem., US)
Istrono (Chem., Werke J. Dimitrow, CS)	Propathene (ICI, GB)	Extrel, Twistlock, Vistalon(Exxon Chem, US)
Tatren (Petrimex, CS)	Biofol (Chem. Kombinat. Tisza, HU)	Fortilene (Soltex Polymer Corp. US)
Hostalen PP (Hoechst, DE)	Afax, Moplen, Valtec (Himont, IT)	Liteplate S (Hercules, US)
Platilon (Deutsche ATOchem., DE)	Bifax (Showa denko, JP)	Profax (Himont, US)

Table 3.4 *Continued*

2. Polypropylene (PP)		
Trovidur (Huls-Troisdorf, DE)	Eperon (Kanegafuchi Chem., JP)	Rexene (El Paso Chem., US)
Ultralen (Lonza Werke, DE)	Noblen (Mitsubishi Petrochemical, JP)	Tenite (Eastman Chemical, US)
Vestolen P (Huls, DE)	Novatec (Mitsubishi Chem., JP)	
Apryl, Lacqtene P (Atochem., FR)	PolyPro, Sunlet (Mitsui Petrochem., JP)	
3. Polyurethane (PU)		
	General	
Ucefix, Uceflex (UCB, BE)	Europolymers (Avalon Chemical Co., GB)	Urafil (Akzo-Wilson-Fiberfil, US)
Fabeltan (Tubize Plastics, BE)	Jectothane (Dunlop Holdings, GB)	Hi-Tuff (J.P. Stevens & Co., US)
Caprolan, Elastolen, Elastolan (Elastogran Polyurethane, DE)	Pemuflex (Pemu Chemolimpex, HU)	Esteloc, Estane, Roylar (B.F. Goodrich Chemical Co., US)
Desmopan (Bayer, DE)	Uthane (Urethanes India, IN)	Irogran, Plastothane (Morton Thiokol, US)
Luroflex (Lehmann u. Voss Co., DE)	Pelprene (Toyobo Co., Resins Div., JP)	Proplastic (Pro Lam, US)
Oldopren (Busing u. Fasch & Co., DE)	Durane (Swanson, US)	Q-Thane (Quinn & Co., US)
Durelast (B & T polymers, GB)		
	Medical special	
Angioflex (Abiomed Danvers, MA)	Mitrathane (PolyMedica Burlington, MA, US)	Corplex (Corvita Miami, FL, US)
Biomer (Ethicon Somerville, NJ, US)	Pellethane (Dow Chemical La Porte, TX, US)	Unithane 80F (NICPBP Beijing, China)
Cardiothane (Kontron Everett, MA, US)	Surethane (Cardiac Control Palm Coast, FL, US)	Corethane (Corvita Miami, FL, US)
Chronoflex (PolyMedica Burlington, MA, US)	Tecoflex (Thermedics Inc Woburn, MA, US)	PU 10 (Univ. NSW, Australia)
Hemothane (Sams, Div 3M Ann Arbor, MI, US)	Toyobo TM5 (Toyobo Co. Osaka, Japan)	
4. Polytetrafluoroethylene (PTFE)		
Hostaflon TF (Hoechst, DE)	Neoflon (Daikin Ind., JP)	RT duroid (Rogers Corp., US)
Pamflon (Norton Pampus, DE)	Polyflon (Daikin Kogyo Co., JP)	Rulon (Dixon Ind. Corp., US)
Foraflon (ATOCHEM, FR)	Ferrotron, Fluorosint (Polymer Corp., US)	Salox (Allegheny Plastics, US)
Soreflon (Pechiney U.K., FR)	Fluoroloy (Flurocatbon, US)	Teflon (Du Pont de Numours, US)
Gaflon (Plastic Omnium, FR)	FluoroMet (Raymark, US)	Turcite (W.S. Shamban & Co., US)
Fluon (ICI, GB)	Goretex (W.L. Gore Assoc., US)	Tygaflor (American Cyanamid Aerospace, US)
Algoflon (Montedison, IT)	Halon (Ansimont, US)	Xylon (Whitford Corp., US)

Table 3.4 *Continued*

5. Polyvinylchloride (PVC)		
Benvic (Solvay, BE)	Corvic, Vynide, Welvic (ICI, GB)	Rosevil (Chem. Kombinat Borzesti, RO)
Plastilit, Selchim, Solvic (Solvay & Cie., BE)	Ongrovil (Barsodi Veggi Komb., HU)	Ensolite (Uniroyal Chem., US)
Vipopham (Lonza, CH)	Ravinil, Sicron, Vipla, Viplast (EniChem, IT)	Ethyl (Ethyl Corp., Polymer Div., US)
Astralon, Trocal, Trosiplast, Trovidur, Vestolit (Huls-Troisdorf, DE)	Vixir (S.I.R. (Montedison), IT)	Fiberloc, Geon (B.F. Goodrich, US)
Decelith (VEB Ellenburger Chemiewerk, DE)	Hishiplate (Mitsubishi Plastics Ind., JP)	Pliovic, Vinacel, Vycell (Goodyear, US)
Vinnol (Wacker Chemie, DE)	Kureha, Viclon (Kureha Chem. Ind., JP)	Vygen (General Tire & Rubber Co., US)
Genopak, Genotherm, Hostalit (Hoechst, DE)	Vinychlon (Mitsui Toatsu Chem., JP)	Vynaloy (B.F. Goodrich Chem. Co., US)
Armodur (Rhone-Poulenc, FR)	Vinylfoil (Mitsubishi Gas Ind., JP)	Hipnil (Hemijska Industria, YU)
Bipeau, Orgavyl, Polycal (ATOCHEM., FR)	Varlan (DSM, NL)	Jugotherm, Juvinil (Jugovinil, YU)
Ekavyl (PCUK, FR)	Norvinyl, Pevikon (Norsk Hydro, NO)	Zadrovil (Polikem, YU)
Carina, Duraflex (Shell Intern. Chem Co., GB)	Oltivil (Chem. Komb. Pitesti, RO)	
6. Polyamide (PA)		
	PA 6	
Fabenyl (Tubize Plastics, CH)	Maranyl (ICI, GB)	Akulon (Engineering Plastics of AKZO Plastics, NL)
Grilon (Ems Chemie, CH)	Latamid (L.A.T.I., IT)	Capron (Allied Signal Engn. Plastics, US)
Durethan B (Bayer, DE)	Nivionplast (EniChem, IT)	Plaskon (Plaskon Moldings Div., US)
Ultramid B (BASF, DE)	Renyl (Snia Technopolimeri, IT)	Zytel (Du Pont de Nemours, US)
Orgamide (ATOCHEM, FR)	Amilan, Amilon (Toray Ind., JP)	
Technyl C (Rhone-Poulenc Specialites Chimiques, FR)	Torayca (Toray Ind., JP)	
	PA 66	
Durethan A (Bayer, DE)	Leona (Asahi Chemical Ind., JP)	Minlon (Du Pont de Nemours, US)
Technyl A (Rhone-Poulenc Specialites Chimiques, FR)	Torayca (Toray Ind., JP)	Zytel (Du Pont de Nemours, US)
Maranyl A (ICI, GB)	Akulon (Engineering Plastics of AKZO Plastics, NL)	
7. Polyacrylates		
Umaplex (Synthesia, CS)	Asterite (ICI, GB)	Sumipex (Sumitomo Chem. Co., JP)
Acrifix (Rohm, DE)	Diakon (ICI, GB)	Casoglas (Casolith, NL)
Lucryl (BASF, DE)	Perspex (ICI, GB)	Acrylite (Cy/Ro Industries, US)

Table 3.4 *Continued*

7. Polyacrylates		
Degaplast (Degussa, DE)	Unilok (British Vita Co., GB)	Lucite (Du Pont de Nemours, US)
Deglas, Dewglas (Degussa, DE)	Vetredil (Vetril, IT)	Corian (Du Pont de Nemours, US)
Dewoglas (Degussa, DE)	Vedril (Montedison, IT)	Crofon (Du Pont de Nemours, US)
Paraglas (Degussa, DE)	Acrypanel (Mitsubishi Rayon Co., JP)	Electroglas (Glasflex Corp., US)
Plexidur, Plexiglas (Rohm, DE)	Delmer, Depet (Asahi Chem. Ind., JP)	Exolite (Cyro Industries, US)
Resarit (Resart, DE)	Eska (Mitsubishi Rayon, JP)	Gardlite (Southern Plastics Co., US)
Vestiform (Huls, DE)	Palapet (Kyowa Gas Chem., JP)	Oroglas (Rohm & Haas Co., US)
Altuglas (Altulor, Orekem, FR)	Shinkolite (Mitsubishi Rayon Co., JP)	Swedcast (Swedlow, US)
8. Polyacetal (POM)		
	Homopolymers	
Delrin (Du Pont, US)	Tenal (Asahi Chemical Ind., JP)	
	Copolymers	
Celcon, Hostaform (Hoechst, DE)	Duracon, Alkon, and Kematal (Daicel Polyplastic Co., JP)	Ultraform (BASF, DE)
9. Polycarbonate (PC)		
Sparlux (Solvay & Cie., BE)	Sinvet (EniChem, IT)	Lexan (General Electric Plastics, US)
Durolon (Policarbonateos do Brazil, BR)	Novarex (Mitsubishi Chem. Ind., JP)	Merlon (Mobay Chemical Corp.. US)
Makrolon (Bayer, DE)	Panlite (Teijin Chemicals, JP)	Polycarbafil (Akzo-Wilson-Fiberfil, US)
Orgalan (ATOCHEM, FR)	Xantar (DSM, NL)	Polygard (Polytech, US)
Star-C (Ferro Eurostar, FR)	Calibre (Dow Chemical Corp., US)	Stat-Kon (LNP Corp., US)
Royalite (British Vita Co., GB)	Ekonol (Carborundum Co., US)	
10. Polyethyleneterephthalate		
	(PET)	
Crastin (Ciba Geigy, CH)	Melinar, Melinite (ICI, GB)	Petlon (Mobay Chem. Corp., US)
Grilpet (Ems Chemie, CH)	Arnite (Akzo Engng. Plastics, NL)	Petra (Allied Signal, US)
Impet (Hoechst, DE)	Etar (Eastman Chem. Intern., US)	Ropet (Rohm & Hass Co., US)
Ultradur (BASF, DE)	Mindel (Amoco Performance Products, US)	Rynite (Du Pont de Nemours, US)
11. Polyetheretherketone		
	(PEEK)	
	Victrex PEEK (ICI, UK)	

Table 3.4 *Continued*

12. Polysulphone		
Ultrason S (BASF DE)	Stabar (ICI, UK)	Udel (Amoco Performance Products, US)
Sumilik FST (Sumitomo, Chem. Co., JP)		

REFERENCES

Black, J. (ed.) (1992), in *Biological Performance of Materials: Fundamentals of Biocompatibility*, Second edition, Marcel Dekker. Inc, New York.

Brydson, J.A. (ed.), *Plastics Materials,* Butterworths Scientific, fourth edition, 1982; fifth edition, 1989.

Carhart, R.O. (1985) Polycarbonate, in *Engineering Thermoplastics, Properties and Applications*, Margolis, J.M. (ed.), Chapter 3, pp. 29–82.

Chapman, R.D. and Chruma, J.L. (1985) Nylon plastics, in *Engineering Thermoplastics, Properties and Applications*, Margolis J.M. (ed.), pp. 83–122.

Charrier, J.M. (ed.) (1990) *Polymeric Materials and Processing: Plastics, Elastomers and Composites,* Hanser.

Domininghaus, H. (ed.) (1993) *Plastics for Engineers, Materials Properties, Applications,* Car-Hanser Verlag.

Goodman, S.B. and Fornasier, V.L. (1992) Clinical and experimental studies in the biology of aseptic loosing of joint arthroplastics and the role of polymer particles, in *Particulate Debris from Medical Implants: Mechanisms of Formation and Biological Consequences,* ASTM ATP 1144, K.R. St John, (ed), American Society for Testing and Materials, Philadelphia, pp. 27–37.

Harper, C.A. (eds) (1992) *Handbook of Plastics, Elastomers, and Composites*, McGraw-Hill.

How, T.V. (1992) Mechanical properties of arteries and arterial grafts, in *Cardiovascular Biomaterials,* Hastings, G.W. (ed.), Springer-Verlag, London, pp. 1–35.

Jones, A.J. and Denning, N.T. (1988) in *Polymeric Biomaterials: Bio- and Eco-compatible Polymers, A Perspective for Australia,* Department of Industry, Technology and Commerce.

Lilley, P.A., Blunn, G.W., and Walker, P.S. (1993) Wear performance of PEEK as a potential prosthetic knee joint material, in *7th International Conference on Polymers in Medicine and Surgery,* 1–3 September 1993, Leeuwenhorst Congress Center, Noordwijkerhout, The Netherlands, pp. 320–326.

Margolis, J.M. (1985) *Engineering Thermoplastics: Properties and Applications*, Dekker, New York.

Mascia, L. (1989), in *Thermoplastics: Materials Engineering*, Second Edition, Elsevier Applied Science, London and New York.

McMillin, C.R. (1994) Elastomers for biomedical applications, *Rubber Chem. and Tech.* **67,** 417–446.

Park, J.B. and Lakes, R.S. (1992) *Biomaterials, an Introduction*, Second Edition, Plenum Press, New York and London.

Rubin, I.I. (ed.) (1990), *Handbook of Plastic Materials and Technology*, John Wiley & Son.

Staudinger, H. (1932) *Die Hochmolekularen Organischer Verbindungen*, Julius Springer.

Stokes, K., McVenes, R., and Anderson, J.M. (1995) Polyurethane elastomer biostability, *J. Biomaterials Applications*, **9,** 321–355.

Szycher, M. (1991) in *Blood Compatible Materials and Devices: Perspectives Towards the 21st Century*, Sharma, C.P. and Szycher, M. (eds), Technomic Publishing CO., Inc., Lancaster, Basel, pp. 33–85.

Teoh, S.H., Lim, S.C., Yoon, E.T., and Goh, K.S. (1994) A new method for *in vitro* wear assessment of materials used in mechanical heart valves, in *Biomaterials Mechanical Properties*, ASTM STP 1173, H.E. Kambic and A.T. Yokobori, Jr. Eds., American Society for Testing and Materials, Philadelphia, pp. 43–52.

Teoh, S.H., Lim, S.C., Yoon, E.T., and Goh, K.S. (1994a) A new method for *in vitro* wear assessment of materials used in mechanical heart valves, in *Biomaterials Mechanical Properties*, ASTM STP 1173, H.E. Kambic and A.T. Yokobori, Jr. (eds), American Society for Testing and Materials, Philadelphia, pp. 43–52.

Teoh, S.H., Martin, R.L., Lim, S.C., *et al.* (1990) Delrin as an occluder material, *ASAIO Transactions*, **36,** M417–421.

Watson, M., Cebon, D., Ashby, M., Charlton, C., and Chong, W.T. (eds) (1994) *Cambridge Materials Selector V2.02*, National University of Singapore, Granta Design Ltd.

Wenz, L.M., Merritt, K., Brown, S.A., and Moet, A. (1990) In-vitro biocompatibility of polyetheretherketone and polysulphone composites, *J. Biomed. Maters Res.*, *24,* 207–215.

Ziegler, K.E. (1955) *Angew. Chem.* **67**(426), 541.

4 Biomedical elastomers

J.W. Boretos and S.J. Boretos

4.1 INTRODUCTION

Elastomers are described as materials that possess pronounced elasticity and rebound. They can be tough, relatively impermeable to air and water and exhibit resistance to cutting, tearing and abrasion. Often they are modified by compounding to increase their hardness and strength. Or, conversely, they can be soft, compliant and absorbent to water if the need exists. In some instances their properties can closely simulate that of the tissues which they must contact. As biomedical materials they may have originated from commercial formulations or been custom designed from basic chemistry. Those that have been judged as biocompatible have made significant contributions towards the development of successful medical devices. Literally, every basic elastomer has been evaluated at some time for its possible suitability in contact with the body. This would include such materials as natural rubber, styrene rubber, polybutyl rubber, silicone rubber, acrylate rubber, Hypalon®, polyurethanes, fluorinated hydrocarbon rubbers, polyvinyl chloride, thermoplastic vulcanizates and others. Of these, only special medical grade formulations of silicone, polyurethane, polyvinyl chloride and thermoplastic elastomer have continued to be commercially successful.

There are important differences between materials and differences among similar materials within a given generic class. These differences are due to the chemical composition of the polymer, the molecular configuration of the polymer and the presence of functional groups. For instance, polyurethanes of a polyester base were initially tried and found unstable for implantation whereas polyether based polyurethanes were decidedly

Handbook of Biomaterial Properties. Edited by J. Black and G. Hastings.
Published in 1998 by Chapman & Hall, London. ISBN 0 412 60330 6.

more stable. Elastomers with aromatic structures behave differently than the polymer having aliphatic structure. Not every material is suitable for every application. Some have been found to perform successfully under static conditions but fail or perform undesirably under dynamic situations. Often, the design of a device and the demands upon it will determine if the elastomer chosen is the proper selection. Therefore the material and its use are inseparable. They must be evaluated together. Merely passing an array of physical and biological tests do not confer success. Biocompatibility is an essential element of medical grade elastomers. A set of compatibility tests determine the general physiological acceptability of an elastomer. These consist of passing USP Class VI tests. Additional testing may be required depending upon the device, its area of application and the time it is in contact with tissues. A Master File is often registered by the manufacturer of the basic elastomer with the FDA to attest to its properties, composition and response to biological testing. Demands on medical device manufacturers have never been more stringent. Regulatory pressures, more indepth testing, the threat of litigation plus the constraints of health care cost containment are affecting all aspects of the design and development process and the availability of some biomedical elastomers. A variety of elastomeric materials are available to meet the design challenges presented by medical devices. However, there is still a need for even better materials.

The elastomers that are listed here should be considered in light of their suitability for a specific application. The properties tables should serve as a guide to design options for those in the early stages of the development process. Keep in mind that these properties listed in the tables and the compatibility standings are only indicative of the performance characteristics that an elastomer may exhibit.

4.2 TYPES OF ELASTOMER

Biomedical elastomers can be classified as to whether they are thermoplastic or thermosetting in nature. Thermoplastic biomedical elastomers are gaining in commercial importance and in some cases replacing traditionally used vulcanized versions. Thermosetting elastomers are irreversibly crosslinked and have had the longest history of medical use. Both groups will be described citing representative medical elastomers that are either commercially available or that may replace elastomers that have been recently withdrawn from the market.

4.2.1 Thermoplastic elastomers

Thermoplastic elastomers (TPEs) are a special class of materials that process similarly to other thermoplastic polymers, yet possess many of the desirable properties of thermoset elastomers. Some TPEs are elastomeric alloys consisting of crosslinked particles of rubber surrounded by a thermoplastic matrix. Others consist of block copolymers and are typified by polyurethanes and styrene polymers.

Depending upon which thermoplastic elastomer is chosen, physical properties can vary over a wide range. They can be either hard, or soft, flexible or stiff, elastic or rigid. For the most part, they are smooth to the touch, yet will form tight seals to surfaces they contact. They can be processed using conventional techniques and equipment and in automated modes. Medical applications consist of such examples as pacemaker lead wire coatings, artificial hearts, and catheters. A wide variety of sundry uses have contributed to patient care and consists of bulbs and bladders, serum caps and tubes, cushions, diaphragms, electrical connectors, flexible medical wire coatings, gaskets, needle shields, pharmaceutical closures, seals, stoppers, tubing, and valves. Most of the TPEs can be sterilized using gas, steam and radiation with very little change in their molecular structures or properties (Table 4.13).

Thermoplastic vulcanizates

Thermoplastic vulcanizates are a separate class of thermoplastic elastomers (TPEs) with Santoprene® as the representative biomedical elastomer.

Santoprene®

This thermoplastic vulcanizate is an olefin based elastomer; an elastomeric alloy. It is totally synthetic and does not contain any natural rubber thereby avoiding many of the allergic reaction problems associated with natural rubber latex. It exhibits outstanding flex-fatigue resistance, low temperature flexibility (-40 °C) and resistance to tearing and abrasion. Its resistance to plastic deformation under tensile and compression stress is another of its features. Santoprene® is reported to be superior to natural rubber in some situations and replaces silicone elastomers in others. It has found use in peristaltic pump tubing, syringe plungers, seals, and caps, tracheal and enteral tubing, vial closures and pump seals, disposable anesthetic hoses, intravenous delivery systems, and other hospital devices. Santoprene® has met USP Class IV requirements for *in vivo* biological reactivity and conforms to the Tripartite Biocompatibility Guidance standards. However, the manufacturer does not recommend Santoprene® for use as part of human implants. The material may be injection molded, extruded, blow molded and thermoformed. For details on physical properties, processing and biocompatibility see Tables 4.1, 4.2, 4.13 and 4.14.

Table 4.1 Typical Properties of Thermoplastic Vulcanizates

Product and Manufacturer	*Product no.*	*Specific gravity ASTM D-792*	*Durometer hardness shore ASTM D-2240*	*Tensile strength, psi ASTM D-412*	*Elongation, percent ASTM D-412*	*Modulus ASTM D-412 psi*	*Modulus ASTM D-412 %*	*Tear strength pli,die C ASTM D-624*	*Compression set, percent ASTM D-395*
Santoprene®	281–45	0.97	45A	435	300	175	100	80	11
Rubber,	281–55	0.97	55A	640	330	250	100	108	23
	281–64	0.97	64A	1,030	400	340	100	140	23
Advanced	281–73	0.98	73A	1230	460	520	100	159	26
Elastomer	281–87	0.96	87A	2,300	520	1,010	100	278	29
Systems	283–40	0.95	40 D	2,750	560	1,250	100	369	32

Table 4.2 Typical Properties of Copolyester Elastomers, PCCE

Product and Manufacturer	*Product no.*	*Specific gravity ASTM D-792*	*Durometer hardness shore ASTM D-2240*	*Tensile strength, psi ASTM D-412*	*Elongation, percent ASTM D-412*	*Modulus ASTM D-412 psi*	*Modulus ASTM D-412 %*	*Tear strength pli,die B ASTM D-624*	*Compression set, percent ASTM D-395*
Ecdel™	9965							—	
Elastomer,	9966	1.13	95 A	3,500	380	16,000	100	100	40
Eastman Chemical Co.	9967							135	

Table 4.3 Typical Properties of Polyurethane-based Elastomers

		Property							
Product and Manufacturer	*Product no.*	*Specific gravity ASTM D-792*	*Durometer hardness shore ASTM D-2240*	*Tensile strength, psi ASTM D-412*	*Elongation, percent ASTM D-412*	*Modulus ASTM D-412 psi*	*Modulus ASTM D-412 %*	*Tear strength pli,die C ASTM D-624*	*Compression set, percent ASTM D-395*
Biospan segmented polyurethane, The Polymer Technology Group, Inc.	Biospan®		75A	6000	850	575	100		
	Biospan® D		70 D	6000	1000	550	100		
	Biospan® S		70 D	5500	1050	450	100		
Hydrothane™, Poly Medica Biomaterials, Inc.	Dry		93 A	7800	580				
	Very dry		95 A	5800	475				
	Wet		85 A	5600	500				
Medicaflex™, Advanced Resin Technology	MF-5000	1.15	50 A	3000	500	300	100		
	MF-5001	1.15	55 A	3000		300	100		
	MF-5040	1.15	60 A	5000	700	300	100		
	MF-5041					300	100		
	MF-5056	1.15	65 A	5000	750	500	100		
	MF-5057					550	100		
	MF-5062	1.14	60 A	5000	800	500	100		
Pellethane™ 2363 series, Dow Chemical Co.	2363-55D	1.15	55 D	6900	390	2500	100	650	25
	2363-55DE	1.15	53 D	6500	450	2300	100	600	30
	2363-65D	1.17	62 D	6460		2900	100	1100	30
	2363-75D	1.21	76 D	5810	380		1470		
	2363-80A	1.13	81 A	5200	550	880	100	470	25
	2363-80AE	1.12	85 A	4200	650	890	100	420	30
	2363-80A R0120	1.30	81 A	6860	670	970	100		
	2363-90A	1.14	90 A	5850	500	1700	100	570	25
	2363-90AE	1.14	90 A	6000	550	1475	100	540	
PolyBlend™ 1000 and PolyBlend™ 1100, Poly Medica Biomaterials, Inc.	PB1000–650		65 D to 75 D	6500	350	5300	100	—	—
	PB1100–55	1.02	55 A	2150	800	135	100	140	55–66
	PB1100–60	1.02	60 A	2400		210	100	150	50–60
	PB1100-75	1.02	75 A	3250	575	420	100	240	45–50
	PB1100-80	1.02	80 A	4600	590	555	100	330	25–30
Tecoflex®, Thermedics, Inc.	EG60D	1.09	51 D	7829	363	2000	100		
	EG60D-B20	1.32	55 D	7484	370				
	EG65D	1.10	60 D	8074	335	2500	100		
	EG65D-B20	--	63 D	6986	321				
	EG68D	1.10		8686	332				
	EG72D	1.11	67 D	7739	307	3400	100		
	EG80A	1.04	72 A	5640	709	400	100		

Table 4.3 *Continued*

Product and Manufacturer	*Product no.*	*Property* Specific gravity ASTM D-792	Durometer hardness shore ASTM D-2240	Tensile strength, psi ASTM D-412	Elongation, percent ASTM D-412	Modulus ASTM D-412 psi	Modulus ASTM D-412 %	Tear strength pli,die C ASTM D-624	Compression set, percent ASTM D-395
Thermedics,	EG80A-B20	1.24	73 A	5571	715				
Inc.	EG85A	1.05	77 A	6935	565	700	100		
	EG85A-B20	1.25	83 A	5282	632				
	EG85A-B40	1.51	84 A	5093	559				
	EG93A	1.08	87 A	7127	423	1100	100		
	EG100A	1.09	94 A	8282	370	1800	100		
	EG100A-B20	1.29	93 A	7104	369				
	EG100A-B40	1.54	96 A	5607	360				
	1055D	1.16	54 D	9600	350	2500	100		
Tecothane®	1065D	1.18	64 D	10 000	300	3200	100		
	1074A	1.10	75 A	6000	530	530	100		
	1075D	1.19	75 D	8300	240	3600	100		
Thermedics,	1085A	1.12	85 A	7000	450	800	100		
Inc.	1095A	1.15	94 A	9400	400	1600	100		
	2055D	1.36	55 D	9000	360	2700	100		
	2065D	1.38	67 D	8500	300	3100	100		
	2074A	1.30	77 A	5500	580	510	100		
	2075D	1.40	77 D	7600	230	3000	100		
	2085A	1.32	87 A	6600	550	800	100		
	2095A	1.35	97 A	8200	450	1600	100		
	5187	1.20	87 A	6000	500	750	100	500	12
Texin™	5265	1.17	65 D	6000	460	3300	100	1200	20
	5286	1.12	86 A	6000	550	700	100	500	16
Miles, Inc.	5370	1.21	70 D	6000	180	4500	100	900	
	DP7-3002		88 A	2208	579	815	100	399	—
	DP7-3003	—	50 D	3714	458	1049	100	564	
	DP7-3004		55 D	4783	392	1766	100	819	

Table 4.4 Typical Properties of Polycarbonate-based Polyurethane

Product and Manufacturer	*Product no.*	*Property*						
		Specific gravity ASTM D-792	*Durometer hardness shore ASTM D-2240*	*Tensile strength, psi ASTM D-412*	*Elongation, percent ASTM D-412*	*Modulus ASTM D-412 psi*	*Modulus ASTM D-412 %*	*Tear strength pli,die C ASTM D-624*
	PC-3555D	1.15	60 D	7000	350	1500	100	
Carbothane™,	PC-3555D-B20	1.36	57 D	8300	380	1600	100	
	PC-3572D	1.15	71 D	8500	300	4100	100	
Thermedics,	PC-3572D-B20	1.35	71 D	8400	310	3400	100	
Inc.	PC-3575A	1.15	73 A	4400	500	380	100	
	PC-3575A-B20		73 A	3500	600	410	100	
	PC-3585A	1.15	84 A	6500	390	640	100	
	PC-3585A-B40	1.68	89 A	3800	521	700	100	
	PC-3595A	1.15	95 A	6500	520	900	100	
	PC-3595A-B20	1.36	96 A	8300	390	1100	100	
Chronoflex™ AR, Poly Medica Biomaterials, Inc.	Chronoflex™ AR		70 A	7500	500	700	100	
Corethane®	TPE 55D	1.211	55 D	7000–8500	365–440	1850–2200	100	
and	TPE 75D	1.216	75 D	7000–9100	255–320	5300–5700	100	
	TPE 80A	1.179	80 A		400–490	770–1250		
Corhesive™, Corvita Corp.	Corhesive™ (cured)	1.179	80 A	6500–7500	400–900	770–1250	100	
Texin™ 5370, Miles, Inc.	5370	1.21	70 D	6000	180	4500	100	900

Copolyester ether elastomer

Ecdel™.

This copolyester ether TPE is essentially polycyclohexanedimethyl-cyclohexanedicarboxylate (PCCE). It is reported to possess the chemical resistance, toughness and inertness yet exhibits elastic flexibility over a broad temperature range. Ecdel™ is an unusual elastomer since it has a crystalline structure. Quenching during molding can reduce its crystallinity and impart increased clarity. The material is being used for uniquely designed intravenous bags with built-in bottle necks and fasteners. The material can be injection or blow molded and extruded into film or sheet; but only Ecdel™ 9967 may be processed into tubing. This TPE is also manufactured under the name CR3 by Abbott Labs (Tables 4.2, 4.12, 4.13, and 4.14).

Table 4.5 Typical Properties of Polypropylene-based Elastomers

		Property					
Product and Manufacturer	*Product no.*	*Specific gravity ASTM D-792*	*Durometer hardness, shore ASTM D-2240*	*Tensile strength, psi ASTM D-412*	*Elongation, percent ASTM D-412*	*Tear strength pli, die B ASTM D-624*	*Compression set, percent ASTM D-395*
Sarlink® medical grade DSM Thermoplastic Elastomers, Inc.	3260	0.95	60 A	870	619	183	42

Polyurethane-based elastomers

Polyurethanes are another class of TPEs. They are a large family of chemical compounds that can consist of ether-based, ester-based, polycarbonate-based or polypropylene-based varieties. A number of copolymers are also included;. polyurethanes are combinations of macroglycols and diisocyanates that have been polymerized into tough and elastic materials. TPE polyurethanes have been used for peristaltic pump tubing, parenteral solution tubing and catheters. The tables list the majority of those that are commercially available. Among others are those either of limited supply, available for proprietary use only or that have been successful, but recently discontinued such as:

- Hemothane Sarns Div. of 3M. Restricted to proprietary use.
- Biomer Ethicon, Inc. No longer available through this source.
- Surethane Cardiac Control Systems, Inc. Redissolved Lycra® thread. Some formulations may have a few percent PDMS blended with it. Limited availability.
- Pellethane™ 2360 Dow Chemical, USA. This material is no longer available for medical implant use (see also Pellethane™).
- Angioflex ABIOMED, Danvers, Mass. Restricted to proprietary use.
- Cardiothane Kontrol, Inc. A silicone-urethane interpenetrating polymer network. Limited availability.

Internationally, polyurethanes for medical use have been developed by Italy, China and Japan.

Biospan®

This TPE is a segmented polyurethane and is reported to be not significantly different from biomer in chemistry and molecular weight. It is a polytetra-methyleneoxide-based aromatic polyurethane urea with mixed aliphatic and cycloaliphatic diamine chain extenders. A copolymer of

Table 4.6 Typical Properties of Plasticized Polyvinyl Chloride

Product and Manufacturer	*Product no.*	*Specific gravity ASTM D-792*	*Durometer shore ASTM D-2240*	*Tensile strength, psi ASTM D-412*	*Elongation, percent ASTM D-412*	*Modulus ASTM D-412 psi*	*Modulus ASTM D-412 %*
	3511TX-02	1.12	35 A	1110	525	235	100
Elastichem™	4011TX-02	1.16	40 A	1300	500	266	100
PVC,	5011TX-02	1.16	50 A	1650	465	426	100
Colorite	5511TX-02	1.18	55 A	1790	465	455	100
Plastics Co.	6011TX-02	1.18	60 A	1936	465	488	100
	7011TX-02	1.21	70 A	2667	400	952	100
	7511TX-02	1.22	75 A	3000	360	1400	100
	8011TX-02	1.23	80 A	3646	330	2025	100
	0–1234	1.21	58 A	1400	400	600	100
Ellay™ PVC,	0–1290	1.26	83 A	2750	275	1500	100
	0–1541	1.23	81 A	2400	300	1400	100
	0–1554	1.21	70 A	2000	400	950	100
Ellay, Inc.	0–2112	1.24	82 A	2650	320	1200	100
	0–2129	1.24	83 A	2670	310	1500	100
	0–2202	1.54	75 A	2360	270	1190	100
	0–2609	1.20	68 A	1950	410	800	100
	0–2610	1.24	83 A	2460	295	1450	100
	0–2623	1.24	82 A	2550	325	1350	100
	0–2631	1.19	65 A	1800	390	650	100
	0–3110	1.22	74 A	2100	355	1000	100
	0–3115R	1.20	68 A	1900	400	800	100
	0–3119	1.22	75 A	2150	350	1100	100
	0–3138R	1.22	75 A	2200	350	1075	100
	0–3140R	1.25	87 A	2850	330	1600	100
	0–3147	1.28	95 A	3100	250	2350	100
	0–3149R	1.23	78 A	2400	340	1150	100
	0–3154	1.19	65 A	1750	410	725	100
	0–3155R	1.20	68 A	1850	390	780	100
	0–3166R	1.25	85 A	2700	320	1650	100
	0–3195	1.27	90 A	2950	280	2210	100
	0–3200	1.18	60 A	1600	450	525	100
Ellay™ PVC,	0–3201	1.21	70 A	2000	340	800	100
	0–3224R	1.21	77 A	2300	345	1100	100
	0–3231R	1.26	88 A	3000	280	1800	100
Ellay, Inc.	0–4106R	1.25	85 A	2650	300	1600	100
	0–4108	1.25	85 A	2750	300	1600	100
	0–4109R	1.25	85 A	2800	310	1700	100
	0–4113	1.31	100 A	3960	184	3200	100
	0–4114	1.20	67 A	1900	400	780	100
	0–4115	1.26	87 A	2800	295	1650	100
	0–4116R	1.27	90 A	2950	265	2100	100

Table 4.6 *Continued*

Product and Manufacturer	Product no.	Specific gravity ASTM D-792	Durometer shore ASTM D-2240	Tensile strength, psi ASTM D-412	Elongation, percent ASTM D-412	Modulus ASTM D-412 psi	%
Ellay, Inc.	0–4120	1.21	68 A	2180	400	830	100
	0–4121	1.23	81 A	2550	325	1400	100
	0–4122	1.33	110 A	4500	135	4180	100
	0–4124R	1.28	95 A	3050	250	2200	100
	0–4125	1.24	80 A	3150	355	1310	100
	0–4129	1.18	63 A	1670	430	620	100
	0–4132	1.21	70 A	2000	395	900	100
	0–4135	1.23	80 A	2550	320	1260	100
	0–4140	1.23	80 A	2500	330	1250	100
	0–4150	1.26	88 A	2900	290	2200	100
	0–5210C	1.26	82 A	2300	225	1250	100
	BB–69	1.23	78 A	2200	340	1150	100
	EH–222C	1.21	70 A	2050	365	1100	100
	ES–2967ZPH	1.22	75 A	2300	360	1200	100
Geon® PVC,	121AR	1.4		2800	380		
	213	1.4		2205	379	1010	100
B. F. Goodrich Co.	250×100			1700–1850	430–460	400–500	100
Multichem™ PVC, Colorite Plastics Co.	6014	1.15	60 A	1640	540	400	100
	7014	1.19	70 A	2040	600	625	100
	8014	1.22	80 A	2100	500	1000	100
	8514	1.24	85 A	2250	530	880	100
Teknor™ PVC, Teknor Apex Co.	3300–45 NT	1.13	45 A	1100	480	325	100
	3300–50 NT	1.14	50 A	1220	460	370	100
	3300–55 NT	1.16	55 A	1500		520	100
	3300–60 NT	1.17	60 A	1550	450	560	100
	3300–68 NT	1.18	68 A	1850	430	690	100
	3300–75 NT	1.20	75 A	2150	420	900	100
	3300–80 NT	1.21	80 A	2400		1,320	100
	3300–85 NT	1.23	85 A	2800	380	1,560	100
	3300–90 NT	1.25	90 A	3100	340	2,100	100
	3310–50 NT	1.35	50 A	1000	430	330	100
	3310–55 NT	1.35	55 A	1100	410	400	100
	3310–60 NT	1.35	60 A	1300	400	480	100
	3310–65 NT	1.35	65 A	1500	390	590	100
	3310–70 NT	1.35	70 A	1770	380	700	100
	3310–75 NT	1.35	75 A	1900	370	800	100
	3310–80 NT	1.35	80 A	2200	360	1,050	100
	3310–85 NT	1.35	85 A	2500	340	1,470	100
	3310–90 NT	1.35	90 A	2900	330	1,900	100

Table 4.6 *Continued*

Product and Manufacturer	Product no.	Specific gravity ASTM D-792	Durometer shore ASTM D-2240	Tensile strength, psi ASTM D-412	Elongation, percent ASTM D-412	Modulus ASTM D-412 psi	%
Teknor Apex Co.	90A471R–60NT	1.16	60 A	1500	450		
	90A471R–65NT	1.17	65 A	1750	440		
	90A471R–70NT	1.18	70 A	1900	430		
	90A471R–75NT	1.20	75 A	2150	420		
	90A471R–80NT	1.23	80 A	2690	380		
	90A471R–85NT	1.23	85 A	2800			
	90A471R–90NT	1.27	90 A	3350	360		

diisopropylamino-ethyl methacrylate and decyl methacrylate are added as a stabilizer. The material is supplied as 25% solids in dimethyl acetamide solvent (Tables 4.3, 4.12, 4.13, and 4.14).

Biospan®-S

This is a silicone modified analog of Biospan® with a different stabilizer. It possesses a silicone-rich surface to enhance thromboresistance while maintaining the bulk properties of Biospan® (Tables 4.3, 4.12, 4.13, and 4.14).

Biospan®-D

This is another version of Biospan® with surface modification by an oligomeric hydrocarbon covalently bonded to the base polymer during synthesis. The additive has a pronounced effect on the polymer surface chemistry but little effect on the bulk properties of the base polymer according to the manufacturer (Tables 4.3, 4.12, 4.13, and 4.14).

Hydrothane™

Hydrothane™ is a TPE hydrogel belonging to the polyurethane family of polymers. Hydrothane™ is an aliphatic material with water absorption capabilities ranging from 5 to 25% by weight while still maintaining high tensile strength and elongation. Because of its water absorption capacity, Hydrothane™ is reported to be bacteria-resistant and lubricious. The polymer can be processed by conventional extrusion and injection molding techniques. It can also be dissolved in dimethyl acetamide solvent to produce a 25% solids solution suitable for dip-coating and other solution processing techniques (Tables 4.3, 4.12, and 4.13).

Table 4.7 Typical Properties of Styrene-based Thermoplastic Elastomers

		Property							
Product and Manufacturer	*Product no.*	*Specific gravity ASTM D-792*	*Durometer hardness shore ASTM D-2240*	*Tensile strength, psi ASTM D-412*	*Elongation, percent ASTM D-412*	*Modulus ASTM D-412 psi*	*Modulus ASTM D-412 %*	*Tear strength pli,die B ASTM D-624*	*Compression set, percent ASTM D-395*
	R70-001	0.90	50 A	1200	900	150	100		16
C-Flex®,	R70-003	0.90	70 A	1280	760	340	100		25
	R70-005	0.90	30 A	1400	950	100	100		11
	R70-026	0.90	90 A	1830	650	1,010	100		
Consolidated	R70-028	0.90	35 A	990	800	120	100		13
Polymer	R70-046	0.90	34 A	1320	940	110	100	135	12
Technologies,	R70-050	0.90	48 A	1250	880	170	100	100	18
Inc.	R70-051	0.90	74 A	1140	680	370	100	150	28
	R70-058	0.94	70 A	2080	660	300	100	120	55
	R70-057	0.92	40 A	1220	890	100	100	90	33
	R70-068	0.93	50 A	1630	850	140	100	110	38
	R70-072	0.90	60 A	1270	780	240	100		20
	R70-081	0.90	45 A	1440	920	120	100		17
	R70-082	0.90	61 A	1270	860	230	100	130	19
	R70-085	0.90	50 A	1380	750	200	100		17
	R70-089	0.90	45 A	1640	700				
	R70-091	0.90	50 A	1280	780	130	100		
	R70-116	0.90	30 A	1105	810	100	100	84	24
	R70-190	0.90	5 A	270	1010	20	100		
	R70-214	0.90	18 A	450	780				
	D-2103	0.94	70 A	4300	880	400	300	205	
Kraton®,	D-2104	0.93	27 A	1700	1350	200	300	180	
	D-2109	0.94	44 A	950	800	300	300	160	
Shell	G-2701	0.90	67 A	1600	800	480	300	260	
Chemical	G-2703	0.90	63 A	1200	670	470	300	230	
Co.	G-2705	0.90	55 A	850	700	400	300	140	38
	G-2706	0.90	28 A	850	950	130	300	140	
	G-2712	0.88	42 A	840	820	250	300	140	

Medicaflex™

The Lambda series of Medicaflex is a polyurethane-based TPE polymer that exhibits low modulus characteristics with high tear strength and abrasion resistance. Those listed in the tables have passed USP Class VI compatibility tests and have been used as replacements in some natural rubber latex and silicone rubber applications. The polymer has been applied to uses such as catheters, tubing and films where softness, low durometer hardness, low modulus or high elongation are needed (Tables 4.3, 4.12, and 4.13).

Pellethane™ polyurethane elastomers

The 2363 series Pellethane™ TPE elastomers have a wide range of durometer hardness and are noted for their high tensile and tear strength and abrasion resistance. Chemically they are classed as polytetramethylene glycol ether polyurethanes. The ether series is the most widely used for medical applications although polyester versions of Pellethane™ are useful for some applications. None of these polymers have the disadvantage of containing plasticizers which can migrate out of the polymer over time resulting in reduction in physical properties. Medical tubing made from Pellethane™ polymer is widely used. These TPEs are unaffected by ethylene oxide gas, gamma radiation and electron beam sterilization procedures. Pellethane™ can be processed by injection molding and extrusion. For details on physical properties, processing and biocompatibility (Tables 4.3, 4.12, and 4.13).

Notice Regarding Long-Term Medical Implant Applications

The Dow Chemical Company does not recommend Pellethane™ elastomers for long-term medical implant applications in humans (more than 30 days). Nor do they recommend the use of Pellethane™ elastomers for cardiac prosthetic devices regardless of the time period that the device will be wholly or partially implanted in the body. Such applications include, but are not limited to, pacemaker leads and devices, cardiac prosthetic devices such as artificial hearts, heart valves, intra-aortic balloon and control systems, and ventricular bypass assist devices. The company does not recommend any non-medical resin (or film) product for use in any human implant applications.

PolyBlend™ polyurethane

This TPE has been described as an aromatic elastoplastic polyurethane alloy. It possesses a low coefficient of friction, low extractables, and dimensional stability. Hardness ranges from 65 to 75 Shore D. The material is classified for short-term (29 days or less) implantation. Clear and radiopaque formulations are available. Tubing should be annealed at 80°C for four hours to reduce crystallinity (Tables 4.3, 4.4, 4.12, and 4.14).

Tecoflex® polyurethane

Tecoflex is an aliphatic polyether-based polyurethane that is available in clear and radiopaque grades. They are reaction products of methylene bis (cyclohexyl) diisocyanate (HMDI), poly (tetramethylene ether glycol) (PTMEG), and 1,4 butane diol chain extender. The manufacturer claims that the aliphatic composition of Tecoflex® eliminates the danger of forming methylene dianiline (MDA) which is potentially carcinogenic. MDA can be generated from aromatic polyurethanes if they are improperly processed or overheated. Tecoflex has been reported to crack under stress when implanted, long-term, in animals. An advantage of Tecoflex is that it softens considerably within minutes of insertion in the body. This feature can offer patient comfort for short-term applications such as catheters and enteral tubes; it is also reported to reduce the risk of vascular trauma (Tables 4.3, 4.12, and 4.13).

Tecothane®

Tecothane® is an aromatic polyether-based TPE polyurethane polymer. It has processibility and biocompatibility characteristics similar to Tecoflex® except that it is an aromatic rather than an aliphatic polyurethane. Tecothane® is synthesized from methylene diisocyanate (MDI), polytetramethylene ether glycol and 1,4 butanediol chain extender. By varying the ratios of the reactants, polymers have been prepared ranging from soft elastomers to rigid plastics. The manufacturer of Tecoflex® and Tecothane® point out that there is not much difference between medical-grade, aliphatic and aromatic polyether-based polyurethanes with regard to chemical, mechanical and biological properties. However, they caution that with improper processing of Tecothane® (e.g., high moisture content or steam sterilization) it is possible to form measurable amounts of methylene dianiline (MDA), a listed carcinogen. The use of ethylene oxide or gamma radiation are suitable sterilizing agents that do not affect the chemical or physical properties (Tables 4.3, 4.12, and 4.13).

Texin™

There are four basic polymer formulations of Texin polyurethane TPE that may be suitable for medical applications. They range in hardness and flexural modulus. Texin elastomers are produced by the reaction of diisocyanate with a high molecular weight polyester or polyether polymer and a low molecular weight diol. The polyethers (products 5286 and 5265) offer greater hydrolytic stability and stress crack resistance. The polyester-based polyurethane (product 5187) and the polyester polyurethane/polycarbonate blend (product 5370) possess high impact strength and high stiffness along with useful low-temperature properties. Texin is not recommended for implants of greater than 30 days duration. Texin should not be sterilized by autoclave or use of boiling water. Other advantages offered by Texin TPUs are that plasticizers are not necessary to achieve flexibility, the amount of extractables are low, and they possess high tensile strength, high tear strength, and high abrasion resistance. Texin polyurethanes are hydroscopic and will absorb ambient moisture. They can be processed by extrusion and injection molding if thoroughly dried beforehand. As with all chemical systems, the proper use and handling of these materials can not be over-emphasized (Tables 4.3, 4.12, and 4.13).

Texin™ 5370 is a blend of polyester-based polyurethane and polycarbonate. It offers high impact strength and high stiffness. Steam sterilization or boiling should be avoided (Tables 4.3, 4.12, and 4.13).

Polycarbonate-based polyurethanes

Carbothane™.
This medical grade TPE polyurethane is the reaction product of an aliphatic diisocyanate, a polycarbonate-based macrodiol, and a chain terminating low molecular weight diol (Tables 4.4, 4.12, and 4.13).

ChronoFlex™ AR.
Available as a dimethyl acetamide solution, this segmented, aromatic, polycarbonate-based TPE polyurethane was designed to mimic Ethicon Corporation's Biomer. The polymer is made from the addition of diphenylmethane 4,4′-diisocyanate to a polycarbonate diol followed by addition of a mixture of chain extenders and a molecular weight regulator. The polymer is believed to be resistant to environmental stress cracking such as that experienced by other polyurethanes coated onto pacemaker leads (Tables 4.4, 4.12, and 4.13).

Coremer™
Specifically designed as an 80 Shore A durometer TPE, this is a diamine chain extended version of Corethane®. Coremer™ solution cast films have a low initial modulus and high flex fatigue life. Information as to long-term biostability is not available at this time (Tables 4.4 and 4.13).

Corethane®
A polycarbonate TPE polyurethane that claims biostability is achieved through its replacement of virtually all ether or ester linkages with carbonate groups. The soft segment is composed of a polycarbonate diol formed by the condensation reaction of 1,6-hexanediol with ethylene carbonate. The polycarbonate diol is converted to a high molecular weight polyurethane by the reaction with 1,4-methylene bisphenyl diisocyanate (MDI) and 1,4-butanediol. It is reported to be resistant to environmental stress cracking as experienced with insulation on pacemaker lead wires. The polymer can be extruded, injection molded or compression-molded, and can be bonded with conventional urethane adhesives and solvents (Tables 4.4, 4.12, 4.13, and 4.14).

Corhesive™
Corhesive™ is a solvent-free, two-component reaction adhesive system for use with polyurethanes, plasma treated silicones and certain metals (Tables 4.4, 4.12, 4.13, and 4.14).

Polypropylene-based elastomers

Sarlink®
This is a polypropylene-based TPE that has been used as a replacement for medical stoppers previously made from butyl rubber. Sarlink® has the characteristics typical of rubber vulcanizates such as elasticity, flexibility, high coefficients of friction and softness. Sarlink® combines gas impermeability without concern for contamination of biological medium. Applications for medical grade Sarlink® are inserts on syringe plungers, reusable injection caps, vacuum assisted blood sampling tubes, plus flexible grade tubing. The number of stoppers produced from Sarlink annually number in the billions. The material can be injection molded, blow molded, extruded, calendered, and thermoformed on standard processing equipment. It can be thermal bonded or adhesive bonded (Tables 4.5, 4.12, and 4.13).

Polyvinyl chloride elastomers

Polyvinyl chloride polymer is polymerized from vinyl chloride monomers. It is a hard material which can be made soft and flexible through the addition of a plasticizer or a copolymer. As such, it resembles an elastomer and can be included with other TPEs. Also optionally added to PVC are fillers, stabilizers, antioxidants and others. A typical PVC plasticizer for medical products is di(2-ethylhexyl) phthalate (also known as dioctyl phthalate, DOP). Some producers of PVC also offer non-phthalate formulations. PVC has been used extensively for blood bags, blood tubing, endotracheal tubes, catheters and fittings, urology tubes, intravenous tubing, respiratory devices and dialysis sets. Leaching of the plasticizer can offer difficulties if the application is not short-term. Medical grade PVC is available from B.F. Goodrich under the name Geon® RX, Elastichem™ PVC, Ellay™ PVC, Multichem™ PVC, Teknor™ PVC, AlphaGary and others. PVC polymers have also been incorporated as additives to polyurethane to alter the properties of the latter.

Elastichem™ PVC.
This polyvinyl chloride compound family is highly elastomeric and exhibits a dry non-tacky surface even at hardnesses as low as 40 Shore A durometer. Their rubber-like resilience, high elongation and low permanent set and fatigue resistance offer advantages over conventional formulations (Tables 4.6, 4.12, and 4.13).

Ellay™ PVC.
Compounds from Ellay Corp. are available with Shore hardness ranges from 55 A to 100 A. The polymers have been applied to medication

delivery systems, blood collection, processing and storage, gastro-urological devices and collection systems. Product numbers ending in 'R' are special radiation resistant grades (Tables 4.6, 4.12 and 4.13).

Geon® PVC.

Geon® PVC is associated with vinyl examination gloves. For this use, Geon® recommends a combination of Geon® 121 AR and 213. For a more 'latex type' feeling, Goodtouch 250×100 is recommended. Typical film samples have passed patch insult tests when worn against the skin for extended periods (Tables 4.6, 4.12 and 4.13).

Multichem™ PVC

This line of PVC polymers consist of alloys of PVC in combination with other polymers. They display notable dynamic properties and resistance to migration and extraction. These non-toxic PVC compounds (includes Multichem™ and Elastichem™) have over 25 years of experience in the medical field (Tables 4.6, 4.12 and 4.13).

Teknor™ Apex PVC

This extrudable PVC has found use as tubing for blood transport and delivery systems, dialysis and enteral feeding systems, oxygen delivery systems, catheters, and drainage systems. Product numbers containing an R are special radiation resistant grades (Tables 4.6, 4.12 and 4.13).

Styrene-based elastomers

C-Flex® TPE.

C-Flex® thermoplastic elastomers are based on styrene/ethylene-butylene/styrene block copolymers. C-Flex® polymers designated as 'medical grade' are clear and can be processed using conventional extrusion and injection molding equipment. They have been tested using Good Laboratory Practices and have successfully passed USP Class VI, biocompatibility tests. Translucent versions have high rebound values at ultimate elongation. Medical tubing, ureteral stents, blood pumps, feeding tubes and nephrostomy catheters are successful uses of this material (Tables 4.7, 4.12 and 4.13).

Kraton®

Kraton® elastomer consists of block segments of styrene and rubber monomers and are available as Kraton® D and G series. The D series is based on unsaturated midblock styrene-butadiene-styrene copolymers whereas the G series is based on styrene-ethylene/butylene-styrene copolymers with a stable saturated midblock. Listed among the attributes of both series are such features as low extractables, dimensional stability, vapor and gas transmission properties, ease of sterilization, softness and clarity. They exhibit elastomeric flexibility coupled with thermoplastic processibility (Tables 4.7, 4.12, 4.13).

4.2.2 Crosslinked elastomers

Natural rubber

Natural rubber (cis-polyisoprene) is strong and one of the most flexible of the elastomers. The material has been used for surgeon's gloves, catheters, urinary drains and vial stoppers. However, because it has the potential to cause allergic reactions thought to be due to the elution of entrapped natural protein, this elastomer is being used less now than in the past. Safer substitutes are being selected.

Silicone elastomers

Silicone elastomers have a long history of use in the medical field. They have been applied to cannulas, catheters, drainage tubes, balloon catheters, finger and toe joints, pacemaker lead wire insulation, components of artificial heart valves, breast implants, intraocular lenses, contraceptive devices, burn dressings and a variety of associated medical devices. A silicone reference material has been made available by the National Institutes of Health to equate the blood compatibility of different surfaces for vascular applications. This material is available as a silica-free sheet. Contact the Artificial Heart Program, NHBLI, NIH, Bethesda, Md. for further information.

The silicone elastomers most commonly used for medical applications are the high consistency (HC) and liquid injection molding (LIM) types. The former is most often peroxide cured and the latter platinum cured although there are variations. Both materials are similar in properties. LIM offers greater advantages to the medical device molder and is gaining in popularity. This form of silicone may become the molder's material of choice within the next few years.

High consistency (HC) silicone elastomer

High consistency silicone elastomer consists of methyl and vinyl substituted silicones with aromatic and fluorinated functional groups in some formulations. For the most part, they are peroxide crosslinked. Items are usually compression or transfer molded (Tables 4.8).

Liquid injection molding (LIM) silicone elastomer

Liquid injection molding (LIM) with liquid silicone rubber (LSR) is fast

Table 4.8 Typical Properties of High Consistency (HC) Silicone Elastomers

Product and Manufacturer	*Product no.*	*Property* Specific gravity ASTM D-792	Durometer hardness, shore ASTM D-2240	Tensile strength, psi ASTM D-412	Elongation, percent ASTM D-412	Tear strength pli, die B ASTM D-624
	40039	1.12	35 A	1600	1200	200
Applied Silicone	40040	1.15	50 A	1500	900	220
Medical Implant	40041	1.20	66 A	1200	900	260
Grade,	40042	1.20	78 A	1200	600	280
Applied Silicone	40043	1.12	23 A	1100	1500	160
Corp.	40044	1.12	33 A	1600	1015	150
	40045	1.15	51 A	1400	600	190
	40046	1.20	66 A	1200	500	250
	40063	1.20	70 A	1400	850	280
	MED-2174	1.15	52 A	1200	715	200
NuSil Silicone,	MED-2245	1.13	41 A	1300	700	140
	MED-4515	1.15	52 A	1350	450	90
NuSil Technology	MED 4516	1.21	72 A	1175	370	80
	MED-4735	1.10	35 A	1310	1250	200
	MED 4750	1.15	50 A	1350	810	230
	MED 4755	1.14	57 A	1375	800	300
	MED 4765	1.20	65 A	1100	900	240
	MED-4770	1.17	70 A	1375	700	300
	MDX4-4210	1.10	25 A	550	350	50
Silastic ®	Q7-4535	1.10	33 A	1200	1015	160
Medical Materials,	Q7-4550	1.14	51 A	1375	600	170
	Q7-4565	1.20	66 A	1000	550	210
Dow Corning	Q7-4720	1.10	23 A	1200	1100	150
Corp.	Q7-4735	1.10	35 A	1050	1200	200
	Q7-4750	1.14	50 A	1300	900	230
	Q7-4765	1.14	50 A	1300	900	230
	Q7-4780	1.22	78 A	850	600	190

becoming the technique of choice for processing silicone elastomers. Modifications of conventional injection molding equipment are required. For example, pumps to handle two components being injected simultaneously are required. The heaters on the injection barrel and nozzle are replaced by water cooled jackets. The mold is heated in the range of 300 to 400°F. Because the (LSR) flows easily, injection pressures are low (800 to 3000 psi). Elastomeric items cure rapidly in the mold (e.g., a 7 gram part will crosslink in about 15 seconds at 350 °F). Many formulations rely on platinum as a crosslinker. Perhaps in the future, the majority of silicone rubber molded parts will be made in this fashion. Appropriate equipment is commercially available.

Table 4.9 Typical Properties of Liquid Injection Molding (LIM) Silicone Elastomers

Product and Manufacturer	*Product no.*	*Specific gravity ASTM D-792*	*Durometer hardness, shore ASTM D-2240*	*Tensile strength, psi ASTM D-412*	*Elongation, percent ASTM D-412*	*Tear strength pli, die B ASTM D-624*
Applied Silicone Medical Implant Grade, Applied Silicone Corp.	40023	1.11	10 A	500	750	80
	40024	1.11	20 A	800	600	140
	40025	1.12	30 A	950	600	150
	40026	1.12	40 A	980	450	170
	40027	1.13	50 A	1000	400	190
	40028	1.13	60 A	1100	350	220
	40029	1.10	30 A	900	300	80
	40071	1.14	70 A	1200	350	220
	40072	1.10	25 A	650	400	60
	40082	1.10	40 A	900	250	110
NuSil Silicone, NuSil Technology	MED-6210	1.04	50 A	1000	100	35
	MED-6233	1.03	50 A	1200	300	75
	MED-6382	1.13	45 A	400	200	
	MED-6820	1.05	40 A	750	125	25
Silastic® Medical Materials, Dow Corning Corp.	Q7-4840	1.12	40 A	950	425	150
	Q7-4850	1.14	50 A	1350	550	225
	Q7-6860	1.16	60 A	1300	450	250

Tables 4.8, 4.9, 4.10 and 4.11 list the silicones made by Applied Silicone Corp., Dow Corning Corp., and NuSil Technologies. Table 4.12 lists their biocompatibility status and Table 4.13 recommended sterilization methods. Dow Corning no longer offers the following materials for general sale:

- Silastic MDX 4–4515
- Silastic MDX 4–4515
- Silastic Q7–2245
- Dow Corning Q7–2213

Further, they have discontinued the sale of all implant grade materials.

Other silicones

Silicones and polyurethanes have been used to produce denture liner materials and maxillofacial prostheses. Most of these materials are silicone based, e.g., Flexibase, Molloplast-B, Prolastic, RS 330 T-RTV, Coe-Soft, Coe-Super Soft, Vertex Soft, PERform Soft, and Petal Soft. Other custom

Table 4.10 Typical Properties of Elastomeric Dispersions

Product and Manufacturer	*Product no.*	*Property*						
		Specific gravity ASTM D-792	*Durometer hardness shore ASTM D-2240*	*Tensile strength, psi ASTM D-412*	*Elongation, percent ASTM D-412*	*Modulus ASTM D-412 psi*	*Modulus ASTM D-412 %*	*Tear strength pli,die B ASTM D-624*
Applied Silicone Medical Implant Grade, Applied Silicone Corp.	40000	1.10	35 A	1800	800		185	
	40001	1.18	32 A	1200			200	
	40002	1.08	24 A	800	700		60	
	40016	1.10	35 A	1800	800		185	
	40021	1.08	24 A	1000			100	
	40032	1.19	40 A		500		120	
NuSil Silicone, NuSil Technology	MED-2213	1.13	Shore 00, 82	1300	700	190	200	140
	MED-6400	1.08	32 A	1250		325	300	150
	MED2-6400	1.08	32 A	1250	800			
	MED-6600	1.10	20 A	1000		275	300	90
	MED2-6600	1.10	25 A	1000	750	325	300	
	MED-6605	1.08	25 A	900	1000	75	175	100
	MED3-6605	1.08	25 A	900	1000	100	200	125
	MED-6607	1.10	40 A	900	650	—		130
	MED-6640	1.12	30 A	1650	1100	150	100	280
	MED2-6640	1.12	30 A	1750		100	100	275
	MED2-6650	1.15	35 A	1100	750	200	300	
Silastic® Medical Materials, Dow Corning Corp.	Q7-2630	—	Shore 00, 70	800	900	50	200	—

Product no.	*Form*	*viscosity cp.*	*Solvent System Used*	*Cure System*	*Chemical Type*
40000	35% solids, 1 part	2000	Xylene	Platinum addition	Methyl vinyl siloxane
40001				Phenyl vinyl siloxane	
40002	32% solids, 1 part	500		Acetoxy	Dimethyl siloxane
40016	27% solids, 1 part	2000	1,1,1 trichloro-ethane	Platinum addition	Methyl vinyl siloxane
40021	32% solids, 1 part	500	Xylene	Acetoxy	Dimethyl siloxane
40032	21% solids, 1 part	800	1,1,1 trichloro-ethane	Platinum addition	Fluorovinyl methyl siloxane
MED-2213	15% solids, 1 part	7000	1,1,1 trichloro-ethane		Dimethyl-methyl vinyl siloxane

Table 4.10 *Continued*

Product no.	*Form*	*viscosity cp.*	*Solvent System Used*	*Cure System*	*Chemical Type*
MED-6400	35% solids, 2 part, 1:1	600	Xylene	Platinum addition	
MED2-6400	25% solids, 2 part, 1:1	800	1,1,1 trichloro-ethane		Vinyl methyl siloxane
MED-6600	35% solids, 2 part	300	Xylene		
MED2-6600		1600	1,1,1 trichloro-ethane		
MED-6605	30% solids, 1 part	800	Xylene	Acetoxy	
MED3-6605	22% solids, 1 part	1250	1,1,1 trichloro-ethane		Dimethyl siloxane
MED-6607	33% solids, 1 part	5500	VM&P naphtha	Oxime	
MED-6640	25% solids, 2 part	7000	Xylene		Methyl vinyl siloxane
MED2-6640	15% solids, 2 part	5000	1,1,1 trichloro-ethane	Platinum addition	
MED2-6650	20% solids, 2 part	3000			Fluorovinyl methyl siloxane
Q7-263010% solids		—	Q7–2650	Acetoxy	Dimethyl siloxane

Table 4.11 Typical Properties of Silicone Elastomeric Adhesives

Product and Manufacturer	*Product no.*	*Specific gravity ASTM D-792*	*Durometer hardness shore ASTM D-2240*	*Tensile strength, psi ASTM D-412*	*Elongation, percent ASTM D-412*	*Tear strength, die B, pli ASTM D-624*	*Adhesive strength (to silicone) pli*
Applied Silicone Medical Implant Grade,	40064						18+
	Medical Grade RTV Silicone Adhesive	1.08	24 A	850	750	70	18
Applied Silicone Corp.	Medical Grade High Strength RTV Silicone Adhesive			950	770		18
NuSil Silicone, NuSil Technology	MED-1137	1.07	29 A	550	450		
Silastic® Medical Materials Dow Corning Corp.	Medical Adhesive A	1.06	29 A	450	400	30	20+
	355 Medical Grade Pressure Sensitive	1.40					

Product no.	*Cure Conditions*	*Comments*
40064	Produces acetic acid. Cures @ RT with atmospheric moisture, 20 to 60% RH.	Bonds silicones to each other and some synthetics, metals.
Medical Grade RTV Silicone Adhesive	24 hours @ 25°C, aged 24 hours @ RT.	Bonding silicone to polyester, etc.
Medical Grade High Strength RTV Silicone Adhesive		High strength bonds to polyester, nylon, polyurethane and metals.
MED-1137	Produces acetic acid. Cure 3 days @ RT with atmospheric moisture, 20 to 60% RH.	Bonding silicones to each other & some synthetics/metals. When fully cured resembles some conventional silicone elastomers.
Medical Adhesive A	Produces acetic acid, requires 50% RH & 7 days to cure.	Bonding silicone rubber to itself. Useful for cast films or parts from dispersions.
355 Medical Grade Pressure Sensitive	Non-curing dispersion – becomes adhesive as solvent evaporates.	Adheres to skin for use with ileostomy and colostomy appliances.

Table 4.12 Biocompatibility of Various Elastomers

Classification	*Product and Manufacturer*	*Product no.*	*Biocompatibility Status**				
			Hemolysis	*Pyrogenicity*	*Intracutaneous Injection*	*Systemic Injection*	*Skin Sensitization*
	Santoprene®	281–45	passed	passed	passed	passed	passed
Thermoplastic	Rubber,	281–55	passed	passed	passed	passed	passed
elastomer		281–64	passed	passed	passed	passed	passed
	Advanced	281–73	passed	passed	passed	passed	passed
	Elastomer	281–87	passed	passed	passed	passed	passed
	Systems	283–40	passed	passed	passed	passed	passed
PCCE	Ecdel™ Elastomer,	9965	passed		passed	passed	
copolyester	Eastman Chemical Co.	9966					
elastomer	Biospan® Segmented,						
Polyurethane-based elastomers	Polyurethane, The Polymer Technology Group, Inc.	Biospan®	passed	passed	passed	passed	passed
	Hydrothane™, Poly Medica Biomaterials, Inc.	Hydrothane™					
Medicaflex™,	Advanced Resin Technology	MP-5000 MF-5001 MF-5040 MF-5041 MF-5056 MF-5057 MF-5062		passed	passed	passed	
	Pellethane™ 2363 series, Dow Chemical Co.	Pellethane™ 2363 series		passed	passed	passed	
	PolyBlend™ 1000 , and PolyBlend™ 1100 Poly Medica Biomaterials, Inc.	PolyBlend™ 1000 and PolyBlend™ 1100					

Product no.	*Biocompatibility Status**				
	Intramuscular				
	10 days	*30 days*	*90 days*	*Tissue Cell Culture*	*Comments*
281–45					
281–55		passed	passed	passed	Passed USP Class VI testing, Tripartite testing, mouse embryo toxicity testing and Ames Mutagenicity testing.
281–64					
281–73					
281–87					
283–40					
9965				passed	
9966					
Biospan®				passed	
Hydrothane™					See text for status.

Table 4.12 *Continued*

	*Biocompatibility Status**				
	Intramuscular				
Product no.	*10 days*	*30 days*	*90 days*	*Tissue Cell Culture*	*Comments*
MF-5000		passed		passed	
MF-5001		passed		passed	Passed USP Class VI testing.
MF-5040				passed	
MF-5041		passed		passed	
MF-5056				passed	
MF-5057				passed	
MF-5062					
Pellethane™					Passed USP Class VI testing.
2363 series		passed		passed	See text for status.
PolyBlend™					See text for status.
1000 and					
PolyBlend™					

			*Biocompatibility Status**				
Classification	*Product and Manufacturer*	*Product no.*	*Hemolysis*	*Pyrogenicity*	*Intracutaneous Injection*	*Systemic Injection*	*Skin Sensitization*
	Tecoflex®,	EG60A	passed		passed	passed	
Polyurethane-	and	EG80D					
based	Tecothane®,	1055D					
elastomers		1065D					
		1074A	passed		passed	passed	
	Thermedics, Inc.	1075D					
		1085A					
		1095A					
	Texin™,						
		Texin™		passed	passed	passed	
	Miles, Inc.						
		PC-3555D					
Polycarbonate-	Carbothane™,	PC-3572D					
based		PC-3575A	passed		passed	passed	
polyurethanes	Thermedics, Inc.	PC-3585A					
		PC-3595A					
	ChronoFlex™ AR,						
	Poly Medica	ChronoFlex™	passed	passed	passed	passed	
	Biomaterials, Inc.	AR					
	Coremer™,	Coremer™					
	Corethane®,	TPE 55D			passed	passed	passed
	and	TPE 75D		passed			
		TPE 80A	passed		passed	passed	passed
	Corhesive™,	Corhesive™	passed	passed	passed	passed	passed
	Corvita Corp.						
	Sarlink®	Sarlink®					
Polypropylene-	medical grade,	medical grade					
based	DSM Thermoplastic						
elastomers	Elastomers, Inc.						

Table 4.12 *Continued*

	*Biocompatibility Status**				
	Intramuscular			*Tissue Cell*	
Product no.	*10 days*	*30 days*	*90 days*	*Culture*	*Comments*
EG60A EG80D 1055D 1065D 1074A 1075D 1085A 1095A					
Texin™		passed		passed	Passed USP Class VI testing. See text for status.
PC-3555D PC-3572D PC-3575A PC-3585A PC-3595A					
ChronoFlex™ AR		passed		passed	Passed USP Class VI testing.
Coremer™					See text for status.
TPE 55D	passed	passed	passed	passed	
TPE 75D				passed	
TPE 80A	passed	passed	passed	passed	
Corhesive™	passed	passed	passed	passed	
Sarlink® medical grade					See text for status.

			*Biocompatibility Status**				
Classification	*Product and Manufacturer*	*Product no.*	*Hemolysis*	*Pyrogenicity*	*Intracutaneous Injection*	*Systemic Injection*	*Skin Sensitization*
Polyvinyl chloride elastomers	Elastichem™ PVC, Colorite Plastics Co.	Elastichem™ PVC					
Ellay™ PVC,	Ellay™ PVC Ellay, Inc.		passed	passed	passed		
	Geon® PVC, B. F. Goodrich Co.	Geon® PVC					
	Multichem™ PVC, Colorite Plastics Co.	Multichem™ PVC					
	Teknor™ PVC, Teknor Apex Co.	3300–45 NT 3300–50 NT 3300–55 NT 3300–60 NT 3300–68 NT 3300–75 NT					
		3300–80 NT		passed	passed	passed	passed

Table 4.12 *Continued*

Classification	*Product and Manufacturer*	*Product no.*	*Biocompatibility Status** *Hemolysis*	*Pyrogenicity*	*Intracutaneous Injection*	*Systemic Injection*	*Skin Sensitization*
	Teknor™ PVC,	3300–85 NT		passed	passed	passed	passed
		3300–90 NT					
	Teknor Apex Co.	3310–50 NT					
		3310–55 NT					
		3310–60 NT					
		3310–65 NT					
		3310–70 NT					
		3310–75 NT					
		3310–80 NT					
		3310–85 NT					
		3310–90 NT					
		90A471R–60NT		passed	passed	passed	
		90A471R–65NT		passed	passed	passed	
		90A471R–70NT		passed	passed	passed	
		90A471R–75NT		passed	passed	passed	
		90A471R–80NT		passed	passed	passed	
		90A471R–85NT		passed	passed	passed	
		90A471R–90NT		passed	passed	passed	

Product no.	*Biocompatibility Status** *Intramuscular* *10 days*	*30 days*	*90 days*	*Tissue Cell Culture*	*Comments*
Elastichem™ PVC					See text for status.
Ellay™ PVC		passed		passed	Passed USP Class VI testing.
Geon® PVC					See text for status.
Multichem™ PVC					See text for status.
3300–45 NT				passed	
3300–50 NT				passed	
3300–55 NT				passed	
3300–60 NT				passed	
3300–68 NT				passed	
3300–75 NT				passed	
3300–80 NT		passed		passed	Passed USP Class VI testing.
3300–85 NT				passed	Passed USP Class VI testing.
3300–90 NT				passed	
3310–50 NT				passed	
3310–55 NT				passed	
3310–60 NT				passed	
3310–65 NT				passed	
3310–70 NT				passed	
3310–75 NT				passed	

Table 4.12 *Continued*

Product no.	*Intramuscular* 10 days	*Intramuscular* 30 days	*Intramuscular* 90 days	*Tissue Cell Culture*	*Comments*
3310–80 NT				passed	
3310–85 NT				passed	
3310–90 NT				passed	
90A471R–60NT		passed			
90A471R–65NT		passed			Passed USP Class VI testing.
90A471R–70NT		passed			Passed USP Class VI testing.
90A471R–75NT		passed			Passed USP Class VI testing.
90A471R–80NT		passed			Passed USP Class VI testing.
90A471R–85NT		passed			Passed USP Class VI testing.
90A471R–90NT		passed			Passed USP Class VI testing.

*Biocompatibility Status** (applies to columns after Product no. in both tables)

Classification	*Product and Manufacturer*	*Product no.*	*Hemolysis*	*Pyrogenicity*	*Intracutaneous Injection*	*Systemic Injection*	*Skin Sensitization*
		R70–001	passed	passed	passed	passed	
Styrene-based	C-Flex®,	R70–003	passed	passed	passed	passed	
elastomers		R70–005	passed	passed	passed	passed	
	Consolidated Polymer	R70–026	passed	passed	passed	passed	
	Technologies, Inc.	R70–028	passed	passed	passed	passed	
		R70–046	passed	passed	passed	passed	
		R70–050	passed	passed	passed	passed	
		R70–051	passed	passed	passed	passed	
		R70–058	passed	passed	passed	passed	
		R70–067	passed	passed	passed	passed	
		R70–068	passed	passed	passed	passed	
		R70–072	passed	passed	passed	passed	
		R70–081	passed	passed	passed	passed	
		R70–082	passed	passed	passed	passed	
		R70–085	passed	passed	passed	passed	
		R70–089	passed	passed	passed	passed	
		R70–091	passed	passed	passed	passed	
		R70–116	passed	passed	passed	passed	
		R70–190	passed	passed	passed	passed	
		R70–214	passed	passed	passed	passed	
		D–2103	passed	passed	passed	passed	
	Kraton®,	D–2104	passed	passed	passed	passed	
		D–2109	passed	passed	passed	passed	
	Shell	G–2701	passed	passed	passed	passed	
	Chemical Co.	G–2703	passed	passed	passed	passed	
		G–2705	passed	passed	passed	passed	
		G–2706	passed	passed	passed	passed	
		G–2712	passed	passed	passed	passed	

Table 4.12 *Continued*

	*Biocompatibility Status**				
	Intramuscular			*Tissue Cell*	
Product no.	*10 days*	*30 days*	*90 days*	*Culture*	*Comments*
R70–001	passed	passed	passed	passed	
R70–003	passed	passed	passed	passed	C-Flex testing data is available from manufacturer.
R70–005					
R70–026	passed	passed	passed	passed	
R70–028	passed	passed	passed	passed	
R70–046	passed	passed	passed	passed	
R70–050	passed	passed	passed	passed	
R70–051	passed	passed	passed	passed	
R70–058	passed	passed	passed	passed	
R70–067	passed	passed	passed	passed	
R70–068	passed	passed	passed	passed	
R70–072	passed	passed	passed	passed	
R70–081	passed	passed	passed	passed	
R70–082	passed	passed	passed	passed	
R70–085	passed	passed	passed	passed	
R70–089	passed	passed	passed	passed	
R70–091	passed	passed	passed	passed	
R70–116	passed	passed	passed	passed	
R70–190	passed	passed	passed	passed	
R70–214	passed	passed	passed	passed	
D-2103	passed	passed	passed	passed	
D-2104	—	passed	—	passed	Passed USP Class VI testing.
D-2109		passed		passed	Passed USP Class VI testing.
G-2701		passed		passed	Passed USP Class VI testing.
G-2703		passed		passed	Passed USP Class VI testing.
G-2705		passed		passed	Passed USP Class VI testing.
G-2706		passed		passed	Passed USP Class VI testing.
G-2712		passed		passed	Passed USP Class VI testing.

			*Biocompatibility Status**				
Classification	*Product and manufacturer*	*Product no.*	*Hemolysis*	*Pyrogenicity*	*Intracutaneous Injection*	*Systemic Injection*	*Skin Sensitization*
Polydimethylsiloxane	Applied Silicone Medical Implant Grade, Applied Silicone Corp.	Applied Silicone Medical Implant Grade					
	NuSil Silicone, NuSil Technology	NuSil Silicone					
		MDX4–4210		passed	passed	passed	passed
	Silastic®	Q7–4535	passed	passed	passed	passed	
	Medical Materials,	Q7–4550	passed	passed	passed	passed	
		Q7–4565	passed	passed	passed	passed	
	Dow Corning Corp.	Q7–4720	passed	passed	passed	passed	
		Q7–4735	passed	passed	passed	passed	

Table 4.12 *Continued*

Classification	*Product and Manufacturer*	*Product no.*	*Biocompatibility Status** *Hemolysis*	*Pyrogenicity*	*Intracutaneous Injection*	*Systemic Injection*	*Skin Sensitization*
Polydimethyl-siloxane	Silastic ®	Q7–4750	passed	passed	passed	passed	
	Medical Materials,	Q7–4765	passed	passed	passed	passed	
		Q7–4780	passed	passed	passed	passed	
	Dow Corning Corp.	Q7–4840	passed	passed	passed	passed	
		Q7–4850	passed	passed	passed	passed	passed
		Q7–6860	passed	passed	passed	passed	
		Medical Adhesive A		passed	passed	passed	passed
		355 Medical Grade Pressure Sensitive		passed	passed	passed	passed

Product no.	*Biocompatibility Status** *Intramuscular* *10 days*	*30 days*	*90 days*	*Tissue Cell Culture*	*Comments*
Applied Silicone Medical Implant Grade					Applied Silicone testing data is available from manufacturer.
NuSil Silicone					See text for status.
MDX4–4210	passed	passed		passed	See text for status.
Q7–4535	passed	passed			See text for status.
Q7–4550	passed	passed			See text for status.
Q7–4565	passed	passed			See text for status.
Q7–4720				passed	See text for status.
Q7–4735	passed		passed		See text for status.
Q7–4750	passed				See text for status.
Q7–4765	passed				See text for status.
Q7–4780	passed				See text for status.
Q7–4840	passed				See text for status.
Q7–4850		passed		passed	See text for status.
Q7–6860	passed				See text for status.
Medical Adhesive A					See text for status.
	passed	passed	passed		See text for status.
355 Medical Grade Pressure Sensitive	passed	passed	passed	passed	See text for status.

* Biocompatibility based on comparison with USP negative controls
Note: It is the user's responsibility to adequately test or determine that these materials are suitable or safe for any application.

Table 4.13 Sterilization Methods for Elastomers

Product		*Steam/autoclave*	*Cobalt 60*	*Ethylene oxide*	*Cold solution*
Biospan		OK	—	OK	—
Biospan D		—	—	—	—
Biospan S		—	—	—	—
C-Flex	R70–001	OK	OK	OK	—
	R70–003	OK	OK	OK	—
	R70–005	no	OK	OK	—
	R70–026	OK	no	OK	—
	R70–028	no	OK	OK	—
	R70–046	no	OK	OK	—
	R70–050	OK	OK	OK	—
	R70–051	OK	OK	OK	—
	R70–072	OK	OK	OK	OK
	R70–081	OK	OK	OK	—
	R70–082	OK	OK	OK	—
	R70–085	OK	OK	OK	—
	R70–089	NR	OK	OK	—
	R70–091	NR	OK	OK	—
	R70–116	no	OK	OK	—
	R70–190	no	OK	OK	—
	R70–214	no	OK	OK	—
Carbothane		with caution	—	OK	—
ChronoFlex		—	—	—	—
Coremer		—	OK	OK	OK
Corethane	80A	—	OK	OK	OK
	55D	—	OK	OK	OK
	75D	—	OK	OK	OK
Corhesive		—	—	—	—
Ecdel elastomers		OK	no	OK	—
Hydrothane			—	—	—
—					
Kraton	G-series	—	OK	—	—
	D-series	—	—	OK	—
Medicaflex		no	OK	OK	—
Natural rubber, gum		OK	OK	OK	—
Natural rubber, latex		with caution	OK	OK	—
Pellethane		no	OK	OK	—
Poly blend		—	—	—	—
Poly blend 1100		—	—	—	—
PVC	Elastichem	OK	OK	OK	—
	Ellay	OK	OK	OK	—
	Geon	—	—	—	—
	Multi-Chem	OK	OK	OK	—
	Teknor	OK	OK	OK	—
	in general	Flexible PVC, OK rigid PVC, no	with caution	OK	—
Santoprene		OK	OK	OK	OK
Sarlink 3260		—	—	—	—

Table 4.13 *Continued*

Product		*Steam/autoclave*	*Cobalt 60*	*Ethylene oxide*	*Cold solution*
Silicone	High consistency	OK	OK	OK	—
	LIM	OK	OK	OK	—
	Adhesives	OK	OK	OK	—
	Dispersions	OK	OK	OK	—
Tecoflex		with caution	OK	OK	with caution
Tecothane		—	OK	OK	with caution
Texin		no	OK	OK	—

Caution: with some aromatic polyurethanes methylene dianiline (MDA) can be generated with steam sterilization.

Table 4.14 Water Absorption of Various Elastomers

Classification	*Product and manufacturer*	*Product no.*	*Water absorption, percent (after 24 hours) ASTM-D 570*
Thermoplastic vulcanizate	Santoprene® Rubber,	281–55	6.0
		281–64	
	Advanced Elastomer Systems	281–87	0.0
		283–40	
PCCE copolyester elastomer	Ecdel™ Elastomer,	9965	
		9966	0.4
	Eastman Chemical Co.	9967	
Polycarbonate-based polyurethanes	Corethane®,	TPE 80A	1.2
		TPE 55D	0.9
	Corvita Corp.	TPE 75D	0.8
	Corhesive™, Corvita Corp.		1.2
Polyurethane-based elastomers	Biospan® segmented	Biospan®	1.5
	polyurethane,	Biospan® D	1.3
	The Polymer Technology Group, Inc.	Biospan® S	1.5
	PolyBlend™ 1000, and	PB1000–650	<
	PolyBlend™ 1100	PB1100–55	
		PB1100–60	<0.4
	Poly Medica	PB1100–75	
	Biomaterials, Inc.	PB1100–80	
Silicone rubber			0.1–0.5
Silicone type A adhesive			<0.2

made elastomers have been applied to maxillofacial prostheses, e.g., Cosmesil, Silastic® 4–4210, Silastic® 4–4515, Silicone A-102, Silicone A-2186, Silskin II, Isophorone polyurethane, and Epithane-3. Denture liners with acrylic and silicone include Coe-Soft, Coe Super-Soft, Vertex Soft, Molloplast-B and Flexibase.

Dispersions

Solvent solutions of polyurethane elastomers and silicone elastomers are given in Table 4.10. These materials are helpful in casting thin films and odd or complex shapes.

4.3 ESTABLISHING EQUIVALENCE

Specific polymeric materials traditionally used for medical applications have been recently withdrawn from the medical market. Silicone elastomers are among those withdrawn. To maintain continued supply of vital implants, methods of determining equivalence for withdrawn elastomers with new or existing ones has been adopted by the FDA in the form of an FDA Guidance Document.

4.3.1 FDA Guidance document for substitution of equivalent elastomers

The FDA will allow manufacturers to change sources of silicone elastomers (and others) if they can show that the replacement material is 'not substantially different' from materials described in existing approved applications. The device manufacturer is still required to certify that the processes of fabrication, cure and sterilization it uses in the manufacture of its device are appropriate for the new material and that the device will perform as intended. Premarket notification submission under section 510(k) of the Federal Food, Drug, and Cosmetic Act (21 USC 360(k) and 21 CFR 807.81(a)(3)(i), or a supplemental premarket approval application under 21 USC 360(k) section 515 and 21 CFR 814.39 is necessary when change could significantly affect the safety or effectiveness of the device. These submissions are required to be submitted and approved before the device may be marketed with the change.

There are a number of tests necessary for comparison of silicone elastomers as indicated by 'Guidance for Manufacturers of Silicone Devices Affected by Withdrawal of Dow Corning Silastic® Materials' (Federal Register, Vol. 58, No. 127, Tuesday, July 6, 1993/ Notices, 36207). They compare the physical, chemical and biological properties of the bulk poly-

Table 4.15 Equivalent Silicone Elastomers for Existing Dow Corning Silicones

Dow Corning Silicone*	*NuSil‡ Silicone Equivalent*	*AppliedΔ Silicone Equivalent*	*Medical Grade Silicone Description*
Medical Adhesive A	MED-1137	40064	Medical RTV Adhesive, Acetoxy System (see also Rehau, Table 4.16)
Q7-4535	MED-4535	40044	High Consistency, 35 Durometer, Peroxide Cure
Q7-4550	MED-4550	40045	High Consistency, 50 Durometer, Peroxide Cure
Q7-4565	MED-4565	40046	High Consistency, 65 Durometer, Peroxide Cure
Q7-4720	MED-4720	40043	High Consistency, 20 Durometer, Platinum Cure
Q7-4735	MED-4735	40039	High Consistency, 35 Durometer, Platinum Cure
Q7-4750	MED-4750	40040	High Consistency, 50 Durometer, Platinum Cure
Q7-4780	MED-4780	40042	High Consistency, 80 Durometer, Platinum Cure
MDX4–4210	MED-42111	40072	Liquid Silicone, 25 Durometer, Platinum Cure
		40029	Liquid Silicone, 30 Durometer, Platinum Cure
Q7-4840	MED-4840	40026	Liquid Silicone, 40 Durometer Platinum Cure
Q7-4850	MED-4850	40027	Liquid Silicone, 50 Durometer, Platinum Cure
Q7-4865	MED-4865		Liquid Silicone, 65 Durometer, Platinum Cure
DC-360	MED-360	40047	Medical Grade Silicone Fluid, 1000 cps.
	Specify	40073	Medical Grade Silicone Fluid, 350 cps.
	viscosity	40074	Medical Grade Silicone Fluid, 20 cps.

* Dow Corning Corp., Midland, Ml. ‡ NuSil Silicone Technology, Carpinteria, CA
Δ Applied Silicone Corp., Ventura, CA Note: It is the user's responsibility to adequately test or determine that these materials are suitable or safe for any application.

Table 4.16 Equivalent Silicone Elastomers for Withdrawn Dow Corning silicones

Dow Corning Sillicone*	*NuSil‡ Silicone Equivalent*	*AppliedΔ Silicone Equivalent*	*Medical Grade Silicone Description*
MDX4–4515	MED-4515	40045	50 Durometer, peroxide cure
MDX4–4516	MED-4516	40046	60 Durometer, peroxide cure
Q7–2245	MED-2245	40009	40 Durometer, platinum cure
Q7–2213	MED-2213	40016	Dispersion in 1, 1, 1 trichloroethane
Rehau 1511¥		40076	Medical RTV adhesive, acetoxy system

* Dow Corning Corp., Midland, MI. ‡ NuSil Silicone Technology, Carpinteria, CA.
Δ Applied Silicone Corp., Ventura, CA. ¥ Rehau AG and Co., Rehau, Germany.
Note: It is the user's responsibility to adequately test or determine that these materials are suitable or safe for any application.

mers as they are received from the supplier and also compare the molded elastomer as it exists in the final medical device.

4.3.2 Equivalent silicone elastomers

Two manufacturers, NuSil Technology and Applied Silicone Corp., are providing equivalent silicone materials for the Dow Corning products that have been withdrawn. Tables 4.15 and 4.16 gives reported comparisons.

Table 4.17 Relevant ASTM Standards

D 395	Test Method for Rubber Property – Compression Set
D 412	Test Method for Vulcanized Rubber, Thermoplastic Rubbers and Thermoplastic Elastomer – Tension
D 471	Test Method for Rubber Property – Effect of Liquids
D 570	Test Method for Water Absorption of Plastics
D 624	Test Method for Tear Strength of Conventional Vulcanized Rubber and Thermoplastic Elastomer
D 638	Test method for Tensile Properties of Plastics
D 792	Test Method for Specific Gravity (Relative Density) and Density of Plastics by Displacement
D 797	Test Methods for Rubber Property – Young's Modulus at Normal and Subnormal Temperatures
D 1630	Test Method for Rubber Property – Abrasion Resistance (NBS Abrader)
D 1708	Test method for Tensile Properties of Plastics by Use of Microtensile Specimens
D 1790	Test method for Brittleness Temperature of Plastic Film by Impact
D 1938	Test method for Tear Propagation Resistance of Plastic Film and Thin Sheeting by a Single-Tear Method
D 2240	Test Method for Rubber Property – Durometer Hardness
D 2702	Standard Practice for Rubber Chemicals – Determination of Infrared Absorption Characteristics
D 3418	Test Method for Transition Temperatures of Polymers by Thermal Analysis
D 3593	Test Method for Molecular Weight Averages and Molecular Weight Distribution of Certain Polymers by Liquid Size-Exclusion Chromatography (Gel Permeation Chromatography, GPC) Using Universal Calibration
D 5023	Test Method for Measuring the Dynamic Mechanical Properties of Plastics Using Three Point Bending
D 5026	Test Method for Measuring the Dynamic Mechanical Properties of Plastics in Tension
E 355	Standard Practice for Gas Chromatography, Terms and Relationships
E 1356	Test Method for Glass Transition Temperatures by Differential Scanning Calorimetry or Differential Thermal Analysis
F 604	Classification for Silicone Elastomers Used in Medical Applications
F 619	Standard Practice for Extraction of Medical Plastics
F 720	Standard Practice for Testing Guinea Pigs for Contact Allergens: Guinea Pig Maximization Test
F 748	Standard Practice for Selecting Generic Biological Test Methods for Materials and Devices
F 749	Standard Practice for Evaluating Material Extracts by Intracutaneous Injection in the Rabbit
F 750	Standard Practice for Evaluating Material Extracts by Systemic Injection in the Mouse
F 813	Standard Practice for Direct Contact Cell Culture Evaluation of Materials for Medical Devices
F 895	Standard Practice for Agar Diffusion Cell Culture Screening for Cytotoxicity
F 981	Standard Practice for Assessment of Compatibility of Biomaterials (Non-porous) for Surgical Implants with Respect to Effect of Materials in Muscle and Bone

4.4 STERILIZATION OF ELASTOMERS

4.4.1 Sterilization methods

Not all materials respond alike when subjected to various means of sterilization. Some are heat sensitive, some will absorb sterilization fluids, some will be affected by molecular changes when subjected to radiation sterilization and others will absorb and hold irritating gases for extended periods of time. Table 4.13 gives sterilization methods that have been judged most appropriate for each elastomer. The consequences of using an inappropriate method can be loss in physical properties and an adverse biological response.

4.5 RELEVANT ASTM STANDARDS

Standard methods of testing elastomers used for medical applications are given by specific ASTM test methods. Physical and biological tests are provided here to serve as references for the data cited in the tables and listed in Table 4.17. They are also designated in the FDA Guidance Document.

4.6 BIOCOMPATIBILITY

Table 4.12 on biocompatibility of various elastomers is intended to show the status of *in vitro* and *in vivo* testing. The successful outcome of these tests can serve as guides to potentially acceptable performance of an elastomeric product in a medical device under development. However, the use of elastomeric products in medical devices is the responsibility of the device manufacturer who must establish their safety and efficacy with the FDA.

4.7 SOURCES

- AlphaGaryAlphaGary, Leominster, MA
- Applied SiliconeApplied Silicone Corp., Ventura, CA
- Biospan®Polymer Technology Group, Inc., Emeryville, CA
- C-Flex®Consolidated Polymer Technologies, Inc., Largo, FL
- Carbothane™Thermedics, Inc., Woburn, MA
- ChronoFlex™PolyMedica Industries, Inc., Woburn, MA
- Coremer™Corvita Corp., Miami, FL
- Corethane®Corvita Corp., Miami, FL

- Corhesive™Corvita Corp., Miami, FL
- Ecdel™Eastman Chemical Co., Kingsport, TN
- Elastichem™Colorite Plastics Co., Ridgefield, NJ
- Ellay™Ellay, Inc., City of Commerce, CA
- Geon®B.F. Goodrich Co., Chemical Group, Cleveland, OH
- Hydrothane™PolyMedica Industries, Inc., Woburn, MA
- Kraton®Shell Chemical Co., Oak Brook, IL
- Medicaflex™Advanced Resin Technology, Manchester, NH
- Multichem™Colorite Plastics Co., Ridgefield, NJ
- Natural rubberExxon Chem. Co., Buffalo Grove, IL Goodyear Tire and Rubber Co., Akron, OH
- NuSil SiliconeNuSil Technology, Carpinteria, CA
- Pellethane™Dow Chemical Co., Midland, MI
- PolyBlend™PolyMedica Industries, Inc., Woburn, MA
- Santoprene®Advanced Elastomer Systems, St Louis MO
- Sarlink®DSM Thermoplastic Elastomers, Inc., Leominster, MA
- SilasticDow Corning Corp., Midland, MI
- Tecoflex®Thermedics, Inc., Woburn, MA
- Tecothane®Thermedics, Inc., Woburn, MA
- Teknor™Teknor Apex Co., Pawtucket, RI
- Texin™Miles, Inc., Pittsburgh, PA

5 Oxide bioceramics: inert ceramic materials in medicine and dentistry

J. Li and G.W. Hastings

5.1 INTRODUCTION

Single oxide ceramics, e.g. aluminium oxide (Al_2O_3, alumina) and zirconium dioxide (ZrO_2, zirconia), are bioceramics of an inert nature. An inert ceramic does not form a bonding to bone similar to those bioceramics of bioactive nature. Alumina bioceramics are in the pure aluminium oxide form, whereas zirconia bioceramics are partially stabilized by additional oxides, e.g. yttrium oxide, calcium oxide or magnesium oxide.

Oxide ceramics exhibit superior mechanical properties, corrosion and wear resistance. Since the oxides are the highest oxidation state of the metal, they are stable even in the most invasive industrial and biomedical environments. Alumina and zirconia are utilized as load-bearing hard tissue replacements and fixation implants in dentistry and surgery.

5.2 SHORT HISTORY

Although the use of alumina as implants can be traced back to the 1930s as described by Hulbert *et al.* (1) (Table 5.1), the extensive use of alumina since the 1980s has depended on new powder processing technology enabling grain size reduction of the sintered ceramics from 10 micrometers

Handbook of Biomaterial Properties. Edited by J. Black and G. Hastings.
Published in 1998 by Chapman & Hall, London. ISBN 0 412 60330 6.

down to 2 micrometers (Figure 5.1, microstructure of alumina). This significantly improves the performance of the alumina ceramic hip balls. Alumina and partially stabilized zirconia are currently in extensive use as implants in consequence of their high strength, excellent corrosion and wear resistance and stability, non-toxicity and biocompatibility *in vivo*. A summary of alumina- and zirconia-based implants is presented in Table 5.2. The most established example is in the total hip endoprosthesis with a combination of metallic stem, ceramic ball and ultra high molecule weight polyethylene (UHMWPE) acetabular cup. A ten year clinical success rate better than 90% is reported for the cemented total hip endoprosthesis.

Dental implants of polycrystalline alumina were suggested by Sandhaus in Germany (4). Type Tübingen was produced by Frialit in the 1970s. These devices have not been generally accepted, due to the fracture failure of the implants, particularly for those of polycrystalline type produced in

Table 5.1 Evaluation of oxide ceramic implants: alumina and zirconia

1932	First suggestion of application of alumina ceramics in medicine	Rock (2)
1963	First orthopaedic bone substitute application	Smith (3)
1964	First dental implant of alumina	Sandhaus (4)
1970	French hip prosthesis: Alumina ceramic ball and cup	Boutin (5)
1974	German hip prosthesis	Mittelmeier (6)
1977	28 mm alumina ball	Shikita (7)
1981	Alumina total knee prosthesis	Oonishi *et al.* (8)
1982	FDA approval for non-cemented alumina ceramic cup and ball and CoCrMo-stem of Mittelmeier type	
1986	First zirconia ball of 32 mm	Lord *et al.* (9)
1993	First dental implant of zirconia	Akagawa *et al.* (10)
1995	First zirconia dental post	Meyenberg *et al.* (11)
1996	First zirconia inlay	Johansson (12)

Table 5.2 Biomedical applications of oxide ceramics

Materials	*Applications*	*References*
Alumina	Hip ball & cup	Clarke and Willmann (13)
	Knee joint	Oonishi *et al.* (8)
	Bone screws	
	Dental implant	Kawahara (14)
	Dental crowns & brackets	Sinha *et al.* (15)
Zirconia	Hip ball	Christel (16)
	Dental implants	Akagawa *et al.* (10)
	Dental post, brackets and inlay	(10,11), Keith *et al.* (17)

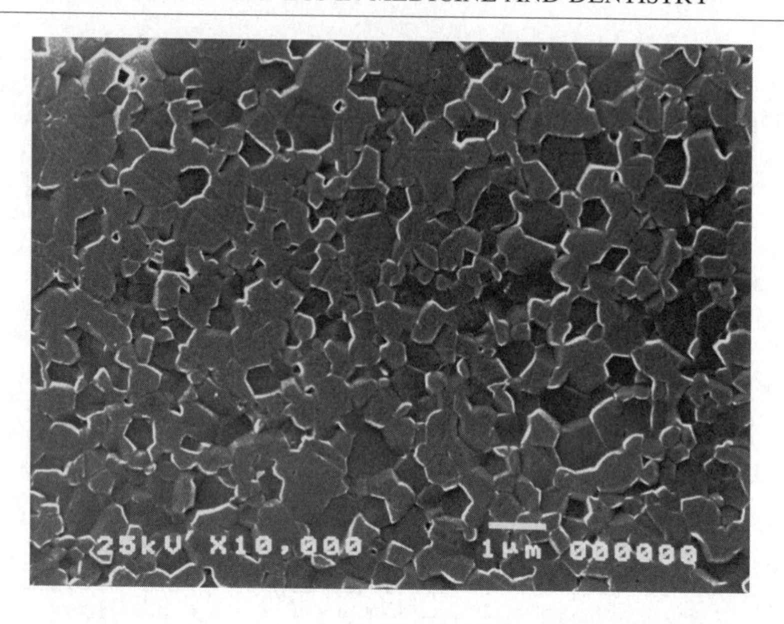

Figure 5.1 SEM micrograph of dense alumina, etched in boiling H_3PO_4 for 6 minutes to show the microstructure.

the early 1970s. The single crystal sapphire type, introduced in Japan by Kawahara in the 1970s (18) is, however, still being used and a recent 10-year clinical follow-up report from Sweden showed a 92% success rate (19) for the single crystal dental implants.

Alumina and zirconia ceramics are also being used for alveolar ridge reconstruction (20), maxillofacial reconstruction, as ossicular bone substitutes (21), and in ophthalmology (22), knee prosthesis (8), bone screws as well as other applications as dental biomaterials, such as dental crown core, post, bracket and inlay (23,24).

5.3 MATERIAL PROPERTIES AND PROCESSING

5.3.1 Materials properties

Although alumina is chemically more stable it is mechanically weaker than zirconia, and the phase changes or transformation mechanisms in zirconia produce a unique ceramic material having much higher strength and higher fracture toughness compared with alumina and other ceramics. The excellent mechanical properties of zirconia allow the design of hip balls of smaller diameter in order to reduce the wear of the UHMWPE cup with expected increased long-term clinical performance as a result.

The chemical stability of alumina is related to its phase stability, whereas the phase changes of zirconia result in degradation in strength and wear resistance. Release of substances from zirconia and alumina implants to the surrounding tissue is very low and neither local nor systemic effects have been reported.

Aluminium oxide: alumina

Aluminium oxide is produced by heating its hydrates. At least seven forms of alumina have been reported, but six of these forms have traditionally been designated 'gamma alumina'. When heated above 1200°C, all other structures are irreversibly transformed to the hexagonal alpha-alumina, corundum, a close-packed arrangement of oxygen ions. Thus alpha-alumina is the only stable form above 1200°C and by far the most commonly used of structural ceramics. Alpha-alumina is thermodynamically stable and is crystallographically identical with the single crystal ruby and sapphire ceramics. Each aluminium ion is surrounded by six oxygen ions, three of which form a regular triangle on one side, the other three form a similar triangle on the other side, with the two planes of the triangles being parallel and the triangles being twisted 180° (25).

Physical and mechanical properties
Table 5.3 and 5.4. Resulting from a strong chemical bond between the Al and O ions, as expected from the value of heat of formation (-400K cal/mol), Al_2O_3 has a high melting point, the highest hardness among known oxides, and high mechanical strength (26).

Chemical properties
Alumina is chemically stable and corrosion resistant. It is insoluble in water and very slightly soluble in strong acids and alkalies. Therefore, practically no release of ions from alumina occurs at a physiological pH level, 7.4.

Wear resistance
Arising from the chemical stability and high surface finish and accurate dimensions, there is a very low friction torque between the alumina femoral heads and the acetabular cup, leading to a low wear rate. Combinations of ceramic head/UHMWPE cup and ceramic head/ceramic cup were tested and compared to the metal head/UHMWPE cup. The wear resistance of the ceramic head/UHMWPE cup combination over metal/UHMWPE has improved from 1.3 to 34 times in the laboratory and from three to four times clinically (27,28). No alumina wear particles from retrieved ceramic/UHMWPE were found, whereas UHMWPE wear particles from microns to millimetres in size were found in the retrieved

Table 5.3 Engineering Properties of Alumina and Zirconia (At 25 °C)*

Property	Al_2O_3	ZrO_2**
Physical		
Crystallography	Hexagonal	Tetragonal***
a (Å)	4.76	3.64
c (Å)	13.0	5.27
Space group	D^6_{Ba}	$P4_2/nmc$
Melting point (°C)	2040	2680
Density (g/cm³)	3.98	6.08
Grain size (μm)	1–6	0.54
Hardness (GPa)	22	12.2
Modulus of elasticity, (GPa)	366	201
Poisson's ratio	0.26	0.30
Thermal coefficient of expansion 25–200 °C	6.5	10.1
Mechanical		
Flexural strength (MPa)	551	1074
Compressive Strength (MPa)	3790	7500
Tensile strength (MPa)	310	420
Fracture toughness (MPa m$^{1/2}$)	4.0	6–15

* Sources: refs 26, 44 and 45
** Zirconia presented is the yttria-partially stabilized material
*** Most of the medical-grade zirconia is partially stabilized tetragonal zirconia

Table 5.4 Properties of medical-grade ceramic materials according to the standards and the manufacturer's technical date – alumina and zirconia

Property	*Alumina according to ISO-6474 ASTM F 603–83 DIN 58 8353*	*Frialit bioceramic alumina*	*Zirconia according to ISO/DIS 13356*	*Prozyr® zirconia*
Purity (%)	>99.5	>99.5	>99.5*	>95
Density (g/cm³)	>3.9	>3.98	≥6.0	6
Porosity (%)	0	**	0	0
Grain size (μm)	<4.5	>2.5	≤0.6	<1
Microhardness (GPa)	23	23	—	13
Young's modulus (GPa)	380	380	—	220
Flexural strength (MPa)	>400	>450	>900	≥920
Biaxial flexural strength (MPa)	250	—	>550	—
Impact strength (cm MPa)	>40	>40	—	124
Fracture toughness (MPa m$^{1/2}$)			—	10
Wear resistance (mm³/h)	0.01	0.001	—	—
Corrosion resistance (mg/m²d)	<0.1	<0.1	—	—

* ZrO_2+HfO_2+Y_2O_3
** Not available.

surrounding tissues. However, from the ceramic/ceramic combination, ceramic particles resembling 'fine grains and great fragments in the ranges from 0.5 to 10 micrometers diameter, with the predominant size of about 1 micrometer' were found in the surrounding tissue (29). The advantage of ceramic/ceramic combination over ceramic/UHMWPE is, therefore, doubtful. For wear tests, we refer to ISO-6474 ASTM F-603.

Clinical performance

The fracture of ceramic balls in ceramic: UHMWPE combination has been virtually zero. Fritsch and Gleitz (30) published a failure analysis on 4341 alumina ceramic heads articulating with 2693 alumina ceramic and 1464 polymer sockets implanted over 20 years (1974 to 1994), and concluded that the use of ball type neckless heads brought the fracture rate close to zero. The success rate of 10 years follow-up is normally above 90% for the 'elderly' patient population. Stem and cup loosening are the causes of failure, where the consistent wear debris from UHMWPE and bone cement remain the problems.

Zirconium dioxide: zirconia

Zirconia ceramics are termed polymorphic because they undergo several transformations on cooling from a molten state to room temperature. It exhibits three well-defined polymorphs, the monoclinic, tetragonal and cubic phases and a high pressure orthorhombic form also exists. The monoclinic phase is stable up to about 1170°C where it transforms to the tetragonal phase, stable up to 2370°C, while the cubic phase exists up to the melting point 2680°C. A large volume change of 3 to 5% occurs when zirconia is cooled down and transforms from the tetragonal to the monoclinic phase.

Partially stabilized zirconia (PSZ) and tetragonal zirconia polycrystals (TZP)

The volume change due to phase transformation is sufficient to exceed elastic and fracture limits and causes cracking of the zirconia ceramics. Therefore, additives such as calcia (CaO), magnesia (MgO) and/or yttria (Y_2O_3) must be mixed with zirconia to stabilize the material in either the tetragonal or the cubic phase. PSZ is a mixture of cubic and tetragonal and /or monoclinic phases, whereas TZP is 100% tetragonal (phase diagram Figure 5.2). Both PSZ and TZP are suggested for medical implant applications. Yttria-TZP ceramics have a strength and fracture toughness approximately twice that of alumina ceramics used in the biomedical field. This makes zirconia heads less sensitive to stress concentrations at the points of contact with metal cones.

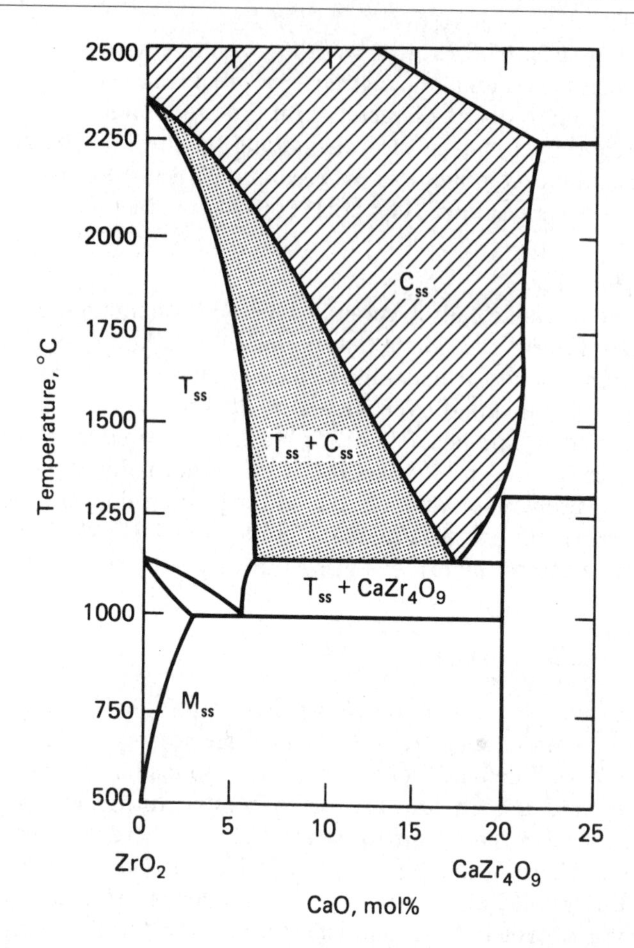

Figure 5.2(a) Part of the equilibrium phase diagram for the system ZrO_2–CaO. C_{ss} refers to the cubic solid-solution phase, Tss to the tetragonal solid-solution phase, and Mss to the monoclinic solid-solution phase (ref. 21).

Physical and mechanical properties

Zirconia ceramics have a high density because of heavy zirconium ions, and a low microhardness and elastic modulus, together with high strength and fracture toughness compared to other ceramics including alumina. The superior mechanical strength provides the possibilities for producing ceramic ball heads of size below 32 mm.

Fracture toughness mechanisms:

Garvie *et al.* were the first to realize the transformation toughening mechanism for zirconia ceramics. Increase of both strength and fracture

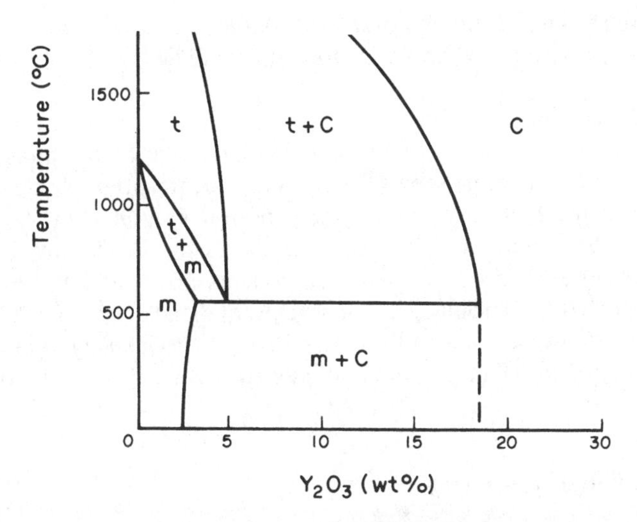

Figure 5.2(b) Y_2O_3–ZrO_2 phase diagram: the addition of less than 5% of Y_2O_3 to ZrO_2 allows the sintering of a fully tetragonal material (t=tetragonal phase; m=monoclinic phase; c=cubic phase) (ref. 16).

toughness can be obtained by utilizing the tetragonal-monoclinic phase transformation of metastable tetragonal grains induced by the presence of the stress field ahead of a crack (31). The volume change and the shear strain developed in the martensitic reaction were recognized as opposing the opening of the crack and therefore acting to increase the resistance to crack propagation.

Wear resistance and chemical stability:
The published results of *in vitro* wear tests demonstrated that zirconia has a superior wear resistance. Saikko (32) showed no wear of zirconia femoral heads on his hip simulator wear test against 10.9 mm UHMWPE cup, and Praveen Kumar *et al.* (33) demonstrated the high wear resistance of zirconia against UHMWPE and the superiority of zirconia ceramics even over alumina ceramics in terms of low wear and low friction. A significant reduction in the wear rate of zirconia ball heads compared to the metal ball heads was reported on a pin-on-disc wear test and on a hip simulator (34). However, there are two potential limitations for the use of zirconia as bioceramics: degradation and radiation. It is known that the phase transformation is accelerated in aqueous environment, but little is known about how this phase transformation will occur in biological environment, particularly under dynamic loadings. A warning against steam resterilization has been issued in the UK. Radioactive U-235 impurity was detected in some 'pure zirconia', both alpha- and gamma-irradiation were

measured from zirconia femoral balls. Although the radioactivity was low, more work is required to verify this matter (13).

Clinical performance
The surface degradation of the zirconia balls due to the phase transformation under loading seems to be a problem, although no significant change in mechanical strength was reported in some long-term *in vivo* and *in vitro* studies (35,36). Seriously, catastrophic failure of modular zirconia ceramics femoral head components after total hip arthroplasty was reported (37). Since zirconia femoral heads have a short clinical history and few clinical results are available, more investigation is required to eliminate the factors which impair the clinical stability of zirconia ceramics under loading.

5.3.2 Materials processing

An advanced ceramic is processed in such a way that the structure of the materials on different levels, including atomic, electronic, grain boundary, microstructural and macrostructural, is under strict control. In the manufacturing processes, emphasis is placed on producing dense ceramics with a fine microstructure. However, other factors such as chemical composition, the nature and distribution of the impurities, crystal structure, grain size, and defects are also of importance to the performance of the ceramic materials. Three basic processes are involved in the production of fine ceramic components, namely: 1. powder technology, 2. densification or sintering and 3. machining. Both alumina and zirconia hip balls are produced by compacting fined-grained powder (green bodies), and sintering at 1500–1700 °C and finally grinding or lapping to obtain a high surface finish and sphericity ($Ra<0.02\ \mu m$).

5.4 BIOCOMPATIBILITY OF OXIDE BIOCERAMICS

No materials placed within a living tissue can be considered to be completely inert. However, oxide bioceramics, by their very nature, do not suffer from corrosion or degradation in biological environments, as metals or plastics do. Ceramics, having molecular structures completely different from those of living tissues, are generally stable inside the living body and provide a high degree of acceptance by the apposition to the surrounding tissue as shown by *in vitro* and *in vivo* studies Ichikawa *et al.* observed no adverse soft tissue responses to zirconia and alumina implants after 12 months of implanation (38). Takamura *et al.* reported that alumina and zirconia did not possess chronic toxicity to mice (39), whereas Steflik *et al.* found a biological seal at the alumina dental implant and epithelium interface (40). However, oxide bioceramics do not form a chemical bond to bone tissue and are therefore defined as inert biomaterials. Oxide bioceramics are defined as inert biomaterials.

The ASTM standards (F 748/82, 763/82) and ISO standards No 10993 have set the guidance for biological testing of biomaterials for orthopaedic application. The materials should be tested in soft tissue as well as in hard tissue environments, for both short-term and long-term experiments. A summary of recommended biological testing is presented in Table 5.5. Both alumina and zirconia have shown non-toxicity and good biocompatibility according to the tests. Testing results for zirconia made by a French Company are shown in Table 5.6. Although some serious problems occurred with zirconia balls, the basic biocompatibility of the zirconia remains. Soft tissue and bone responses to zirconia and alumina were studied in our lab: no adverse tissue reaction to these ceramics were found. The patterns of tissue-materials interface after 1 month implantation in muscle and femur of rat are shown in Figure 5.3.

Table 5.5 Guidance for Biologic Evaluation Tests of the Implant Device in Contact to bone Tissue (According to ISO 10993–1:1992 (E))

	Contact duration		
Biological tests	*A-limited (>24 h)*	*B-prolonged (<24 h to 30 days)*	*C-permanent (<30 days)*
Cytotoxity	x	x	x
Sensitisation	x	x	x
Irritation/Intracutaneous reactivity	x	x	x
Irritation/Intracutaneous	x		
Genotoxicity		x	x
Implantation		x	x
Chronic toxicity			x
Carcinogenicity			x

The related tests see ISO standards from No. 10993–1 to 10993–6

Table 5.6 Biological evaluations of zirconia ceramics (Prozyr®, Ceramiques Desmarquest, France)

Biocompatibility	*Standard used*	*Results*
Short-term *in vivo* biocompatibility	ASTM F 763/82	Very good
In vitro biocompatibility	ASTM F 748/82	
Cell culture cytotoxicity	PRS 90.702	Good cytocompatibility
Mutagenicity	Ames test Micronucleus test	No mutagenic activity
Systemic injection acute toxicity	ASTM F 750/82	According to standard
Intracutaneous injection	ASTM F 749/82 ASTM F720/81	No irritation
Sensitization	Magnusson	No sensitization

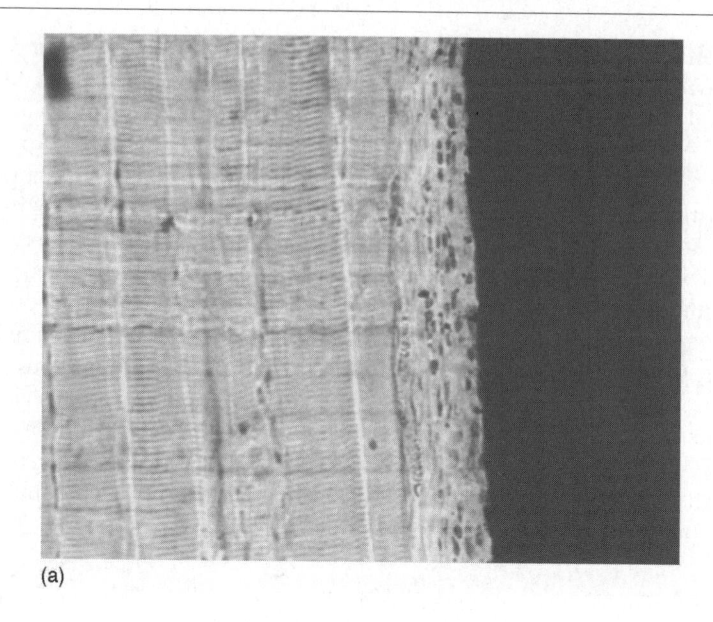

Figure 5.3(a) Optical micrograph of alumina and soft tissue interface.

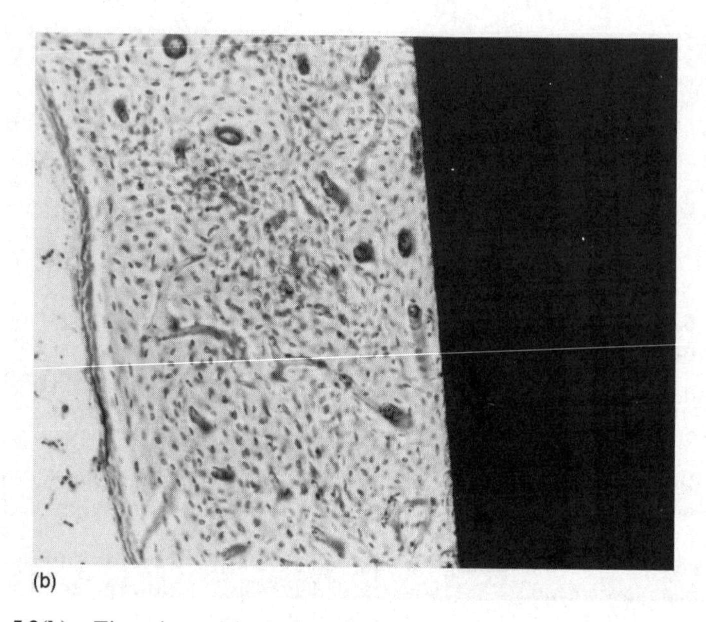

Figure 5.3(b) Zirconia and bone interface 1 month after implantation. Arrows are pointing to the interfaces.

Table 5.7 Ceramic manufacturers known for their bioceramic productions

Manufacturer	*Country*	*Primary Materials*	*Secondary Materials*	*Trade Names Al_2O_3 (ZrO_2)*
Astroment	USA	ZrO_2	Al_2O_3	
Ceraver	France	Al_2O_3	ZrO_2	
Cerasiv	Germany	Al_2O_3	ZrO_2	Biolox
Desmarquest	France	ZrO_2		(Proyzr)
HiTech	France	ZrO_2	Al_2O_3	
Kyocera	Japan	Al_2O_3	ZrO_2	Bioceram
Metoxit	Switzerland	ZrO_2		
Morgan Matroc	England	ZrO_2	Al_2O_3	
NGK	Japan	ZrO_2		
Biocare	Sweden	Al_2O_3		Procera
Unitek	USA	Al_2O_3		Transcend 2000
Maillefer	Switzerland	ZrO_2		

5.5 APPLICATIONS

5.5.1 Orthopaedic applications

The dominating application of alumina and zirconia is as hip balls as well as cups of total femoral prosthesis. The neckless hip balls are the most popular design. In 1981, Oonishi *et al.* (8) reported on the use of an alumina ceramic total knee prosthesis. High alumina ceramic middle ear implants (Frialit) are used clinically in Europe since 1979 (21). An opthalmological implant device consisting of a combination of a single crystal alumina optional cylinder and a polycrystalline alumina holding ring was introduced clinically in 1977 (22). Kawahara (12) has reported extensively on single crystal alumina bone screws.

5.5.2 Dental applications

Alumina and zirconia ceramics have been utilized for root analogue, endosteal screws, blades and pin-type dental implants. The root and blade form dental implants used during the 1970s tended to fracture after a few years in function (41,42) (Brose *et al.*, 1987, Driskell, 1987). Although initial testing of these polycrystalline alumina materials showed adequate mechanical strength, the long-term clinical results demonstrated functional limitations related to material properties and implant design. However, single crystalline alumina showed mechanical strength superior to that of polycrystalline alumina. It allows a much higher load. One-stage dental implants of single crystalline alumina are used clinically with a high success rate. McKinnery (43) had also reported on single crystal alumina blade and screw dental implants. Dental implants of zirconia have not been widely used clinically although zirconia has a similar mechanical strength and a much higher fracture toughness in addition to lower cost of production compared to single crystalline alumina. The term dental implant is used only for materials in contact with bone and soft tissue (14). Alumina and zirconia are also used in other dental applications, alumina ceramic crowns, Procera®(23), zirconia dental post, (10) and recently a dental inlay of zirconia was introduced (11). Orthodontic brackets made of oxide ceramics were also produced, tested and used clinically. Unfortunately, tooth surface damage was observed when the brackets were taken away (15). Modification of the debonding technique is under developing.

5.6 MANUFACTURERS AND THEIR IMPLANT PRODUCTS

Clarke and Willmann (13) make a comprehensive summary about the bioceramic manufacturers (Table 5.6). Some dental companies are included.

5.7 PROBLEMS AND FUTURE PROSPECTS

Hip balls of polycrystalline alumina have a minimum size limitation to ca. 28 mm due to strength limitations. A reduced ball size might have two positive effects on the applications: reduced wear and better suitability (smaller) for Asian patients. Although single crystalline alumina might overcome the strength limitation, the cost of manufacturing is unreasonably high and in addition, some processing problems remain. Zirconia, on the other hand, has a high strength and high fracture toughness, but it suffers from potential biodegradation. Therefore, the future research and development will focus on the understanding of degradation mechanisms of zirconia in the body and the improvement of stability of this material. Of course, combinations, such as alumina/zirconia composite and even non-oxide ceramic, such as nitrides and carbides, ought also to be investigated.

REFERENCES

1. Hulbert, S.F., Bokros, J.C., Hench, L.L., Wilson, J. and Heimke, G. In *Ceramics in Clinical Applications*, ed. by Vincenzini, P. Elsevier, Amsterdam, 1987, pp. 3–27.
2. Rock, M. German Patent 583 589, 1933.
3. Smith, L. *Arch. Surg.* 1963; **87**: 653–661.
4. Sandhaus, S. British Patent 1083769, 1967.

5. Boutin, P. *Presse Med.* 1971; **79**: 639.
6. Mittelmeier, H. *Z. Orthop. Ihre Grenzgeb* 1974; **112**: 27.
7. Shikita, T. Paper presented at the XIV World Congress of SICOT, Kyoto, Japan, October 15–20, 1978.
8. Oonishi, H., Okabe, N., Hamaguchi, T. and Nabeshima, T. *Orthopaedic Ceramic Implants 1,* 1981; 11–18.
9. Lord, G. *et al.* Paper presented at the Harrington Arthritis Research Centre Symposium, November 18–21, 1990.
10. Akagawa, Y. *et al. J. Prosthet. Dent.* 1993; **69**: 599–604.
11. Meyenberg, K.H., Luthy, H. and Scharer, P. *J. Esthet. Dent.*, 1995; **7**(2): 73–80.
12. Johansson, B. *Tandläkartidningen* 1996; 14746–749.
13. Clarke, I.C. and Willmann, G. In *Bone implant Interface* ed. H.V. Cameron, Hugh U., Mosby, 1994, pp. 222.
14. Kawahara, H. In *Encyclopedic handbook of biomaterials and bioengineering* ed. by Wise, Donald L. *et al.* Marcel Dekker, Inc., New York, 1995, pp. 1469–1524.
15. Sinha, P.K., Rohrer, M.D., Nanda, R.S. and Brickman, C.D. *American J. Orthodont & Dentofacial Orthop*, 1995; **108**: 455–63.
16. *Christel, P.S.* In *Concise Encyclopedia of Medical & Dental Materials*, ed. by Williams, D.F., Pergamon Press, Oxford, 1990, pp. 375–379.
17. Keith, O., Kusy, R.P. and Whitley, J.Q. *American J. Orthodont. & Dentofacial Orthop.*, 1994; **106**(6): 605–614.
18. Kawahara, H. *Orthopaedic Ceramic Implants 1*, 1981; 1–10.
19. Fartash, B. Single Crystal Sapphire Dental Implants: Experimental and Clinical Studies. PhD thesis, Karolinska Institute, Sweden, 1996.
20. Hammer, N.B., Topazian, R.G., McKinney, P.V. and Hulbert, S.F. *J. Dent. Res.* 1973; **52**: 356–361.
21. Jahnke, K. *Biomaterials in Otology*, Martinus Nijhoff, The Hague, 1984: 205–209.
22. Polack, F.M. and Heimke, G. *Ophthalmology*, 1980; **87**(7): 693–698.
23. Andersson, M. and Odén, A. *Acta Odont. Scand.*, 1993; **51:** 59–64.
24. Kittipibul, P. and Godfrey, K. *American J. Orthodont & Dentofacial Orthopedics*, 1995; **108**(3): 308–315.
25. Heimke, G. In *Metal and Ceramic Biomaterials* Vol I Structure, ed. by Ducheyne, P. and Hastings, G.W. CRC Press Inc., Boca Raton, Florida, 1984, pp. 41–42.
26. Miyayama, M. *et al.* In *Ceramics and Glass, Engineered Materials Handbook* Volume 4, ASM International, 1991, pp. 748–757.
27. Griss, P. In *Functional Behavior of Orthopaedic Biomaterials II*, Ch 2, 1984.
28. Jager M. and Plitz, W. *Triobology of aluminium ceramics, Symposium of Biomaterials*, pp. 114–122, 1981.
29. Willert, H.G. *et al.* In *Implant Retrieval: Material and Biological Analysis*, ed. by Weinstein, A., Gibbons, D., Brown, S. and Ruff, W. 1981.
30. Fritsch, E.W. and Gleitz, M. *Clin. Orthop. & Related Res.*, 1996; **328**: 129–136.
31. Garvie, R.C., Hannink, R.H. and Pascoe, R.T. *Nature*, 1975; **258**: 703.
32. Saikka, V.O. *Acta Orthop. Scand.*, 1995; **66**(6): 501–506.
33. Kumar, P. *et al. J. Biomed. Mater. Res.*, 1991; **25**: 813–828.
34. Derbyshire, B. *et al. Medical Eng. & Phys.*, 1994; **16**(39): 229–36.

35. Shimizu, K. *et al.* J. Biomed. Mater. Res., 1993; **27**: 729–734.
36. Cales, B., Stefani, Y. and Lilley, E. *J. Biomed. Mater. Res.*, 1994; **28:** 619–624.
37. Hummer, C.D., Rothman, R.H. and Hozack, W.J. *J. Arthroplasty*, 1995; **10**(6): 848–850.
38. Ichikawa, Y. *et al. J. Prosthet. Dent.* 1992; **68**: 322–6.
39. Takamura, K. *et al. J. Biomed. Mater. Res.*, 1994; **28**: 583–589.
40. Steflik, D., McKinney Jr R.V. and Koth, D. In *Bioceramics: Materials characteristics versus* in vivo behavior, ed. by Ducheyne, P. and Lemons, J.E. *Ann. N.Y. Acad. Sci.* **523**, pp. 4–18.
41. Brose, M. *et al. J. Dent. Res.*, 1987; **66**: 113.
42. Driskel, T.D. *J. Calif. Dent. Assoc.*, 1987; 16–25.
43. Mckinney, R.V. and Koth, D.L. *J. Prosthet. Dent.*, 1982: **47**: 69–84.
44. Park, J.B. and Lakes, R.S. *Biomaterials: an Introduction*, 2nd edition, Plenum Press, New York, 1992.
45. Bajpai, P.K. and Billotte, W.G. In *The Biomedical Engineering Handbook*, ed. by Bronzino, J.D. CRC Press, 1995, pp. 552–580.

Properties of bioactive glasses and glass-ceramics

6

L.L. Hench and T. Kokubo

Definition of bioactivity:

A bioactive material is one that elicits a specific biological response at the interface of the material which results in the formation of a bond between the tissues and the material. A common characteristic of bioactive glasses, bioactive glass-ceramics, and bioactive ceramics is that their surface develops a biologically active hydroxy carbonate apatite (HCA) layer which bonds with collagen fibrils. The HCA phase that forms on bioactive implants is equivalent chemically and structurally to the mineral phase of bone. It is that equivalence which is responsible for interfacial bonding[1–3].

6.1 BIOACTIVE BONDING

Bioactive materials develop an adherent interface with tissues that resist substantial mechanical forces. In many cases the interfacial strength of adhesion is equivalent to or greater than the cohesive strength of bone. The interfacial strength of a bioactive implant bonded to bone is 15–40 times greater than the interfacial adherence of non-bioactive materials (such as Al_2O_3) (Table 6.1 and Figure 6.1), tested in the same animal model (rabbit tibia) (Figure 6.2)[4].

Handbook of Biomaterial Properties. Edited by J. Black and G. Hastings.
Published in 1998 by Chapman & Hall, London. ISBN 0 412 60330 6.

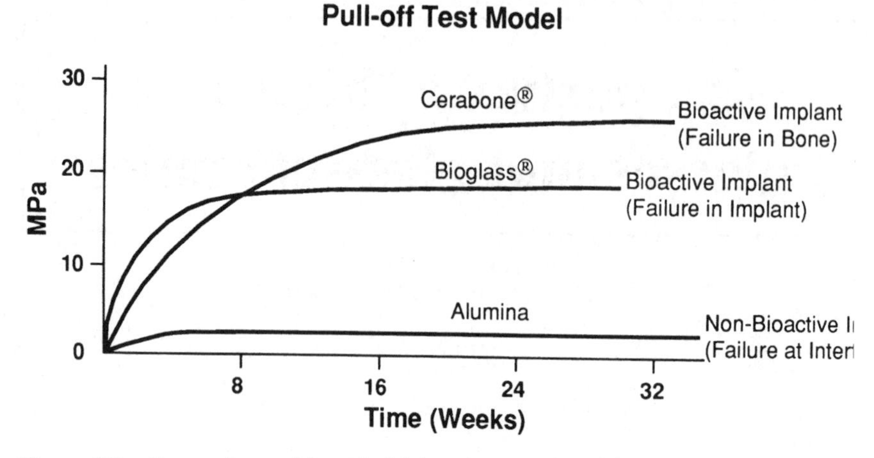

Figure 6.1 Comparison of interfacial bond strengths of bioactive implants with non-bonding implants (alumina) using 'pull off' detaching test [4,5].

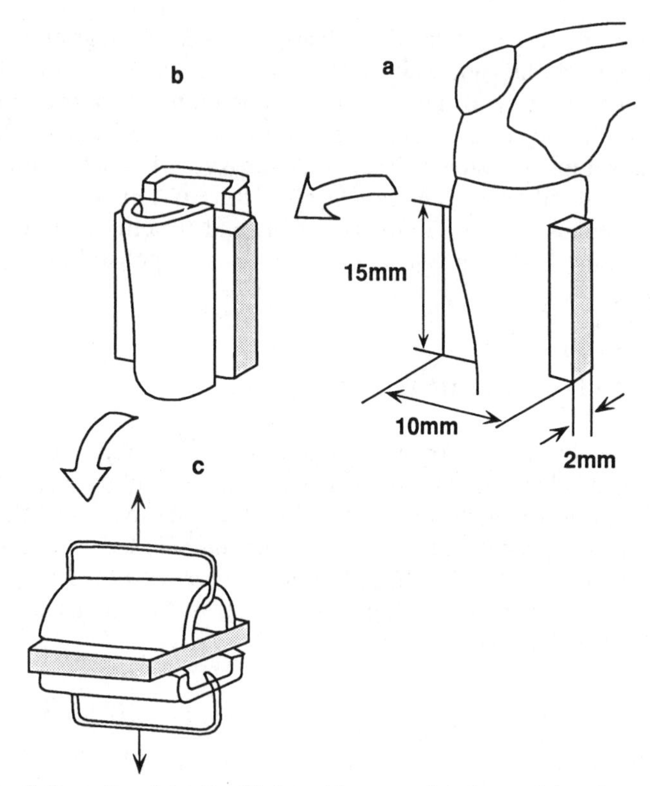

Figure 6.2 Schematic of 'pull off' detaching test for determining bone-implant bonding (based upon T. Yamamuro, ref. 4).

Table 6.1 Failure Loads of Bioceramics by Detaching (Pull-Off) Test

Materials	*Failure Load (kg)* 8 Weeks	24 Weeks	*Location of Fracture*
Dense sintered alumina[1,2]	0.13 ± 0.02		Interface
Bioglass® 45S5-type glass[1,2]	2.75 ± 1.80		within material
Ceravital® KGS-type glass-ceramic[3]	3.52 ± 1.48	4.35 ± 1.45	within material
Cerabone® A-W glass-ceramic[1,2]	7.44 ± 1.91	8.19 ± 3.6	within bone
Dense sintered hydroxyapatite[1,2]	6.28 ± 1.58	7.77 ± 1.91	within material
Dense sintered β-$3CaO \cdot P_2O_5$[4]	7.58 ± 1.97		not specified
Natural polycrystalline calcite[5]	4.11 ± 0.98		within material

1. T. Nakamura, T. Yamamuro, S. Higashi, T. Kokubo and S. Ito (1985) A New Glass-Ceramic for Bone Replacement: Evaluation of its Bonding to Bone Tissue, *J. Biomed. Maters Res.* **19**, 685–698.
2. T. Nakamura, T. Yamamuro, S. Higashi, Y. Kakutani, T. Kitsugi, T. Kokubo and S. Ito, 1985, A New Bioactive Glass-Ceramic for Artificial Bone, in *Treatise on Biomedical Materials, 1*, T. Yamamuro, ed., Research Center for Medical Polymers and Biomaterials at Kyoto University, Kyoto, Japan, pp. 109–17.
3. S. Kotani, T. Yamamuro, T. Nakamura, T. Kisugi, Y. Fujmita, K. Kawanabe, T. Kokubo and C. Ohtsuki (1990) The Bone-Bonding Behavior of Two Glass-Ceramics (KGS and A-W GC), in *Bioceramics*, Vol. 2, G. Heimke, ed., German Ceramic Society, Cologne, pp. 105–112.
4. S. Kotani, Y. Fujita, T. Kitsugi, T. Nakamura, T. Yamamuro, C. Ohtsuki and T. Kokubo (1991) Bone Bonding Mechanisms of β-tricalcium Phosphate, *J. Biomed. Maters. Res.* **25**, 1303–15.
5. Y. Fujita, T. Yamamuro, T. Nakamura, S. Kotani, C. Ohtsuki and T. Kokubo (1991) The Bonding Behavior of Calcite to Bone, *J. Biomed. Maters. Res.* **25**, 1991–2003.
6. T. Yamamuro (1993) A/W Glass-Ceramic: Clinical Applications, in *Introduction to Bioceramics*, eds L.L. Hench and J. Wilson, World Scientific Publishing Co., London, 1993, pp. 89–104.

6.2 BIOACTIVE COMPOSITIONS

Bioactive materials are composed of very specific compositional ranges of Na_2O, CaO, P_2O_5 and SiO_2 due to the importance of these compounds in the *in vivo* formation of hydroxy carbonate apatite (HCA) bone mineral (Table 6.2) [1,2]. All compositions either form a HCA layer on their surface or partially dissolve (resorb) as HCA crystals are formed during the mineralization of osteoid. The rate of formation of HCA and bone depends upon the composition of the material (Figure 6.3) with bioactive glasses and glass-ceramics containing < 52% SiO_2 being the most rapid. The time difference in time dependence of interfacial bond strength (Figure 6.1) is due to the different rates of growth of the interfacial HCA layer. The bioactivity index of a materials (I_B) is defined as:

$$I_B = 100/t_{0.5bb}$$

I_B is obtained from Figure 6.3, and is proportional to the reciprocal of the time required for one half (0.5) of the interface to be bonded to bone. I_B values are shown in Table 6.2 for the various bioactive implants.

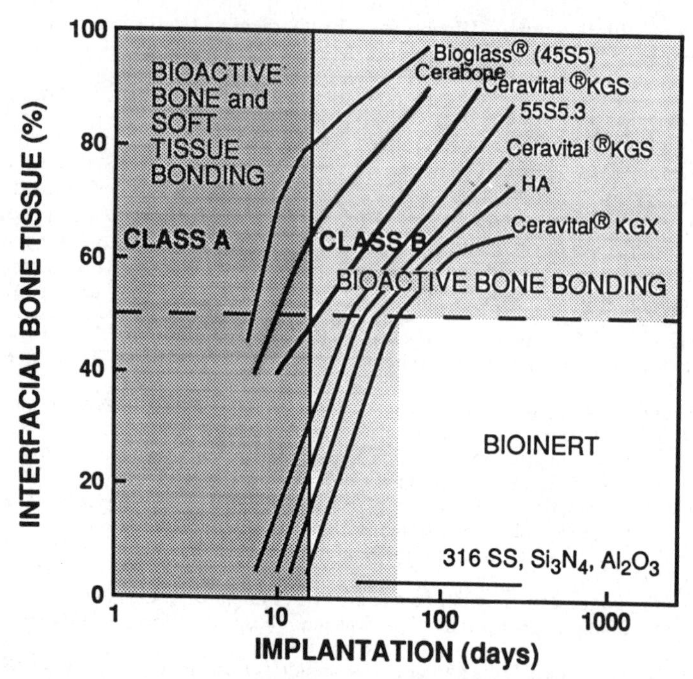

Figure 6.3 Time dependence of interfacial bone formation for various types of bioceramic implants.

The compositional dependence of bonding of bone to various bioactive glasses is illustrated in Figure 6.4 for the Na_2O–CaO–SiO_2 system, with a constant 6 weight percent P_2O_5 and in Figure 6.5 for the CaO–P_2O_5–SiO_2 system. Figure 6.4 also shows iso I_B values for the Na_2O–CaO–P_2O_5–SiO_2 system. When $I_B = 0$ there is no interfacial bond with bone; i.e., the material develops a non-adherent fibrous capsule and is nearly bioinert.

6.3 PHYSICAL PROPERTIES

Table 6.2 summarizes the physical properties of the bioactive glasses, glass-ceramics, and ceramics in clinical use, with references. The bioactive glasses are single phase amorphous materials which have high I_B values (rapidly form a bone bond) but have low mechanical strength and toughness. These materials should be used in particulate form (as powders), as coatings, or in low load bearing applications, as listed in Table 6.3. Bioactive glass-ceramics are multi-phase materials with a fine, homogeneous grain size and good mechanical strength and toughness[5] and intermediate I_B values. They can be used in moderate load bearing

Table 6.2 Composition and Mechanical Properties of Bioactive Ceramics Used Clinically

Composition	*Bioglass®[1] 45S5*	*S53P4[2]*	*Glass-ceramic[3] Ceravital®*	*Glass-ceramic[4] Cerabone® A-W*	*Glass-ceramic[5] Ilmaplant® L1*	*Glass-ceramic[6] Bioverit®*	*Sintered[7,8,9] hydroxypatite $Ca_{10}(PO_4)_6(OH)_2$ > 99.2%*	*Sintered[10,11] β-$3CaO \cdot P_2O_5$ > 99.7%*
Na_2O	24.5 wt%	22.6 wt%	5–10 wt%	0 wt%	4.6 wt%	3–8 wt%		
K_2O	0		0.5–3.0	0	0.2	3–8 wt%		
MgO	0		2.5–5.0	4.6	2.8	2–21		
CaO	24.5	21.8	30–35	44.7	31.9	10–34		
Al_2O_3	0		0	0	0	8–15		
SiO_2	45.0	53.9	40–50	34.0	44.3	19–54		
P_2O_5	6.0	1.7	10–50	16.2	11.2	2–10		
CaF_2	0			0.5	5.0	F 3–23		
B_2O_3	0							
Phase	Glass	Glass	Apatite	Apatite ($Ca_{10}(PO_4)_6(O,F_2)$)	Apatite	Apatite	Apatite ($Ca_{10}(PO_4)_6(OH)_2$)	Whitlockite (β-$3CaO \cdot P_2O_5$)
			Glass	β-Wollastonite ($CaO \cdot SiO_2$)	β-Wollastonite	Phlogopite ($(Na_1K)Mg_3(AlSiO_{10})F_2$)		
				Glass	Glass	Glass		
Density (g/cm^3)	2.6572			3.07		2.8	3.16	3.07
Hardness (Vickers) (HV)	458 ± 9.4			680		500	600	
Compressive strength (MPa)			500	1080		500	500–1000	460–687
Bending strength (MPa)	42(Tensile)			215	160	100–160	115–200	140–154
Young modulus (GPa)	35		100–150	118		70–88	80–110	33–90

Table 6.2 *Continued*

Composition	*Bioglass®[1] 45S5*	*S53P4[2]*	*Glass-ceramic[3] Ceravital®*	*Glass-ceramic[4] Cerabone® A-W*	*Glass-ceramic[5] Ilmaplant® L1*	*Glass-ceramic[6] Bioverit®*	*Sintered[7,8,9] hydroxypatite $Ca_{10}(PO_4)_6(OH)_2$ > 99.2%*	*Sintered[10,11] β-3CaO · P_2O_5 > 99.7%*
Fracture toughness, K_{IC}(MPa $m^{1/2}$)				2.0	2.5	0.5–1.0	1.0	
Slow crack growth, n				33			12–27	
Index of bioactivity I_B[12]	12.5	3.8	5.6	7.5 (est)			3.1	

1. L.L. Hench and E.C. Ethridge, Biomaterials, An Interfacial Approach, p. 137, Academic Press, New York, 1982.
2. ö.H. Andersson, K.H. Karlsson, K. Kangasniemi, and A. Yli-Urpo, Models for Physical Properties and Bioactivity of Phosphate Opal Glasses, *Glastech. Ber.*, **61**, 300–305 (1988).
3. H. Bromer, K. Deutscher, B. Blenke, E. Pfeil and V. Strunz, Properties of the Bioactive Implant Material Ceravital®, in *Science of Ceramics*, Vol. 9, 1977, pp. 219–223.
4. T. Kokubo, Mechanical Properties of a New Type of Glass-Ceramic for Prosthetic Applications, in *Multiphase Biomedical Materials*, T. Tsuruta and A. Nakajima, eds, VSP, Utrecht, Netherlands, 1989.
5. G. Berger, F. Sauer, G. Steinborn, F.G. Wishsmann, V. Thieme, St Kohler and H. Dressel, Clinical Application of Surface Reactive Apatite/Wollastonite Containing Glass-Ceramics, in Proceedings of XV International Congress on Glass, Vol. 3a, O.V. Mazurin, eds, Nauka, Leningrad, 1989, pp. 120–126.
6. W. Vogel and W. Holland, The Development of Bioglass® Ceramics for Medical Applications, *Angew Chem. Int. Ed. Engl.* **26**, 527–544 (1987).
7. M. Jarcho, C.H. Bolen, M.B. Thomas, J. Bobick, J.F. Kay and R.H. Doremus, Hydroxyapatite Synthesis and Characterization in Dense Polycrystalline Form, *J. Mater. Sci.* **11**, 2027–2035 (1976).
8. M. Akao, H. Aoki, and K. Kato, Mechanical Properties of Sintered Hydroxyapatite for Prosthetic Applications, *J. Mater. Sci.* **16**, 809–812 (1981).
9. G. Dewith, H.J.A. Van Dijk, N. Hattu and K. Prijs, Preparation, Microstructure and Mechanical Properties of Dense Polyerystalline Hydroxyapatite, *J. Mater. Sci.* **16**, 1592–1598 (1981).
10. M. Jarcho, R.L. Salsbury, M.B. Thomas and R.H. Doremus, Synthesis and Fabrication of β-tricalcium Phosphate (Whitlockite) Ceramics for Potential Prosthetic Applications, *J. Mater. Sci.* **14**, 142–150 (1979).
11. M. Akao, M. Aoki, K. Kato and A. Sato, Dense Polycrystalline β-tricalcium Phosphate for Prosthetic Applications, *J. Mater. Sci.* **17**, 343–346 (1932).
12. L.L. Hench, Bioactive Ceramics, in *Bioceramics: Materials Characteristics Versus In Vivo Behavior*, P. Ducheyne, J.E. Lemons, eds, *Annuals of the NY Academy of Sciences*, u**523**, 1988, pp. 54–71

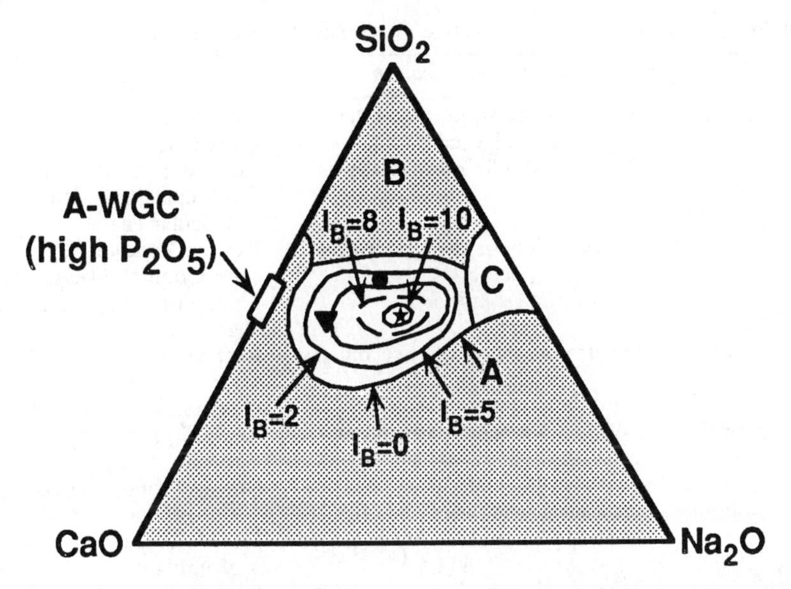

Figure 6.4 The compositional dependence of bone bonding to bioactive glasses (region A) containing 6 weight % P_2O_5. Soft tissue bonding occurs for compositions with l_B values > 8 (see text). Region B: non-bioactive compositions. Glasses in Region C are resorbable. (Based upon chapters 1 and 3 in ref. 1.)

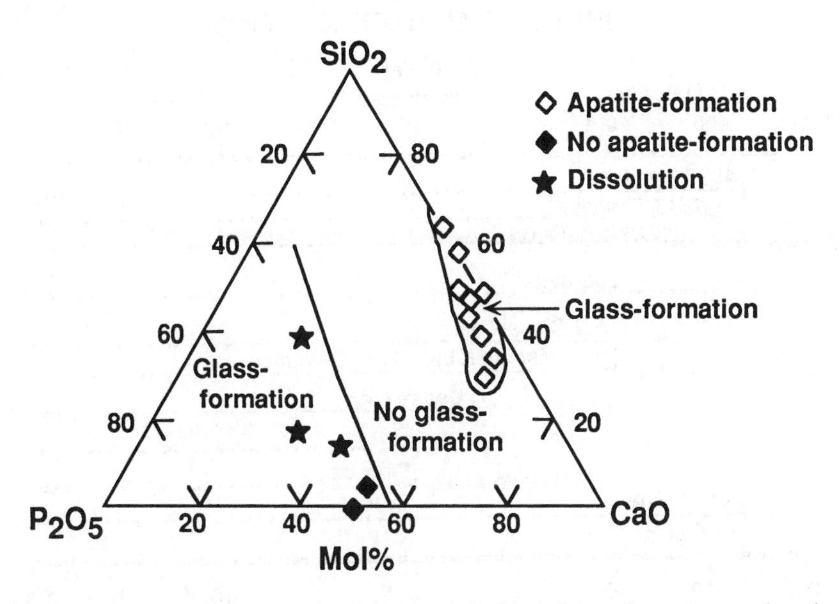

Figure 6.5 Compositional dependence of bioactivity for glasses in the $CaO–P_2O_5–SiO_2$. (Based upon T. Kokubo, ref. 5.)

Table 6.3 Clinical Uses of Bioactive Glasses and Glass-Ceramics

Material	*Form*	*Application*	*Function*
45S5 Bioglass®	Bulk	Endosseous alveolar ridge maintenance	Space filling and tissue bonding
	Bulk	Middle ear prostheses	Restore conductive hearing by replacing part of ossicular chain
	Powder	Repair of periodontal defects	Restore bone lost by periodontal disease and prevent epithelial down growth
	Powder	Fixation of revision arthroplasty	Restore bone loss due to loosening of hip prostheses
Cerabone® (A/W glass-ceramic)	Bulk	Vertebral prostheses	Replace vertebrae removed in tumor surgery
		Iliac crest prostheses	Replace bone removed for autogenous graft
	Coating	Fixation of hip prostheses	Provide bioactive bonding of implant
S53P4	Bulk	Orbital floor prostheses	Repair damaged bone supporting eye
	Powder	Cranial repair	Repair bone lost due to trauma

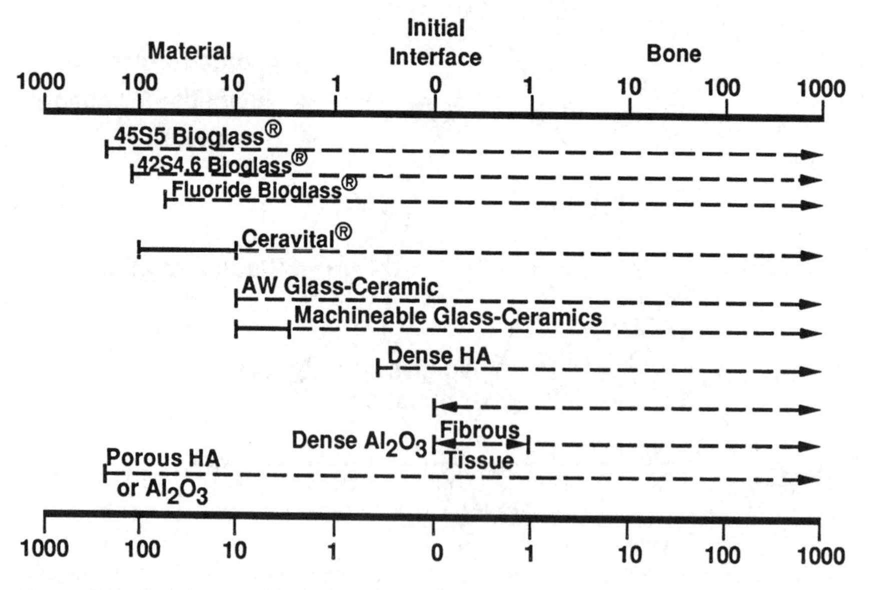

Figure 6.6 Thickness of interfacial bonding layers for various bioceramics.

applications as bulk materials (Table 6.3). Polycrystalline bioactive ceramics, such as synthetic hydroxyapatite (HA), have moderate strengths and relatively low I_B values and should be used as particulate or in non-load bearing applications. Compositions with the highest I_B values develop interfacial bonding layers (Figure 6.6) composed of both hydrated silica gel layers and Ca, P-rich layers. Compositions with low to moderate I_B values form thinner bonding zones composed primarily of Ca-P-rich compounds. Non-bonding implants have a non adherent fibrous tissue layer at the implant interface.

REFERENCES

1. Hench, L.L. and Wilson, J. (eds) (1993) *Introduction to Bioceramics*, World Scientific Publishers, London and Singapore, pp. 1–24.
2. Gross, U., Kinne, R., Schmitz, H.J. and Strunz, V. (1988) The response of bone to surface active glass/glass-ceramics. *CRC Critical Reviews in Biocompatibility*, **4,** 2.
3. Yamamuro, T., Hench, L.L. and Wilson, J. (eds) (1990) *Handbook of Bioactive Ceramics, Vol 1: Bioactive Glasses and Glass-Ceramics*, CRC Press, Boca Raton, FL.
4. Yamamuro, T. (1993) A/W glass-ceramic: clinical applications, in *Introduction to Bioceramics* (eds L.L. Hench and J. Wilson), World Scientific Publishers, London and Singapore, pp. 89–104.
5. Kokubo, T. (1993) A/W glass-ceramic: processing and properties, in *Introduction to Bioceramics* (eds L.L. Hench and J. Wilson), World Scientific Publishers, London and Singapore, pp. 75–88.

7 Wear

M. LaBerge

7.1 INTRODUCTION

Biomaterials used in the fabrication of implants are subjected to wear. Wear of biomaterials and devices has been shown to be detrimental to their long term success resulting in implant retrieval and revision. One of the most dramatic impacts of the wear of biomaterials and its consequences is observed with artificial joints. As stated by Jacobs *et al.*, (1994) wear has emerged as a central problem limiting the long-term longevity of total joint replacements. Ultra-high-molecular-weight polyethylene (UHMWPE) wear debris has been shown by many authors to trigger an osteolytic reaction which leads to implant loosening (Mittlmeier and Walter, 1987). Wear is a process resulting in the progressive loss of material involving many diverse mechanisms and phenomena which are often unpredictable (Table 7.1). The wear process of materials is predominantly governed by their mechanical and/or chemical behavior. More often than not, the wear processes listed in Table 7.1 do not act independently. However, even though several wear mechanisms are involved, it is often the case that one particular mechanism dominates (Dowson, 1981).

Unfortunately surface wear of an implant results from its use, and therefore, cannot be avoided or eliminated. Because wear is a limiting factor in the successful outcome and lifetime of an implant, it is of the utmost importance to characterize the wear resistance of materials used in implant design, and the effect of the design on wear. The volume of material removed from surfaces in specific tribosystems as a result of wear processes has been described phenomenologically and estimated by different models (Table 7.2). Several experimental wear studies have been

Handbook of Biomaterial Properties. Edited by J. Black and G. Hastings. Published in 1998 by Chapman & Hall, London. ISBN 0 412 60330 6.

Table 7.1 Wear Mechanisms

Wear Mechanisms	*Definition*
Adhesive Wear	Characterized by the transfer of material from one surface to another surface during relative motion. This type of wear is a consequence of adhesive forces acting at the junction of surface asperities. The transferred fragments may either be permanently or only temporarily attached to the other surface. Adhesive wear has been denoted as being the most commonly detected mechanism of wear, unfortunately it is also the least preventable (Dowson, 1981).
Abrasive Wear	Results from a hard asperity damaging or ploughing the surface of a softer material. The presence of hard particles may be due to the original material properties of one of the surfaces or loose debris particles which have become entrapped between the two sliding surfaces and/or embedded into one of the surfaces expediting abrasive wear. Generally, the resistance to abrasion can be related to the hardness of the material, however, this relationship is not directly proportional (Suh, 1986).
Delamination Wear	Involves material removal subsequently to plastic deformation, crack nucleation, and propagation in the subsurface (Jahanmir and Suh, 1977; Suh, 1986)
Fatigue Wear	Associated with cyclic stress variations and therefore, the lifetime of the material is dependent on the number of cycles. Cyclic deformation of the contacting surfaces leads to the initiation and propagation of microcracks (Rowe, 1980). Subsurface crack initiation generally occurs in the region of maximum shear stress which will depend upon the geometry of the materials
Fretting Wear	Generated by a relative oscillatory tangential movement of small amplitudes (damage can be caused by movement with amplitudes as small as 0.125 μm) which may occur between two surfaces in contact subjected to vibration (Waterhouse, 1992).
Corrosive Wear	Observed when the environment interacts chemically or electrochemically with one or both of the surfaces. Therefore, the wear rate is dependent on the environmental conditions affecting the chemical reactivity of the surfaces. This type of wear mechanism is important for biomaterials since they function in an extremely harsh environment, the human body (Black, 1988).

conducted to (1) predict the amount of material removed in specific conditions, (2) compare the effect of different fabrication and sterilization processes on materials, (3) produce wear debris to be used in biocompatibility studies, and (4) characterize the behavior of a new material destined for biomedical applications. Overall wear tests are primarily conducted to ascertain the basic mechanisms of wear for a particular

Table 7.2 Selected Wear Models

Wear Process	*Model*	*Specifications*
Adhesive Wear# (Archard, 1980)	**Archard Equation:** $W_{ad} = \frac{V}{L} = K \frac{F_N}{H}$ W_{ad} = wear rate (worn volume per unit sliding distance) K = wear coefficient V = volume of wear L = sliding distance F_N = normal load H = hardness of the softer material	• Use hardness as the only material property, even though K depends on various properties of both materials • Implies that wear rate is proportional to real contact area in plastic contacts and may not be applicable for cases involving elastic contacts
(Hornbogen, 1975)	**Hornbogen equation:** $W_{ad} = N^2 \frac{P_Y E' F_N^{1.5}}{K_{IC}^2 H^{1.5}}$ W_{ad} = wear rate K_{IC} = fracture toughness P_y = yield strength N = work hardening factor E′ = equivalent elastic modulus $E' = 1/[(1 - \nu_1^2)/E_1 + (1 - \nu_2^2)/E_2]$	• Based on a comparison of the strain occurring during asperity interactions with the critical strain at which crack growth is initiated. If the applied strain is smaller than the critical strain, the wear rate is independent of toughness, and follows Archard's

Table 7.2 *Continued*

Wear Process	*Model*	*Specifications*
Abrasive Wear (Rabinowicz, 1965)	**Rabinowicz model:** $W_{ab} = \frac{V}{L} = \frac{K\,F_N}{\pi\,H} \tan\theta$ W_{ab} = wear rate (worn volume per unit sliding distance) K = wear coefficient V = volume of wear L = sliding distance F_N = normal load H = hardness of the softer material $\tan\theta$ = weighted average of the $\tan\theta$ values of all the individual cones θ = average slope of the asperities	• Assumes that asperities of the harder surface are conical
(Zum Gahr, 1982)	**Zum Gahr model:** $W_{ab} = \frac{f_{ab}}{K_1 K_2 \tau_c} \frac{\cos\rho \sin\theta}{[\cos(\theta/2)]^{0.5} \cos(\theta - \rho)} F_N$ W_{ab} = wear rate f_{ab} = model factor (1 for microcutting) K_1 = relaxation of normal and shear stress K_2 = texture factor (1 for fcc metals) t_c = shear stress for dislocation movement ρ = friction angle at abrasive-material interface	• Considers the processes of microcutting, microploughing, and microcracking in the abrasive wear of ductile metals. • This model includes the effects of • work hardening • ductility • homogeneity of strain • crystal anisotropy

Table 7.2 *Continued*

Wear Process	*Model*	*Specifications*
Fatigue Wear (Halling, 1975)	**Halling model:** $W_{fa} = K \frac{\eta \gamma}{\epsilon_1^2 H} F_N$ W_{fa} = wear rate η = line distribution of asperities γ = constant defining particle size e_1 = strain to failure in one loading cycle H = hardness of the softer material K = wear coefficient	• Incorporates the concept of fatigue failure as well as simple plastic deformation failure.
Corrosive Wear (Quinn, 1980; Quinn *et al.*, 1983)	**Quinn Model:** $W_{corr} = \frac{dA_c \exp[-Q/(R_c T_c)]}{3\epsilon^2 \rho^2 \nu H} F_N$ W_{corr} = wear rate ρ = density of material A_c = Arrhenius constant Q = activation energy R_c = gas constant T_c = contact temperature d = asperity contact diameter ν = sliding velocity e = critical thickness of reaction layer	• Explains wear in steel and assumes that surface asperity layers formed tribochemically are detached at a certain critical thickness

Note
- The wear factor (k) is a measure of the rate at which a given combination of materials wears in the environment of the test. K is widely used for comparative purposes.
- According to Dowson (1995), if the mean contact stresses are not too high the wear of polymer against a hard surface (metal or ceramic) is obtained with fair accuracy with the relationship V = kFL.
- K is directly influenced by the roughness average (Ra) of the metallic counterface for the contact UHMWPE–stainless steel in water under reciprocating pin-on-plate conditions given by the relationship $k = 4.0 \times 10^{-5}$ Ra $^{1.2}$(Dowson *et al.*, 1985).

combination of materials, or the more restrictive yet equally elusive determination of the rate of wear to facilitate the estimation of their 'clinical' life. Experimental results are highly dependent on the geometry of the contact, the lubricant, the tribological conditions including velocity and load, and material properties (Suh, 1986). Therefore, experimental protocols aimed at investigating the wear properties of biomaterials should be designed to assess or predict their behavior in simulated clinical conditions (Dumbleton, 1981).

7.2 *IN VITRO* WEAR TESTING

Although wear is a very complex process, apparatuses are available which allow for the accumulation of data resulting in an estimate of the wear resistance of a combination of materials or a device. Preliminary material studies will commonly be performed on laboratory wear benches while devices will be evaluated with simulators. Numerous *in vitro* and *in vivo* studies have been conducted to evaluate the wear properties of biomaterial tribosystems (Table 7.3). Over the years, different wear apparatuses (Table 7.4) and protocols have been used for this purpose. Only one standard procedure under the American Society for Testing and Materials (ASTM F-732–82, reapproved 1991) for Reciprocating Pin-on-Flat Evaluation of Friction and Wear Properties of Polymeric Materials for Use in Total Joint Prostheses) describes the testing protocol for characterizing the wear resistance of material combinations to be used in the design of implants. Several investigators have used modified or adapted versions of this standard to assess the wear resistance of bearing surfaces for orthopaedic applications (Streicher, 1991; Schmidt *et al.*, 1995; Jin *et al.*, 1993; Medley *et al.*, 1995; Brown *et al.*, 1976; Rose and Radin, 1982; Fisher and Dowson, 1991, Agrawal *et al.*, 1993). Other ASTM protocols pertinent to the evaluation of wear performance of engineering materials are listed in Table 7.5. Wear resistance is usually reported in terms of wear rate, either linear or volumetric, with different units such as volume lost per 10^6 cycles, mass loss per 10^6 cycles, or linear displacement per 10^6 cycles. A complete walking cycle is represented by two steps. One cycle on a reciprocating pin-on-flat system is obtained by two passes (return to starting point), while one cycle on a rotating pin-on-disc system corresponds to one revolution. It is assumed that a normal individual will make two million steps per year while an active subject may make more than 10 million steps (Dumbleton, 1981) at a maximum frequency of 1 Hz. Investigators have also reported wear rates as cubic millimeters (volume) per millimeter (sliding distance) (mm^3/mm). The volume is calculated by measuring the mass loss and using the density of the polymer as a conversion factor. Tables 7.6 and 7.7 present a critical selection of wear data available for biomaterial tribosystems useful to the orthopaedic design community. Both friction coefficient and wear rate are used as design parameters. Unless independently monitored, friction coefficients are usually acquired during wear tests. The static coefficient of friction is calculated using the force required to initiate motion. The kinetic coefficient of friction may vary during a test for a constant velocity and should be calculated from averaged force readings during the duration of the test. ASTM Standard G115–93 proposes a guide for Measuring and Reporting Friction Coefficients (ASTM, 1993) which is designed to assist investigators in the selection of an appropriate method for measuring the frictional properties of materials.

Table 7.3 Biomaterial Combinations Tribologically Characterized

Material combinations	*Test apparatus*
Stainless steel UHMWPE	Pin -on disc; joint simulator (McKellop *et al.*, 1981; Dowson *et al.*, 1988; Kumar *et al.*, 1991)
Co–Cr-alloys UHMWPE	Pin-on-disc; joint simulator (McKellop *et al.*, 1978; McKellop *et al.*, 1981; Rose *et al.*, 1984; Saikko, 1993)
Titanium alloys UHMWPE	Pin-on-disc; joint simulator (Miller *et al.*, 1974; McKellop *et al.*, 1978; McKellop and Rostlünd, 1990)
Alumina UHMWPE	Pin-on-disc; joint simulator (Semlitsch *et al.*, 1977; McKellop *et al.*, 1981; Saikko, 1993)
Zirconia UHMWPE	Pin-on-disc; joint simulator (Saikko, 1993; Kumar *et al.*, 1991)
CoCrMo CoCrMo	Pin-on-disc; joint simulator (Galante, 1973; Semlitsch *et al.*, 1977; Streicher *et al.*, 1990; Medley *et al.*, 1995; Chan *et al.*, 1996)
CoCrMo Delrin	Disc-on-flat (Clarke *et al.*, 1982)
CoCrMo Alumina	Joint simulator (Saikko *et al.*, 1993)
Ti6A14V Alumina	Joint simulator (Saikko *et al.*, 1993)
Alumina Alumina	Wear and friction benches; joint simulator (Galante *et al.*, 1973; Boutin *et al.*, 1972; Semlitsch *et al.*, 1977)
Polyurethane low modulus elastomers) Metal	Reciprocating friction benches; joint simulator (Gladstone and Medley, 1990; Jin *et al.*, 1993; Auger *et al.*, 1993; Chow *et al.*, 1994; Auger *et al.*, 1995; Graham *et al.*, 1995)
Dental resins Enamel	Pin-on-flat (Suzuki *et al.*, 1996)

Table 7.4 *In vitro* Measurement wear machines

Wear Apparatus Type	*Comments*
Pin-on-disc or pin-on-plate	Useful in studying basic wear mechanisms. Steady and well controlled operating conditions. Fails to replicate the reciprocating motion observed in joints
Reciprocating pin-on-plate	Simulates the reciprocating motion observed *in vivo* and fatigue loading (loading and unloading).
Joint simulators (knee and hip simulators)	Improved understanding of the wear processes encountered in prostheses.

Table 7.5 *In vitro* Friction and Wear Measurement Standards*

ASTM Standard	*Title*
B460	Test Method For Dynamic Coefficient Of Friction And Wear Of Sintered Metal Friction Materials Under Dry Conditions (vol. 2.05, p. 223–225, 1989)
B461	Test Method For Frictional Characteristics Of Sintered Metal Friction Materials Run In Lubricants (vol. 2.05, 1989)
C808	Guidelines For Reporting Friction And Wear Test Results Of Manufactured Carbon And Graphite Bearing And Seal Materials (vol. 15.01, p. 243–344, 1989)
D1894	Test Method For Static And Kinetic Coefficients Of Friction Of Plastic Film And Sheeting (vol. 8.01, p. 439–444, 1995)
D3028	Test Method For Kinetic Coefficient Of Friction Of Plastic Solids (vol. 8.02, p. 225–233, 1995)
D3108	Test Method For Coefficient Of Friction, Yarn To Solid Material (vol. 7.01, p. 758–766, 1995)
D3334	Method Of Testing Fabrics Woven From Polyolefin Monofilaments (vol. 7.01, p. 516–520, 1989)
D3412	Test Method For Coefficient Of Friction, Yarn-To-Yarn. (vol. 7.02, p. 10–14, 1995)
F732	Practice For Reciprocating Pin-On-Flat Evaluation Of Friction And Wear Properties Of Polymeric Materials For Use In Total Joint Prosthesis (vol. 13.01, p. 183–188, 1995)
G40	Terminology Relating to Wear and Corrosion (vol. 3.02, p. 145–151, 1995)
G77	Test Method for Ranking Resistance of Materials to Sliding Wear Using Block-on-Ring Wear Test (vol. 3.02, p. 302–315, 1995)
G83	Test Method for Wear Testing with a Crossed-Cylinder Apparatus (vol. 3.02, p. 339–344, 1995)
G99	Test Method for Wear Testing with a Pin-on-Disk Apparatus (vol. 3.02, p. 380–390, 1995)
G115	Standard Guide For Measuring And Reporting Friction Coefficients (vol. 13.01, p. 472–481, 1995)

* American Society for Testing and Materials, Annual Book of ASTM Standards, Philadelphia, PA.

Table 7.6 Friction coefficients of various implant materials from *in vitro* studies

Material contact	*Average (or range) friction coefficient*	*Testing apparatus*	*Tribological conditions*	*References*
Stainless steel (316LVM) + UHMWPE	0.07–0.13	Pin-on-disk	● Load = 3.45 M Pa ● Velocity = 50 × 10^6 mm/yr ● Lub#: serum ● Duration: 2 years test ● 28–32 °C	McKellop *et al.* (1978)
Stainless steel (316L) + UHMWPE	0.078	Pin-on-disk	● Load = 3 MPa ● Velocity = 60 mm/s ● Lub: bovine serum, 40–50 ml ● 24–26 °C	Kumar *et al.* (1991)
Stainless steel (100CR6 – German) + UHMWPE (Chirulene–German)	0.17 (a) 0.10 (b) 0.16 (c) 0.14 (d)	Ball-on-disk vibrotribometer (Optimol SRV – German)	● 10 mm diameter ball ● Oscillation = 10 Hz; 1.65 mm amplitude ● Load = 50 and 300 N ● Lub: (a) none; (b) human synovial fluid; (c) yellow bone marrow; (d) red bone marrow ● 37 °C	Gavrjushenko (1993)
Stainless steel + UHMWPE	0.03–0.09	Reciprocating flat-on-flat	● Load = 445N ● Velocity = 100 cycles/min ● Lub: bovine serum ● Duration: 3.7 × 10^6 cycles	McKellop *et al.* (1981)
Stainless steel + UHMWPE (Charnley)	0.05	Dual hip simulator	● Velocity = 30 cycles/min ● Load = 250 kg ● Duration: 1000 h ● Lub: serum ● Room temperature	Simon *et al.* (1973)

Table 7.6 *Continued*

Material contact	*Average (or range) friction coefficient*	*Testing apparatus*	*Tribological conditions*	*References*
Stainless steel (Ortron 90) + UHMWPE (ASTM F 648)	0.034	Single channel hip joint simulator	● Range of motion = 30° ● Lub: Deionized water @ 37 °C ● Load = 1–4 kN ● Angular Velocity = 0.6–2.4 rad/s	Saikko (1992)
Stainless steel (316L) + UHMWPE	0.040	Single channel hip joint simulator	● Range of motion = 30° ● Lub: Deionized water @ 37 °C ● Load = 1–4 kN ● Angular velocity = 0.6–2.4 rad/s	Saikko (1992)
Stainless steel (316L) + UHMWPE (ASTM F 648)	0.03–0.09	Twelve channel friction and wear machine FW-12	● Conforming, flat-on-flat configuration ● Velocity = 100 cyc./min ● Pressure = 6.90 MPa ● Duration: 3.7 × 10^6 cycles ● Lub: bovine calf serum w/55 sodium azide	McKellop (1981)
CoCrMo (Protasul-2) + UHMWPE	Dry 0.13 Lub: 0.21	Rolling-sliding apparatus	● Velocity = 25 m/min ● Pressure = 30N/cm^2 ● Duration: 20 h ● Lub: none or distilled water ● Room temperature	Semlitsch *et al.* (1977)
Co–Cr + UHMWPE	0.05–0.11	Pin-on-disk	● Load = 3.45 M Pa ● Velocity = 50 × 10^6 mm/yr ● Lub: serum ● Duration: 2 years test ● 28–32 °C	McKellop *et al.* (1978)

Table 7.6 *Continued*

Material contact	*Average (or range) friction coefficient*	*Testing apparatus*	*Tribological conditions*	*References*
Co–Cr + UHMWPE	00.07–0.25	Pin-on-flat	● Axial load = 223 N ● Duration 250 000 cycles ● Lub: bovine serum	Tateishi *et al.* (1989)
Co–Cr–Mo (Vitallium) + UHMWPE	0.08–0.15	Pin-on-flat	● Contact pressure = 4.8 MPa ● Frequency = 1 Hz ● Sliding dist. = 50 mm ● Lub: distilled, deionized H_2O ● 37.1 °C	Saikko (1993)
Co–Cr–Mo (ASTM F799) + UHMWPE (GUR 415)	0.060–0.093	Reciprocating motion friction bench (line/flat)	● Maximum stress = 6 MPa ● Lub: 86% Glycerine ● Frequency = 1 Hz ● Duration: 500 000 cycles ● Sliding Dist. = 100 mm/cycle	Ruger (1995)
Co–Cr–Mo (Muller) + UHMWPE	0.018–0.045	Durham hip function simulator	● Range of motion = 20° ● Lub: Carboxymethyl Cellulose ● Dynamic load = 2000 N ● Frequency = 1 Hz	Unsworth *et al.* (1988)
Co–Cr–Mo (Vitallium) + UHMWPE (ASTM F 648)	0.057	Single channel hip joint simulator	● Range of motion = 30° ● Load = 1–4 kN ● Angular velocity = 0.6–2.4 rad/s ● Lub: deionized water @ 37 °C	Saikko (1992)
Co–Cr–Mo (Zimalloy) + UHMWPE (ASTM F 648)	0.038–0.063	Single channel hip joint simulator	● Range of motion = 30° ● Load = 1.4 kN ● Angular velocity = 0.6–2.4 rad/s ● Lub: deionized water @ 37 °C	Saikko (1992)

Table 7.6 *Continued*

Material contact	*Average (or range) friction coefficient*	*Testing apparatus*	*Tribological conditions*	*References*
Co–Cr–Mo (ASTM F75) + UHMWPE	0.044	Hip simulator machine	• Lub: synovial fluid • Peak load = 150 kg	Walker *et al.* (1973)
Co–Cr–Mo (ASTM F 799) + UHMWPE (ASTM F 648)	0.052–0.070	Single channel hip joint simulator	• Range of motion = 30° • Load = 1.4 kN • Angular velocity = 0.6–2.4 rad/s • Lub: deionized water @ 37 °C	Saikko (1992)
CoCrMo + UHMWPE (Charnley-Muller)	0.06	Dual hip simulator	• Velocity = 30 cycles/min • Load = 250 kg • Duration: 100 h • Lub: serum • Room temperature	Simon *et al.* (1973)
Co–Cr–Mo + UHMWPE	0.05–01.1	Twelve channel friction and wear machine FW-12	• Conforming, flat-on-flat configuration • Velocity = 100 cyc./min • Pressure = 6.90 MPa • Duration: 3.7×10^6 cycles • Lub: bovine calf serum w/55 sodium azide	McKellop (1981)
Co–Cr–Mo + UHMWPE	0.06–0.07 (a,c) 0.10–0.12 (b,d)	Hip joint simulator	• Load 2.5 kN static load • Lub: (a) serum, (b) serum albumin, (c) synovial fluid, (d) veronate buffer	Weightman *et al.* (1972)
Co–Cr–Mo + UHMWPE	0.04–0.06	Hip joint simulator	• Load 2.5 kN static load • Velocity: 30 cycles/min • Duration: 1.8 million cycles • Lub: serum	Weightman *et al.* (1973)

Table 7.6 *Continued*

Material contact	*Average (or range) friction coefficient*	*Testing apparatus*	*Tribological conditions*	*References*
Co–Cr–Mo + UHMWPE	0.03–0.05	Pin-on-disk	● Load = 100 N ● Lub: Ringer's solution ● Velocity = 0.05 m/s ● Duration: 48 h	Ungethum and Refior (1973)
Ti–6Al–4V + UHMWPE	0.04–0.26	Pin-on-flat	● Axial load = 223 N ● Duration: 250 000 cycles ● Lub: bovine serum	Tateishi *et al.* (1989)
Ti–6Al–4V + UHMWPE	0.05–0.121	Reciprocating flat on-flat	● Load = 445 N ● Velocity = 100 cycles/min ● Lub: bovine serum ● Duration: 4.1×10^6 cycles	McKellop *et al.* (1981)
Ti–6Al–4V (Ion implanted) + UHMWPE (ASTM F 648)	0.058	Single channel hip joint simulator	● Range of motion = 30° ● Lub: deionized water @ 37 °C ● Load = 1–4 kN ● Angular velocity = 0.6–2.4 rad/s	Saikko (1992)
Ti–6Al–4V ELI (ASTM F 136) + UHMWPE (ASTM F 648)	0.123–0.133	Single channel hip joint simulator	● Range of motion = 30° ● Lub: deionized water @ 37 °C ● Load = 1–4 kN ● Angular velocity = 0.6–2.4 rad/s	Saikko (1992)
Alumina + UHMWPE	0.06–0.10	Reciprocating flat-on-flat	● Load = 223 N ● Velocity = 60 cycles/min ● Lub: bovine serum	McKellop *et al.* (1981)
Alumina + UHMWPE	0.056	Pin-on-disk	● Load = 3 MPa ● Velocity = 60 mm/s ● Lub: bovine serum, 40–50 ml ● 24–26 °C	Kumar *et al.* (1991)

Table 7.6 *Continued*

Material contact	*Average (or range) friction coefficient*	*Testing apparatus*	*Tribological conditions*	*References*
Alumina (Vitox) + UHMWPE	0.06–0.18	Pin-on-flat	• Contact pressure = 4.8 MPa • Frequency = 1 Hz • Sliding dist. = 50 mm • Lub: distilled, deionized H_2O • 37.1 °C	Saikko (1993)
Alumina + UHMWPE	0.06–0.25	Pin-on-flat	• Axial load = 223 N • Duration: 250 000 cycles • Lub: bovine serum	Tateishi *et al.* (1989)
Alumina + UHMWPE	Dry: 0.16 Lub: 0.05	Rolling-sliding apparatus	• Velocity = 25 m/min • Pressure = 30 N/cm^2 • Duration: 20 h • Lub: none or distilled water • Room temperature	Semlitsch *et al.* (1977)
Alumina (BIOLOX) + UHMWPE (ASTM F 648)	0.022–0.062	Single channel hip joint simulator	• Range of motion = 30° • Lub: deionized water @ 37 °C • Load = 1–4 kN • Angular velocity = 0.6–2.4 rad/s	Saikko (1992)
Alumina (ASTM F 603) + UHMWPE (ASTM F 648)	0.050	Single channel hip joint simulator	• Range of motion = 30° • Lub: deionized water @ 37 °C • Load = 1–4 kN • Angular velocity = 0.6–2.4 rad/s	Saikko (1992)
Zirconia (Y–PSZ) + UHMWPE	0.049	Pin-on-disk	• Load = 3 MPa • Velocity = 60 mm/s • Lub: bovine serum, 40–50 ml • 24–26 °C	Kumar *et al.* (1991)

Table 7.6 *Continued*

Material contact	*Average (or range) friction coefficient*	*Testing apparatus*	*Tribological conditions*	*References*
Zirconia (Zyranox) + UHMWPE	0.05–0.16	Pin-on-flat	• Contact pressure = 4.8 MPa • Frequency = 1 Hz • Sliding dist. = 50 mm • Lub: distilled, deionized H_2O • 37.1 °C	Saikko (1993)
Zirconia + UHMWPE (ASTM F 648)	0.059	Single channel hip joint simulator	• Range of Motion = 30° • Lub: deionized water @ 37 °C • Load = 1–4 kN • Angular velocity = 0.6–2.4 rad/s	Saikko (1992)
Stainless steel (100CR6 – German) + Stainless steel (100CR6 – German)	0.6 (a) 0.26 (b) 0.106 (c) 0.1 (d)	Ball-on-disk vibrotribometer (Optimol SRV – German)	• 10 mm diameter ball • Oscillation = 10 Hz; 1.65 mm amplitude • Load = 50 & 300 N • Lub: (a) none; (b) human synovial fluid; (c) yellow bone marrow; (d) red bone marrow • 37 °C	Gavrjushenko (1993)
Co–Cr–Mo + Co–Cr–Mo	0.03–0.04	Pin-on-disk	• Load = 100 N • Lub: Ringer's solution • Velocity = 0.05 m/s • Duration: 48 h	Ungethum and Refior (1974)
CoCrMo (Protasul-2) + CoCrMo (Protasul-2)	Dry: 0.4 Lub: 0.35	Rolling-sliding apparatus • Duration: 20 h	• Velocity = 25 m/min • Pressure = 30 N/cm^2 • Lub: none or distilled water • Room temperature	Semlitsch *et al.* (1977)

Table 7.6 *Continued*

Material contact	*Average (or range) friction coefficient*	*Testing apparatus*	*Tribological conditions*	*References*
Co–Cr–Mo + Co–Cr–Mo	0.12–0.13 (a,b,c) 0.22 (d)	Hip joint simulator	● Load 2.5 kN static load ● Lub: (a) serum, (b) serum albumin, (c) synovial fluid, (d) veronate buffer	Weightman *et al.* (1972)
Co–Cr–Mo + Co–Cr–Mo	0.13–0.14	Hip joint simulator	● Load 2.5 kN static load ● Velocity: 30 cycles/min ● Duration: 1.8 million cycles ● Lub: serum	Weightman *et al.* (1973)
Co–Cr–Mo (ASTM F75)	0.16	Hip simulator machine	● Lub: synovial fluid ● Peak load = 150 kg	Walker *et al.* (1973)
CoCrMo + CoCrMo (McKee–Farrar)	Serum & synovial fluid: 0.12 Saline: 0.22	Dual hip simulator	● Velocity = 30 cycles/min ● Load = 250 kg ● Duration: 1000 h ● Lub: serum & synovial fluid or saline ● Room temperature	Simon *et al.* (1973)
CoCrMo + CoCrMo (McKee–Farrar)	0.13	Dual hip simulator	● Velocity = 30 cycles/min ● Load = 250 kg ● Duration: 1000 h ● Lub: serum ● Room temperature	Simon *et al.* (1973)
Alumina + alumina	0.26–0.35	Pin-on-disk	● Load = 100 N ● Lub: Ringer's solution ● Velocity = 0.05 m/s ● Duration: 48 h	Ungethum and Refior (1974)
Alumina + alumina	Dry: 0.71 Lub: 0.09	Rolling-sliding apparatus	● Velocity = 25 m/min ● Pressure = 30 N/cm^2 ● Duration: 20 h ● Lub: none or distilled water ● Room temperature	Semlitsch *et al.* (1977)

Table 7.7 Wear Rates of Various Material Combination from *in vitro* Studies

Material Contact	*Wear rate*	*Wear Coefficient*	*Tribological Conditions*	*Wear Mechanisms*	*References*
Stainless steel (316LVM) + UHMWPE	0.4 mm/yr	NA	● Pin-on-disk ● Lub*: bovine serum ● Duration: 2 yrs test ● Load = 3.45 MPa ● Velocity = 50×10^6 mm/yr ● 28–32 °C	Smooth polymer, metal – scraches.	McKellop *et al.*, (1978)
Stainless steel (316L) + UHMWPE	0.17–0.23 $mm^3/10^6$	NA	● Reciprocating flat-on-flat ● Load = 445 N ● Velocity = 100 cycles/min ● Lub: bovine serum ● Duration = 3.7×10^6 cycles	Surface scratching.	McKellop *et al.* (1981)
Stainless steel (316L) + UHMWPE	NA	27.7×10^{-7} mm^3/Nm	● Pin-on-disk ● Lub: bovine serum, 40–50 ml ● Load = 3 MPa ● Velocity =60 mm/s ● 24–26 °C	Original machine marks gone, new wear marks.	Kumar *et al.* (1991)
Stainless steel (316L) + Machined UHMWPE (HiFax 1900)	Machined UHMWPE: 3.23 in/in $\times 10^{-9}$ Molded UHMWPE: 1.70 in/in $\times 10^{-9}$	NA	● Annular disk on flat pin ● Range of motion = 110° ● Sliding velocity = 43.3 in/min ● Stress = 500 psi ● Lub: Ringer's solution	UHMWPE transfer film.	Miller *et al.* (1974)
Stainless steel + UHMWPE (Charnley)	Max. depth of wear: 0.15 mm	NA	● Dual hip simulator ● Velocity = 30 cycles/min ● Load = 250 kg ● Duration: 1000 g ● Lub: serum ● Room temperature	Evidence of brittle fracture.	Simon *et al.* (1973)

Table 7.7 *Continued*

Material Contact	*Wear rate*	*Wear Coefficient*	*Tribological Conditions*	*Wear Mechanisms*	*References*
Stainless steel (316L)	UHMWPE: 0.20 $mm^3/10^6$ cycles UHMWPE 0.65 μm/year	NA	● Twelve channel friction and wear machine FW-12 ● Conforming, flat-on-flat configuration ● Velocity = 100 cyc./min ● Pressure = 6.90 MPa ● Duration: 3.7×10^6 cycles ● Lub: bovine calf serum w/55 sodium azide	Quantification of wear separately from creep deformation. Adhesive/abrasive wear emphasizes over fatigue wear.	McKellop (1981)
Stainless steel + UHMWPE	UHMWPE: 40 $mg/10^6$ cycles	NA	● Ten station hip simulator ● Range of motion = 46° ● Lub: Bovine blood serum @37° C ● Load = Oscillating 0–2030 N ● Frequency = 1 Hz ● Duration: 1×10^6 cycles	Highly loaded region of UHMWPE smooth & shiny, peeling, pitting.	Eyerer *et al.* (1987)
Stainless steel + UHMWPE	NA	1.62×10^{-7} mm^3/Nm	● Ball and socket simulator ● Ra < 0.016 ● Sterilized with 2.5 Mrad g rad ● Lub: bovine serum with sodium azide ● Load = 2000 N ● Speed = 100 mm/sec	Uniform superficial scratches, occasional deeper marks. Metal particles, acrylic cement particles.	McKellop & Rostlünd (1990)
Cast Co-Cr-Mo pins (ASTM F-75) + UHMWPE (GUR 415 plate)	PE thickness change: 64 ± 13 μm	NA	● Reciprocating pin-on-flat ● Sterilized with 2.5 Mrad ● Lub: deionized water ● 36 MPa Line contact stress ● Frequency = 2.1 Hz ● Stroke length = 15 mm ● Duration = 2×10^6 cycles ● Final friction = 0.079 ± 0.001	Abrasive wear of PE. Transfer of PE on Co–Cr pins. Oxidative wear of Co–Cr pins.	Poggie *et al.* (1992)

Table 7.7 *Continued*

Material Contact	*Wear rate*	*Wear Coefficient*	*Tribological Conditions*	*Wear Mechanisms*	*References*
Wrought Co-Cr pins (ASTM F-90) + UHMWPE GUR 415 plate	PE thickness change: 71 ± 25 μm	NA	● Reciprocating pin-on-flat ● Sterilized with 2.5 Mrad ● Lub: deionized water ● 36 MPa Line contact stress ● Frequency = 2.1 Hz ● Stroke length = 15 mm ● Duration = 2×10^6 cycles ● Final friction = 0.101 ± 0.019	Abrasive wear of PE. Trnasfer of PE on Co–Cr pins. Oxidative wear of Co–Cr pins.	Poggie *et al.* (1992)
Co–Cr–Mo (Protasul-2) + UHMWPE	CoCrMo: 0.1 mg/20h UHMWPE: 1 mg/20h	NA	● Rolling–sliding wear and friction apparatus ● Velocity ● 25 m/min ● Pressure = 30 N/cm^2 ● Duration: 20 h ● Dry condition ● Room temperature	NA	McKellop *et al.* (1978)
Co–Cr–Mo (hot pressed) + UHMWPE	0.5 mm/yr	NA	● Pin-on-disk ● Lub: bovine serum ● Duration: 2 yrs test ● Load = 3.45 M Pa ● Velocity = 50×10^6 mm/yr ● 28–32° C	Smooth polymer, metal – scratches.	Tateishi *et al.*, (1989)
Co-Cr + UHMWPE	1.05 mg/10^6 cycles	NA	● Pin-on-flat ● Lub: distilled, deionized water ●Contact pressure: 4.8 MPa ● Frequency = 1 Hz ● Sliding dist. = 50 mm ● 37.1 °C	Transfer of PE to Co–Cr Surface. Adhesive wear.	Saikko (1993)

Table 7.7 *Continued*

Material Contact	*Wear rate*	*Wear Coefficient*	*Tribological Conditions*	*Wear Mechanisms*	*References*
Co-Cr-Mo (passivated) + UHMWPE (HiFax 1900)	Machined UHMWPE: 3.23 in/in × 10^{-9} Molded UHMWPE: 1.50 in/in × 10^{-9}	NA	● Annular disk on flat pin ● Range of motion = 110° ● Sliding velocity = 43.3 in/min ● Stress = 500 psi ● Lub: Ringer's solution ● Twelve channel friction and	UHMWPE transfer film. Quantification of wear	Miller *et al.* (1974)
Co-Cr-Mo + UHMWPE	UHMWPE: 0.17 $mm^3/10^6$ cycles 0.55 μm/year	NA	wear machine FW-12 ● Conforming, flat-on-flat configuration ● Velocity = 100 cyc./min ● Pressure = 6.90 MPa ● Duration: 3.7 × 10^6 cycles ● Lub: bovine calf serum w/55 sodium azide	separately from creep deformation. Adhesive/abrasive wear emphasizes over fatigue wear.	McKellop (1981)
Co–Cr–Mo + UHMWPE	UHMWPE: 68 mg/10^6 cycles	NA	● Ten station hip simulator ● Range of motion = 46° ● Lub: bovine blood serum @37° C ● Load = Oscillating 0–2030 N ● Frequency = 1 Hz ● Duration: 1 × 10^6 cycles	Highly loaded region of UHMWPE smooth & shiny. Peeling. Pitting.	Eyerer *et al.* (1987)
Co-Cr-Mo + UHMWPE (Charnley–Muller)	Max. depth of wear: 0.08 mm	NA	● Dual hip simulator ● Velocity = 30 cycles/min ● Load = 250 kg ● Duration: 1000 hours ● Lub: serum ● Room temperature	Evidence of brittle fracture.	Simon *et al.* (1973)

Table 7.7 *Continued*

Material Contact	*Wear rate*	*Wear Coefficient*	*Tribological Conditions*	*Wear Mechanisms*	*References*
Co-Cr-Mo + UHMWPE (Charnley)	0.15mm/1.8×10^6 cycles	NA	● Hip joint simulator ● 2.5 kN static load ● Lub: bovine serum ● Duration: 1.8 × 10^6 cycles ● Velocity = 30cycles/min	Creep, abrasion, adhesion. Max cup wear depth.	Weightman *et al.* (1972)
Co-Cr-Mo + UHMWPE (Charnley–Muller)	0.075 mm/ 1.8×10^6 cycles	NA	● Hip joint simulator ● 2.5 kN static load ● Lub: bovine serum ● Duration: 1.8×10^6 cycles ● Velocity = 30cycles/min	Creep, abrasion, adhesion. Max cup wear depth.	Weightman *et al.* (1972)
Co-Cr-Mo + UHMWPE (Duo-Patella)	1.8 mg/10^5 cycles	NA	● Knee joint simulator ● 700 lb peak load ● Velocity = 33 cycles/min ● Duration: 10^5 cycles ● Lub: double spun bovine serum	Creep and fatigue cracks evident.	Rose *et al.* (1984)
Co-Cr-Mo + UHMWPE (Ewald)	1.1 mg/10^5 cycles	NA	● Knee joint simulator ● 700 lb peak load ● Velocity = 33 cycles/min ● Duration: 10^5 cycles ● Lub: double spun bovine serum	Creep and fatigue cracks evident.	Rose *et al.* (1984)
Co-Cr-Mo + UHMWPE (Spherocentric)	0.3 mg/10^5	NA	● Knee joint simulator ● 700 lb peak load ● Velocity = 33 cycles/min ● Duration: 10^5 cycles ● Lub: double spun bovine serum	Creep and fatigue cracks evident.	Rose *et al.* (1984)

Table 7.7 *Continued*

Material Contact	*Wear rate*	*Wear Coefficient*	*Tribological Conditions*	*Wear Mechanisms*	*References*
Co–Cr–Mo + UHMWPE (Geomedic)	0.4 mg/10^5 cycles	NA	● Knee joint simulator ● 700 lb peak load ● Velocity = 33 cycles/min ● Duration: 10^5 cycles ● Lub: double spun bovine serum	Creep and fatigue cracks evident.	Rose *et al.* (1984)
Co–Cr–Mo + UHMWPE (Geometric)	0.3 mg/10^5 cycles	NA	Knee joint simulator ● 700 lb peak load ● Velocity = 33 cycles/min ● Duration = 10^5 cycles ● Lub: double spun bovine serum	Creep and fatigue cracks evident.	Rose *et al.* (1984)
Ti–6Al–4V + UHMWPE	0.47 mg/10^6 cycles	NA	● Pin-on-flat ● Axial load = 223 N ● Duration: 250 000 cycles ● Lub: bovine serum	Surface scratching.	Tateishi *et al.* (1989)
Ti-6Al-4V + UHMWPE	0.3 mm/yr	NA	● Pin-on-disk ● Lub: bovine serum ● Duration: 2 yrs test ● Load = 3.45 MPa ● Velocity = 50×10^6 mm/yr ● 28–32 °C	Abrasion by cement particles.	McKellop *et al.* (1978)
Ti-6Al-4V Pins + UHMWPE GUR 415 plate	PE thickness change: 59 ± 12 μm	NA	● Reciprocating pin-on-flat ● Sterilized with 2.5 Mrad ● Lub: deionized water ● 36 MPa Line contact stress ● Frequency = 2.1 Hz ● Stroke length = 15 mm ● Duration = 2×10^6 cycles ● Final friction = 0.112 ± 0.007	Adhesive transfer of PE on cylinders. Oxidative wear of Ti-6Al-4V. Abrasive wear of PE.	Poggie *et al.* (1992)

Table 7.7 *Continued*

Material Contact	*Wear rate*	*Wear Coefficient*	*Tribological Conditions*	*Wear Mechanisms*	*References*
Ti-6Al-4V (nitrided) + UHMWPE	0.9 mm/yr	NA	● Pin-on-disk ● Lub: bovine serum ● Duration: 2 yrs test ● Load = 3.45 MPa ● Velocity = 50×10^6 mm/yr ● 28–32 °C	No scratches present.	McKellop *et al.* (1978)
Ti–6Al–4V (passivated) + UHMWPE (HiFax 1900)	Machined UHMWPE: 0.84–2.07 in/in $\times 10^{-9}$	NA	● Annular disk on flat pin ● Range of motion = 110° ● Sliding velocity = 43.3 in/min ● Stress = 500 psi ● Lub: Ringer's solution	UHMWPE transfer film.	Miller *et al.* (1974)
Ti-6Al-4V (nitrided) + UHMWPE (HiFax 1900)	Machined UHMWPE: 1.83 in/in $\times 10^{-9}$	NA	● Annular disk on flat pin ● Range of motion = 110° ● Sliding velocity = 43.3 in/min ● Stress = 500 psi ● Lub: Ringer's solution	UHMWPE transfer film.	Miller *et al.* (1974)
Ti-6Al-4V (not passivated) + UHMWPE (HiFax 1900)	Machined UHMWPE: 1.55 in/in $\times 10^{-9}$	NA	● Annular disk on flat pin ● Range of motion = 110° ● Sliding velocity = 43.3 in/min ● Stress: 500 psi ● Lub: Ringer's solution	UHMWPE transfer film.	Miller *et al.* (1974)
Ti-6Al-4V + UHMWPE	0.04–0.11 $mm^3/10^6$	NA	● Reciprocating flat-on-flat ● Load = 445 N ● Velocity = 100cycles/min ● Lub: bovine serum ● Duration: 4.1×10^6 cycles	Surface scratching.	McKellop *et al.* (1981)

Table 7.7 *Continued*

Material Contact	*Wear rate*	*Wear Coefficient*	*Tribological Conditions*	*Wear Mechanisms*	*References*
Ti-6Al-4V (implanted with nitrogen) + UHMWPE	NA	1.9×10^{-7} mm^3/Nm	● Ball and socket simulator ● Ra < 0.016 ● Sterilized w/ 2.5Mrad g rad ● Lub: bovine serum w/ sodium azide ● Load = 2000 N ● Speed = 100 mm/sec	Uniform superficial scratches, occasional deeper marks. Metal particles, acrylic cement particles.	McKellop & Rostlünd (1990)
Ti-6Al-4V (conventional) + UHMWPE	NA	1.98×10^{-7} mm^3/Nm	● Ball and socket simulator ● Ra < 0.016 ● Sterilized w/ 2.5Mrad g rad ● Lub: bovine serum w/ sodium azide ● Load = 2000 N ● Speed = 100 mm/sec	Uniform superficial scratches, occasional deeper marks. Metal particles, acrylic cement particles.	McKellop & Rostlünd (1990)
Alumina + UHMWPE	NA	18.2×10^{-7} mm^3/Nm	● Pin-on-disk ● Lub: bovine serum, 40–50 ml ● Load = 3 M Pa ● Velocity = 60 mm/s ● 24–26 °C	Original machine marks worn, smoother.	Kumar *et al.* (1991)
Alumina + UHMWPE	0.26 $mg/10^6$ cycles	NA	● Pin-on-flat ● Axial load = 223 N ● Duration: 250 000 cycles ● Lub: bovine serum	NA	McKellop *et al.* (1981)
Alumina + UHMWPE	0.04 $mg/10^6$ cycles	NA	● Pin-on-flat ● Lub: distilled, deionized water ● Contact pressure: 4.8 MPa ● Frequency = 1 Hz ● Sliding dist. = 50 mm ● 37.1°C	Minimal wear.	Saikko (1993)

Table 7.7 *Continued*

Material Contact	*Wear rate*	*Wear Coefficient*	*Tribological Conditions*	*Wear Mechanisms*	*References*
Alumina + UHMWPE	Alumina: 0.1 mg/20h UHMWPE: 0.1 mg/20h	NA	● Rolling-sliding wear and friction apparatus ● Velocity = 25 m/min ● pressure = 30 N/cm^2 ● Duration: 20 h ● Dry condition ● Room temperature	NA	Semlitsch *et al.* (1977)
Zirconia + UHMWPE	0.03 mg/10^6 cycles	NA	● Pin on flat ● Lub: distilled, deionized water ● Contact pressure: 4.8 MPa ● Frequency = 1 Hz ● Sliding dist. = 50 mm ● 37.1°C	Minimal wear.	Saikko (1993)
Solid ytrria ZrO_2 pins + UHMWPE GUR 415 plate	PE thickness change: 33 ± 13 μm	NA	Reciprocating pin-on-flat ● Sterilized with 2.5 Mrad ● Lub: deionized water ● 36 MPa Line contact stress ● Frequency = 2.1 Hz ● Stroke length = 15 mm ● Duration = 2 × 10^6 cycles ● Final friction = 0.033 ± 0.005	Abrasive wear from the surface roughness characteristic and adhesive wear.	Poggie *et al.* (1992)
ZrO_2 surface on Zr–2.5Nb pins + UHMWPE GUR 415 plate	Pe thickness change: 25 ± 20 μm	NA	● Reciprocating pin-on-flat ● Sterilized with 2.5 Mrad ● Lub: deionized water ● 36 MPa Line contact stress ● Frequency = 2.1 Hz ● Stroke length = 15 mm ● Duration = 2 × 10^6 cycles ● Final friction = 0.040 ± 0.008	Abrasive wear from the surface roughness characteristics and adhesive wear.	Poggie *et al.* (1992)

Table 7.7 *Continued*

Material Contact	*Wear rate*	*Wear Coefficient*	*Tribological Conditions*	*Wear Mechanisms*	*References*
Zirconia (Y–PSZ) + UHMWPE	NA	10.7×10^{-7} mm^3/Nm	● Pin-on-disk ● Lub: bovine serum, 40–50 ml ● Load = 3 M Pa ● Velocity = 60 mm/s ● 24–26 °C	Original machine marks still visible.	Kumar et al. (1991)
Co–Cr–Mo + Co-Cr-Mo	$2–10 \times 10^{-9}$ mm/mm	NA	● Disc on plate ● Lub: water ● 37 °C	NA	Galante (1973)
Co-Cr-Mo (Protasul-2) + Co-Cr-Mo (Protasul-2)	Roller: 23 mg/20 h Slider: 23 mg/20h	NA	● Rolling-sliding wear and friction apparatus ● Velocity = 25 m/min ● Pressure = $30N/cm^2$ ● Duration: 20 h ● Dry condition ● Room temperature	NA	Semlitsch *et al.* (1977)
Co-Cr-Mo + Co-Cr-Mo (McKee–Farrar)	Max. depth of wear: 0.01 mm	NA	● Dual hip simulator ● Velocity = 30 cycles/min ● Load = 250 kg ● Duration: 1000 h ● Lub: serum ● Room temperature	Adhesive and abrasive types of wear.	Simon *et al.* (1973)
Co-Cr-Mo (Protasul-2) + Co-Cr-Mo (Protasul-2)	● initial wear: 10–20 mm ● linear wear: 2–4 mm/10^6 cycles	NA	● Stanmore Mk III hip simulator ● 37 mm diameter head ● Frequency = 1/2 Hz ● Load = 300–3500 N ● Duration: min. 2.5×10^6 movements/test ● Lub: Ringer's solution w/30% calf serum	Equal amount of wear on both compoents. Preferential wear direction, with pronounced grooving.	Streicher *et al.* (1990)

Table 7.7 *Continued*

Material Contact	*Wear rate*	*Wear Coefficient*	*Tribological Conditions*	*Wear Mechanisms*	*References*
Co–Cr–Mo + Co-Cr-Mo (McKee-Farrar)	0.013 mm/ 1.8×10^6 cycles	NA	● Hip joint simulator ● 2.5 kN static load ● Lub: bovine serum ● Duration: 1.8×10^6 cycles ● Velocity = 30 cycles/min	Abrasion, scratching. Max cup wear depth.	Weightman *et al.* (1972)
Co-Cr-Mo (Protasul-21WF) + Co-Cr-Mo (Protasul-21WF)	● initial wear: 10–20 mm ● linear wear: 2–4 mm/10^6 cycles	NA	● Stanmore Mk III hip simulator ● 28 & 32 mm heads ● Frequency = 1//2 Hz ● Load = 300–3500 N ● Duration: min. 2.5×10^6 movements/test ● Lub: Ringer's solution w/30% calf serum	Equal amount of wear on both components. Preferential wear direction, with pronounced grooving.	Boutin (1972)
Alumina + alumina	1.2×10^{-7} mm/mm	NA	● Disc on plate ● Lub: water ● 37 °C	NA	Semlitsch *et al.* (1977)
Stainless steel (316 S16) + PTFE	2.26 mm/yr	3.4×10^{-5} mm^3/Nm	● Pin-on-flat ● Lub: bovine serum ● Ra = 0.0 mm ● Load=40 n/pin ● Speed = 2 p rad/s ● Sliding dist. = 0.24 m/s	No creep. Particles present.	Dowson & Wallbridge (1985)
Stainless Steel + Delrin 500	31 mm/yr	NA	● Pin-on-flat ● Velocity = 100 mm/sec ● Load = 6.9 N/mm^2 ● Lub: serum ● Room temperature ● 4.8 yrs effective use	NA	Clarke (1982)

Table 7.7 *Continued*

Material Contact	*Wear rate*	*Wear Coefficient*	*Tribological Conditions*	*Wear Mechanisms*	*References*
Stainless steel + Polyester	521 mm/yr	NA	● Pin-on-flat ● Velocity = 100 mm/sec ● Load = 6.9 N/mm^2 ● Lub: serum ● Room temperature ● 4.8 yrs effective use	NA	Clarke (1982)
Stainless steel + Alumina (Protek)	(mg/cyc) SS: 176, 146, 212 Al_2O_3: 0.3, 2.1, 0.2	NA	● Five station hip simulator (Helsinski) ● 32 mm head ● Frequency = 1.08 s^{H_3} ● Load = 35 kN ● Duration: $3{\times}10^6$ cycles ● Lub: distilled, deionized water ● 37 °C	Corrosion of stainless steel heads.	Saikko *et al.* (1992)
Stainless steel + Alumina (Thackray)	(mg/cyc) SS: 50.9, 62.4, 46.0 Al_2O_3: 0.8, 1.0, 0.7	NA ● 22.2 mm head	● Five station hip simulator (Helsinski) ● Frequency = 1.08 s^{H_3} ● Load = 35 kN ● Duration: $3{\times}10^6$ cycles ● Lub: distilled, deionized water ● 37 °C	Corrosion of stainless steel heads.	Saikko *et al.* (1992)
Co–Cr–Mo + Alumina (Link)	(mg/cyc) CoCrMo: 39.7, 48.2. 94.0 Al_2O_3: 1.5, 0.5, 0.0	NA	● Five station hip simulator (Helsinski) ● 32 mm head ● Frequency = 1.08 s^{H_3} ● Load = 35 kN ● Duration: $3{\times}10^6$ cycles ● Lub: distilled, deionized water ● 37 °C	NA	Saikko *et al.* (1992)

Table 7.7 *Continued*

Material Contact	*Wear rate*	*Wear Coefficient*	*Tribological Conditions*	*Wear Mechanisms*	*References*
Co–Cr–Mo + Alumina (Howmedica)	(mg/cyc) CoCrMo: 2.6, 4.7, 4.3 Al_2O_3: 0.1, 0.0, 0.0	NA	● Five station hip simulator (Helsinski) ● 32 mm head ● Frequency = 1.08 s^{H_3} ● Load = 35 kN ● Duration: 3×10^6 cycles ● Lub: distilled, deionized water ● 37 °C	NA	Saikko *et al.* (1992)
Co–Cr–Mo + Delrin 550	37.5 mm/yr	NA	● Disk-on-flat ● Velocity = 10^6 mm/sec ● Load = 3.7 N/mm^2 ● Lub: water ● 37 °C	NA	Clarke (1982)
Si_3N_4 + UHMWPE	0.27 mg/10^6 cycles	NA	● Pin on flat ● Lub: distilled, deionized water ● Contact pressure: 4.8 MPa ● Frequency = 1 Hz ● Sliding dist. = 50 mm ● 37.1 °C	NA	Saikko (1993)

* Lub = lubricant.

7.3 CLINICAL WEAR

Methods have been proposed by Griffith *et al.* (1978) and Deavane *et al.* (1995) to radiographically measure linear wear in UHMWPE acetabular cups of total hip replacements. The overall penetration of a femoral head (Tables 7.8 and 7.9) into a UHMWPE acetabular cup is a consequence of both creep and wear, where creep is predominantly observed for the first million loading cycles (Dowson, 1995). Atkinson *et al.* (1980) estimated that the total UHMWPE residual compression due to creep in total hip replacements after x can be estimated by:

$$\text{Residual compression} = 94 + 33\,(x\text{-}1)\ \mu\text{m}$$

This relationship has served as a guide to the significance of UHMWPE creep for total hip arthroplasty (Dowson, 1995). Another important issue in the tribological behavior of polymers used as bearing surfaces is their viscoelastic-plastic character. For example, due to this time dependent stress–strain response, the measured hardness varies continuously as a function of indentation time. Therefore, in certain conditions the wear behavior of these materials cannot accurately be characterized in terms of wear coefficient alone and is often defined in terms of wear factor and Pv limit. The wear factor is described as $K' = V/PS = V/Pvt$ where V is the wear volume, v the sliding velocity, P the normal load, and t the sliding time. The Pv limit or factor (which is equal to load times velocity) defines the onset of failure of polymeric surfaces. Pv limits have to be specified in terms of a limiting load at a given sliding velocity or limiting velocity at a given load. These values will depend on the test conditions (Suh, 1986).

7.4 COMBINED WEAR AND FATIGUE

Materials used in the design of medical devices are subjected to high stresses and high cycle loading. This very demanding loading condition results in failure of metals, ceramics, and polymers. The fatigue process depends on stress rather than load, therefore partly explaining the success of congruent total hip replacements and thick polymeric bearing components (7–10 mm thick) which allows for a larger contact area (Black, 1988). Fatigue cracking of polymers such as UHMWPE results in delamination wear following crack growth. In a corrosive environment like the human body, the fatigue wear process of metal surfaces will be coupled with corrosive wear since tensile stress increases chemical reactivity. Fretting wear caused by micromotion is commonly observed in implants. Modular implants used in orthopaedics are potentially degraded by fretting corrosion/wear which plays a deleterious role in the degradation process of

Table 7.8 Clinical Penetration into UHMWPE Cups for Metallic Femoral Heads

Reference	*UHMWPE penetration rate*	*Clinical*
Griffith *et al.*, 1978	• 0.07 mm/year average (range 0.06 mm/year to 0.24 mm/year)	491 acetabular cups 8.3 year follow-up (range 7 to 9 years)
Livermore *et al.*, 1990	• 0.13 mm/yr average (range 0 to 0.39 mm/year) for 22 mm head size • 0.08 mm/yr average (range 0 to 0.3 mm/year) for 28 mm head size • 0.10 mm/yr average (range 0 to 0.32 mm/year) for 32 mm head size	Follow-up at least 9.5 years after implantation (227 of the 22 mm femoral head size; 98 of the 28 mm size; and 60 of the 32 mm head size)
Isaac *et al.*, 1992	• 0.21 mm/year (range 0.005 to 0.6 mm/year)	87 acetabular cups 9 year service life (range <1 to 17.5 years)
Wroblewski *et al.*, 1992	• 0.022 mm/year (range 0.010 to 0.034 mm/year)	Four explained acetabular cups with no apparent deterioration of the finish of the femoral head 20 year mean service life (range 17 years to 23 years)

Table 7.9 Clinical Penetration into UHMWPE Cups for Alumina Ceramic Heads

Reference	*Femoral Head*	*Average Penetration Rate*
Oonshi *et al.*, 1989	Alumina	0.098 mm/year (6 year follow-up; 28-mm cups)
Oonshi *et al.*, 1989	Alumina (g irradiated UHMWPE)	0.072 mm/year (6 year follow-up; 28-mm cups)
Okumura *et al.*, 1990	Alumina	0.084 mm/year
Egli *et al.*, 1990	Alumina	0.080 mm/year (38 acetabular cups over a period of 6.7 years)
Zichner and Willert, 1992	Alumina	0.100 mm/year

articulating surfaces. Hoeppner and Chandrasekaran (1994) reviewed the fretting of orthopaedic implants and its implication in implant failure emphasizing the complexity of implant surface change in use.

7.5 SOLVING THE WEAR PROBLEM

Historically, the evaluation of the tribological behavior of biomaterials has resulted in the development of new materials or the use of surface treatments to improve their frictional and wear properties (Long and Rack, 1996). As such, the assessment of the poor tribological properties of Ti-6Al-4V as compared to other metallic bearing alloys (e.g. Co–Cr alloys) articulating against UHMWPE has triggered the use of surface treatments to enhance the hardness and the wear resistance of the alloy. Among numerous processes including plasma vapor deposition (PVD) coating (TiN, TiC) and thermal treatments (nitriding, surface hardening), ion implantation (N+) has been the most widely accepted surface treatment. Table 7.10 reports friction and wear data obtained for treated Ti alloys.

Another approach to improve the wear performance of total joint replacements is through lubrication optimization. In this respect, the use of elastomeric bearing surfaces (Table 7.3), also known as cushion bearings, has been proposed (Table 7.11). Despites providing an improved lubrication in simulated physiological conditions through elastohydrodynamic lubrication (Auger *et al.*, 1993; Graham *et al.*, 1995; Auger *et al.*, 1995), these materials have shown a poor fatigue behavior both *in vivo* and *in vitro* (LaBerge *et al.*, 1991; Chow *et al.*, 1994; Caravia *et al.*, 1993). However, only limited data on wear performance and wear mechanisms of cushion bearings are available (Table 7.11).

7.6 CONCLUSION

The wear and frictional properties of materials are dependent on tribological conditions of the tribosystem. Their investigation involves many parameters such as wear rate, wear mechanisms, transition between initial and steady-state wear, and generation and geometry of wear debris. The physical and mechanical properties of the materials, the environmental and operating conditions, and the geometry of the wearing bodies are determining factors for these parameters. Another important tribological attribute that should be reported along with wear data is the coefficient of friction. The use of different lubricants combined with the operating conditions (load, velocity) will result in different coefficients of friction and consequently different lubrication mechanisms of the tribosystem. The wear mechanisms and wear data are partly governed by the lubrication of the tribosystem.

By definition, a tribosystem is a dynamic system that can potentially change over time emphasizing the importance of wear monitoring during testing. It is of utmost importance to fully define and report the tribological conditions during testing. The confidence in the quality of the wear data is not only related to the tribological conditions, material properties, material combinations, and experimental method including device used for testing, but also to the number of tests conducted and number of specimens evaluated, level of statistical significance, and duration of

Table 7.10 Friction and Wear Data for Titanium Orthopaedic Alloys

Titanium alloy	*Available Tribological Conditions*	*Friction Data*	*Wear Data*	*Reference*
Ti–6Al–7Nb	• Pin-on-disk • Lub: 30% serum • Abrasive PMMA pin • 3.45 MPa/ 25 mm/sec	Friction coefficient 0.100 (N+) 0.078 (TiN) 0.051 (Oxygen Diffusion hardening (ODH))	$k = 3.32 \times 10^7$ (N+) $k = 2.11 \times 10^7$ (TiN) $k = 1.35 \times 10^7$ (ODH)	Semlitsch *et al.*, 1992
Ti5Al–2.5Fe	• pin-on-disk • 0.9% NaC1 • UHMWPE disk • 5ON	NA	depth of wear track on disc 18–44 μm (polished metal) 12–24 μm (oxidized metal)	Zwicker *et al.*, 1985
Ti5Al–2.5Fe	• Ball-in-socket • 0.9% NaCl • UHMWPE socket • 100–2500 N	Friction moment 0.5–1.0 Nm (oxidized, induction hardened)		Zwicker *et al.*, 1985
Ti–15Mo–5Zr–3A1	• NaC1 solution	Friction coefficient 0.82 (β alloy)	3 times that of stainless steel 316L	Steinemann *et al.*, 1993
Ti-12Mo-6Zr-2Fe	• Pin-on-disk • Deionized water • Abrasive PMMA pin • 100 g/ 74 mm/sec	Friction coefficient 0.30–0.44	NA	Wang *et al.*, 1993
Ti-12Mo-6Zr-2Fe	• Pin-on-disk • Deionized water • UHMWPE pin • 500 g/ 73 mm/sec	Friction coefficient 0.04	NA	Wang *et al.*, 1993

Table 7.10 *Continued*

Titanium alloy	*Available Tribological Conditions*	*Friction Data*	*Wear Data*	*Reference*
Ti-6Al-4V (N+)	● Ball-in-socket (hip simulator) ● 32 mm metal ball; γ irradiated ● UHMWPE cups ● Filtered calf serum ● 2000N; 1 Hz ● One million cycles	NA	Wear rate of UHMWPE 39.5 ± 0.6 mm^3/106 cycles (N + Ti6A14V) (metallic wear reduced compared to conventional Ti6A14V)	McKellop and Róstlünd, 1990
Ti-6Al-4V	● Ball-in-socket (hip simulator) ● 32 mm metal ball; γ irradiated ● UHMWPE cups ● Filtered calf serum ● 2000N; 1 Hz ● One million cycles	NA	Wear rate of UHMWPE 38.8 ± 1.0 mm^3/106 cycles (Conventional Ti6A14V)	McKellop and Róstlünd, 1990

Table 7.11 Tribological Properties of Compliant Surface Materials In Joint Replacements

Elastomer (pin)	*Tribological conditions*	*Coefficient of friction*	*Wear factor*	*Reference*
Polyurethane (Tecoflex™ EG93A)	• 2.5 mm thick layer injection molded onto polysulfone (pin with a 30 degree cone angle) • Stainless steel flat counterpart (RA=0.01-0.025 μm) • Tri-pin-on-disk • Load: 100 N • Speed: 0.24 m/sec • Stress: Approx. 5 MPa • Lub: distilled water	• Start-up friction: 0.2 • Steady-state friction: 0.003–0.008	• For Ra metal of 0.01: 9.2 × 10-9 mm^3 Nm • For Ra metal of 0.02: 8.1 × 10-8 mm^3 Nm	Jin *et al.*, 1993

the test. When these parameters are not reported, it is difficult to compare wear data obtained with different protocols. This often leads to an inconclusive analysis and disagreements. In this respect, the standardization of testing protocols for wear of biomaterials and devices as well as how they are reported can significantly improve the wear literature. This literature review clearly indicates that there is no convention for wear-testing systems as well as for reporting wear data.

ACKNOWLEDGEMENTS

The author thanks John Killar, Aude Leroy-Gallissot, Tara McGovern, Jonette M. Rogers, Tracy Tipton, and Jennifer Woodell for their assistance in preparing this chapter.

ADDITIONAL READING

1. Clarke, I.C. and McKellop, H.A. (1986) Wear Testing in *Handbook of Biomaterials Evaluation* (A.F. von Recum, Ed.) Macmillan Publishing Co., New York. pp. 114–130.
   A concise review of testing protocols used for wear testing of cardiovascular, orthopaedic, and dental implants. Introduces some of the technical parameters involved in the understanding and measurement of wear performance.
2. Dowson, D. (1995) A comparative study of the performance of metallic and ceramic femoral head components in total replacement hip joints. *Wear*, **190,** 171–183.
   Historical review of tribological studies of metallic and ceramic bearing surfaces used for total hip arthroplasty (THA). Presents an objective assessment of wear mechanisms, wear measurement, laboratory studies, and clinical observations for THA.
3. Dumbleton, J.H. (1981) *Tribology of natural and artificial joints.* Elsevier, New York.
   An excellent critical review of testing parameters and conditions for wear and friction of orthopaedic materials. Includes an in-depth analysis of the polyethylene response to wear testing.
4. McKellop, H., Clarke, I., Markolf, K. and Amstutz, H. (1981) Friction and wear properties of polymer, metal, and ceramic prosthetic joint materials evaluated on a multichannel screening device. *J. Biomed. Mat. Res.*, **15,** 619–653.
   Compilation of laboratory tribological studies of currently used orthopaedic bearing materials. Presents a critical discussion of work by others and that of the authors. Data presented in this manuscript are commonly referred to by the orthopaedic tribology community.
5. Suh, N.P. (1986) *Tribophysics.*, Prentice-Hall, Inc. Englewood Cliffs, NJ.
   Engineering analysis of friction and wear of materials. Gathers and presents an overview of the author's own work and others on basic engineering principles that should be included in tribological study design and analysis.

REFERENCES

1. Agrawal, C.M., Micallef, D.M., Wirth, M.A., Lankford, J., Dearnaley, G. and McCabe, A.R. (1993) The effects of diamond-like-carbon coatings on the friction and wear of enhanced UHMWPE-metal couples. *Trans 21st Annual Meet of the Society For Biomaterials*, Birmingham, AL. **26,** 10.
2. Archard, J.F. (1980) Wear theory and mechanisms. in *Wear Control Handbook* (M.B. Peterson and W.O. Winer, eds) American Society of Mechanical Engineers, New York, pp. 35–80.
3. Atkinson, J.R., Dowling J.M. and Cicek, R.Z. (1980) Materials for internal prostheses: the present position and possible future developments. *Biomaterials*, **1,** 89–96.
4. Auger, D.D., Dowson, D., Fisher, J. and Jin, M.Z. (1993) Friction and lubrication in cushion form bearings for artificial hip joints. *Proc. Instn Mech. Engrs*, **207,** 25–33.
5. Auger, D.D., Dowson, D. and Fisher, J. (1995) Cushion form bearings for total knee joint replacement Part 1: design, friction, and lubrication. *Proc. Inst. Mech. Engrs*, **209,** 73–81.
6. Black, J. (1988) *Orthopaedic Biomaterials in Research and Practice*. Churchill Livingstone, NY, p. 255.
7. Boutin, P. (1972) Arthroplastie total de la hanche par prothèse en alumina frittée, *Revue de Chirurgie Orthopédique et Réparatrice de l'Appareil Moteur*, **58,** 229.
8. Brown, K.J., Atkinson, J.R., Dowson, D. and Wright, V. (1976) The wear of ultra high molecular weight polyethylene and a preliminary study of its relation to the *in vivo* behaviour of replacement hip joints. *Wear*, **40,** 255–264.
9. Caravia, L., Dowson, D. and Fisher J. (1993) Start up and steady state friction of thin polyurethane layers. *Wear*, **160,** 191–197.
10. Chan, F. W., Medley, J.B., Krygier, J.J., Bobyn, J.D., Podgorsak, G.K. and Tanzer, M. (1996) Wear performance of cobalt–chromium metal–metal bearing surfaces for total hip arthroplasty. *Trans. 42nd Annual Meeting of the Orthopaedic Research Society*, **21 (2),** p. 464.
11. Chow, A.B., Medley, J.B. and LaBerge, M. (1994) Mechanical and tribological analyses of elastomeric surface layers in load bearing implants. *Trans of 20th Annual Meeting of the Society for Biomaterials*, Boston, MA. p. 434.
12. Clarke, I.C. (1982) Wear-screening and joint simulation studies vs. materials selection and prosthesis design. *CRC Crit. Rev. in Biomed. Eng.*, **8,** 29–91.
13. Clarke, I.C. and McKellop, H.A. (1986) Wear Testing in *Handbook of Biomaterials Evaluation*. (A.F. von Recum Ed.) Macmillan Publishing Co., New York. pp. 114–130.
14. Deavane, P.A., Bourne, R.B., Rorabeck, C.H., Hardie, R.M. and Horne, J.G. (1995) Measurement of polyethylene wear in metal-backed acetabular cups. *Clin. Orthop. Rel. Res.* **319,** 303–316.
15. Dowson, D., El-Hady Diab M.M., Gillis B.J. and Atkinson, J.R. (1985) Influence of counterface topography on the wear of ultra high molecular weight polyethylene under wet conditions. Am. Chem. Soc. Symposium Series No. 287, in *Polymer wear and its control*, Ed. Lieng-Huang Lee. Ch. 12, pp. 171–187.

16. Dowson, D.B. and Jobbins, B. (1988) Design and development of a Versatile hip joint simulator and a preliminary assessment of wear and creep in Charnley total replacement hip joints, *Engineering in Medicine*, **17,** 111–117.
17. Dowson, D. and Wallbridge N.C. (1985) Laboratory wear tests and clinical observations of the penetration of femoral heads into acetabular cups in total replacement hip joints I: Charnley prosthesis with polytetrafluoroethylene acetabular cups. *Wear*, **104,** 203–215.
18. Dowson, D. (1981) Basic Tribology in *An Introduction to the Bio-mechanics of Joints and Joint Replacement*. Mechanical Engineering Publications, Ltd, London, England, pp. 49–60.
19. Dowson, D. (1995) A comparative study of the performance of metallic and ceramic femoral head components in total replacement hip joints. *Wear*, **90,** 171–183.
20. Dumbleton JH. (1981) *Tribology of natural and artificial joints*. Elsevier, NY; pp. 94–103, 110–148, 183–214.
21. Egli, A., Weber, B.G., Sieber, H., Semlitsch, M. and Dörre, E. (1990) Experience with the pairing of polyethylene/ceramic materials in hip endoprostheses, *Ultra-High Molecular Weight Polyethylene as Biomaterial in Orthopaedic Surgery*. (H.-G. Willert, G.H. Bucchorn, and P. Eyerer (eds)), Hoffrefe and Huber, Göttingen, pp. 154–158.
22. Eyerer, P., Kurth, M., McKellop, H.A. and Mittlmeier, T. (1987) Characterization of UHMWPE Hip cups run on joint simulators, *Journal of Biomedical Materials Research* **21,** 275–291.
23. Fisher, J and Dowson, D. (1991) Tribology of total artificial joints. *Proc. Instn Mech. Engrs*, **205,** 73–79.
24. Galante, J. and Rostoker, W. (1973) Wear in total hip protheses, *Acta Orthopaedica Scandinavica* (Supplement), **145,** 1–46.
25. Graham, R.M., Joseph, P.F., Dooley, R.L. and LaBerge, M. (1995) Effect of lubricant viscosity and bearing surface stiffness on the lubrication mechanism of a point contact as a total hip arthroplasty model. *Transactions of the Society For Biomaterials*, **23,** 124.
26. Gavrjushenko, N.S. (1993) Recommendations with respect to the improvement of lubrication quality of synovial fluid in artificial joints. *Proc. Instn. Mech. Engs* **207,** 111–114.
27. Griffith, MJ, Seidenstein MK, Williams, D. and Charnley, J. (1978) Socket wear in Charnley low friction arthroplasty of the hip. *Clin. Orthop. Rel. Res.* **137,** 36–47.
28. Halling, J.A. (1975) contribution to the theory of mechanical wear. *Wear*, **34,** 239–249.
29. Hoeppner, D.W. and Chandrasekaran, V. (1994) Fretting in orthopaedic implants: a review. *Wear*, **173,** 189–197.
30. Hornbogen, E. (1975) The role of fracture toughness in the wear of metals. *Wear*, **33,** 251–259.
31. Isaac, G.I., Wroblewski, P.J., Atkinson, J. R. and Dowson, D. (1992) Tribological study of retrieved hip prostheses. *Clin. Orthop. Rel. Res.* **276,** 115–125.
32. Jacobs J.J., Shanbhag A., Glant T.T., Black J. and Galante J.O. (1994) Wear debris in total joint replacements. *J Am. Acad. Orthop. Surg.*, **2,** 212–220.

33. Jahanmir, S and Suh, N.P. (1977) Mechanics of subsurface void nucleation in delamination wear. *Wear*, **44,** 17–38.
34. Jin, Z.M., Dowson, D. and Fisher, J. (1993) Wear and friction of medical grade polyurethane sliding on smooth metal counterfaces. *Wear*, **162–164,** 627–630.
35. Kumar P., Oka, M., Ikeuchi, K., Shimizu, K., Yamamuro, T., Okumura, H., Kotoura and Y. (1991) Low wear rate of UHMWPE against zirconia ceramic (Y–PSZ) in comparison to alumina ceramic and SUS 316L alloy. *J. Biomed. Mater. Res.*, **25,** 813–828, 1991.
36. LaBerge, M., Kirkley, S. Chow, A., Medley, J.B. and Brox, W.T. (1991) Biotribological Study of the Contact Elastomer-Cartilage. *Proceedings of the Combined Meeting of Orthopaedic Research Societies* (USA, Japan, Canada), Banff, Alberta, Canada, June, 1991.
37. Livermore, J., Ilstrup, D. and Morrey, B. (1990) Effect of femoral head size on wear of the polyethylene acetabular component. *J. Bone Joint Surg.*, **72A,** 518–528.
38. Long, M and Rack, H.J. Titanium alloys in total joint replacement – A review. Submitted to *Biomaterials*. March 1996.
39. McKellop, H. (1981) Wear of artificial joint materials II. Twelve-channel wear-screening device: correlation of experimental and clinical results. *Engg in Med.*, **10(3),** 123–136.
40. McKellop, H, Clarke, I, Markolf, K. and Amstutz, H. (1981) Friction and wear properties of polymer, metal, and ceramic prosthetic joint materials evaluated on a multichannel screening device. *J. Biomed. Mat. Res.*, **15,** 619–653.
41. McKellop, H.A., Clarke, I.C., Markolf, K.L. and Amstutz, H.C. (1978) Wear characteristics of UHMW polyethylene: A method for accurately measuring extremely low wear rates, *J. Biomed. Mater. Res.*, **12,** 895–927.
42. McKellop, H.A., Clarke I.C., Markolf K.L. and Amstutz H.C. (1981) Friction and wear properties of polymer, metal, and ceramic prosthetic joint materials evaluated on a multichannel screening device, *J. Biomed. Mater. Res.*, **15,** 619–653.
43. McKellop, H.A., Rostlünd, T.V. (1990) The wear behavior of ion-implanted Ti-6A1-4V against UHMW polyethylene, *J. Biomed. Mater. Res.*, **24,** 1413–1425.
44. McKellop, H., Clarke, I.C., Markolf, K.L., Amstutz, H.C. (1978) Wear characteristics of UHMW polyethylene. Method to accurately measuring extremely low wear rates. *J. Biomed. Mater. Res.* **12,** 895–927.
45. Medley, J.B., Krygier, J.J., Bobyn, J.D., Chan, F.W., Tanzer, M. (1995) Metal-metal bearing surfaces in the hip: Invetigation of factors influencing wear. *Trans. Orthop. Res. Soc.*; **20**(2), 765.
46. Miller, D.A., Ainsworth, R.D., Dumbleton, J.H., Page, D., Miller, E.H. and Chi Shen (1974) A comparative evaluation of the wear of ultra-high-molecular weight polyethylene abraded by Ti-6A1-4V; *Wear*, **28,** 207–216.
47. Mittlmeier, T. and Walter, A. (1987) The influence of prosthesis design on wear and loosening phenomena. *CRC Critical Reviews in Biocompatibility*. **3,** 319–419.
48. O'Connor, D.O., Burke, D.W., Bragdon, C.R., Ramamurti, B.S. and Harris, W.H. (1995) Dynamic frictional comparisons of different femoral head sizes and different lubricants. *Trans 21st Annual Meeting of the Society For Biomaterials*, San Francisco, CA, **28,** 230.

49. Okumara, H., Yamamuro, P., Kumar, T., Nakamura, T. and Oka, M. (1989) Socket wear in total hip prosthesis with alumina ceramic head. *Bioceramics*, **1,** 284–189.
50. Oonishi, H. and Takayama, Y. (1989) Comparisons of wear of UHMW polyethylene sliding against metl and alumina in total hip prostheses. *Bioceramics*, **1,** 272–277.
51. Poggie, R.A., Wert, J.J., Mishra, A.K. and Davidson, J.A. (1992) Friction and wear characterization of UHMWPE in reciprocating sliding contact with Co–Cr, Ti–6Al–4V, and Zirconia implant bearing surfaces; in wear and friction of elastomers. ASTM STP 1145. R. Denton and M.K. Keshavan, Eds., American Society For Testing and Materials, Philadelphia, pp. 65–81.
52. Quinn, T.F.J. (1983) A review of oxidational wear. Parts I and II. *Tribology International*, **16**: 257–271, 305–315.
53. Quinn, T.F.J., Rowson, D. and Sullivan J.L. (1980) Application of the oxidational theory of mild wear to the sliding wear of low-alloy steel. *Wear*, **65,** 1–20.
54. Rabinowicz, E. (1965) *Friction and Wear of Materials*. John Wiley and Sons, New York. pp. 53–58.
55. Rose, R.M. and Radin, E.L. (1982) Wear of polyethylene in total hip prostheses. *Clin. Orthop. Rel. Res.*, **170,** 107–115.
56. Rose, R.M., Ries, M.D., Paul, I.L., Crugnola, A.M. and Ellis, E. (1984) On the true wear rate of ultrahigh molecular weight polyethylene in the total knee prosthesis, *J. Biomed. Mater. Res.*, **18,** 207–224.
57. Rowe, C.N. (1980) Lubricated wear, in *CRC Handbook of Lubrication*. Boca Raton, FL:CRC Press; pp. 209–225.
58. Ruger, L.M., Love, B.J., Drews, M.J., Hutton, W.C. and LaBerge, M. (1996) Effect of antioxidant on the tribological properties of gamma sterilized ultra high molecular weight polyethylene. *Proc. Fifth World Biomaterials Congress*. Toronto, Canada. May 29–June 2.
59. Saikko, V., Paavolainen, P., Kleimola, M. and Slatis, P. (1992) A five-station hip joint simulator for wear rate studies, *Proc. Instn Mech. Engrs, Part H*, **206,** 195–200.
60. Saikko, V. (1992) Simulator study of friction in total replacement hip joints, *Proceedings of the Institution of Mechanical Engineers Part H: Journal of Engineering in Medicine*, **206,** 201–211.
61. Saikko, V. (1993) Wear and friction properties of prosthetic joint materials evaluated on a pin on flat apparatus, *Wear*, **166,** 169–178.
62. Schmidt, M.B., Lin, M. and Greer, K.W. (1995) Wear performance of UHWMPE articulated against ion implanted CoCr. *Trans 21st Annual Meeting of the Society For Biomaterials*, San Francisco, CA. **28,** 230.
63. Semlitsch, M., Lehmann, M., Weber, H., Doerre, E. and Willert, H.G. (1977) New prospects for a prolonged functional life-span of artificial hip joints by using the material combination polyethylene/aluminium oxide ceramic/metal. *J. Biomed. Mater. Res.*, **11,** 537–552.
64. Semlitsch, M.F., Weber, H., Streicher, R.M. and Schön, R. (1992) Joint replacement components made of hot-forged and surface treated Ti-6Al-7Nb alloy. *Biomaterials* **13**, 781–788.

65. Simon, S.R. and Radin, E.L. (1973) Lubrication and wear of the Charnley, Charnley-Muller, and McKee-Farrar prostheses with special regard to their clinical behavior, *Proc. 1st Scient. Meet. Hip Society*, Saint Louis, Chap.5, 33–45.
66. Steinemann, S.G., Mäusli P-A, Szmukler-Moncler, S., Semlitsch, M., Pohler, O., Hintermann, H.E. and Perren, S.M. (1993) Beta-titanium alloy for surgical implants. Titanium '92 Science and Technology. *The Minerals, Metals & Materials Society*, **2,** 689–2, 696.
67. Streicher, R.M., Schon, R. and Semlitsch, M. (1990) Investigation of the tribological behaviour of metal-on-metal combinations for artificial hip joints, *Biomed. Tech.*, **35(5),** 3–7.
68. Streicher, R.M. (1991) Ceramic surfaces as wear partners for polyethylene in *Bioceramics* (Bonfiled, W., Hastings, G.W., Tanner, K.E. Eds), Butterworth–Heinemann Ltd, London, England, **4,** 9.
69. Suh, N.P. (1986) *Tribophysics*. Prentice-Hall, Inc., Englewood Cliffs, New Jersey. pp. 3–11, 195–222.
70. Suzuki, S., Suzuki, S.H. and Cox, C.F. (1996) Evaluating the antagonistic wear of restorative materials. *J. Am. Dental. Ass.* **127,** 74–80.
71. Tateishi, T., Terui, A. and Yunoki, H. (1990) Friction and wear properties for biomaterials for artificial joint, *Bioceramics*, **2,** 145–151.
72. Ungethum, M. and Refior, H.J. (1974) Ist Aluminiumoxidkeramik als Gleirlagerwekstoff fur Totalendoprothesen geeignet? *Archiv für Orthopadische und Unfall-Chirurgie*, **79**: 97.
73. Unsworth, A., Pearcy, M.J., White, E.F.T. and White, G. (1988) Frictional properties of Artificial Hip Joints. *Engineering in Medicine*, **17,** 101–104.
74. Walker, P.S. and Bullough, P.G. (1973) The effects of friction and wear in artificial joints. *Orthopeadic Clinics of North America*, **4,** 275–293.
75. Wallbridge, H., Dowson, D. and Roberts, E.W. (1983) A study of the wear characteristics of sliding pairs of high density polycrystalline aluminum oxide with particular reference to their use in total replacement in human joints. *Engg in Med.*, **12(1),** 23–28.
76. Wang, K., Gustavson, L. and Dumbleton, J. (1993) The characterization of Ti-12Mo-6Zr-2Fe. A new biocompatible titanium alloy developed for surgical implants. Beta Titanium in the 1990s. *The Minerals, Metals & Materials Society*, **2,** 49–60.
77. Waterhouse, R.B. (1992) Fretting wear. *Friction, Lubrication and Wear Technology*, **18,** 242–256.
78. Weightman, B., Simon, S., Paul, L.I., Rose, R. and Radin, E.L. (1972) Lubrication mechanisms of hip joint replacement prostheses, *Journal of Lubrication Technology* (Trans. American Society of Mechanical Engineers) **94,** 131.
79. Weightman, B., Paul, I.L., Rose, R.M. Simon, S.R. and Radin, E.L. (1973) A comparative study of total hip replacement prostheses, *Journal of Biomechanics*, **6,** 299.
80. Wright, K., Dobbs, H. and Scales, J. T. (1982) Wear studies on prosthetic materials using pin on disc-machines, *Biomaterials*, **3,** 41–48.

81. Wroblewski, B.M., McCullagh, P.J. and Siney P.D. (1992) Quality of the surface finish of the head of the femoral component and the wear of the socket in long-term results of the Charnley low-friction arthroplasty. *Engg in Med.* **20,** 181–183.
82. Zichner, L.P. and Willert, H.G. (1992) Comparison of alumina–polyethylene and metal–polyethylene in clinical trials. *Clin. Orthop. Rel. Res.* **282,** 86–94.
83. Zum Gahr, K-H. (1982) Abrasive Wear of ductile materials. *Z. f. Metallkd.,* **73,** 267–276.
84. Zwicker, J. Etzold, U, and Moser, T. (1985) Abrasive properties of oxide layers on TiA15Fe2.5 in contact with high density polyethylene. Titanium '84 Science and Technology. *Deutsche Gesellschaft Für Metallkunde E.V.*, **2,** 1343–1350.

8 Degradation/resorption in bioactive ceramics in orthopaedics

H. Oonishi and K. Oomamiuda

8.1 INTRODUCTION

Bioceramics have now been widely used as bone replacement materials in orthopaedic surgery. In particular, calcium phosphate ceramics have been applied as bioactive ceramics with bone bonding capacities.

Biological responses such as bone bonding and the biodegradation properties of these materials are very important in clinical applications. Any convincing conclusion has not yet been reached as to whether these materials are biodegradable or not, although it has been discussed for a long time.

Degradation is an important characteristic for biomaterials, and it is considered to have a large influence on the bone bonding properties. This degradation characteristic must be considered from the following two view points. These are the solution mediated dissolution process and the cell-mediated process (phagocytosis).

This chapter overviews the literature regarding the biodegradation processes of bioactive calcium phosphate ceramics from the viewpoint of *in vitro* physico-chemical dissolution processes and *in vivo*/*in vitro* biological degradation processes.

In this chapter, each calcium phosphate material is abbreviated as follows:

Handbook of Biomaterial Properties. Edited by J. Black and G. Hastings.
Published in 1998 by Chapman & Hall, London. ISBN 0 412 60330 6.

DCPD ; Dicalcium phosphate dihydrate $[CaHPO_4.2H_2O]$
DCPA ; Dicalcium phosphate anhydrate $[CaHPO_4]$
OCP ; Octacalcium phosphate $[Ca_8H_2\ (PO_4)_6.5H_2O]$
TCP ; Tricalcium phosphate $[Ca_3\ (PO_4)_2]$
HAp ; Hydroxyapatite $[Ca_{10}\ (PO_4)_6\ (OH)_2]$
TTCP ; Tetracalcium phosphate $[Ca_4\ (PO_4)_2O]$

8.2 *IN VITRO* PHYSICO-CHEMICAL DISSOLUTION PROCESSES

Dissolution of a solid material continues until an equilibrium condition is reached, followed by a saturated condition where a solid and a liquid remain in equilibrium. Solubility is defined as the maximum concentration of solute *in the solution under* the equilibrium condition. This concept of solubility is very convenient to know how much the material has actually dissolved. However, it is not convenient for showing general solubility of the material since its value depends on the pH of the solution.

Therefore, a thermodynamic equilibrium constant known as the solubility product constant K_{sp} is used for slightly soluble salts. This solubility product constant is useful for understanding the dissolution characteristics, because its value does not change in either acid or basic solutions under the same conditions of temperature, pressure and ionic strength.

For example, HAp dissolves in water as follows;

$$\{Ca_{10}\ (PO_4)_6\ (OH)_2\}_{solid} \rightleftarrows 10Ca^{2+} + 6PO_4^{3-} + 2OH^-$$

Therefore, its solubility product constant K_{sp} is calculated as follows;

$$K_{SP\ (HAp)} = [Ca^{2+}]^{10}\ [PO_4^{3-}]^{6}\ [OH^-]^{2}$$

where values in brackets represent ionic activities.

There are many reports on solubility product constants of calcium phosphate compounds obtained by the above equation, and these values are shown in Table 8.1.

Chow [18] calculated, based on these data, the solubility isotherms at 37 °C over a wide pH range (Figure 8.1). These solubility isotherms were shown as the function of the concentration of calcium and phosphate ions in a saturated solution of each calcium phosphate salt. The relative stability of calcium phosphate salts at various values of pH can be obtained by these solubility isotherms. At a given pH, a salt with its isotherm lying below that of another salt is less soluble and more stable than the other. Therefore, HAp is the most stable and least soluble salt among these salts in the range of pH below approximately 4.2 where DCPA is the least soluble. Similarly, TTCP is the least stable and most soluble salt in the range of pH below 8.5, above which pH DCPD is the most soluble.

Table 8.1 Solubility product constants of calcium phosphate compounds at 25°C

Compound	*Abbreviation*	*Formula*	*p KSP*	*Reference*
Dicalcium phosphate dihydrate	DCPD	$CaHPO_4 \cdot 2H_2O$	6.59	1,2
			6.63	3
Dicalcium phosphate anhydrous	DCPA	$CaHPO_4$	6.90	2, 4
Octacalcium phosphate	OCP	Ca_8H_2	96.6	5
		$(PO_4)_6 \cdot 5H_2O$	98.6	6
α-Tricalcium phosphate	α-TCP	α-$Ca_3(PO_4)_2$	25.5	7
β-Tricalcium phosphate	β-TCP	β-$Ca_3(PO_4)_2$	28.9	2, 8
			29.7	3
Hydroxyapatite	HAp	$Ca_{10}(PO_4)_6(OH)_2$	115.5	2, 9, 10
			115–117	11
			117	12–15
			122	16
			125	17
Tetracalcium phosphate	TTCP	$Ca_4(PO_4)_2O$	38	15

pK_{sp}: the negative logarithm of K_{sp}.

Newesely [19] and Monma and Kanazawa [20] reported that α-TCP was converted to HAp by hydration as follows;

$$3Ca_3\ (PO_4)_2 + Ca^{2+} + 2OH^- \rightarrow Ca_{10}\ (PO_4)_6(OH)_2$$

However, this phase diagram can apply only in a thermodynamic equilibrium for the ternary system of $Ca(OH)_2$–H_3PO_4–H_2O, and it shows only a general tendency under *in vivo* conditions where various different ions are involved. Furthermore, this relation is also considered to be influenced by the experimental conditions and the characteristics of the material used in the experiments.

Most of the implanted materials used in the investigations were TCP and HAp. It has been reported in earlier investigations that TCP dissolves more rapidly than HAp in various solutions [21].

Jarcho [22] compared the relative dissolution rates of dense HAp and TCP. The dissolution rate of TCP was 12.3 times higher than that of HAp in buffered lactic acid solution (0.4 M, pH 5.2), and was 22.3 times higher than that of HAp in buffered EDTA solution (0.05 M, pH 8.2). Klein *et al.* [23] carried out dissolution tests on HAp and β-TCP with various values of porosity in buffered lactic acid solution. The dissolution rate of β-TCP was three times higher than that of HAp. And it was concluded that the degradation rates of these materials were determined by neck dissolution rate and neck geometry, the latter factor being dependent on the crystallography and stoichiometry of the material and of the sintering conditions. Ducheyne *et al.* [15] compared the dissolution rate and the precipitation rate of the following six calcium phosphates in calcium and

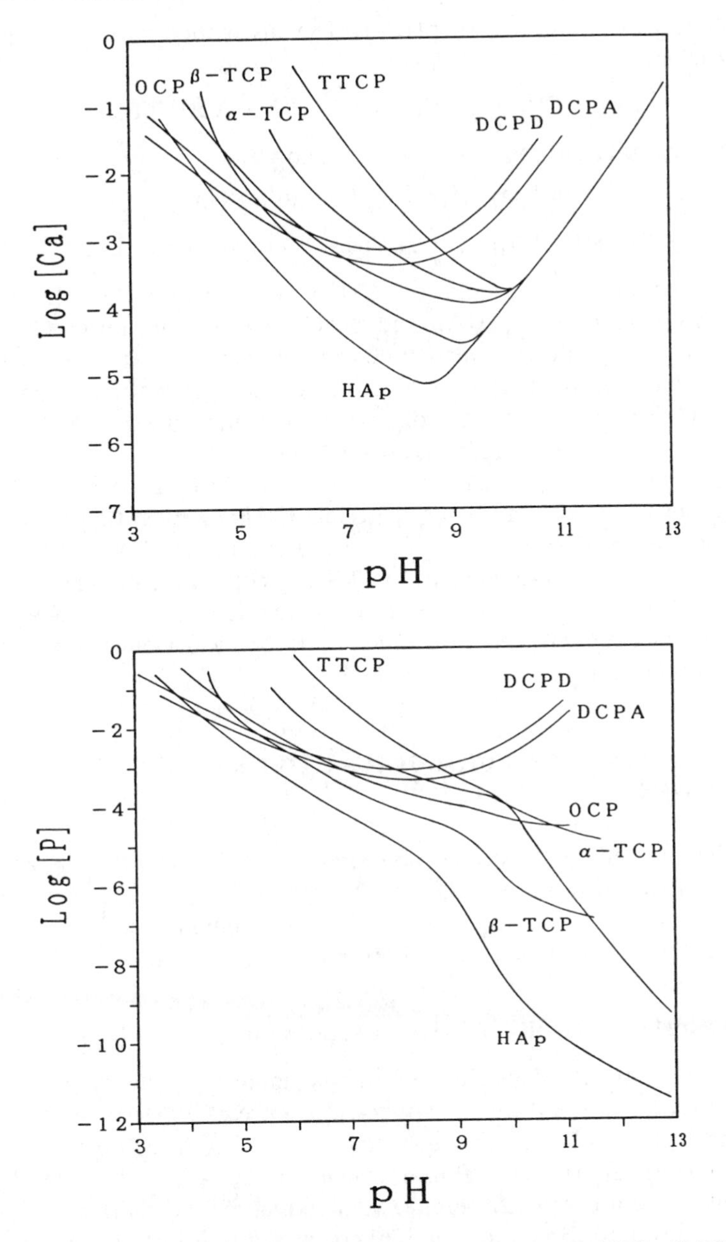

Figure 8.1 Solubility phase diagram for the ternary system $Ca(OH)_2$–H_3PO_4–H_2O at 37°C [18].

phosphate free solution with pH 7.3. The dissolution rate increased in the following order:

HAp < CDAp < OHAp < β-TCP < α-TCP < TTCP

and the precipitation rate increased as follows:

β-TCP < (HAp and α-TCP) < CDAp

(CDAp; Ca-deficient HAp, OHAp; dehydroxylated HAp)

The precipitate that formed on CDAp was apatitic; on the other hand, the precipitates on HAp and β-TCP had a much lower Ca/P. In TTCP, the precipitate was calcium deficient carbonate containing hydroxyapatite. Niwa *et al.* [24] evaluated the concentration of calcium and phosphate ions being slightly dissolved in saline solution from HAp sintered at the temperature range from 250 to 1250 °C. It was concluded that the sintering temperature was closely related to the crystallinity and the amount of dissolution of the material. Maximan *et al.* [25] compared the dissolution rate of plasma spray coated amorphous HAp and poorly crystallized HAp by exposure to Hank's physiological solutions (pH 7.2 and 5.2). The poorly crystallized HAp coating showed faster resorption, greater surface film precipitation and greater chemical changes than amorphous HAp coating.

8.3 *IN VIVO/IN VITRO* BIOLOGICAL DEGRADATION PROCESSES

Biological degradation processes have been investigated either by animal experiments *in vivo* and clinical applications or by cell cultures *in vitro*. These results were obtained by observing the remaining implanted materials and the behavior of each cell around the materials.

8.3.1 Animal experiments and clinical applications

Most of the implanted calcium phosphate materials that were used in animal experiments and clinical applications were TCP, HAp and calcium phosphate glasses. Table 8.2 shows major reports of these investigations.

Most of the reports on TCP have concluded that TCP is biodegradable although there are some differences depending on the characteristics of the materials used. Bhaskar *et al.* [26] concluded that this biodegradation of TCP was caused by the phagocytosis of the mesenchymal cells. Cameron *et al.* [28] stated that the ingestion by giant cells did play a significant role in the degradation of TCP although passive dissolution occurred. Klein *et al.* [32, 33] stated that the micro-pores played an important role in the biodegradation rate of TCP. The degradation of TCP started mostly

Table 8.2 Biodegradation of calcium phosphate compounds *in vivo*.

Implanted material (sintering temp., porosity or density)	*Implantation*	*Duration*	*Biodegradation*	*Reference*
• TCP (plug)	Tibia of rats	14 weeks	Progressive decrease	26
• TCP (pellet)	Tibia of rats	48 days	95% of implant was degradated	27
• β-TCP (porous plug) [36%]	Femur of dogs	4 months	Considerable resorption	28
• TCP and TTCP (porous cylinder) [45%]	Tibia of dogs	10 months	TCP; resorbed TTCP; unchanged	29
• TCP (block)	Vertebrae cervicales of dogs	22 weeks	Partially resorbed (implants were crushed)	30
• HAp and β-TCP (ten types of micro and macro porous cylinder)	Tibia of rabbits	9 months	HAp: no resorption TCP: more or less degradable	31
• β-TCP (seven types of micro and macro porous cylinder)	Tibia of rabbits	12 months	Microporous>macroporous reduced by addition of Mg^{2+}, F^{-}	32,33
• HAp and TCP (porous block) [HAp: 1300 °C – 56%, TCP: 1150 °C – 50%]	Femur of dogs	50 weeks	HAp: no resorption TCP: 25–30% (in 22 weeks)	34
• Coral (porites) – HAp (porous block)	Mandible of dogs	1 year	29% of implant	35
• Coral (goniopora) – HAp (porous block)	Tibia of dogs	1 year	No bioresorption	36
• Coral (porites and goniopora) – HAp (porous block)	Animal studies Clinical application	12 months 15 months	Minimal No degradation	37,38
• Coral (goniopora) – HAp and TCP [36%]	Animal experiments Clinical application	1 year 4 years	Coral-HAp: not apparent TCP: observed in many cases	39
• HAp (three types of dense block) [900 °C – 97%, 1200 °C – 97 and 99.9%]	Dorsal muscle and tibia of rats	6 months	No degradation (no difference in three types)	40
• HAp (porous blocks) [1300 °C, 56%]	Femur of dogs	3.5 years	Negligible	41
• HAp (porous blocks) [900 and 1200 °C, 86%]	Tibia of dogs	2 years	Slow bioresorption (900 °C>1200 °C)	42
• HAp (macro and micro porous blocks) [macroporosity: 26%, microporosity: 5%]	Middle ear of rats	1 year	Resorption by 15–20 μm during the first yr.	43,44

Table 8.2 *Continued.*

Implanted material (sintering temp., porosity or density)	*Implantation*	*Duration*	*Biodegradation*	*Reference*
• DCPD, DCPA, OCP, α- and β-TCP, HAp, amorphous HAp Bioglass (granule sizes of 100–300 and 10 μm)	Femur of rabbits	12 weeks	(α- and β-TCP) < (DCPD, DCPA, TTCP) < (amorphous HAp, OCP)	45
• MBCP (macroporous blocks) [40–50%] (60%HAp + 40% β – TCP)	Animal experiments	18 weeks	Initially fast (~1 month)	46
	Clinical application	16 months		
• Plasma sprayed HAp (cylindrical plug)	Tibia of rabbits	3 months	Loss of coating thickness	47
• Plasma sprayed HAp, TTCP, MWL (cylindrical rod) (crystallinity of HAp: 10, 60, 95%)	Femur of rats	4 weeks	60%-HAp and TTCP: distinct bulk degradation, 10%-HAp: gradual surface degradation 95%-HAp and MWL: negligible	48
• Plasma sprayed HAp, FAp, MWL (cylindrical plug)	Femur and humerus of goats	25 weeks	HAp: considerable and progressive reduction, MWL: considerable reduction in thickness, FAp: no degradation or dissolution	49
• Bioglass (SiO_2–P_2O_5–CaO–Na_2O system)	Femur of rats	6 weeks	Silica-rich layer and Ca-P rich layer formation	51
• A-W glass-ceramics (MgO–CaO–SiO_2–P_2O_5–CaF_2 system)	Tibia of rabbits	25 weeks	Ca-P rich layer formation	53

from the medulla by solution mediated disintegration processes, and fine particles released were phagocytosed and removed by macrophages in the medulla to the lymph nodes. Renooij *et al.* [35] reported that HAp was not affected by biodegradation processes, while TCP was subject to extensive bioresorption. Resorption debris from TCP was found in mononuclear phagocytes and multinuclear osteoclastlike cells. Although multinuclear cells were occasionally seen near the surface of HAP, cells carrying HAP debris were never observed. And it was supposed that TCP was transformed into HAp in a physiologic environment.

Concerning the biodegradation of HAp, there are reports in the case of no degradation, slow or partial degradation and for the degradable case. The differences in these results are dependent on the experimental conditions such as the characteristics of the materials, animal species, implanted sites and methods of observation.

Holmes *et al.* [35–39] carried out investigations using HAp which was derived from marine coral and reported the results as follows. Significant biodegradation occurred when implanted in load bearing sites such as mandibles, while minimal biodegradation was observed in cortical bone of radius and no apparent evidence of biodegradation was observed in cancellous bone of tibia. In clinical applications, radiographic observations did not show any irrefutable evidence of biodegradation and history of biopsies showed no conclusive evidence of biodegradation, while osteoclasts were occasionally seen along the implant surface. In contrast to these results, degradation of TCP appeared to occur by passive dissolution and osteoclastic resorption, and in many cases it was radiographically observed in clinical trials, especially where the implant was applied in a diaphyseal onlay fashion. Denissen *et al.* [40] reportered no degradation of three different dense HAp varying in its density. Similarly, Hoogendoorn *et al.* [41] reported through their long-term study that porous HAp did not undergo biodegradation during 3.5 years of implantation, while giant multinucleated cells were occasionally seen in pores near the bone and ceramic surface.

On the other hand, Kurosawa *et al.* [42] observed the degradation of highly porous HAp in their experiments, and concluded that this degradation was caused in two ways; the mechanical collapse of the material and the ingestion of fine particles released from the HAp surface by multinuclear giant cells. Similarly, Blitterswijk *et al.* [43, 44] observed in their implantation experiments with dense and macroporous HAp that the deposition of calcium, partially in the form of calcium phosphate, was found on the implant surface, and the resorption of the implant occurred as the result of phagocytosis by mono- and multi-nuclear cells. Oonishi *et al.* [45] compared bioactivity for bone formation in several kinds of bioceramics. These materials were divided into three groups; bioinert ceramics (alumina), surface bioactive ceramics (HAp and Bioglass), and resorbable bioactive ceramics (DCPD, DCPA, OCP, α-TCP, β-TCP, TTCP and amorphous HAp). In resorbable bioactive ceramics, bioactivity or bioresorbability might increased in the following order:

(α- and β-TCP) < (DCPD, DCPA and TTCP)
< (amorphous HAp and OCP)

Daculsi *et al.* [46] stated that the bioresorption of macroporous biphasic calcium phosphate consisting of HAp and β-TCP was conducted by multinucleated cells (osteoclastlike cells) and was related to the β-TCP content of this material. Bruijin *et al.* [48] and Dhert *et al.* [49] compared the degradation of plasma spray coated TTCP, MWL (magnesium whitlockite) and three types of HAp with various degrees of crystallinity. It was revealed that both TTCP and semi-crystalline HAp underwent distinct bulk degradation and amorphous HAp showed a gradual surface degradation, while the degradation was negligible with the highly crystalline HAp and MWL. Biodegradation appeared to be related to bone apposition, since more bone seemed to be present on amorphous HAp and TTCP, as compared to highly crystalline HAp and MWL. The degrading surface of TTCP and amorphous HAp coatings was most likely a dynamic zone in which dissolution and reprecipitation occurs. This zone was therefore thought to be favourable for rapid bone formation and bonding. At the interface between bone and MWL, a seam of unmineralized bone-like tissue was frequently seen, and a substantial amount of aluminum was detected in the MWL coating and the unmineralized bone-like tissue, which might cause the impaired mineralization.

Since the discovery of Bioglass by Hench *et al.* [50], various kinds of bioactive glasses and glass ceramics have been developed and applied clinically. Hench *et al.* [51] summarized their study on Bioglasses which were based on the SiO_2–P_2O_5–CaO–Na_2O system. When a bioactive glass was immersed in an aqueous solution, three general processes occurred; leaching, dissolution and precipitation. In these reactions, hydrated silica was formed on the glass surface, resulting in a silica-rich gel layer, and then a calcia-phosphate-rich layer was formed on or within the gel layer. This layer was initially amorphous and later crystallized to a hydroxycarbonate apatite structure to which bone could bond. Kokubo *et al.* [52] developed A-W glass-ceramics which was based on the MgO–CaO–SiO_2–P_2O_5–CaF_2 system. In this material, oxyfluorapatite [$Ca_{10}(PO_4)_6(O,F_2)$] and β-wollastonite [Cao · SiO_2] both in the form of rice grain-like particles were dispersed in an MgO–CaO–SiO_2 glass matrix. In their experiments [53] it was shown that a thin layer, rich in Ca and P, was formed on the surface of this material. This Ca, P-rich layer was identified as a layer of apatite, and this material was observed to be closely connected to the surrounding bone through this apatite layer without any distinct boundary. The same type of apatite layer was formed on the surface of this material exposed to the simulated body fluid, and consisted of carbonate-containing hydroxyapatite of defective structure and small crystallites. It was concluded that this apatite layer played an essential role in forming the chemical bond of all bioactive materials which bonded to bone.

8.3.2 Cell cultures

To study biodegradation and interfacial bonding phenomena, *in vitro* cell culture systems have been developed. Gregoire *et al.* [54] investigated the influence of calcium phosphate on human bone cell activities and demonstrated that the isolated human bone cells were capable of ingesting HAp and β-TCP granules. And the capacity for ingesting a synthetic mineral component clearly suggested that bone cells were able to participate in the degradation of calcium phosphates. Gomi *et al.* [55] showed that osteoclasts are capable of resorbing sintered HAp *in vitro* and that the fusion of osteoclast mononuclear precursors was influenced by substratum rugosity. Similarly, Ogura *et al.* [56] demonstrated that osteoclast-like cells were capable of resorbing unsintered calcium phosphate substrata *in vitro*. Bruijn *et al.* [57–59] carried out a series of cell culture tests on various plasma sprayed calcium phosphate compounds and reported the results as follows. Rat bone marrow cells were cultured on plasma sprayed HAp. The cells formed a mineralized extracellular matrix that exhibited several characteristics of bone tissue. Two distinctly different interfacial structures were observed on HAp. An electron-dense layer which was rich in glycosaminoglycans was regularly present. A collagen-free amorphous zone was frequently seen interposed between the electron-dense layer and HAp. In cell culture tests on three types of plasma sprayed HAp varying in degree of crystallinity, an electron-dense layer was clearly visible on a stable, non-degrading crystalline HAp and was frequently observed at the interface of semi-crystalline HAp. An amorphous zone was regularly seen at degrading surfaces of semi-crystalline and poorly crystallized HAp. It was concluded that the crystallinity of plasma sprayed HAp was an important parameter which influenced the establishment of the bony interface and might, as a result, have an effect on the bone formation rate and bonding strength between HAp and bone tissue. Similarly, rat bone marrow cells were cultured on various plasma sprayed calcium phosphate coatings. Mineralized extracellular matrix was formed on HAp, TCP and TTCP in 2 weeks, and was formed on FAp (fluorapatite) in 8 weeks. It was only occasionally observed in some area on MWL, which phenomenon might have been due to aluminium impurities in the coating. It was concluded that plasma sprayed calcium phosphates would display different bone-bonding and biodegradation properties, depending on their chemical composition and crystal structures.

Table 8.3 Biodegradation of calcium phosphate compounds *in vitro*

Substrate (sintering temp., porosity or density)	*Strain*	*Incubation*	*Biodegradation*	*Reference*
HAp and β-TCP (granule, <50 μm)	Human bone cell	7 days	Human bone cell are capable of ingesting HAP and TCP granules	54
HAp (dense disc; three types of surface rugosities) [1130°C]	Rat bone marrow cell	8 days	Osteoclast-like cells are capable of resorbing HAp	55
HAp (dense disc; three types of porosity [dried at 200 °C, unsintered]	Rat bone marrow cell	7 days	Osteoclast-like cells are capable of resorbing HAp	56
Plasma sprayed HAp (crystallinity; 15, 43, 69%)	Rat bone marrow cell	18 days	15 & 43%: rapidly degrated 69%; degradation rate was reduced	58
Plasma sprayed HAp, FAp, TCP, TTCP, MWL	Rat bone marrow cell	2 weeks	Different bone-bonding and biodegradation properties	59

8.4 SUMMARY

No convincing conclusion has been reached as to the biodegradation mechanisms of bioactive ceramics. Many researchers have reported different results, as described above. These discrepancies are considered to be caused by the fact that materials used for the experiments were different, and that experimental methods and analytical methods were also different. Therefore, when these reported results are compared, it is important to consider the characteristics of the material used (chemical compositions, impurity, crystallinity, dense or porous, micro- or macro-porous, porosity), experimental methods used (*in vivo* or *in vitro*, animal species, implanted duration, implanted sites, load bearing or not), and analytical methods used (radiographic, optical microscopic, electron microscopic). Futhermore, a good understanding of the characteristics of the materials to be used becomes important when bioactive ceramics are used clinically.

REFERENCES

1. L.C. Chow and W.E. Brown, *J. Dent. Res.*, **54,** 65–16, 1975.
2. F.C.M. Driessens, J.W.E. van Dijk and J.M.P.M. Borggreven, *Calcif. Tissue Res.*, **26,** 127–136, 1978.
3. J.L. Meyer, and, E.D. Eanes, *Calcif. Tissue Res.*, **25,** 59–68, 1978.
4. H.McDowell, W.E. Brown and J.R. Sutter, *Inorg. Chem.*, **10,** 1638–1643, 1971.
5. M.S. Tung, N. Eidelman, B. Sieck and W.E. Brown, *J. Res. Nat. Bur. Stand.*, **93,** 613–624, 1988.
6. J.L. Shyu, L. Perez, S.J. Zawacki, J.C. Heughebaert and G.H. Nancollas, *J. Dent. Res.*, **62,** 398–400, 1983.
7. B.O. Fowler and S. Kuroda, *Calcif. Tissue Int.*, **38,** 197–208, 1986.
8. T.M. Gregory, E.C. Moreno, J.M. Patel and W.E. Brown, *J. Res. Nat. Bur. Stand.*, **78(A),** 667–674, 1974.
9. E.C.Moreno, T.M. Gregory and W.E. Brown, *J. Res. Nat. Bur. Stand.*, **72(A),** 773–782, 1968.
10. J.S. Clark, *Can. J. Chem.*, **33,** 1696–1700, 1955.
11. R.M.H. Verbeek, H. Steyaer, H.P. Thun and F. Verbeek, *J. Chem. Soc. Faraday Trans. 1*, **76,** 209–219, 1980.
12. R. Chuong, *J. Dent. Res.*, **52,** 911–914, 1973.
13. A.N. Smith, A.M. Posner and J.P. Quirk, *J. Coll. Inter. Sci.*, **54,** 176–183, 1976.
14. H.McDowell, T.M. Gregory and W.E. Brown, *J. Res. Nat. Bur. Stand.*, **81(A),** 273–281, 1977.
15. P. Ducheyne, S. Radin, L. King, K. Ishikawa and C.S. Kim, *Bioceramics* vol.4, eds W. Bonfield, G. W. Hastings and K.E. Tanner, Butterworth-Heinemann, London, UK, pp. 135–144, 1991.
16. M.B. Fawzi, J.L. Fox, M.G. Dedhiya, W.I. Higuchi and J.J. Hefferren, *J. Coll. Inter. Sci.*, **67,** 304–311, 1978.

17. M.S. Wu, W.I. Higuchi, J.L. Fox and M. Friedman, *J. Dent. Res.*, **55,** 496–505, 1976.
18. L.C. Chow, *J. Ceram. Soc. Japan*, **99,** 954–964, 1991.
19. H. Newesely, *J. Oral Rehab.*, **4,** 97–104, 1977.
20. H. Monma and T. Kanazawa, *Yogyo-Kyokai-Shi*, **84,** 209–213, 1976.
21. R.W. Mooney and M.A. Aia, *Chem. Rev.*, **61,** 433–462, 1961.
22. M. Jarcho, *Cli. Orthop. Rel. Res.* **157**, 259–278, 1981.
23. C.P.A.T. Klein, A. A. Driessen and K. de Groot, *Biomaterials,* **5,** 157–160, 1984.
24. J. Niwa, S. Takahasi and M. Sohmiya, *Fineceramics*, **2,** 25–32, 1981.
25. S.H. Maximan, J.P. Zawadsky and M.G. Dunn, *J. Biomed. Mater. Res.*, **27,** 111–117, 1993.
26. S.N. Bhaskar, J.M. Brady, L. Getter, M.F. Grower and T. Driskell, *Oral Surg.*, **32,** 336–346, 1971.
27. D.E. Cutright, S.N. Bhaskar, J.M. Brady, L. Getter and W.R. Posey, *Oral Surg.*, **33,** 850–856, 1972.
28. H.U. Cameron, I. Macnab and R.M. Pilliar, *J. Biomed. Mater. Res.*, **11,** 179–186, 1977.
29. K. Köster, H. Heide and R. König, *Langenbecks Arch. Chir.*, **343,** 173–181, 1977.
30. T. Shima, J.T. Keller, M.M. Alvira, F.H. Mayfield and S.B. Dunsker, *J. Neurosurg.*, **51,** 533–538, 1979.
31. C.P.A.T. Klein, A.A. Driessen and K. de Groot, *J. Biomed. Mater. Res.*, **17,** 769–784, 1983.
32. C.P.A.T. Klein, K. de Groot, A.A. Driessen and H.B.M. van der Lubbe, *Biomaterials*, **6,** 189–192, 1985.
33. D.C.P.A.T. Klein, K. de Groot, A.A. Driessen and H.B.M. van der Lubbe, *Biomaterials*, **7,** 144–146, 1986.
34. W. Renooij, H.A. Hoogendoorn, W.J. Visser, R.H.F. Lentferink, M.G.J. Schmitz, H.V. Ieperen, S.J. Oldenburg, W.M. Janssen, L.M.A. Akkermans and P. Wittebol, *Cli. Orthop. Rel. Res.*, **197,** 272–285, 1985.
35. R.E. Holmes, *Plast. & Reconstr. Surg.*, **63,** 626–633, 1979.
36. R.E. Holmes, R.W. Bucholz and V. Mooney, *J. Bone and Joint Surg.*, **68-A,** 904–911, 1986.
37. R.E. Holmes, V. Mooney, R. Bucholz and A. Tencer, *Cli. Orthop. Rel. Res.*, **188,** 252–262, 1984.
38. D.J. Sartoris, D.H. Gershuni, W.H. Akeson, R.E. Holmes and D. Resnick, *Radiology*, **159,** 133–137, 1986.
39. R.W. Bucholz, A. Carlton and R.E. Holmes, *Orthop. Cli. North America*, **18,** 323–334, 1987.
40. H.W. Denissen, K. de Groot, P.Ch. Makkes, A. van den Hooff and P.J. Klopper, *J. Biomed. Mater. Res.*, **14,** 713–721, 1980.
41. H.A. Hoogendoorn, W. Renooij, L.M.A. Akkermans, W. Visser and P. Wittebol, *Cli. Orthop. Rel. Res.*, **187,** 281–288, 1984.
42. H. Kurosawa, T. Iwata, I. Shibuya, K. Murase and Takeuchi, *J. Joint Surg.*, **8,** 1761–1769, 1989.
43. C.A. van Blitterswijk, J.J. Grote, W. Kuijpers, C.J.G. Blok-van Hoek and W. Th. Daems, *Biomaterials*, **6,** 243–251, 1985.

44. C.A. van Blitterswijk, J.J. Grote, W. Kuijpers, W. Th. Daems and K. de Groot, *Biomaterials*, **7,** 137–143, 1986.
45. H. Oonishi, S. Kushitani, T. Sugihara, H. Iwaki, H. Ohashi and E. Tsuji, *Bioceramics* vol. **8,** eds L.L. Hench and J. Wilson, ELSEVIER, New York, 1995.
46. G. Daculsi, N. Passuti, S. Martin, C. Deudon, R.Z. Legeros and S. Raher, *J. Biomed. Mater. Res.*, **24,** 379–396, 1990.
47. J.A. Jansen, J.P.C.M. van de Waerden, J.G.C. Wolke and K. de Groot, *J. Biomed. Mater. Res.*, **25,** 973–989, 1991.
48. J.D. de Bruijn, Y.P. Bovell and C.A. van Blitterswijk, *Calcium Phosphate Biomaterials: Bone-bonding and Biodegradation Properties*, ed. J.D. de Bruijn, Offsetdrukkerij Haveka B.V., Alblasserdam, pp. 79–92, 1993.
49. W.J.A. Dhert, C.P.A.T. Klein, J.A. Jansen, E.A. van der Velde, R.C. Vriesde, P.M. Rozing and K. de Groot, *J. Biomed. Mater. Res.*, **27,** 127–138, 1993.
50. L.L. Hench, R.J. Splinter, W.C. Allen and T.K. Greenlee, *J. Biomed. Mater. Res. Symp.*, **2,** 117–141, 1971.
51. L.L. Hench and B. Andersson, *Advanced Series in Ceramic – Vol. 1 An Introduction to Bioceramics* eds L.L. Hench and J. Wilson, World Scientific, Singapore, pp. 41–62, 1993.
52. T. Kokubo, S. Ito, S. Sasaki and T. Yamamuro, *J. Mater. Sci.*, **21,** 536–540, 1986.
53. T. Kokubo, *Advanced Series in Ceramics – Vol. 1 An Introduction to Bioceramics*, eds L.L. Hench and J. Wilson, World Scientific, Singapore, pp. 75–88, 1993.
54. M. Gregoire, I. Orly and J. Menanteau, *J. Biomed. Mater. Res.*, **24,** 165–177, 1990.
55. K. Gomi, B. Lowenberg, G. Shapiro and J.E. Davies, *Biomaterials*, **14,** 91–96, 1993.
56. M. Ogura, T. Sakae and J.D. Davies, *Bioceramics* vol. 4, eds W. Bonfield, G.W. Hastings and K.E. Tanner, Butterworth-Heinemann, London, UK, pp. 121–126, 1991.
57. J.D. de Bruijn, C.P.A.T. Klein, K. de Groot and C.A. van Blitterswijk, *J. Biomed. Mater. Res.*, **26,** 1365–1382, 1992.
58. J.D. de Bruijn, J.S. Flachl, K. de Groot, C.A. van Blitterswijk and J.E. Davies, *Calcium Phosphate Biomaterials: Bone-bonding and Biodegradation Properties*, ed. J.D. de Bruijn, Offsetdrukkerij Haveka B.V., Alblasserdam, pp. 45–62, 1993.
59. J.D. de Bruijn, C.P.A.T. Klein, K. de Groot and C.A. van Blitterswijk, *Calcium Phosphate Biomaterials: Bone-bonding and Biodegradation Properties*, ed. J.D. de Bruijn, Offsetdrukkerij Haveka B.V., Alblasserdam, pp. 63–78, 1993.

9 Corrosion of Metallic Implants

M.A. Barbosa

9.1 GENERAL ASPECTS

9.1.1 Incidence of corrosion

The surfaces of passive metals are normally attacked at specific points where the oxide film has been destroyed and massive quantities of metal ions are released. Depending on the magnification with which surfaces are observed, various degrees of localized attack can be detected. Sometimes, however, corrosion may not be easily distinguishable from mechanical imperfections associated with manufacturing or handling. Even under the scanning electron microscope (SEM) it is often difficult to distinguish between mechanical indentations and pitting or crevice attack.

After determining the existence of corrosion, the next step is to assess its magnitude. This can be done, by corrosion scores, such as those given in Table 9.1 (Thomas *et al.*, 1988). In this table the 'no surface degradation' score is obtained with a magnification of 60×. If a higher magnification was used some 'non-degraded' surfaces might fall in one of the 'surface degradation' categories. The borderline between 'corroded' and 'non-corroded') surfaces is therefore very much dependent on magnification, as well as on surface preparation, as explained above. With these limitations in mind, it is useful to have an idea of the incidence of corrosion, i.e. of the percentage of implants that suffer some degree of attack. Table 9.2 compares the data obtained by several authors. Vacuum melting

Handbook of Biomaterial Properties. Edited by J. Black and G. Hastings.
Published in 1998 by Chapman & Hall, London. ISBN 0 412 60330 6.

Table 9.1 Grading scale used to evaluate the degree of interface and surface corrosion (*Thomas et al.*, 1988)

0 = no surface degradation visible at 60× magnification
1 = very mild surface degradation visible at 60× magnification
2 = mild surface degradation visible at 60× magnification
3 = moderate surface degradation visible without magnification
4 = heavy surface degradation visible without magnification
5 = very heavy severe surface degradation visible without magnification

Table 9.2 Incidence of corrosion

Implant/material	*Corroded implants*	*Ref*
38 fixation devices/AISI 316L	95%; crevice corrosion	Thomas *et al.*, 88
43 miniplates/AISI 316LVM*	19%; only at the countersinks	Torgersen and Gjerdet, 94
19 miniplates/c.p Ti	0%	Torgersen and Gjerdet, 94

* VM – Vacuum melted

(VM) significantly reduces the susceptibility of 316L stainless steel to attack, while titanium is practically immune. Corrosion, apart from affecting the mechanical performance of the implants, also results in contamination of the tissues with metallic ions.

The detection of ions released from metallic implants is dependent on the technique used. Very minute amounts of ions can be detected by electrothermal atomic absorption spectroscopy (ET-AAS), which goes down to concentrations of the order of ng/g. Electrochemical methods enable the detection of extremely low corrosion current densities, below 1 $\mu A/cm^2$, corresponding to dissolution in the passive state. These rates of corrosion do not modify the aspect of the surface and are not normally considered as surface attack.

9.1.2 Potential-pH (Pourbaix) diagrams

These diagrams indicate the regions of immunity, passivation and corrosion of pure metallic elements in pure water at 25°C. Fig. 9.1 (a, b) gives the potential-pH diagrams of Cr and Ti. Cr is the element responsible for the passive behaviour of stainless steels and Co–Cr–Mo alloys. In Fig. 9.1a passivation by a $Cr(OH)_3$ film is assumed. The film is thermodynamically stable over a wide range of pH and potential values. Below pH 4 the film

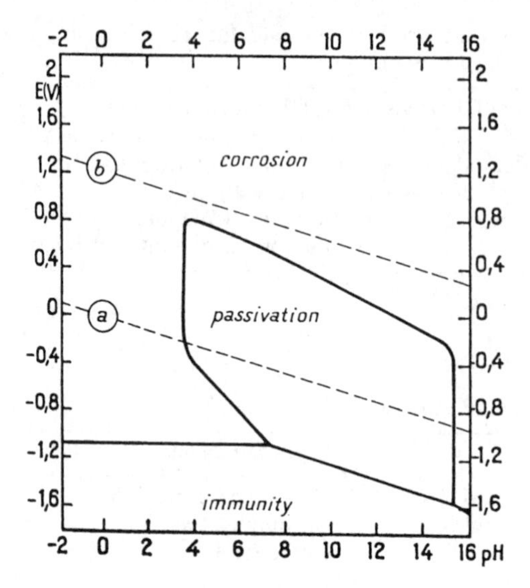

Figure 9.1(a) Theoretical conditions of corrosion, immunity and passivation of chromium, at 25°C. (Pourbaix, 1974.)

is unstable and Cr is corroded. Ti is responsible for the excellent corrosion resistance of Ti–Al–V alloys. In Fig. 9.1b passivation by a hydrated $TiO_2.H_2O$ oxide has been assumed. The passivation region extends to much higher potentials than in the case of Cr. The passive film is unstable below pH 2.5. In both diagrams the dotted lines give the region of stability of water: below line *a* hydrogen is evolved, whereas above line *b* oxygen is released. Normally, the corrosion potentials of implant materials do not reach such extreme values.

In spite of their usefulness in predicting the stability of metals and their oxides, potential–pH diagrams suffer from a number of limitations. They refer to pure metals, not to alloys, and to pure water, not to environments normally found in practical situations. For example, the diversity of chemical species, and particularly the presence of chloride ions in physiological media, is responsible for substantial differences between practical and predicted behaviour. Localized attack, in the form of crevice, pitting and corrosion fatigue, is due to the presence of chloride. Furthermore, the kinetics of metal dissolution or passivation cannot be assessed by these diagrams, which are purely thermodynamic. However, if not misused, potential–pH diagrams can give useful information which must be complemented by other type of date, namely of kinetic nature.

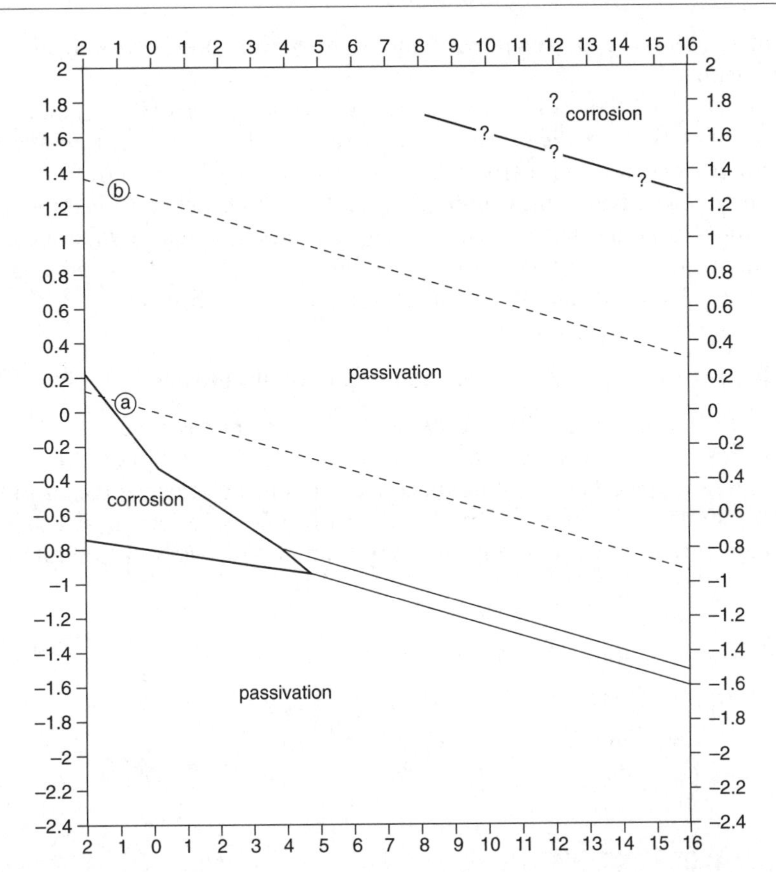

Figure 9.1(b) Theoretical domains of corrosion, immunity and passivation of titanium, at 25°C, considering Tiltz (Pourbaix, 1971).

9.2 ASPECTS RELATED TO THE METAL COMPOSITION

9.2.1 Importance of materials purity in improving the corrosion resistance

The evolution of stainless steel composition can be used to illustrate the importance of materials purity in reducing corrosion susceptibility. Chromium and molybdenum are the key elements in promoting resistance to pitting and crevice attack of stainless steels, but high chromium and molybdenum concentrations are not sufficient to ensure an adequate corrosion resistance. Low concentrations of impurities, like carbon, silicon, phosphorous and sulphur, are required. Type 316L and 316LVM stainless steels are commonly employed to fabricate a variety of fracture fixation devices. They both have low carbon concentration, below 0.03 wt%, which is indicated by the letter L. VM stands for vacuum-melted, a technique that enables the production of metals with very low concentrations of impurities.

A retrieval analysis of Kuntscher intramedullary rods (Cook *et al.* 1990) has shown that significant surface corrosion, inclusion content and carbon content occurred on early materials, which had remained *in situ* for 10 years or longer (maximum 23 years). Significant relationships were obtained for surface corrosion score vs. thin globular oxide inclusion content, and for surface corrosion score vs. sulphide inclusion content. Figure 9.2 shows the data obtained for the former correlation.

9.2.2. Type of metallic material and influence of alloying

Due to the presence of a thin oxide film, titanium has a very high corrosion resistance. However, its low resistance under wear conditions may lead to enormously high titanium concentrations in tissues adjacent to titanium implants (section 9.3.1). Rapid film formation after surface damage is therefore of critical importance to guarantee low levels of titanium ions.

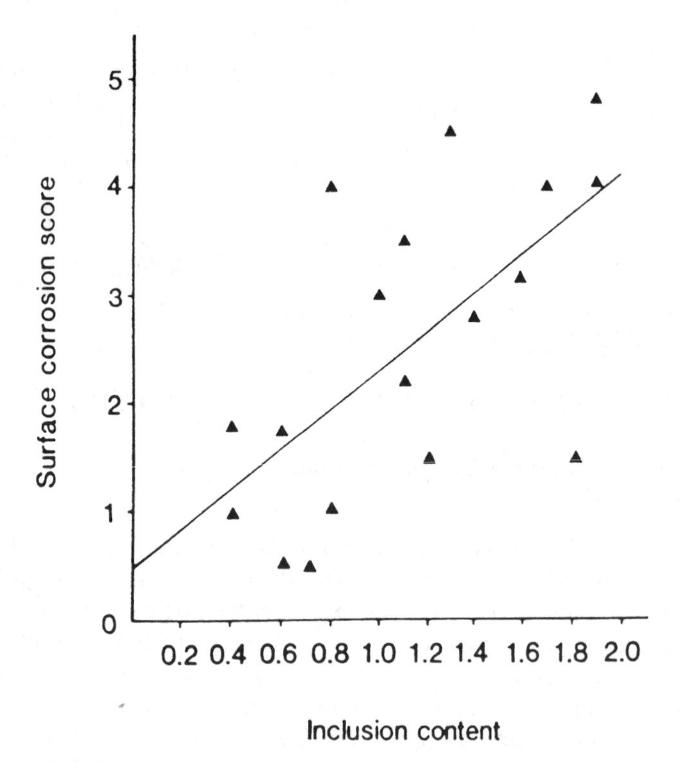

Figure 9.2 Relationship between surface corrosion and thin globular oxide inclusion content. Regression line y= 1.78x+0.52, r= 0.65, n= 18, p <0.05. (Cook *et al.*, 1990.)

The current density (c.d.) required to form a passive film is called the critical c.d. for passivation, i_c. The lower i_c the better. Figure 9.3 shows that Zr, Nb, Ta and Pd decrease i_c, whereas S_n increases it. It has been found (Okazaki *et al.* 1994) that i_c can be related to the percentages of Pd, Ta, Nb, Zr and Sn by the following expression

$$i_c(A.m^{-2} = 10^{-2}\{98\text{-}89.5[\%Pd] - 9.5[\%Ta] - 3.4[\%Nb] - 0.67[\%Zr] + 8[\%Sn]\}$$

A new alloy, Ti–15Zr–4Nb–2Ta–0.2Pd, with better corrosion resistance than the conventional Ti–6Al–4V, was proposed by the same authors.

Replacement of Nb for V, in order to eliminate the possible toxic effects of the latter, has been carried out (Semlitsch *et al.*, 1992). Ti–6Al–7Nb showed a corrosion resistance similar to that of Ti–6Al–4V, as concluded from anodic polarization curves (Figure 9.4).

Although not as widely used as titanium, tantalum has found a number of applications, e.g. in vascular clips, as a suture and to fabricate flexible stents to prevent arterial collapse. The reader is referred to a paper by J. Black (1994), where the material properties are reviewed, together with

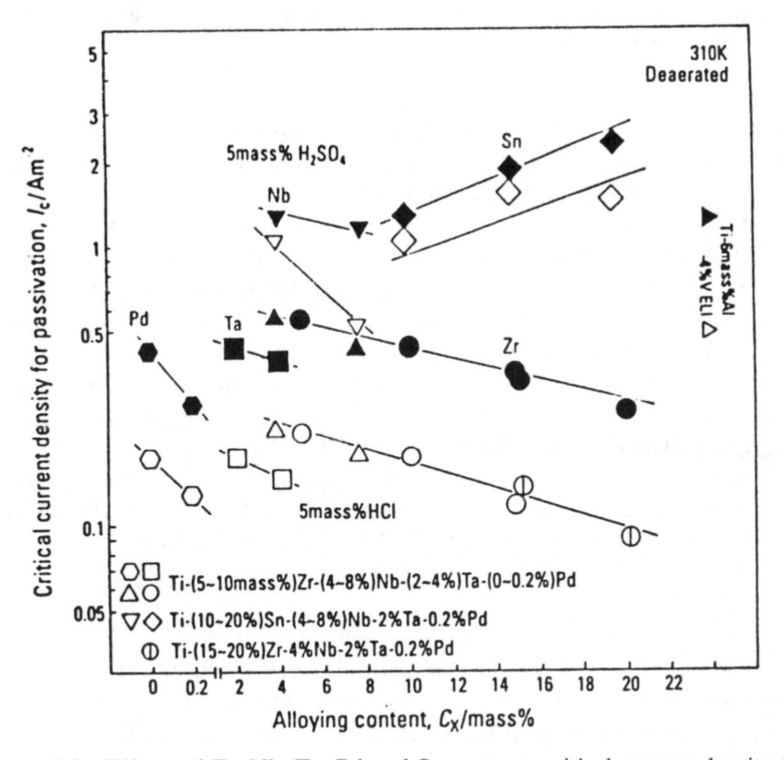

Figure 9.3 Effects of Zr, Nb, Ta, Pd and Sn contents critical current density for passivation in 15% H_2SO_4 and 5% HCl solutions at 310 K. (Okazaki *et al.*, 1994.)

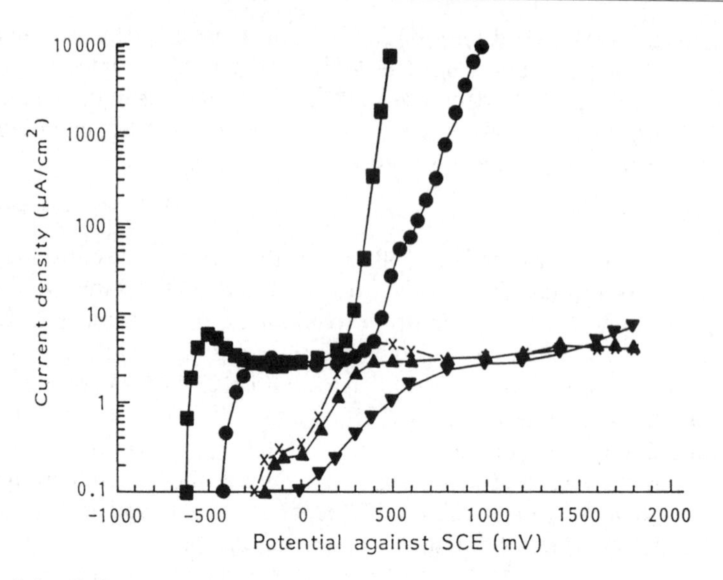

Figure 9.4 Current density/potential curves of five different implant materials in Ringer's solution bubbled through with nitrogen. ■ AISI 316L; ●CoNiCrMo; ▲ Ti6Al-7Nb; ▼ CP-titanium; × Ti-6Al-7Nb/ODH. (Semlitsch *et al.*, 1992.)

the host response and clinical applications. In terms of corrosion resistance, tantalum is at least equivalent to titanium. Its oxide, Ta_2O_5, is very stable over very wide pH and potential ranges, thus explaining the excellent corrosion resistance. According to Black, high cost and difficulties of fabrication are some of the reasons for its limited usage.

Cr and Mo are the major alloying elements responsible for the corrosion resistance of stainless steels. These alloys are also very sensitive to inclusion content, which has led to continuous attempts to reduce impurity concentrations. F138 and F139 are variations of the AISI 316L stainless steel with a lower content of non-metallic inclusions. A duplex stainless steel, 25Cr–7Ni–4Mo–0.25N, shows a better corrosion resistance than conventional austenitic stainless steels (Cigada *et al.*, 1989). The authors have established the following ranking: 23Cr–4Ni<AISI 316L<ASTM F138<22Cr–SNi–3Mo<27Cr–31Ni–3.5Mo<25Cr–7Ni–4Mo–N.

9.2.3 Site for attack

Normally, pitting initiates at non-metallic inclusions. In stainless steels sulphides are particularly prone to attack. Oxide inclusions may also give origin to attack, but they are less active than sulphides. Carbides may also nucleate pitting attack and when they are numerous at grain boundaries they may give rise to intergranular corrosion. However, with surgical grades of stainless steels this type of attack should not occur. Crevice corrosion is also common with stainless steels and less frequent with Co–Cr alloys. Sintered beads of Co–Cr–Mo alloy have been studied by scanning electrochemical microscopy (Gilbert *et al.*, 1993a). At any time, some grains were more active than others, whereas at later stages shifting of the active regions occurred. Titanium is immune to both types of corrosion under static conditions. Sliding between titanium and another material (e.g. cement, polyethylene or bone) may originate severe degradation by corrosive wear.

9.2.4. Combinations of different materials

The need to combine different materials may sometimes arise. An example is the use of hard materials for the head of hip joints in combination with a titanium stem. Titanium has a very high corrosion resistance, but a very poor wear resistance. Therefore, either surface hardening treatments (e.g. ion implantation of nitrogen or surface alloying) or a harder material, e.g. a ceramic, are employed for the femoral head. Ceramics, like alumina or zirconia, do not cause enhanced electrochemical dissolution of the titanium stem because of their low electronic conductivity. However, when another metal (e.g. Co–Cr–Mo alloy) is used instead, the possibility of a galvanic couple between the stem and the head being formed exists. The situation illustrated by this example can be extended to other couples, including those involving carbon. Even in the case of hard coatings galvanic couples between the coating and the substrate may form.

In a first approximation, the safety of couples involving different materials can be preditected by a number of experimental techniques. Table 9.3 summarizes the data obtained by several authors. Notice that the couples between stainless steel and other materials is unsafe. On the contrary, TiAlV/CoCrMo, CoCrMo/C and TiAlV/C combinations may be considered safe. However, repeated fracture of the oxide film at the conical taper region between head and stem of Ti6Al4V/CoCr combinations has been associated with corrosion. Attack also occurred in

Table 9.3 Predicted behaviour of galvanic couples (Barbosa, 1991)

Couple	*Behaviour*
TiAlV/C	Safe
CoCrMo/C	Safe
TiAlV/CoCrMo	Safe
316L S.S./C	Unsafe
316L S.S./TiAlV	Unsafe
316L S.S./CoCrMo	Unsafe

CoCr/CoCr combinations and was proportional to the duration of implantation, as seen in Figure 9.5 (Gilbert *et al.*, 1993b). A larger percentage (34.5%) of cases of corrosion was found with mixed CoCr/TiAlV systems than with CoCr/CoCr systems (7%) (Cook *et al.*, 1994). Corrosion occurred at the interface between head and neck of modular components. No correlation between the presence or extent of corrosion with the time *in situ* was found. In another study the percentage of corroded tapered connections between titanium-alloy stems and cobalt-alloy heads was found to be about 57% (Collier *et al.*, 1991). Titanium-titanium and cobalt-cobalt alloy combinations did not result in interfacial corrosion. 85% of prostheses made of dissimilar materials exhibited corrosion 24 months or more postoperatively. The data indicate that a correlation exists between corrosion and time of implantation.

In view of the above clinical data it is advisable to avoid using dissimilar metals for modular hip prostheses. The occurrence of fretting corrosion at the taper region is responsible for the release of metallic ions that may have cytotoxic effects.

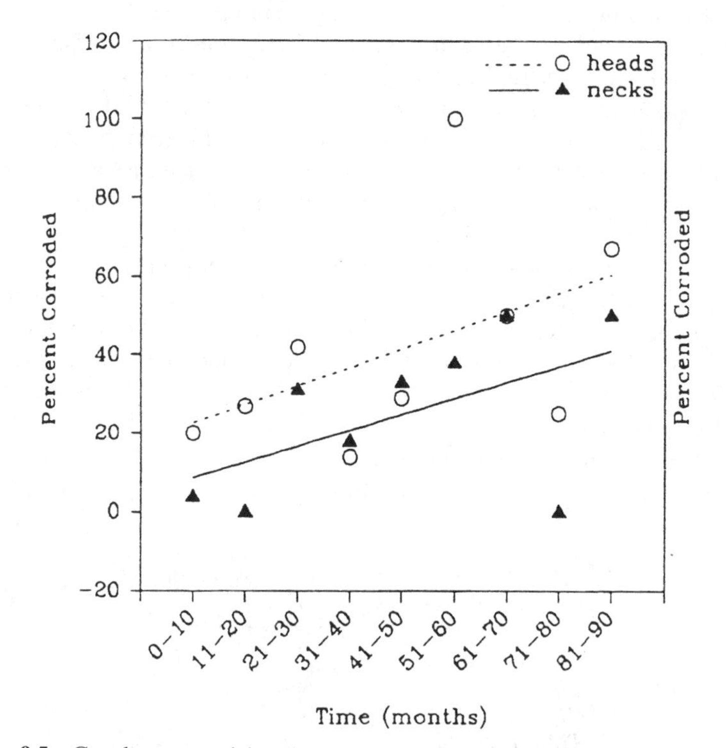

Figure 9.5 Graphs summarizing the percentage of mixed metal components which show signs of moderate to severe corrosion as a function of duration of implanation. The dotted regression line was fit to the data for the heads (○) and the solid line was fit to the data for the necks (▲). (Gilbert *et al.*, 1993b.)

Laboratory galvanic current measurements can be very useful in the pre-screening of materials. For instance, in a study on dental implant bridges it has been reported that silver–palladium, when brazed to titanium, corrodes *in vitro* (Ravnholt and Jensen, 1991), thus eliminating the need to carry out *in vivo* tests.

As a final note it must be stressed that laboratory static tests should only be used to eliminate dangerous metal-metal combinations, and not as an acceptance criterion. Fretting may substantially alter the properties of the interface, by continuously removing the passive oxide film, thereby inducing severe attack of a metal which, otherwise, would remain unaffected.

9.3 ASPECTS RELATED TO THE PHYSIOLOGICAL ENVIRONMENT

9.3.1 Contamination of tissues by corrosion products

Contaminations of tissue with metals may have two origins. The first is the release of ionic species resulting from the process of electrochemical dissolution of the implant. This is normally associated with static corrosion. Under dynamic conditions, and particularly when fretting occurs, small metallic particles detach from the surface, and become embedded in the soft tissue around the implant. The fate of these particles may vary, depending on their size and chemical nature. They may, for instance, undergo a process of corrosion, with the consequent release of metal ions. This process may take place both in the extracellular matrix or as a result of macrophage activity. Table 9.4 gives the concentration of Cr, Ni, Fe and Co in biological samples. It shows that tissues around implants may be orders of magnitude richer in these metallic elements than normal blood or normal bone.

Table 9.4 Concentration of metallic elements in biological samples (Barbosa, 1992)

Sample		*Cr*	*Ni*	*Fe*	*Co*
Normal blood*		2–6 ppb	3–7 ppb	200–680 ppm	0.1–0.2 ppb
Normal bone*		460 ppb	900 ppb	91 ppm	
Tissue around Implants (max)**	316SS	10000 ppm	1400 ppm	20000 ppm	
	Co-Cr-Mo	10200 ppm	1500 ppm	3650 ppm	22000 ppm

* Wet weight; data from Tsalev and Zaprianov, 1983.
** Concentrations in dry tissue; data from Pohler, 1983.
ppm: Parts per million.
ppb: Parts per billion.

Titanium has a tendency to accumulate in tissues. The concentrations can be very high, as indicated in Table 9.5. Titanium was not excreted in the urine of hamsters injected with metal salts (Merritt *et al.*, 1992). Small concentrations were found in the serum, red blood cells and organs. Only 5.5% of the injected titanium was found in the kidneys, liver, lung and spleen tissues. The authors suggest that titanium accumulates at the injection site due to the high stability of the titanium dioxide that is formed at physiological conditions. In the same study nearly all the injected vanadium was recovered in the urine. This behaviour is similar to that of nickel and cobalt, and is related to the formation of highly soluble compounds.

High concentrations of metals were found in capsule and fibrous membranes of loose titanium and Co-Cr stems of total hip prostheses (Dorr *et al.*, 1990). The same work reports elevated metal ion concentrations in synovial fluid and blood whenever cemented and uncemented stems are loose, but no increase when they are fixed. The average values are given in Table 9.6. The standard deviations (not shown) were often very large, of the order of magnitude of the averages.

Polyethylene wear debris may artefactually contribute to high ion readings in periprosthetic tissues, as indicated in Tables 9.7 and 9.8 (Meldrum *et al.*, 1993). The high concentrations found in UHMWPE are due to the manufacturing processes. These tables show that there are statistically significant increases in Co, Al and Ti in the nonarticulated inserts with

Table 9.5 Concentration of titanium in tissues surrounding titanium implants

Tissue	*Concentrations (ppm)*	*Ref.*
Bone	< 2100	Ducheyne, 1984
Soft tissue	2000	Meachim, 1973
Soft tissue	56–3700	Agins, 1988

Table 9.6 Concentration (μg/l) of metals in tissues and blood retrieved during total arthroplasty of cementless stems (Dorr *et al*, 1990)

	TiAlV stems			*CoCr stems*			
Sample	*Ti*	*Al*	*V*	*Co*	*Cr*	*Mo*	*Ni*
SF	556	654	62	588	385	58	32
SF (control)	13	109	5	5	3	21	5
CAP	1540	2053	288	821	3329	447	5789
CAP (control)	723	951	122	25	133	17	3996
FM	20813	10581	1027	2229	12554	1524	13234
Blood	67	218	23	20	110	10	29
Blood (control)	17	12.5	5.8	0.1–1.2	2–6	0.5–1.8	2.9–7.0

SF – synovial fluid; CAP – capsule; FM – fibrous membrane.

respect to bar stock. In retrieved implants, large increases with respect to bar stock were found for Cr, Mo, Ti and V. The role of UHMWPE wear debris would be twofold: irritant to tissues and source of metal ions.

The accumulation of metal ions in periprosthetic tissue is a combination of two sources: the extracellular matrix and the cells themselves. The ability of fibroblasts to incorporate metal cations is a linear function of concentration, up to 50% toxicity concentrations, for Ag^{+}, Au^{4+}, Cd^{2+}, Cu^{2+}, In^{3+}, Ni^{2+}, Pd^{2+} and Zn^{2+} (Wataha *et al.*, 1993), as illustrated in Figure 9.6 for Cu^{2+}, Ni^{2+} and Pd^{2+}. By measuring the slope of the lines in this figure it is possible to estimate the uptake efficiency (Table 9.9). The efficiency is highest for In^{3+} and lowest for Pd^{2+}.

Table 9.7 Cobalt–chrome alloy ion concentrations in UHMWPE *et al.* material and manufactured and retrieved inserts (Meldrum *et al.*, 1993)

	Co	*Cr*	*Mo*	*Ni*
Bar stock, n=3	55±5	330±5	5*	650±5
Manufactured inserts, n=9	440±250	520±440	5*	490±600
Retrieved, n=18(all cemented inserts)	54±42	1,500±1,400	87±120	1,360±1,300

All concentrations are in parts per billion (nanograms/gram).
* This is the minimum detection limit of the spectrometer.

Table 9.8 Titanium alloy ion concentrations in UHMWPE material and manufactured and retrieved inserts (Meldrum, *et al.* 1993)

	AL	*Ti*	*Va*
Bar Stock n=3	5*	5*	5*
Manufactured inserts, n=9	800±200	2300±980	60±95
Retrieved, n=21 (all metal backed)	5*	6700±4500	220±410

All concentrations are in parts per billion (nanograms/gram).
* This is the minimum detection limit of the spectrophotometer.

Table 9.9 Uptake efficiencies of metal cations by fibroblasts (Wataha *et al.*, 1993)

Metal cation	*Uptake efficiency ((fmol/cell)/μM)/h)**
Ag^{+}	23.8
$Au4^{+}$	1.0
$Cd2^{+}$	38.0
$Cu2^{+}$	0.26
$In3^{+}$	45.3
$Ni2^{+}$	0.21
$Pd2^{+}$	0.11
$Zn2^{+}$	0.73

* fmol = femtomoles (10-15 moles).

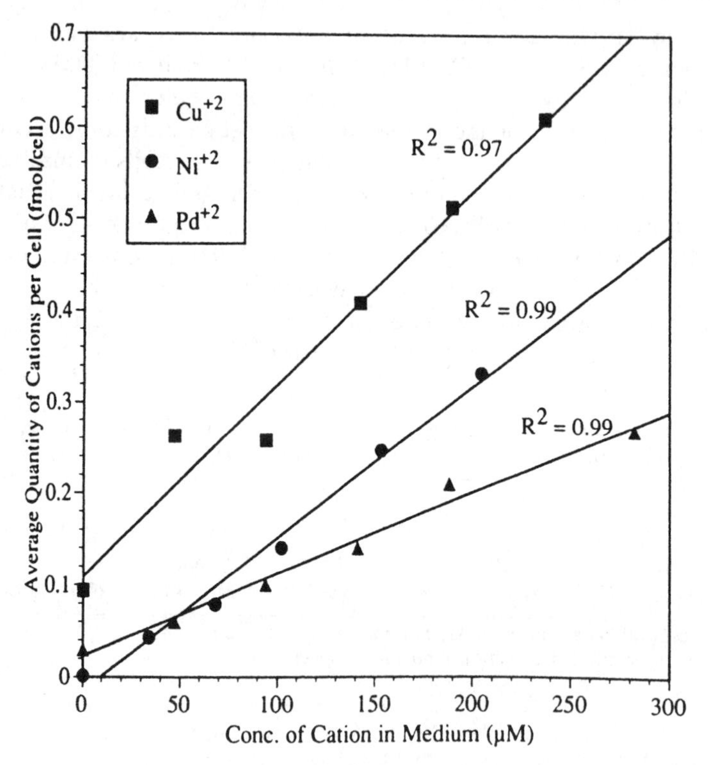

Figure 9.6 Plots of the average uptake of metal cation per cell vs. concentration of the metal cation in the medium for Cu^{2+}, Ni^{2+}, and Pd^{2+}. The least-squares method was used to fit linear curves to the points. (Wataha *et al.*, 1993.)

Two years after implantation of femoral components made of Ti–6Al–4V, the titanium and aluminium concentrations measured in the synovial fluid were higher for cemented components than for the uncemented (200 μm HA, or porous Ti coatings) components (Karrholm *et al.*, 1994). Table 9.10 gives the data for the synovial fluid and the aluminium concentrations in serum and urine. No significant concentrations of vanadium were found in any of the samples, which was also the case for titanium in serum and urine. Fast clearance of vanadium from the synovial fluid, due to high solubility of vanadium complexes, and formation of stable titanium compounds, e.g. titanium phosphates (Ribeiro *et al.*, 1995), might be reasonable explanations for these findings.

Experiments with metal salts and with stainless steel and Co–Cr–Mo electrodes corroded *in vivo* by applying anodic potentials showed that all the nickel and most of the cobalt were rapidly excreted (Brown *et al.*, 1988). Acceleration of corrosion by the use of anodic potentials obeys similar mechanisms both *in vivo* and in saline when a potential of 500 mV

Table 9.10 Metal concentrations (ng/g) in synovial fluid, serum and urine. Median (range) (Karrholm *et al.*, 1994)

	Cemented	*HA-coated*	*Porous*	*Controls*
Ti/synovial fluid	37 (12–56)	3.5 (0–14)	6.4 (0–7.8)	0 (0–7.5)
Al/synovial fluid	12 (6.7–28)	5.2 (2.6–13)	3.8 (2.9–9.1)	7.3 (1.9–19)
Al/serum	2.1 (0–11)	1.4 (0–5.9)	5.7 (2.1–16)	3.7 (0–17)
Al/urine	6.2 (1.7–17)	4.9 (1.7–7.0)	4.2 (3.7–4.6)	4.6 (2.1–14)

vs. SCE is applied. This is illustrated by the single straight line in Figure 9.7 (weight loss vs. total charge). In particular, this implies that the valency of the released cations is no different in both media, according to Faraday's law.

9.3.2 Problems associated with the chemical analysis of metallic elements in tissues

Acurate analysis of trace elements in tissues is essential to assess the degree of contamination. This is not an easy task, mainly because we are dealing with normal levels of the order of μg/litre. Sampling and sample

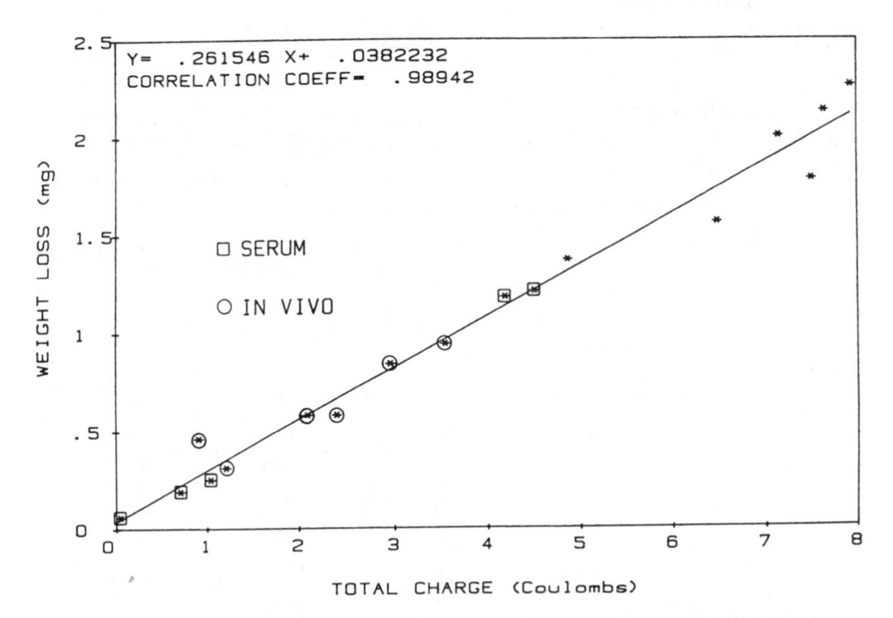

Figure 9.7 Linear regression analysis of weight loss as a function of total charge for stainless steel rods at 500 mV (SCE) for 30 min. Symbols: * = in saline, box = in 10% serum, circle = *in vivo*. (Brown *et al.* 1988.)

preparation are steps prone to serious contaminations, if the necessary precautions are not taken. As indicated in a review by Lugowski *et al.* (1990), reported 'normal' levels of Cr in blood span over four orders of magnitude. Contamination during sampling can be avoided by using PTFE or polyethylene materials for blood collection and sample storage. For cutting tissues a blade made of a material free from the elements to be analysed should be used. For example, in our laboratory we have been using pure titanium blades to cut soft tissues for Cr and Ni analysis. Contamination during sample preparation can be minimized by: (i) adopting a very strict protocol of labware cleaning; (ii) chemical treatment with ultrapure reagents, preferably in a microwave oven to reduce the time necessary for digesting tissues; (iii) use a laminar flow hood to prepare the samples, in order to avoid airborn contamination.

Lugowski has published a number of excellent works where the reader can find very detailed information on the above and other aspects. The degree of precision and accuracy to be expected when adequate experimental methods are used is indicated in Table 9.11. This table refers to an 'internal' lab blood standard and to a Standard Reference Material (SRM) with vanadium concentration certification. The relative standard deviation (RSD) ranges from ca. 10% for Ni and Co, to ca. 29% for V.

9.3.3 Corrosion in sweat

The main constituents of sweat are chlorides (0.3–3.0 g/l), urea (0.12–0.57 g/l) and lactic acid (0.45–4.5 g/l). When metallic objects come in contact with skin corrosion may occur, and if the corrosion products are toxic or irritating they may originate contact dermatitis. The most common example is dermatitis caused by nickel-containing jewelry. In North America ca. 10% of men and women have a history of nickel dermatitis (Randin, 1988). Although the degree of sensitization may not be directly

Table 9.11 Precision of laboratory standard and precision and accuracy of SRM 909 human serum (Lugowski et al., 1990)

Element	*X (μg/litre)*	*n*	*SD*	*RSD (%)*
Al	1.88	10	0.35	18.8
Co	2.37	9	0.26	10.9
Cr	0.71	8	0.14	19.6
Ni	2.95	8	0.30	10.1
Ti	4.20	7	0.41	9.8
V	0.28	8	0.08	29.4
V in SRM 909 certified value = 2.70±0.56 μg/litre	2.73	13	0.14	5.0

X – concentration; n – number of measurements; SD – Standard deviation; RSD – Relative SD.

related to the amount of metal ions released from an object, due to variability of response from person to person, it is generally considered that a high corrosion resistance gives rise to fewer allergies.

The corrosion resistance of several materials in artificial sweat is given in Table 9.12 (Randin, 1988). The composition (g/l) of the medium used was: 20 NaCl, 17.5 NH_4Cl, 5 urea, 2.5 acetic acid, 15 lactic acid, pH 4.7. The table gives the corrosion potential, E_{corr}, in O_2- and N_2-saturated medium, the pitting potential, E_{pit}, and the corrosion rate, i_{corr}, measured by the Tafel extrapolation method. i_{corr} is given only for those alloys which are in the active state. For the other alloys E_{pit} is given. The following materials were found to corrode in the active state: Ni, CuNi25, NiAl (50:50, 60:40 and 70:30), WC+Ni, white gold, FN42, Nilo Alby K, NiP. Alloys such as stainless steels, TiC+Mo_2C+Ni, NiTi, Hastelloy X, Phydur, PdNi, and SnNi are in the passive state and may pit under exceptional circumstances. Titanium has an extremely high E_{pit} and therefore cannot pit under normal use.

9.3.4 Influence of proteins on the corrosion resistance

Albumin has a detrimental effect on the corrosion resistance of cast Co–Cr–Mo alloy (Tomás *et al.*, 1994). The breakdown potential in 0.15 M NaCl is 0.40 ± 0.02 V vs. SCE, whereas in 0.15 M NaCl+albumin it is 0.25 ± 0.06 V vs. SCE.

The presence of 5% bovine serum in lactated Ringer's solution (pH=6.5) increases the corrosion rate of Ti–6Al–4V alloy, as shown in the last two columns of Table 9.13 (Lewis and Daigle, 1993b). This table gives data obtained by direct current (d.c.) and alternating current (a.c.) methods. The difference between d.c. and a.c. corrosion rates found in this system is not unusual. The same table also shows that decreasing the pH of lactated Ringer's solution to 1 has a dramatic effect on corrosion rate.

Table 9.14 summarizes data obtained for Co–Cr, 316L stainless steel and titanium. The type of electrochemical technique used has an important influence on the results, which might indicate that the electrode potential determines the beneficial or detrimental effect of proteins on corrosion.

9.3.5 Antibiotic–metal interactions

The interaction between a number of antibiotics (oxytetracycline, tetracycline, tobramycin, clindamycin, cefamandole, bacitracin and chloramphenicol) and surgical metallic materials (316L stainless steel, Co-Cr and commercially pure Ti) has shown that only oxytetracycline exerts an effect on the electrochemical response. For all the materials this antibiotic shifted the corrosion potential of abraded surfaces in the noble direction, as seen in Figure 9.8.

Table 9.12 Main Electrochemical Parameters in ISO Sweat (Randin, 1988)

	$E_{corr}(V_{SHE})$		E_{pit}	$i_{corr}O_2$	$i_{corr}N_2$
Materials	N_2	O_2	V_{SHE}	($\mu A/cm^2$)	($\mu A/cm^2$)
Ni200	-0.16	0.06	---	22	0.18
CuNi25	-0.09	0.06	---	24	<0.1
$Ni_{50}Al_{50}$	-0.17	0.04	1.1		
$Ni_{60}Al_{40}$	-0.20	-0.09	---	3.6	
$Ni_{70}Al_{30}$	-0.07	-0.02	---	2.2	
WC+Ni	-0.11	0.23	---	19	<<0.1
TiC+Mo_2C+Ni	0.25	0.31	0.43		
White gold	-0.01	0.23	---	0.6	<<0.1
FN 42	-0.24	0.07	0.08	~10	2.4
Nilo Alby K	-0.24	-0.09	---	190	0.32
NiTi	0.03	0.12	0.60–1.05		
AISI 303			0.43		
12/12			0.32		
AISI 304	-0.04	0.21	0.32		
AISI 316F	± 0.09	± 0.08	0.50		
316 PX			0.53		
AISI 316L				0.53	
Hastelloy X	-0.06	0.17	>0.89		
Phydur	0.26	0.29	0.46		
NiP	-0.19	-0.02	---	40	-0.1
NiP/450 °C	-0.15	0.09	---	18	
PdNi	0.33	0.45	0.46		
SnNi	0.07	0.08	0.2		
Cr	0.21–0.36	0.26	0.85		
Sandvik 1802	-0.02	0.22	0.61		
Shomac	0.15	0.26	>0.75		
Co	-0.24	-0.15	---	340	~0.1
$Co_{50}Al_{50}$	-0.29	-0.26	---	18	
WC+7% Co	-0.24	-0.10	---	200	~0.1
WC+10% Co	-0.25	-0.12	---	480	~0.1
Stellite 20			>0.75		
Ni			>3.0		

9.4 ASPECTS RELATED TO THE OXIDE AND OTHER SURFACE LAYERS

9.4.1 Effect of anodizing and passivation treatments on the corrosion resistance of titanium

For a detailed description of anodic oxidation of titanium and its alloys the reader may refer to a review by Aladjem (1973).

The oxide on titanium can grow to thicknesses of the order of 100 nm or more by applying anodic currents in suitable electrolytes. H_3PO_4 and NaOH baths have been used for this purpose. The colour of the oxide

Table 9.13 Electrochemical characteristics of Ti6Al4V alloy in three biosimulating solutions (Lewis, 1993b)

Solution	*Ecorr*[a] *(mV)*	βa[b] *(mV per decade)*	βca[c]	*Rp*[d] *(M Ω/cm²)*	*Rc*[e]	*idc*[f] *(nA/cm²)*	*iac*[g]
Lactated Ringer's (pH = 6.5)	185	210	301	2.57	1.00	21	54
Lactated Ringer's (pH = 6.5) + 5% bovine serum	336	187	234	1.45	0.70	31	65
Lactated Ringer's (pH = 1)	147	306	1650	0.33	0.22	340	510

[a] Corrosion potential.
[b] Anodic Tafel slope.
[c] Cathodic Tafel slope.
[d] Polarization resistance; obtained from d.c. results.
[e] Polarization resistance; obtained from a.c. results.
[f] Corrosion current density; obtained from the values for R_p.
[g] Corrosion current density; obtained from the values for R_c.

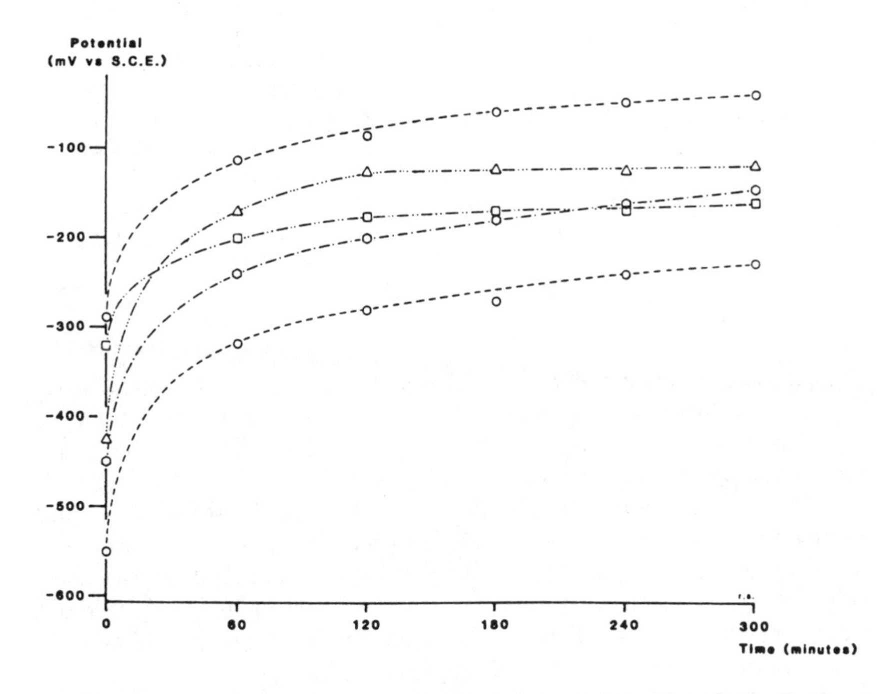

Figure 9.8 Potential-time curves for pure titanium in 0.9% saline with and without additions of oxytetracycline: ○(upper line), as received; ○](lower line), abraded; ◇0.01 mg ml^{-1}; □ 0.1 mg ml^{-1}; △ 1.0 mg ml^{-1}. (von Fraunhofer *et al.*, 1989.)

Table 9.14 The influence of proteins on the corrosion resistance of metals

Material	*Effect*	*Remarks*
F75 Co–Cr–Mo alloy with porous coating of F75 beads	Increased corrosion rate	Accelerated anodic corrosion method: 10% serum (Hughes *et al.*, 1990)
316L stainless steel	Marginal increase in pitting potential	Anodic polarization curves; 10% serum (Chawla *et al.*, 1990)
316L stainless steel	Increased corrosion rate*	Polarization resistance method; static conditions 10% serum (Williams *et al.*, 1988)
cp titanium	Increased corrosion rate	idem
Ti-6Al-4V	Insignificant effect	idem
c.p. titanium	Dual role	Beneficial effect in the absence of breakdown and detrimental when attack takes place; potentiodynamic and galvanostatic experiments; 10% serum (Sousa and Barbosa, 1993)
316L stainless steel	Increased pitting potential	Potentiodynamic and galvanostatic experiments; 10% serum (Sousa and Barbara, 1991)
F75 Co-Cr-Mo alloy	Increased Co and Cr release	Constant potential (500mV vs. SCE); 10% serum (Brown *et al.*, 1988)
316L stainless steel	Decreased weight loss	Constant potential (500mV vs. SCE); 10% serum (Brown *et al.*, 1988)

* Under fretting conditions the corrosion rate decreases.

changes with thickness due to light interference. A gold colour corresponds to a thickness of the order of 10–25 nm whereas a blue colour is normally associated with thicknesses of 30–60 nm. The corrosion resistance of anodized titanium increases as the oxide becomes thicker. This is illustrated in Figure 9.9 (Cigada *et al.* 1992), which shows that films formed in H_3PO_4 are thicker than those formed in air. They are also more protective, since the passive current density in a buffered physiological solution at 38°C is ca. 10% that measured for specimens oxidized in air. The same figure shows that anodizing in NaOH is not so effective in reducing the current density as doing it in H_3PO_4.

The corrosion rate of anodized titanium (solution: 60 ml ethanol, 35 ml water, 10 ml lactic acid, 5 ml phosphoric acid, 5 mg citric acid and 5 mg oxalic acid; 45V, 45s) is much lower than that of passivated titanium (40%

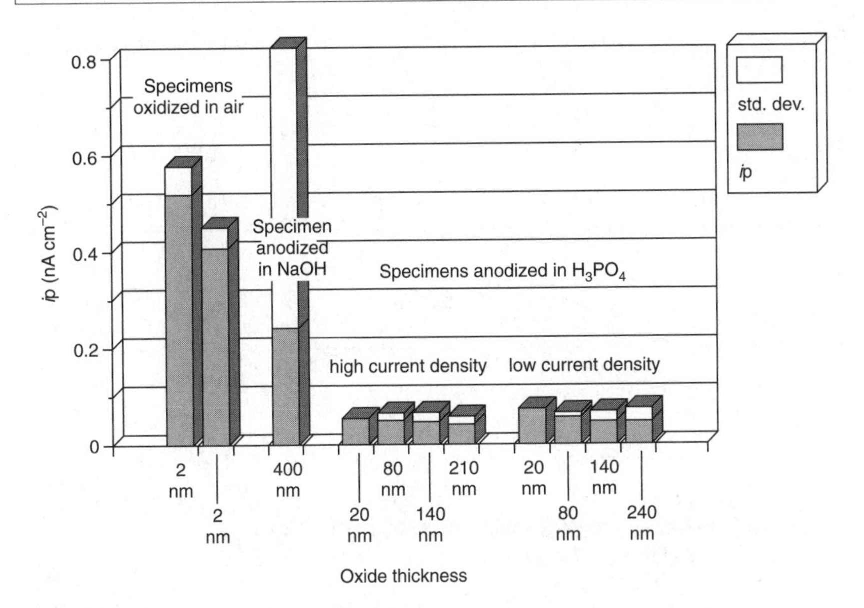

Figure 9.9 Average passivity currents (between 600 and 800 h) and standard deviations in physiological solution of Ti6Al4V specimens, oxidized and anodized in different conditions. (Cigada *et al.* 1992.)

volume nitric acid, room temperature, 30 min.), as indicated in Table 9.15 (Ong *et al.*, 1993). The corrosion potential of the former is also more noble, as indicated in the same table. The average thicknesses are given in Table 9.16. The anodized film is ca. 10 times thicker than the passivated film.

There have recently been reports (Lowenberg *et al.*, 19941 Callen *et al.*, 1995) indicating that passivation of Ti–6Al–4V in HNO_3 increases the release of all three constituent elements in a culture medium (α-Minimal Essential Medium with 15% foetal bovine serum and 10% antibiotics). Table 9.17 exemplifies the results obtained for titanium ions, for three periods of immersion of three days each. The level of Ti is significantly reduced throughout the 9-day experimental period.

Table 9.15 Corrosion results (Ong *et al.*, 1993)

Treatment	*Average E_{corr}±1 SD (mV)*	*Average I_{corr}±1 SD (μA/cm²)*
Non-passivated	-138.4±25.9	0.015±0.01
Passivated	-104.7±22.8	0.003±0.001
Anodized	34.4±17.4	90.0006±0.0001

Table 9.16 Titanium oxide thickness (nm), relative to tantalum pentoxide (Ong *et al.*, 1993)

Treatment	*Mean*	*SD*	*Sample size*
Non-passivated	3.1	0.6	1.8
Passivated	4.1	1.8	1.8
Anodized	43.6	4.9	1.5

Table 9.17 Trace Levels of Ti, Al, and V in culture medium (Callen *et al.*, 1995)

	cpTi Wells		*Ti6Al4V Wells*		
Time points	*Not Passivated*	*Passivated*	*Not Passivated*	*Passivated*	*Control Values*
Ti					
1st	23.696±12.892	15.735±3.354	12.599±3.850	23.338±8.497	4.983±0.977
2nd	12.650±5.275	16.640±4.940	11.050±1.601	24.645±8.419	
3rd	6.444±2.495	8.738±2.983	5.513±1.943	10.486±3.674	
Al					
1st	4.091±0.677	4.133±0.523	8.933±1.187	16.878±4.574	3.476±0.392
2nd	4.694±1.039	5.523±2.784	5.703±0.707	9.656±2.750	
3rd	5.215±1.096	4.149±0.397	4.516±0.384	6.614±1.407	
V					
1st	0.508±0.199	0.366±0.167	6.195±2.191	21.104±8.828	0.246±0.082
2nd	0.255±0.018	0.171±0.051	2.789±1.129	10.096±5.697	
3rd	0	0.330±0.213	0.588±0.334	4.218±2.003	

9.4.2 Effect of coatings and surface treatments on the corrosion resistance of stainless steel and titanium

When metals are used as coatings the possibility of occurrence of galvanic corrosion exists, since cracks or pores in the coating enable the corrosive medium to contact the substrate. Mainly for this reason metallic coatings have not been used in internal implants. However, surface treatments with inert materials have been widely applied and are now in clinical practice. The effect of these and other surface treatments will be addressed in this section.

With the development of ion implantation the plating of practically any element on any substrate opened new perspectives to surface modification of biomaterials. Carbon and nitrogen have been the species most widely employed to modify the corrosion and wear behaviour of stainless steels and titanium alloys. However, the plating of metallic elements, with a view to modifying either the corrosion performance and/or the biological behaviour of metallic implants, is an interesting possibility. This would be particularly valuable in the case of stainless steel substrates. Very little has been reported in this area. Titanium, niobium and tantalum coatings on stainless steel act as anodes, therefore indicating that they may retard the transfer of chromium and nickel into the environment (Gluszek and Masalski, 1992). In the same medium (Ringer's solution) the oxide layers formed on titanium, niobium and tantalum by prolonged (100h) exposure to air are not very stable. Figure 9.10 shows this effect (dotted line). The galvanic current first increases, corresponding to modification/destruction of the original oxide layer, and then decreases, corresponding to increased stability of the film formed in solution. When freshly ground specimens are used (solid line) the galvanic current decreases with time, due to film growth, which follows a logarithmic law [log i $\propto$ (– log t)].

Laser surface alloying (LSA) of Ti6Al4V with Nb, Mo and Zr, in order to increase surface hardness, has shown that the latter element is the most promising (Akgun and Inal, 1994). The hardness increase is almost threefold in comparison to the substrate and identical to that obtained by laser surface melting (LSM). Since a nitrogen atmosphere was used in LSA and LSM, TiN formed during melting appears to be the main reason for the

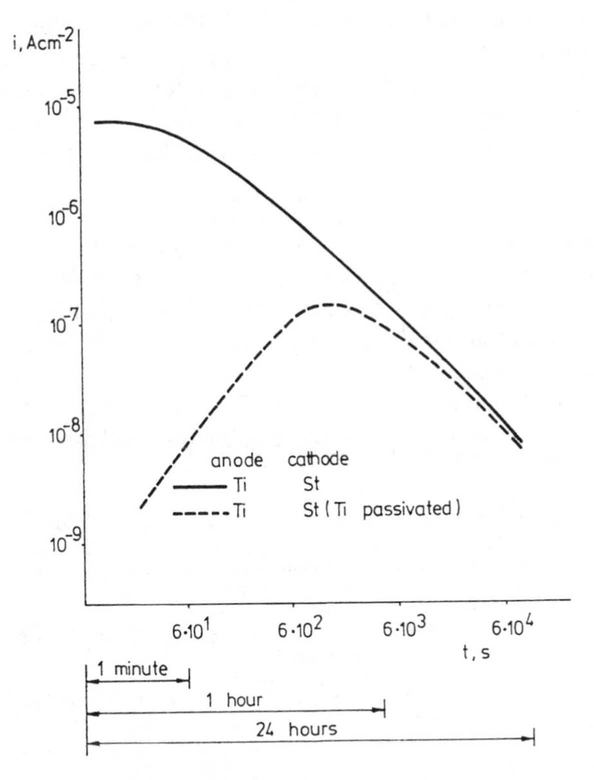

Figure 9.10 Galvanic current density–time relationship for 316L/titanium couple in Ringer's solution. (Gluszek and Masalski, 1992.)

high hardnesses obtained. The hardened zone extends to a depth of over 0.5 mm. Wear and fretting corrosion could be considerably reduced with such surface treatments, but no experimental data are yet available.

Radio-frequency (RF) plasma treatments in air (1.0 torr) produced enhanced ionic release from Co–Cr–Mo and Ti–6Al–4V alloys, without any improvement in biological behaviour (Kummer *et al.*, 1992). Table 9.18 gives the Cr, Co and Ti concentrations obtained after 10 days exposure to cell culture fluid (DMEM with 10% FBS). The RF plasma-treated Ti–Al–V alloy shows a 3-fold increase after the plasma-treatment.

Depassivation of Ti–6Al–4V occurs during planar-planar rubbing against PMMA in Ringer's solution (Rabbe *et al.*, 1994). The free corrosion potential drops to values below -650 mV vs. SCE. This potential is substantially lower than those obtained for nitrogen ion-implanted and ion-nitrided Ti–6Al–4V, which are of the order of, -100 mV vs. SCE. At high doses ($\sim 2\times10^{18}$ ions/cm^2) a TiN layer is formed on ion-implanted surfaces, whereas TiN and Ti_2N form as a result of ion nitriding, thus increasing the hardness of the alloy surface.

Superalloy MA 956 (Fe–20Cr–4.5Al–0.5Ti–0.5Y_2O_3, wt%) possesses the interesting ability of developing a fine α-alumina scale on the surface upon isothermal treatment at 110 °C (Escudero and González-Carrasco, 1994). This layer acts as a coating, being responsible for an improved corrosion resistance of the alloy, as indicated by the anodic polarization curves given in Figure 9.11. No pitting corrosion occurs for potentials up to 700 mV vs. SCE.

Hard ceramic coatings (Al_2O_3 and SiC) deposited by radio-frequency (RF) sputtering on Ti and Co–Cr–Mo alloy resulted in significant corrosion resistance improvement, as seen in Table 9.19 (Sella *et al.*, 1990). The data in this table were obtained by applying a constant potential of 1.4 V vs. SCE and measuring the corrosion current density (c.d.) in artificial saliva. SiC coatings deposited on Ti caused a decrease of c.d. of ca. 300 times. The same coating applied to Co–Cr–Mo was only effective when an intermediate Ti sublayer was used to avoid cracking. An Al–Al_2O_3

Table 9.18 Concentration of Cr, Co and Ti in cell culture fluid after 10 days (Kummer *et al.*, 1992)

	concentration (μ/mL)		
Sample	*Cr*	*Co*	*Ti*
Control	1.1	<2	—
Co–Cr–Mo	96.5	720	—
Co–Cr–Mo/RF	120.5	960	—
Ti-Al-V	—	—	35.6
Ti-Al-V/RF	—	—	102.0

RF = Radio-frequency plasma treated.

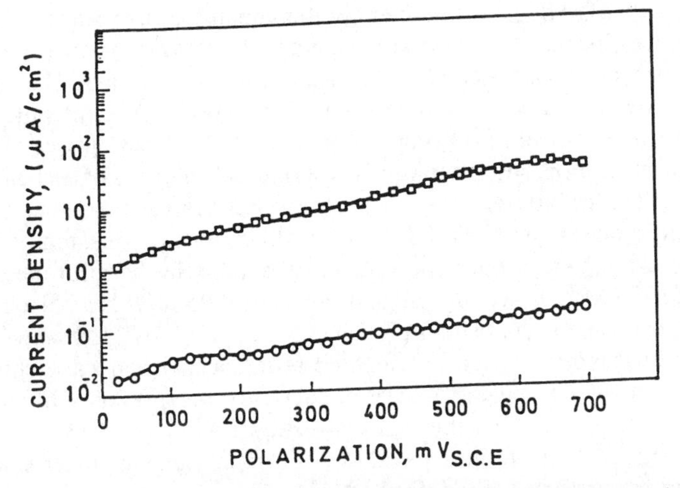

Figure 9.11 Anodic polarization curves for MA956 in the as-received and oxidized conditions after nine months of immersion in Hank's solution. ○ Oxidized; □ as-received. (Escudero and González-Carrasco, 1994.)

cermet sublayer was also very effective in improving the corrosion resistance of Al_2O_3-coated Co–Cr–Mo alloy; the c.d. decreased 200 times when both layers were used. The authors indicate that Al_2O_3 and SiC coatings gave better biocompatibility than Ti and that no signs of corrosion were observed on Al_2O_3-coated dental implants removed after several years of implantation.

Modification of Ti–6Al–4V alloy surfaces by ion implantation with iridium, at fluences of 0.74×10^{16} and 1.48×10^{16} ions/cm^2, corresponding to 2.5 and 5.0 at% Ir peak concentrations, has been reported (Buchanan

Table 9.19 Comparison of the corrosion currents of coated and uncoated metals (*Sella et al., 1990*)

	Corrosion current at E=1.4V/SCE (μA/cm²)
Uncoated metal or alloy	
Ni–Cr	6000–8000
Co–Cr–Mo	8000
Ti	260
Experimental coatings	
SiC (1 μm) on Ti	0.8
SiC (1 μm) on Co–Cr	10000
Ti (1 μm) on Co–Cr	500
SiC (1 μm) + Ti (1 μm) on Co–Cr	28
Al_2O_3 (0.5 μm) on Co–Cr	1800
Al_2O_3 (0.5 μm) + Al–Al_2O_3 cerment on Co–Cr	40

and Lee, 1990). After pre-treatment of the implanted surfaces in 1N H_2SO_4 the surfaces become enriched in Ir (the concentrations are over 60% and may approach 100%), as a consequence of alloy dissolution. The result is a corrosion potential in isotonic saline very close to that of pure Ir, as depicted in Figure 9.12. Owing to the very high corrosion resistance of Ir, its implantation onto titanium is of potential interest, particularly if it becomes significantly enriched on the surface. Galvanic couples formed between Ir and Ti is a possibility that justifies further research.

In an attempt to reduce the release of potentially harmful metal ions from Co–Cr–Mo surgical implants, a thin coating of TiN has been applied via physical vapour deposition (PVD) (Wisbey *et al.*, 1987). *In vitro* corrosion performance has been investigated using electrochemical techniques. The release of Co and Cr ions is reduced by the presence of the TiN coating. Data concerning this study are shown in Figure 9.13.

Thermal heating of titanium at 400 °C or immersion in 30% HNO_3, followed by aging in boiling distilled water for times in the range 6–14 h, greatly reduced the amount of Ti and Al released from Ti–6Al–4V, as shown in Table 9.20 (Browne and Gregson, 1994). The corrosive medium was bovine serum at 37 °C. The table also gives the ion release for two other treatments: immersion in 30% HNO_3, for 10 min., which is the conventional commercial treatment, and immersion for 16h in the same solution followed by rinsing in distilled water (N). The beneficial effect of the first two treatments is attributed to formation of rutile, which is

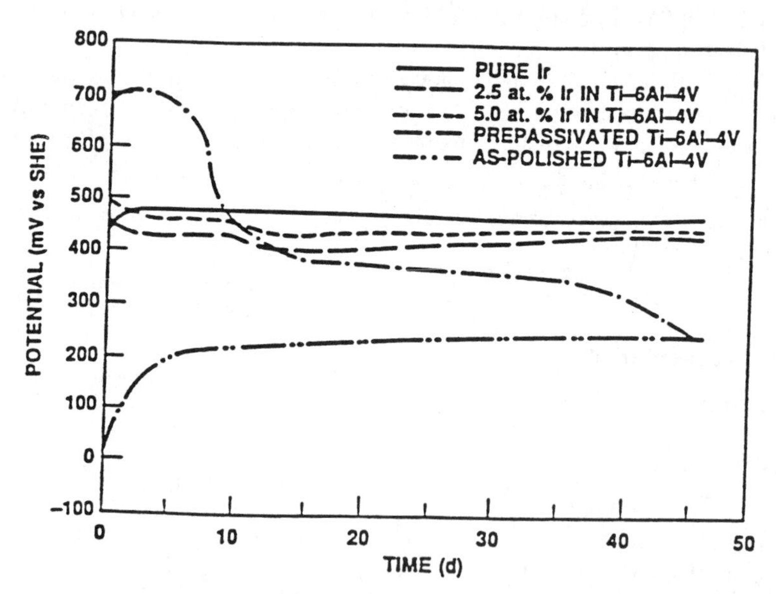

Figure 9.12 Corrosion potential vs. time in aerated isotonic saline. (Buchanan and Lee, 1990.)

more dense and has a closer packed structure, with fewer paths for ion diffusion, than the oxide formed upon passivation in nitric acid.

Commercially pure titanium and Ti–6Al–4V implants ion implanted with nitrogen heal as well as non-treated samples in cortical bone (Johansson *et al.*, 1993), as indicated by the existence of no statistically significant differences in total bone-metal contact.

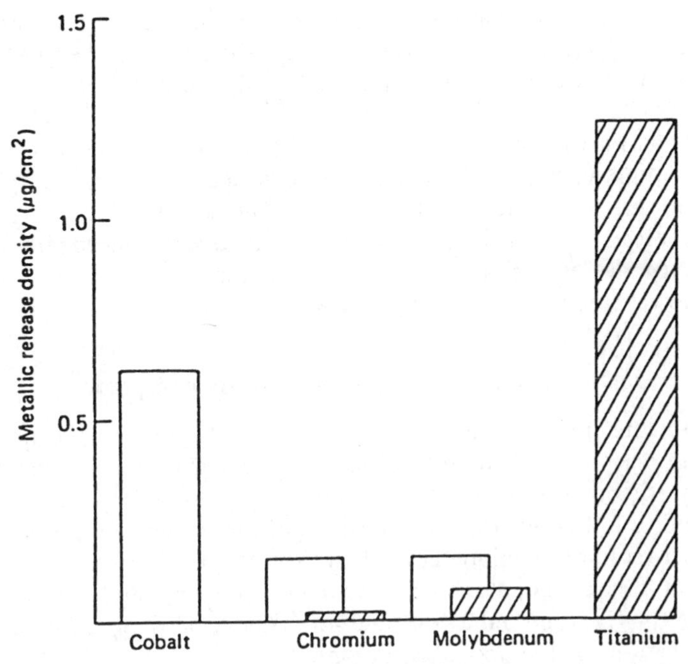

Figure 9.13 Metallic dissolution products released from a polished Co–Cr–Mo alloy after 550 h in 0.17 M NaCl+2.7×10^{-3} M EDTA solution at 37°C. □ uncoated; ■ TiN coated. (Wisbey *et al.*, 1987.)

Table 9.20 Effect of various surface treatments on the dissolution of titanium and aluminium from Ti-6Al-4V alloy (Browne and Gregson, 1994)

	Total ion release (μg/cm²)	
	Titanium 700 h	*Aluminium 700 h*
30% HNO_3 (C)	0.1	0.25
30% HNO_3 (N)	0.11	0.06
400°C (T)	0.03	0.026
Aged 10 h (A)	0.03	0.023

C – Conventional treatment (10 min. immersion).
A – Aging treatment (immersion in destilled water).
N – Immersion in HNO_3 for 16 h.
T – Thermal heating.

9.4.3 Effect of hydroxyapatite coatings on the corrosion resistance of titanium and stainless steels

Most of the data available on this topic refer to hydroxyapatite deposited by plasma spraying. Although compounds may form at the metal/hydroxy-apatite interface, particularly in the case of titanium, their existence has not been unequivocally demonstrated. Titanium phosphates and phosphides, as well as calcium titanates, may exist, but they probably form very thin layers. The large surface roughness, caused by grit blasting of the substrate prior to hydroxyapatite deposition, is another factor that renders identification of any interfacial compounds by surface analysis techniques difficult.

Table 9.21 shows that the corrosion resistance of stainless steel increases upon coating with hydroxyapatite. The presence of calcium phosphate in solution, due to dissolution of hydroxyapatite, seems to be the cause for these changes. The same table indicates that calcium phosphate is detrimental to the corrosion resistance of titanium, both in terms of film breakdown potential and corrosion rate under passive conditions.

9.4.4 Interaction between metal ions and calcium phosphates

Metallic ions may influence the formation of calcium phosphates in different ways. Some inhibit (nickel, tin, cobalt, manganese, copper, zinc, gallium, thalium, molybdenum, cadmium, antimony, magnesium, and mercury), a few stimulate (iron [ferric] and iridium) whereas others have no effect (cerium, titanium, chromium, iron [ferrous], iridium, palladium, platinum, silver, gold, aluminum, and lead) (Okamoto and Hidaka, 1994). Figure 9.14 gives the induction time for calcium phosphate formation vs. concentration for the above metal ions.

Table 9.21 Effect of hydroxyapatite coatings and calcium phosphate solutions on the corrosion resistance of titanium and stainless steel

Material	*Solution*	*Effect*	*Ref.*
316L ss/HA	Saline	Increase in breakdown potential	Hayashi *et al.*, 1990
Ti-6Al-4V/HA	Saline	Decrease in breakdown potential	Hayashi *et al.*, 1990
316L ss	Saline+ Ca phosphate	Increase in breakdown potential	Sousa and Barbosa, 1991
316L ss	Saline+ Ca phosphate	Decrease in corrosion rate (passive state)	Barbosa, 1991b
Ti cp	Saline+ Ca phosphate	Decrease in breakdown potential	Sousa and Barbosa, 1993
Ti cp	Saline+ Ca phosphate	Increase in corrosion rate (passive state)	Barbosa, 1991b

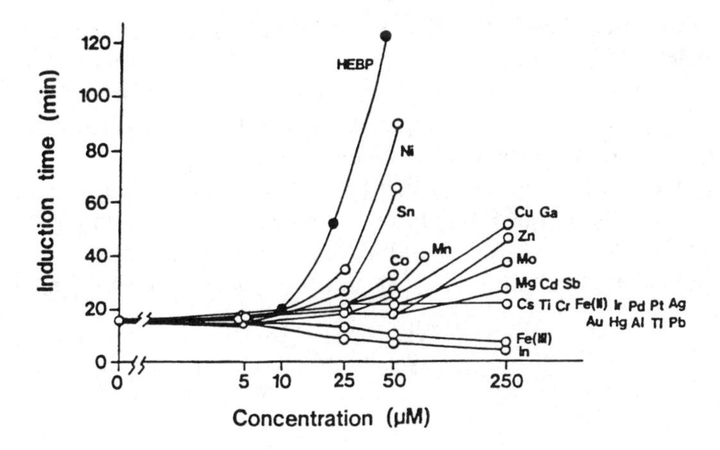

Figure 9.14 The induction time (min) versus concentration of various metal ions (open circle) and HEBP: 1-hydroxyethylidene-1, 1-biphosphonate (closed circle). (Okamoto and Hidaka, 1994.)

Heat treatment of Ti–6Al–4V at 280 °C for 3 h produced a high accumulation of Ca deposited next to screws implanted in rats (Hazan *et al.*, 1993), as indicated in Table 9.22. The oxide was twice as thick as that formed on non-treated screws.

The presence of Ca on the surface of titanium implants after a period *in vivo* is now well established. Ca deposition may be important in influencing protein adsorption, since it has been suggested that glycosaminoglycans adhere to the surface by a Ca–O link rather then via a Ti–N bond (Sutherland *et al.*, 1993).

Aluminium induces demineralization of previously formed bone (Frayssinet *et al.*, 1994), which can be ascribed to formation of stable complex aluminium phosphate compounds (Ribeiro *et al.*, 1995). Aluminium ions may be produced either as a result of dissolution of Ti–6Al–4V alloy or of corrosion of alumina coatings. In pH 4 buffer the release of aluminium ions from alumina is much more significant than at

Table 9.22 Calcium deposition (mg) next to control and heat-treated Ti–6Al–4V implants (Hazan *et al.* 1993)

Time after immersion (days)	*Control*	*Heat treated*
4	–	–
5	–	–
6	2.0±0.2	4.5±6.5
10	3.1±0.5	7.4±1.1
35	4.0±1.0	9.6±1.0

pH 7 (Frayssinet, 1994). V and Ti retard apatite formation and the growth of apatite seeds, as illustrated respectively in Figures 9.15 and 9.16 for V (Blumenthal and Cosma, 1989). The action of V appears to be related to the formation of V-PO_4 complexes, whereas that of Ti may be due to poisoning of active growth sites, as in the case of Al.

Hydroxyapatite coatings applied to porous titanium alloys significantly reduced the titanium and aluminium releases, but had no important effect on vanadium release, as shown in Figure 9.17 (Ducheyne and Healy, 1988). No major change was produced in the ion release kinetics from Co–Cr alloys.

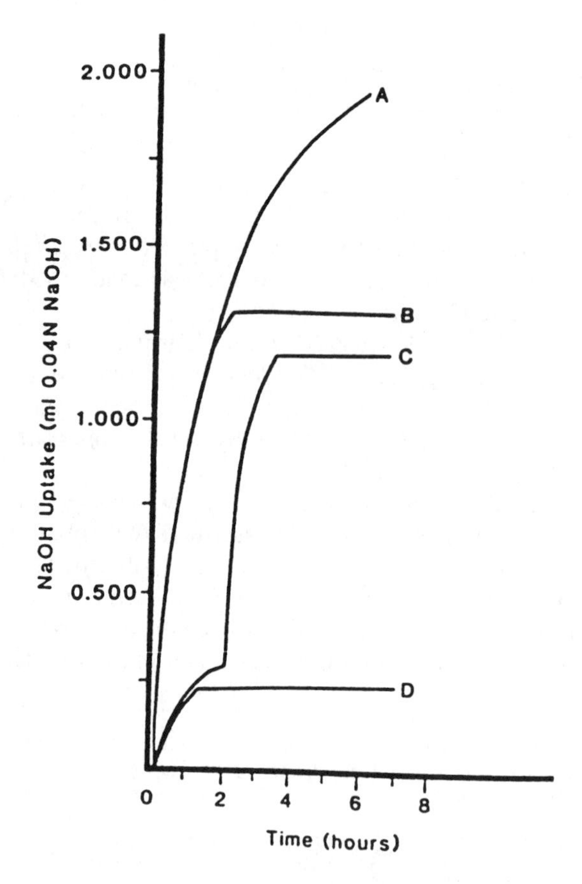

Figure 9.15 The action of V ions in affecting direct HA precipitation, V as VCl_5 in solution at pH 7.4, 0.15 M NaCl, 37°C in a pH-stat. The quantity of HA precipitated is proportional to the extent of OH uptake. Ca concentration is 2.79 mM; PO_4 concentration is 1.87 mM, A= control (no V); B=0.50 mM V; C=1.00 mM V; D=2.00 mM V. (Blumenthal and Cosma, 1989.)

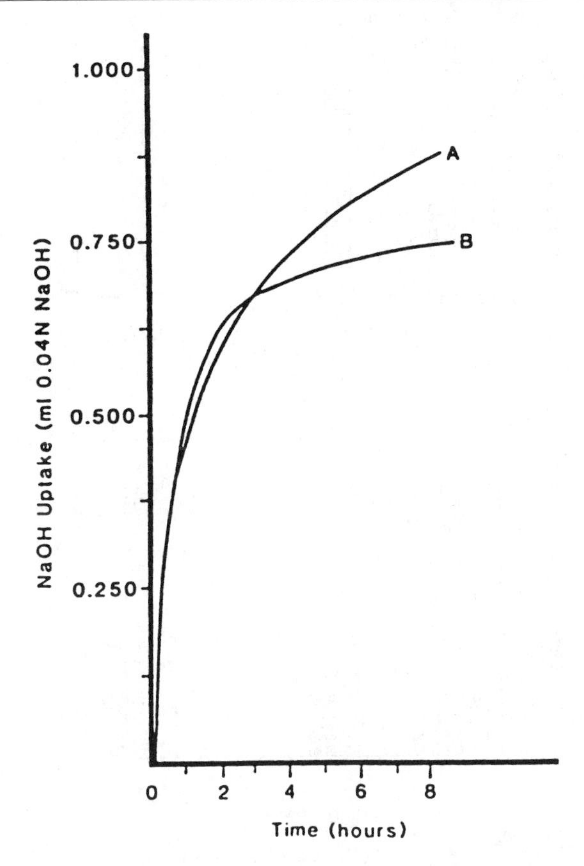

Figure 9.16 The action of V ions on the growth of HA seeds. V as VCl_5 in solution at pH 7.4, 0.15 M NaCl, 37°C in a pH-stat. The amount of HA seeded growth is proportional to the OH uptake. Ca concentration is 1.55 mM; PO_4 concentration is 1.07 mM, Seed crystals were 0.15 mg/mL, and the seeds had a surface area of 110 m^2/g. A = control (no V); B = 1.00 mM V. (Blumenthal and Cosma, 1989.)

9.4.5 Physico-chemical properties of metal oxides

The corrosion resistance of some metals ultimately depends on the presence of a thin oxide film formed by the reaction of the metal with the environment. This is the case of titanium, tantalum, zirconium, molybdenum, aluminium, cobalt, chromium, etc. Table 9.23 gives the physico-chemical properties of the oxides formed on some metals. A low oxide solubility is important to guarantee a low rate of corrosion, since any loss in oxide thickness, due to chemical dissolution, will tend to be balanced by oxidation of the metallic substrate. The oxides should also possess low ionic conductivity.

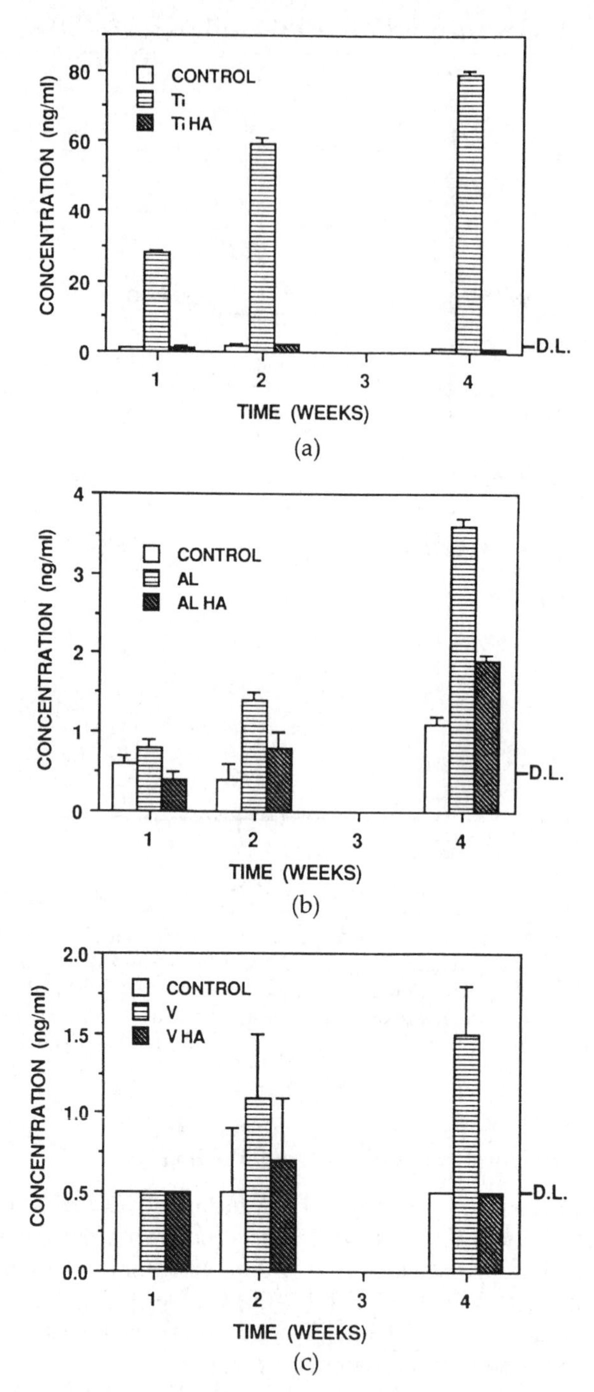

Figure 9.17 (a, b, c) The release of Ti, Al and V from the Ti alloy after 1, 2 and 4 weeks of immersion; D.L. indicates the detection limit of each element. Error bars represent the 95% confidence interval on the means. (Ducheyne and Healy, 1988.)

Table 9.23 Selected physico-chemico properties of metal oxides in water (Tengvall and Lundstrom, 1992)

Order of practical mobility	*Element*	*Water corrosion product*	*pK_a of hydrolysis*	*Solubility at pH 7 (M)*	*Isoelectric point*	*Charge at pH 7*	*Dielectric onst for oxide*	*0.996 Na($FeCN_6^{4-}$ $FeCN_6^{3-}$) polarization resistance, R_p (KΩ/cm²)*	*Essential*	*Soft tissue reaction*	*Corroded in H_2O_2 at pH7*	*Corrosion product*
2	Nb	Nb_2O_5	>20	-10^{-5}	—		280	455	No	Inert?	No	
3	Ta	Ta_2O_5	>20	-10^{-5}	—		12	1430	No	Inert?	No	
4	Au	Au_2O_3	—	7×10^{-2}	>10 (calc.)	++		0.28	No	Sequestration	Yes	Au_2O_3
		$Au(OH)_3$	(pH7)	5×10^{6}							$E_o \simeq 1.04V$	
7	Ti	TiO_2 anat.	+18	3×10^{6}	6.2	—	48	714	No	No	Yes	TiO_2^{2-}
		brook.				—	78					TiO_2
		rutile					110					TiO_2
14	Ag	Ag_2O	+10	10^{4}	(Ag^+)12	++	9		No	Sequestrattion	Yes	AgO^-
		$AgOH$	Ag^++0.7	>1								
19	A1	Al_2O_3 α	14.6	10^{6}	-9	+	5–10		No	Sequestration	?	?
		$Al(OH)_3$ am.	—	10^{-3}								
21	Cr	Cr_2O_3	-1.8($Cr(OH)_2^+$)	10^{-11}	8.4 (Cr^{3+})		12		Yes	Toxicity	Yes	CrO_4^{2-}
		CrO_3		$>10^{-13}$								
		$Cr(OH)_3$	18.6(CrO_2^-)			+				Toxicity	Yes	$HCrO_4^-$
28	Fe	Fe_2O_3	-13.3 (Fe^{2+})	$>10^{-10}$	12.4 (Fe^{2+})	+	100	Stainless steel 316	Yes	Sequestration	Yes	FeO_4^{2-}?
		$Fe(OH)_2$	(pH 9.1)	10^{-1}	8.0 (Fe^{3+})		30–38	4.38				
		$Fe(OH)_3$		10^{-9}								
29	Ni	Ni^{2+}	12.2 (Ni^{2+})	10^{-15}	9.5	+			Yes	Toxicity	Yes	NiO_4^{2-}?
		NiO	(pH 8.9)	10^{-11}								NiO_2
30	Co	Co^{2+}	-12.6	10^{-11}	10.8	+	CoCrNi	Yes	Toxicity	Yes	CoO_2	
		CoO		10^{-12}			3.32					
40	V	V_2O_5	+10.3 (HV_2O^-)	>1	1–2.5 (V^{5+})	-			Yes	Toxicity	Yes	$H_3V_2O_7^-$
		V_2O_4		10^{-4}								$H_2VO_4^-$

9.4.6 Passive films on metallic implants

The oxide film on metallic implants is usually very thin (5–10 nm). It is formed as a result of a spontaneous reaction between the metal and the environment. In spite of the common use of immersion treatments in nitric acid solutions, usually known as passivation treatments, they are not necessary to form an oxide. They are often responsible for an increase in corrosion resistance due to removal of surface contaminations or inclusions, as in the case of stainless steels. As indicated in section 9.4.1, there have been reports suggesting that this acid treatment may decrease the corrosion resistance of titanium.

Generally, the oxide film grows according to a logarithmic law (log thickness proportional to log time), reaching a quasi-stationary thickness very rapidly. Under stationary conditions, film dissolution and film formation rates should be the same. Normally, film thickness increases slowly with time, after an initial period of rapid growth. This is illustrated in Figure 9.18, which depicts film thickening with implantation time (Kasemo and Lausmaa, 1994).

The dissolution kinetics of titanium follows a two-phase logarithmic model (Healy and Ducheyne, 1992, 1993). In the first phase the concentration of OH groups increases. The second phase coincides with the adsorption of P-containing species. Figure 9.19 clearly indicates the presence of a second phase after 400h of immersion. In the initial phase titanium is released either in the form of $Ti(OH)_n^{(4-n)}+$ or $TiO(OH)_2$. In the second phase adsorption of $H_2PO_4^-$

$$Ti(OH)^{3+}(ox) + H_2PO_4^-(aq) \rightarrow Ti_4^+(ox) . HPO_4^{2-}(ad) + H_2O(aq)$$

followed by desorption into the concentration boundary layer

$$Ti^{4+}(ox) . HPO_4^{2-}(ad) \rightarrow Ti\ HPO_4^{2+}(aq) + (ox)\ \text{(charge transfer)}$$

In the bulk electrolyte the complex ion dissociates

$$TiHPO_4^{2+}(aq) + H^+\ (aq) \rightarrow Ti^{4+}(aq) + H_2PO_4\ ^-(aq)$$

and forms a more stable complex

$$Ti^{4+}\ (aq) + 4OH^-\ (aq) \rightarrow Ti(OH)_4\ (aq)$$

In these reactions (ox) represents O_2^{4-} in TiO_2.

This mechanism is consistent with the hypothesis that in the second stage dissolution kinetics is dependent on diffusion within the concentration boundary layer. It is conceivable that in the first stage field assisted dissolution may be the controlling step. In this stage formation of $Ti(OH)_4$ or of hydroxy-cations, e.g. $Ti(OH)_3^+$, has different effects on titanium transport. While $Ti(OH)_4$ does not react with organic molecules, $Ti(OH)_3^+$ can form organometallic complexes which may be transported systemically.

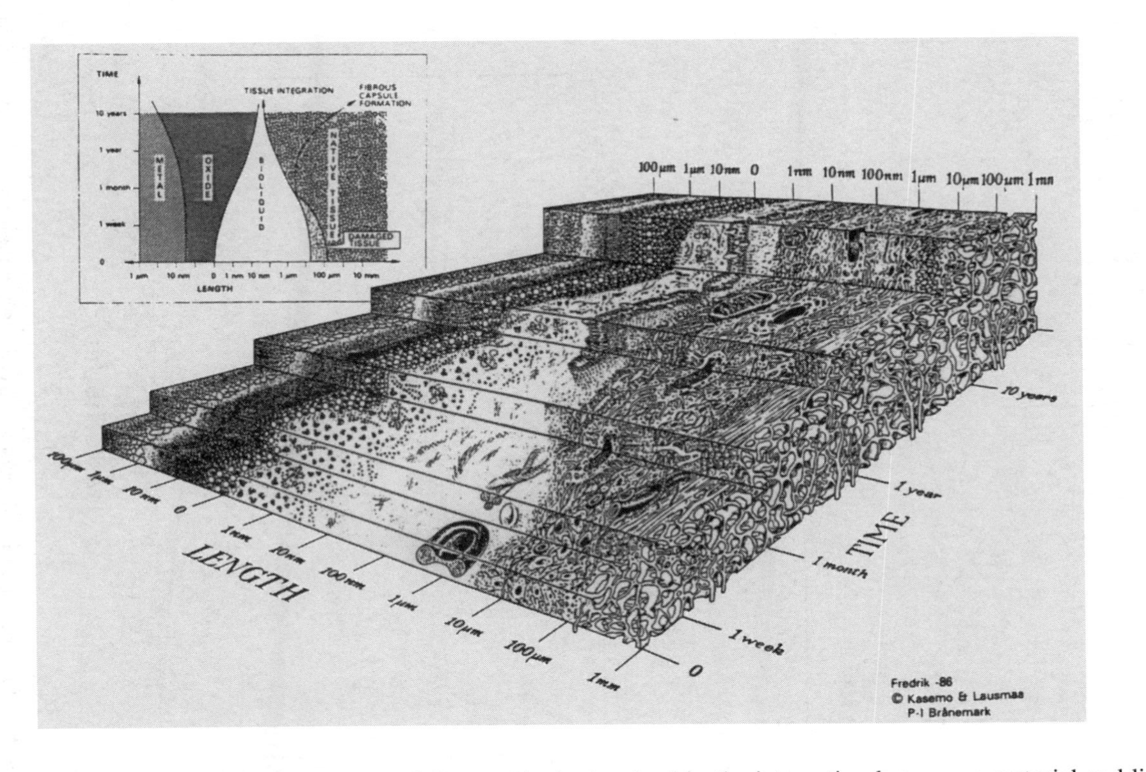

Figure 9.18 An artist's attempt to capture some of the complexity involved in the interaction between a material and living tissue, exemplified here by a titanium implant in bone. Note the wide range of dimensions and time scales that are relevant. (Kasemo and Lausmaa, 1994.)

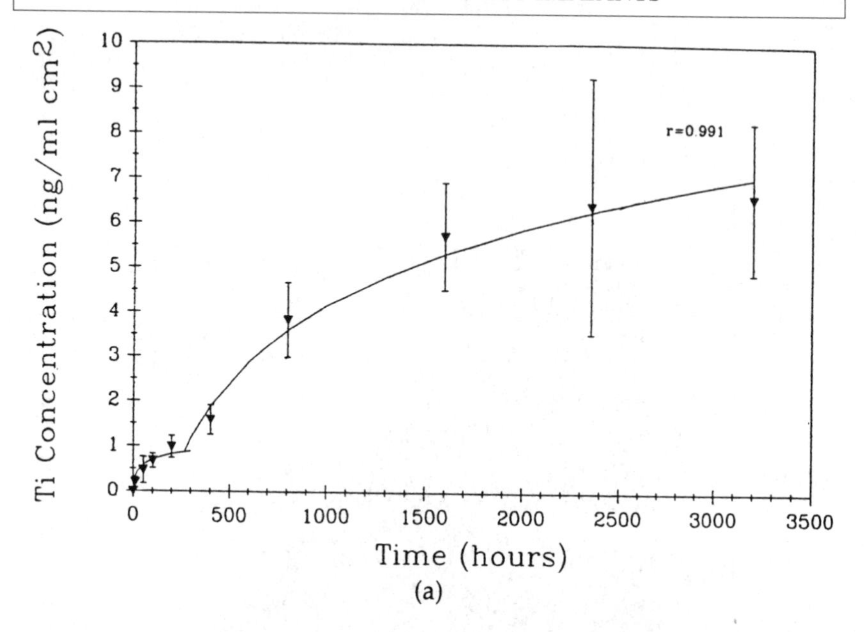

(a)

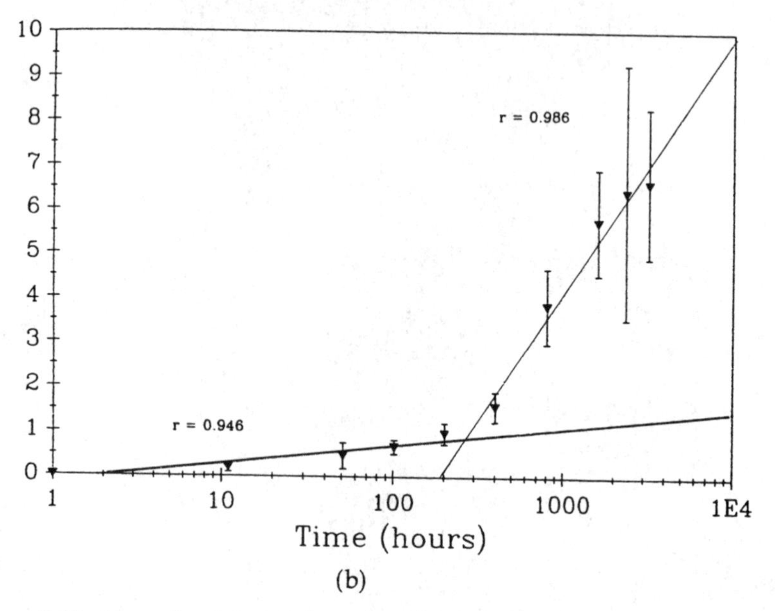

(b)

Figure 9.19 Normalized integral passive dissolution kinetics for titanium thin films immersed in EDTA/SIE (simulated interstitial electrolyte): (a) real time data empirically fitted with two-phase logarithmic law relationship; (b) a semilogarithmic plot of the data demonstrating the two-phase logarithm relationship. The correlation coefficient for the least-squares fit of the linear functions are given. (Healy and Ducheyne, 1992.)

Airborne titanium oxide, TiO_{2-x}, is oxygen defficient but upon immersion in simulated interstitial electrolyte with EDTA (a metal chelating agent) changes to nearly stoichiometric TiO_2 (Healy and Ducheyne, 1993). TiO_2 is also reported to exist on the surface of a new Ti–15Zr–4Nb–2Ta–0.2Pd alloy (Okazaki *et al.*, 1994). The other oxides present were ZrO_2, Nb_2O_5 and Ta_2O_5.

Sterilization by various methods (conventional steam autoclaving, dry heat sterilization in air at 160–180°C, and packaging and sterilization in sealed glass ampoules) originates films with the composition TiO_2. Their thickness is 2–6 nm, depending on the method of sterilization. Heat sterilization increased the thickness of the original oxide by a factor of ca. 2 (Lausmaa and Kasemo, 1990).

Films formed on metallic materials oxidized in pure oxygen at 300° C for 30 min. have the composition shown in Table 9.24 (Oshida, 1992). Strong oxidative conditions may exist *in vivo*, for example due to presence of the superoxide anion, O_2^-, formed by inflammatory cells. The possibility of O_2^- originating hydrogen peroxide, H_2O_2, has led Tengvall *et al.*, (1989) to suggest that hydrogen peroxide may be of great importance to the biological behaviour of titanium. Hydrogen peroxide is responsible for the appearance of an outer layer, formed on top of a TiO_2 layer, composed of titanium oxi-hydroxide or hydrates, non-stoichiometric and rich in water (Pan *et al.*, 1994). The oxide thickness for wet-ground specimens is ca. 3 times that for dry-polished specimens, as shown in Table 9.25. Hydrogen peroxide reduces the oxide thickness and results in enhanced dissolution of titanium, according to the same authors. It is not certain whether titanium acts as a catalyst in the oxidative deterioration of biological molecules, a property which has been established for other metals, e.g. iron, copper, cadmium, chromium, lead, mercury, nickel and vanadium (Stohs and Bagchi, 1995). These metals produce reactive oxygen species, leading to lipid peroxidation, DNA damage, depletion of sulphydryls, apart from modifying calcium homeostasis. Since large concentrations of titanium debris may be found around Ti and Ti-alloy implants (section 9.3.1) the oxidative deterioration of biological molecules induced by the presence of Ti ions is a process that deserves to be studied.

Table 9.24 Type of oxide formed on biomaterials (pure oxygen, 300°C, 30 min.) (Oshida *et al.*, 1992)

Material	*Type of oxide*
Pure Ti	TiO_2 (rutile)
Ti–6Al–4V	TiO_2 with traces of Al_2TiO_5
Ni–Ti, austenitic and martensitic	Mixture of TiO_2 and $NiTiO_3$
316L stainless steel	spinel-type $[(Fe,Ni)O \cdot (Fe,Cr)_2O_3]$[a] and corundum-type oxides $[(Fe,Cr)_2O_3]$[a]

a Possible composition.

Table 9.25 Thickness (nm) of titanium oxide films (Pan *et al.*, 1994)

Source			*Polarized at 0.4 V/SCE*		
H_2O_2 in the PBS (mM)	*Dry-polished*	*Wet-ground*	*0*	*1*	*10*
XPS measurements	1.5	4.6	6.3	6.2	5.8
Capacitance measurements			6.7	5.5	6.0
Literature data	1.2–1.6	4–5	6.6		

The oxide formed on titanium upon passivation in HNO_3 is composed of regions of mixed titanium oxides (anatase and rutile), together with areas of amorphous titanium oxide (Browne and Gregson, 1994). Films formed on anodized titanium may be one order of magnitude thicker than those formed by passivation (section 9.4.1). The film is predominantly constituted by TiO_2, with the presence of carboxyl groups (Ong, 1993). It appears that upon passivation of cp Ti and Ti–6Al–4V alloy the film on the former is thinner (3.2 ± 0.8 nm) than that on the latter (8.3 ± 1.2 nm) (Keller *et al.*, 1994). TiO_2 films are generally amorphous, except in the case of thick films produced by thermal oxidation or anodizing. Table 9.26 summarizes the characteristics (composition, oxide thickness, surface

Table 9.26 Summary of surface characteristics of the four different types of Ti samples (Larsson *et al.*, 1994)

Preparation	*Composition*	*Oxide thickness*	*Surface topography Surface roughness*	*Substrate microstructure Oxide crystallinity*
Clinical reference	TiO_2+45–80% C, traces of Ca, S, Si, P, Cl and Na	4nm	Rough, with grooves, pits and protrusions, ≤ 10 μm R_{rms}=29±4 nm	Plastically deformed, amorphous metal surface Non-crystalline oxide
Electropolished	TiO_2+55–90% C, traces of Ca, S, Si, P, Cl and Na	4–5 nm	Smooth, with occasional pits, ≤ 1 μm R_{rms} = 2.7±0.9 nm	Polycrystalline metal surface Non-crystalline oxide
Electropolished + anodized, 10 V	TiO_2+55–70 %C, traces of Ca, S, Si, and Cl	21 nm	Smooth, with pits and porous regions, ~10 μm R_{rms}=1.5±1 nm	Polycrystalline metal surface Non-crystalline oxide
Electropolished + anodized, 10 V +	TiO_2+~34–40% C, traces of Ca and Cl	180 nm	Heterogeneous, with smooth or porous regions, – 10 μm R_{rms}=16±2nm	Polycrystalline metal surface. Crystalline oxide (anatase)

topography/roughness, and substrate microstructure/oxide crystallinity) of titanium samples subjected to various treatments (Larsson *et al.*, 1994). Electropolished + anodized (1M acetic acid, room temperature) films are thicker than those formed by electropolishing and on 'clinical reference' (machined) surfaces. For 80V the oxide is crystalline.

Table 9.27 summarizes the composition and thickness of oxides formed on a Co–Cr–Mo alloy exposed to 'dry air' and 'wet steam' for 1 h (Lewis, 1993a).

9.4.7 Contact angles of oxide-covered surfaces

When a metallic surface covered by an oxide (either formed naturally or by an appropriate treatment) is placed in contact with the body or a culture medium adsorption of various species, namely proteins, is the prime event. Contact angle, θ, measurements can be used to ascertain the afinity of a liquid to a biomaterial surface, in particular when adsorption occurs, which is revealed by a decrease in θ. Generally speaking, θ is governed by the intermolecular forces between solid and liquid, and in the case of passive metals by the forces between metal oxide and liquid. is a complex function of surface roughness, oxide crystallinity and composition, liquid composition and time. Normally, wettability tends to progress from hydrophobic to hydrophilic. Table 9.28 gives the initial contact angles and the changes in contact angle as a function of time, $d\theta/dt$, for a number of materials (Oshida *et al.*, 1992). Pure Ni and Ti–6Al–AV have the lowest initial contact angle, θ_o, with low $d\theta/dt$; 316L stainless steel and Co–Cr alloy have high θ_o with low $d\theta/dt$; and pure Ti, Ni–Ti alloys and α-alumina have high θ and high $d\theta/dt$. Shot-peening and pre-oxidation (300° C, 30 min.) of the above materials reduced the standard deviation of contact-angle measurements, probably as a result of minimization of microscopic irregularities (Oshida *et al.*, 1993). In this work pure Ti exhibited the highest initial contact angle θ_o, and also the most noble corrosion potential. Both are related to the characteristics of the TiO_2 oxide that covers the metal surface. Note that the value of θ for Al_2O_3 is also high (Table 9.28).

Table 9.27 Composition of oxides formed on a Co–Cr–Mo alloy (Lewis, 1993a)

Medium	*Composition*	*Thickness*	*Remarks*
Dry air	$Co_{14}Cr_5MoO_{21}$	4 nm	May disaggregate into Co, Cr, Mo, CoO, CrO_2 and $Mo_x(OH)_y$ and suboxides of Co, Cr and Mo
Wet steam	$Co_3Cr_6MoO_{20}$	3 nm	May disaggregate into Co, Cr, Mo, $Co(OH)_2$, Cr_2O_3, CoOOH, $CoMoO_4$, $Mo_x(OH)_y$ and suboxides and hydrated species of Co, Cr and Mo

Table 9.28 Initial contact angles and changes in contact angles as function of time of oxidized surfaces of biomaterials after mechanical and buff polishing (Oshida et al., 1992)

	Mechanical polish-oxidizing		*Buff polish-oxidizing*	
	θ_o*(deg)*	$\delta\theta/\delta t$	θ_o*(deg)*	$\delta\theta/\delta t$
Pure Ti	54.24	-0.0046		
Ti6A14V	32.08	-0.0010	30.85	-0.0015
NiTi (m)	69.88	-0.0055	68.92	-0.0053
NiTi (a)	71.88	-0.0048		
316L s.s.	56.46	-0.0024	55.73	-0.0025
Pure Ni	35.72	-0.0016		
Co-Cr alloy	62.04	-0.0023	61.85	-0.0021
α-alumina	60.87	-0.0044		

m – martensite; a – austenite.

Table 9.29 Critical surface tension of Ti surfaces (Kilpadi and Lemons 1994)

Specimen	*Plot*	*Critical Surface Tension,* τ_c *(dyn/cm)*	*Comments*
I	C	—	No liquids were appropriate
	P	46.0±1.08	
	D	42.5±1.08	Only diiodomethane and bromonaphthalene were used
II	C	31.6±0.48	Water was not used in these analyses, as it did not fit with Good's criterion and also did not fall in line with the other liquids
	P	35.4±0.48	Only glycerol and thiodoethanol were used
	D	34.9±0.48	Only diiodomethane and bromonaphthalene were used
III	C	40.0±0.41	
		41.4±0.59	
	D	40.7±0.59	Only diiodomethane and bromonaphthalene were used
IV	C	41.9±0.79	
	P	41.5±1.05D	
	D	42.5±1.05	Only diiodomethane and bromonaphthalene were used
V	C	37.4±0.51	
	P	31.0±0.30	Water was not included
	D	41.8±0.51	Only diiodomethane and bromonaphthalene were used

I – Non-passivated, TFGD-treated, polished machined flats; II – Non-passivated, unsterilized, polished machined flats; III – Passivated, dry-heat-sterilized, polished machined flats; IV – Passivated, dry-heat-sterilized, polished coined flats; V – Passivated, dry-heat-sterilized, unpolished flats; C – Composite (includes all liquids); P – only polar liquids; D – only dispersive liquids. RFGD – Radio Frequency Glow Discharge.

The critical surface tension (CST), which is the highest surface tension of a liquid that completely wets a given surface, is given in Table 9.29 (Kilpadi and Lemons, 1994) for titanium subjected to various surface treatments. Polar (double-distilled water, glycerol and thiodoethanol) and dispersive (diiodomethane, bromonaphthalene, dicyclohexyl and decane) liquids were used in the study. Radio frequency glow discharge (RFGD)-treated samples showed the higher CST. Grain size (70 vs. 23 μm) did not affect the CST of polished, passivated, and dry-heat-sterilized titanium surfaces.

The equilibrium contact angles of cp Ti and Ti–6Al–4V, both passivated in nitric acid, were 52±2° and 56±4°, respectively (Keller *et al.*, 1994). Wettability was measured employing water drops. This similarity in contact angles reflets the similarity in oxide film composition found in the same work. However, the film on the alloy surface was significantly thicker (8.3±1.2 nm) than that on the cp Ti (3.2±0.8 nm).

REFERENCES

O.V. Akgun and O.T. Inal, 'Laser surface modification of Ti-6A1–4V alloy', *Journal of Materials Science*, **29,** 1159–1168 (1994).

A. Aladjem, 'Review Anodic oxidation of titanium and its alloys', *Journal of Materials Science*, **8,** 688–704 (1973).

M.A. Barbosa, 'Corrosion mechanisms of metallic biomaterials', Biomaterials Degradation-Fundamental Aspects and Related Clinical Phenomena, European Materials Research Society Monographs, Vol. **1** (eds. M.A. Barbosa, F. Burny, J. Cordey, E. Dorre, G. Hastings, D. Muster and P. Tranquilli-Leali), pp. 227–257, Elsevier Science Publishers, Amsterdam (1991 **a**).

M.A. Barbosa, 'Electrochemical impedance studies on calcium phosphate–metal interfaces', Bioceramics, Vol. **4** (eds. W. Bonfield, G.W. Hastings and K.E. Tanner), pp. 326–333, Butterworth-Heinemann (1991 **b**).

M.A. Barbosa, 'Surface layers and the reactivity of metallic implants', High-Tech Biomaterials, European Materials Research Society Monographs, Vol. **3** (eds. D. Muster, M.A. Barbosa, F. Burny, J. Cordey, E. Dorre, G. Hastings, and P. Tranquilli-Leali), pp. 257–283, Elsevier Science Publishers B.V., Amsterdam (1992).

J. Black, 'Biological Performance of Tantalum', *Clinical Materials*, **16,** 167–173 (1994)

N.C. Blumenthal and V. Cosma, 'Inhibition of apatite formation by titanium and vanadium ions', *Journal of Biomedical Materials Research: Applied Biomaterials*, **23,** 13–22 (1989).

M. Browne and P.J. Gregson, 'Surface modification of titanium alloy implants', *Biomaterials*, **15,** 894–898 (1994).

S.A. Brown, L.J. Farnsworth, K. Merritt, and T.D. Crowe, '*In vitro* and *in vivo* metal ion release', *Journal of Biomedical Materials Research*, **22,** 321–338 (1988).

R.A. Buchanan and I.S. Lee, 'Surface modification of biomaterials through noble metal ion implantation', *Journal of Biomedical Materials Research*, **24,** 309–318 (1990).

B.W. Callen, B.F. Lowenberg, S. Lugowski, R.N.S. Sodhi, and J.E. Davies, 'Nitric acid passivation of Ti6A14V reduces thickness of surface oxide layer and increases trace element release', *Journal of Biomedical Materials Research*, **29,** 279–290 (1995).

S.K. Chawla, S.A. Brown, K. Merritt, and J.H. Payer, 'Serum protein effects on polarization behavior of 316L stainless steel', *Corrosion* **46**, 147–152 (1990).

A. Cigada, G. Rondelli, B. Vicentini, M. Giacomazzi, and A. Roos, 'Duplex stainless steels for osteosynthesis devices', *Journal of Biomedical Materials Research*, **23,** 1087–1095 (1989).

A. Cigada, M. Cabrini, and P. Pedeferri, 'Increasing of the corrosion resistance of the Ti6A14V alloy by high thickness anodic oxidation', *Journal of Materials Science: Materials in Medicine*, **3,** 408–412 (1992).

J.P. Collier, V.A. Surprenant, R.E. Jensen, and M.B. Mayor, 'Corrosion at the interface of cobalt-alloy heads on titanium-alloy stems', *Clinical Orthopaedics*, **271,** 305–312 (1991).

S.D. Cook, M.R. Brinker, R.C. Anderson, R.J. Tomlinson and J.C. Butler, 'Performance of retrieved Kuntscher intramedullary rods: improved corrosion resistance with contemporary material design', *Clinical Materials*, **5,** 53–71 (1990).

S.D. Cook, R.L. Barrack, G.C. Baffes, A.J.T. Clemow, P. Serekian, N. Dong and M.A. Kester, 'Wear and corrosion of modular interfaces in total hip replacements', *Clinical Orthopaedics*, **298,** 80–88 (1994).

S.D. Cook, R.L. Barrack, A.J.T. Clemow, 'Corrosion and wear at the modular interface of uncemented femoral stems', *The Journal of Bone and Joint Surgery* [Br], **76-B,** 68–72 (1994).

L.D. Dorr, R. Bloebaum, J. Emmanual and R. Meldrum, 'Histologic, biochemical, and ion analysis of tissue and fluids retrieved during total hip arthroplasty', *Clinical Orthopaedics and Related Research*, nr. 261, 82–95 (1990).

P. Ducheyne and K.E. Healy, 'The effect of plasma-sprayed calcium phosphate ceramic coatings on the metal ion release from porous titanium and cobalt-chromium alloys', *Journal of Biomedical Materials Research*, **22,** 1137–1163 (1988).

M.L. Escudero and J.L. González-Carrasco, *In vitro* corrosion behaviour of MA956 superalloy *Biomaterials*, **15,** 1175–1180 (1994).

P. Frayssinet, F. Tourenne, N. Rouquet, G. Bonel, and P. Conté, Biological effects of aluminium diffusion from plasma-sprayed alumina coatings, *Journal of Materials Science: Materials in Medicine*, **5,** 491–494 (1994).

J.L. Gilbert, S.M. Smith and E.P. Lautenschlager, Scanning electrochemical microscopy of metallic biomaterials: reaction rate and ion release imaging modes, *Journal of Biomedical Materials Research*, **27,** 1357–1366 (1993**a**).

J.L. Gilbert, C.A. Buckley, and J.J. Jacobs, *In vivo* corrosion of modular hip prosthesis components in mixed and similar metal combinations. The effect of crevice, stress, motion, and alloy coupling, *Journal of Biomedical Materials Research*, **27,** 1533–1544 (1993**b**).

J. Gluszek and J. Masalski, Galvanic coupling of 316L steel with titanium, niobium, and tantalum in Ringer's solution, *British Corrosion Journal*, **27,** 135–138 (1992).

K. Hayashi, I. Noda, K. Uenoyama, and Y. Sugioka, Breakdown corrosion potential of ceramic coated metal implants, *Journal of Biomedical Materials Research*, **24,** 1111–1113 (1990).

R. Hazan, R. Brener and U. Oron, Bone growth to metal implants is regulated by their surface chemical properties, *Biomaterials*, **14,** 570–574 (1993).

K.E. Healy and P. Ducheyne, The mechanisms of passive dissolution of titanium in a model physiological environment, *Journal of Biomedical Materials Research*, **26,** 319–338 (1992).

K.E. Healy, and P. Ducheyne, Passive dissolution kinetics of titanium *in vitro, Journal of Materials Science. Materials in Medicine*, **4,** 117–126 (1993).

P.J. Hughes, S.A. Brown, J.H. Payer, and K. Merritt, The effect of heat treatments and bead size on the corrosion of porous F75 in saline and serum, *Journal of Biomedical Materials Research*, **24,** 79–94 (1990).

C.B. Johansson, J. Lausmaa, T. Rostlund, and P. Thomsen, Commercially pure titanium and Ti6Al4V implants with and without nitrogen-ion implantation: surface characterization and quantitative studies in rabbit cortical bone, *Journal of Materials Science: Materials in Medicine*, **4,** 132–141 (1993).

J. Karrholm, W. Frech, K.-G. Nilsson and F. Snorrason, Increased metal release from cemented femoral components made of titanium alloy, *Acta Orthop. Scand.*, **65,** 599–604 (1994).

B. Kasemo and J. Lausmaa, Material-tissue Interfaces: the role of surface properties and processes, *Environmental Health Perspectives*, **102,** 41–45 (1994).

J.C. Keller, C.M. Stanford, J.P. Wightman, R.A. Draughn and R. Zaharias, Characterizations of titanium implant surfaces. III, *Journal of Biomedical Materials Research*, **28,** 939–946 (1994).

D.V. Kilpadi and J.E. Lemons, Surface energy characterization of unalloyed titanium implants, *Journal of Biomedical Materials Research*, **28,** 1419–1425 (1994).

F.J. Kummer, J.L. Ricci, and N.C. Blumenthal, RF plasma treatment of metallic implant surfaces, *Journal of Applied Biomaterials*, **3,** 39–44 (1992).

C. Larsson, P. Thomsen, J. Lausmaa, M. Rodahl, B. Kasemo and L.E. Ericson, Bone response to surface modified titanium implants: studies on electropolished implants with different oxide thickness and morphology, *Biomaterials*, **15,** 1062–1074 (1994).

J. Lausmaa and B. Kasemo, Surface spectroscopic characterization of titanium implant materials, *Applied Surface Science*, **44,** 133–146 (1990).

G. Lewis, X-ray photoelectron spectroscopy study of surface layers on orthopaedic alloys. II. Co-Cr-Mo (ASTM F-75) alloy, *Journal of Vacuum Science Technology A*, **11,** 168–174 (1993**a**).

G. Lewis and K. Daigle, Electrochemical behavior of Ti-6Al-4V alloy in static biosimulating solutions, *Journal of Applied Biomaterials*, **4,** 47–54 (1993**b**).

B.F. Lowenberg, S. Lugowski, M. Chipman, and J.E. Davies, ASTM-F86 passivation increases trace element release from Ti6Al4V into culture medium, *Journal of Materials Science: Materials in Medicine*, **5,** 467–472 (1994).

S. Lugowski, D.C. Smith, and J.C. VanLoon, Critical aspects of trace element analysis of tissue samples: a review, *Clinical Materials*, **6,** 91–104 (1990).

R.D. Meldrum, R.D. Bloebaum, and L.D. Dorr, Metal ion concentrations in retrieved polyethylene total hip inserts and implications for artifactually high readings in tissue, *Journal of Biomedical Materials Research*, **27,** 1349–1355 (1993).

K. Merritt, R.W. Margevicius, and S.A. Brown, Storage and elimination of titanium, aluminium, and vanadium salts, *in vivo*, *Journal of Biomedical Materials Research*, **26,** 1503–1515 (1992).

Y. Okamoto and S. Hidaka, Studies on calcium phosphate precipitation: effects of metal ions used in dental materials, *Journal of Biomedicla Materials Research*, **28,** 1403–1410 (1994).

Y. Okazaki, A. Ito, T. Tateishi, and Y. Ito, Effect of alloying elements on anodic polarization properties of titanium alloys in acid solution, *Materials Transactions, JIM*, **35,** 58–66 (1994).

J.L. Ong, L.C. Lucas, G.N. Raikar, and J.C. Gregory, Electrochemical corrosion analyses and characterization of surface-modified titanium, *Applied Surface Science*, **72,** 7–13 (1993).

Y. Oshida, R. Sachdeva, and S. Miyazaki, Changes in contact angles as a function of time on some pre-oxidized biomaterials, *Journal of Materials Science: Materials in Medicine*, **3,** 306–312 (1992).

Y. Oshida, R. Sachdeva, S. Miyazaki, and J. Daly, Effects of shot-peening on surface contact angles of biomaterials, *Journal of Materials Science: Materials in Medicine*, **4,** 443–447 (1993).

J. Pan, D. Thierry, and C. Leygraf, Electrochemical and XPS studies of titanium for biomaterial applications with respect to the effect of hydrogen peroxide, *Journal of Biomedical Materials Research*, **28,** 113–122 (1994).

O.E.M. Pohler, Degradation of metallic orthopaedic implants, in Biomaterials in reconstructive surgery (ed. L.R. Rubin), Chap. 15, The CV Mosby Co., 1983, pp. 158–228.

M. Pourbaix, Atlas of electrochemcial equilibria, NACE/CEBELCOR, 1974.

A. Pourbaix, M. Marek and R.F. Hochman, Comportement electrochimique du titane à bas pH et bas potential d'électrode. *Rapports Techniques CEBELCOR*, **118**, RT 197, (1971).

L.M. Rabbe, J. Rieu, A. Lopez and P. Combrade, Fretting deterioration of orthopaedic implant materials: search for solutions, *Clinical Materials*, **15,** 221–226 (1994).

J.-P. Randin, Corrosion behavior of nickel-containing alloys in artificial sweat, *Journal of Biomedical Materials Research*, **22,** 649–666 (1988).

G. Ravnholt and J. Jensen, Corrosion investigation of two materials for implant supraconstructions coupled to a titanium implant, *Scandinavian Journal of Dental Research*, **99,** 181–186 (1991).

C.C. Ribeiro, M.A. Barbosa, A.A.S.C. Machado, A. Tudor, and M.C. Davies, Modifications in the molecular structure of hydroxyapatite induced by titanium ions, *Journal of Materials Science: Materials in Medicine*, **6,** 829–834 (1995).

C. Sella, J.C. Martin, J. Lecoeur, J.P. Bellier, M.F. Harmand, A. Nadji, J.P. Davidas, and A. Le Chanu, Corrosion protection of metal implants by hard biocompatible ceramic coatings deposited by radio-frequency sputtering, *Clinical Materials*, **5,** 297–307 (1990).

M.F. Semlitsch, H. Weber, R. Streicher and R. Schon, Joint replacement components made of hot-forged and surface-treated Ti-6Al-7Nb alloy, *Biomaterials*, **13,** 781–788 (1992).

S.R. Sousa and M.A. Barbosa, Electrochemistry of AISI 316L stainless steel in calcium phosphate and protein solutions, *Journal of Materials Science: Materials in Medicine*, **2,** 19–26 (1991).

S.R. Sousa and M.A. Barbosa, Corrosion resistance of titanium cp in saline physiological solutions with calcium phosphate and proteins, *Clinical Materials*, **14,** 287–294 (1993).

S.J. Stohs and D. Bagchi, Oxidative mechanisms in the toxicity of metal ions, *Free Radical Biology and Medicine*, **18,** 321–336 (1995).

D.S. Sutherland, P.D. Forshaw, G.C. Allen, I.T. Brown and K.R. Williams, Surface analysis of titanium implants, *Biomaterials*, **14,** 893–899 (1993).

P. Tengvall, L. Lundstrom, L. Sjokvist, H. Elwing, and L.M. Bjurstein, Titanium-hydrogen peroxide interaction: model studies of the influence of the inflammatory response on titanium implants, *Biomaterials*, **10,** 166–175 (1989).

P. Tengvall and I. Lundstrom, Physico-chemical considerations of titanium as a biomaterial, *Clinical Materials*, **9,** 115–134 (1992).

K.A. Thomas, S.D. Cook, A.F. Harding, and R.J. Haddad Jr., Tissue reaction to implant. corrosion in 38 internal fixation devices, *Orthopedics*, **11,** 441–451 (1988).

H. Tomás, A.P. Freire, and L.M. Abrantes, Cast Co–Cr alloy and pure chromium in proteinaceous media: an electrochemical characterization, *Journal of Materials Science: Materials in Medicine*, **5,** 446–451 (1994).

S. Torgersen and N.R. Gjerdet, Retrieval study of stainless steel and titanium miniplates and screws used in maxillofacial surgery, *Journal of Materials Science: Materials in Medicine*, **5,** 256–262 (1994).

D.L. Tsalev and Z.K. Zaprianov, Atomic absorption spectrometry in occupational and environmental health practice, Vol. I, CRC Press, Boca Raton, 1983.

J.A. von Fraunhofer, N. Berberich, and D. Seligson, Antibiotic-metal interactions in saline medium, *Biomaterials*, **10,** 136–138 (1989).

J.C. Wataha, C.T. Hanks, and R.G. Craig, Uptake of metal cations by fibroblasts *in vitro*, *Journal of Biomedical Materials Research*, **27,** 227–232 (1993).

A. Wisbey, P.J. Gregson, and M. Tuke Application of PVD TiN coating to Co-Cr-Mo based surgical implants, *Biomaterials*, **8,** 477–480 (1987).

R.L. Williams, S.A. Brown, and K. Merritt, Electrochemical studies on the influence of proteins on the corrosion of implant alloys, *Biomaterials*, **9,** 181–186 (1988).

10 Carbons

A.D. Haubold, R.B. More and J.C. Bokros

10.1 INTRODUCTION

The biocompatibility of carbon has long been appreciated: ancient man, for example, knew that pulverized charcoal could be placed under the skin without any apparent ill effects (Benson, 1969). The charcoal particles visibly remained indefinitely and thus allowed ancient man the means to decorate himself permanently with tattoos. However, it was not until the mid-1960s that carbon was first considered for use as a structural material in implantable prosthetic devices. During this period, a specific, imperfectly crystalline, man-made, pyrolytic form of carbon was found to be well suited for application in prosthetic heart valves. Because of the outstanding clinical success of pyrolytic carbon in long-term structural components of heart valve prostheses, carbons have assumed a prominent position in our repertoire of biomaterials and have sparked investigation of other forms of carbons for possible *in vivo* use. A number of these forms are listed in Table 10.1. This chapter will be devoted to a discussion of the background and historical uses of carbons in medical devices along with suggestions for future research.

10.1.1 Background

Although only two allotropic crystalline forms of elemental carbon, diamond and graphite occur in nature, carbon also occurs as a spectrum of imperfect crystalline forms that range from amorphous through mixed amorphous, graphite-like and diamond-like to the perfectly crystalline allotropes. Such imperfect crystalline structures are termed turbostatic and

Handbook of Biomaterial Properties. Edited by J. Black and G. Hastings.
Published in 1998 by Chapman & Hall, London. ISBN 0 412 60330 6.

Table 10.1 Carbon Forms

Pyrolytic Carbon	Produced at low or high temperature from the thermal pyrolysis of a hydrocarbon in a fluidized bed. These materials have a laminar, isotropic, granular or columnar structure and may be pure carbon or alloyed with various carbides.
Glassy or Polymeric Carbons	Obtained from the thermal pyrolysis (~1000 °C) of selected polymers and may be monolithic, porous or reticulated.
Artificial Graphites	Produced from a variety of starting materials such as petroleum or naturally occurring cokes and yield bulk structures of varying grain size, crystallite orientation, purity, porosity, strength, and particle size.
Carbon Fibers	Formed from spun polymeric fibers which are subsequently pyrolysed to yield structures of unusual strength and stiffness. The properties are a function of polymer precursor and processing history. More recently, carbon fibers have been grown from the vapor phase.
Charcoal	These are perhaps the oldest and most diverse materials with interesting adsorptive properties and are produced from many organic material spanning the range from wood to coconut shells to animal bones.
Vapor Phase Coatings	Applied, generally at reduced pressures (<1 atm) and often at low temperatures to provide a carbonaceous surface coating that ranges from amorphous to diamond-like with accompanying wide variation in thermal, mechanical and electrical properties.
Composites	Structures have been produced that utilize all of the above materials and even some other binders. Found in this group of materials are carbon fibers infiltrated and held together with pyrolytic carbon, silicon carbide, glassy carbon, PTFE, methyl methacrylate, epoxies, and petroleum pitches as well as combinations thereof. The structures may contain randomly oriented chopped fibers or long filaments oriented in random, 2, 3 and n dimensions.

give rise to considerable variability in physical and mechanical properties (Figure 10.1). Indeed, this ability of carbon to assume either perfectly crystalline or chaotic, turbostatic structures gives rise to confusion when considering physical and mechanical properties. For this reason, it is best to consider carbon as a spectrum of materials and to bear in mind that within this spectrum, a number of unique combinations of structure and physical and mechanical properties occur. This is true with respect to biocompatibility: the fact that one type of pyrolytic carbon has been used successfully in heart valves does not necessarily imply that other forms of pyrolytic carbons or indeed other forms of carbon in general will also prove useful in this or other prosthetic applications. For example, pyrolytic

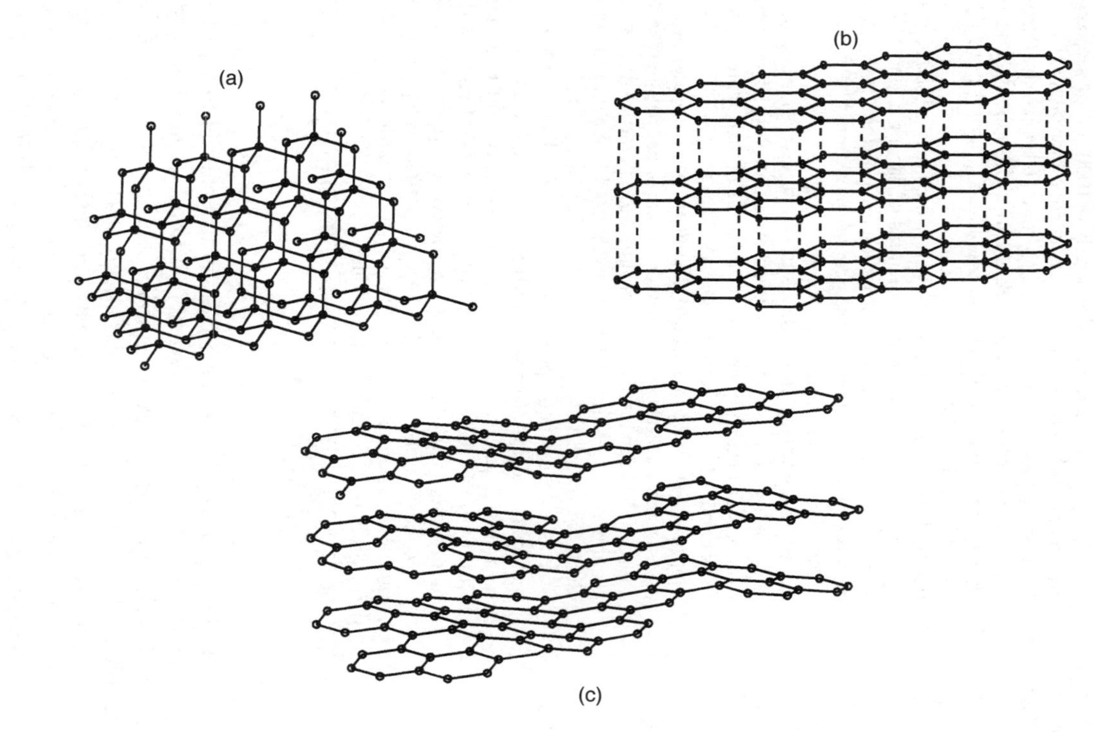

Figure 10.1 Possible atomic arrangements of crystalline carbon: (a) diamond tetrahydral, cyclohexane chair, crystalline structure, (b) graphite planar hexagonal layered structure (c) three-dimensional quasicrystalline turbostatic structure. Biomedical carbons have a turbostatic structure.

and glassy carbon can be finished to have identical appearances, yet the properties of glassy carbon make it unsuitable for use in prosthetic heart valves (Haubold *et al.*, 1981).

For successful use in implantable prostheses a material (1) must retain its properties required for device function in the hostile biological environment and (2) must not provoke adverse effects either locally or systemically. Most of the pure carbons are relatively inert and unlikely to provoke severe tissue reactions, however, only certain pyrolytic carbons have sufficient strength, fatigue resistance, wear resistance and biodegradation resistance to function as long-term implant structural components. In fact, the pyrolytic carbons were deliberately tailored to meet the specific biocompatibility requirements for heart valve component application (Bokros *et al*, 1972; Haubold, 1977). Silicon was added in small amounts (5–12 wt%) as an alloying element in order to form silicon carbide inclusions to assure adequate wear. Furthermore, specific processing parameters were identified in order to produce suitable microstructures and densities, as well as the strength levels required. Glassy carbon, as mentioned above, could not be prepared with adequate strength and wear resistance. Thus, biocompatibility cannot be presumed *a priori* for carbon materials: each particular application has specific demands which require a unique set of properties. While the spectrum of carbon materials encompasses many such properties, the particular material must be engineered to uniquely satisfy all of the properties needed.

10.1.2 Diamond

Diamond, the hardest substance known, has the so called *diamond cubic structure* consisting of a network of regular tetrahedral arrays in which each carbon atom is covalently bonded to four other carbon atoms forming the corners of a regular tetrahedron (Figure 10.1). From X-ray diffraction data, there is a single value, 1.54 Å bond length and a unit cube lattice spacing of 3.56 Å. The entire crystalline array is a single covalently bonded molecule. Because many covalent bonds must be broken to break the crystal, a very large amount of energy is required, therefore, the substance is very hard (Pauling, 1964). There has been an ongoing interest in the use of diamond or diamond-like coatings (May, 1995). However, suitable manufacturing processes do not yet exist that allow economical preparation of diamond type materials in the quantity, quality, shapes and sizes required for durable long term biomedical applications. A specific application uniquely requiring diamond or diamond-like material for clinical success has not been identified as a justification to compel additional research efforts in preparation techniques.

10.1.3 Graphites

Graphite has a layered hexagonal crystal structure. Each atom forms two single bonds and one double bond with its three nearest in-plane neighbors to form sheet-like layers of flat six atom ring arrays (Figure 10.1). Interatomic bond distances are 1.42 Å within the layer and 3.4 Å between each layer. Within each layer, bonding is covalent and between the layers, bonding is of the much weaker van der Waals type. Consequently, the layers are easily separated giving rise to the soft, lubricating properties of graphite.

Naturally occurring graphite is generally found as a isolated small scales or imperfect single crystal precipitates in granite. These small crystals such as those found in Madagascar, Ontario and in New York have dimensions on the order of a few millimeters. Larger graphite masses have been found in China and Korea. Natural graphites are thought to be formed by metamorphosis of sedimentary carbonaceous materials or by reaction with and precipitation from liquid magma. The naturally occurring graphite materials are useful primarily as the starting material for subsequent fabrication of some 'artificial graphites'.

Graphite was first synthesized accidentally by heating carborundum to extreme temperatures. The silicon was driven off leaving a graphite residue. A patent on this production process was granted over 100 years ago. Since then, petroleum and other types of cokes coupled with organic binders have become the major raw materials in the production of a wide variety of carbonaceous conglomerates called artificial graphite.

The manufacturing processes employed today are as varied as are the properties of the resultant materials. Bulk graphites are usually molded, extruded, hot isostatically compacted and may even be formed by combinations of these processes. They may be further reimpregnated with binder subsequent to graphitization (heat-treatment step), infiltrated isothermally or in a thermal gradient with methane or aromatic hydrocarbons. The resultant materials have widely varying properties and purity which can have a profound influence on the interaction of 'graphite' with the living environment.

Because of low strength and low wear resistance, graphite alone is not suitable as a structural member of an implant. But, investigations of colloidal graphite coatings as a blood compatible surface during the mid-1960s led investigators to examine pyrolytic carbon. Pyrolytic carbon, initially developed and used as a coating for nuclear fuel pellets, was found to have excellent blood compatibility, strength, wear resistance and durability for application in long term implants. The historical account leading to the use of LTI (low temperature-isotropic) pyrolytic carbon has been described (Bokros *et al.*, 1972, 1975). Graphite is widely used as a substrate for pyrolytic carbon coatings in heart valve components. In prosthesis applications, graphite is entirely encased in pyrolytic carbon coatings on the order of one mm thickness. Here the stronger, more durable coating stabilizes the interior graphite structures.

10.1.4 Pyrolytic carbons

Pyrolytic carbons of the type developed at General Atomic for use in bioengineering were an off-spring of research directed at developing carbon materials that would be suitable for structural applications in the severe environment of high-temperature, gas-cooled nuclear reactors. The isotropic carbon forms called high-temperature-isotropic carbon were derived from the gas phase nucleation and condensation of droplets formed during the pyrolysis of methane at temperatures in excess of 2000°C where densification can occur by thermally activated processes. The carbons called low-temperature-pyrolytic carbons are formed by the pyrolysis of other hydrocarbons (such as propane and propylene at lower temperatures in the range 1300–1500°C. The carbon materials so produced are not uniquely structured nor are all of them isotropic. Wide and complex variations in properties are possible ranging from weak to very strong, and in structure ranging from laminar and anisotropic, to isotropic, to columnar and granular, the latter also varying in anisotropy. A comprehensive review of the deposition and structure of pyrolytic carbon is given by Bokros (1969)

10.1.5 Glassy carbons

The preparation, structure and properties of glassy, or polymeric carbons has been described in detail by Jenkins and Kawamura (1976). These carbons are derived from a polymer by a slow pyrolysis process which results in a vitreous residue free of macroscopic bubbles.

Fabrication of glassy carbon materials is a relatively straightforward, but time consuming process. A preformed polymeric precursor such as phenol-formaldehyde, polyfurfuryl alcohol, polyvinyl alcohol or oxidized polystyrene is slowly heated in an inert atmosphere to a high temperature in excess of 2000 °C. Heating times may be as short as a day or as long as one month. It is not unusual to encounter exothermic temperature regions that must be traversed very slowly (i.e., 1 °C temperature increase per hour) to avoid the nucleation of bubbles.

There is a volumetric shrinkage of about 50% so the resultant structure formed in this process is a miniature of the precursor preform. The gases generated within the preformed structure must have time to diffuse out and not nucleate bubbles so one dimension of glassy carbon structures is limited to about seven millimeters. Hence materials or objects are limited to thin flat plates or tubes with thin walls. Massive equiaxed structures are not possible unless they are small with dimensions compatible with the diffusional requirements.

10.1.6 Carbon fibers

Carbon fibers, thought by many to be a relatively new material, actually have a long history as evidenced by the issuance of the first patent for incandescent electric lamp filaments (carbon fibers). The patent was issued to Thomas Edison in 1892. Hiram Maxim (the inventor of the machine gun, among other things) was issued a process patent for carbon fibers in 1899. Prior to the 1950s, these fibers had marginal strength and were used primarily for their electrical properties.

High strength carbon fibers were developed in the 1950s for the aerospace industry and military aircraft. The mechanical properties of rayon-based carbon fibers were enhanced using stress graphitization. Since that time, a variety of other precursors have been used including polyacrylonitrile (PAN), specific fractions of asphalt or pitch, lignin, lignosulfonates, hetero and nonheterocyclic aromatic polymers, linear polymers and even coal. The processes for fiber manufacture are as varied as the precursors themselves. In the patent literature, hundreds of processes and variants can be found (Sittig, 1980). Nevertheless, generalizations can be made. The first step in the process is the selection and treatment of a suitable raw material which can be carbonized to a high yield. The second step generally consists of a low temperature (250–500 °C) heat treatment or preoxidation followed by high temperature (up to 2800 °C) carbonization and graphitization steps.

The resultant fibers generally are of three types classified according to their structure and the degree of crystallite orientation. There are the high modulus (50 million psi or above), high strength fibers which, when incorporated into structures, give the highest stiffness per unit weight. Fibers with a lower modulus (about 30 million psi) but still of high strength are the second class of generally available fibers. The lowest modulus (less than 20 million psi) do not have structural applications.

10.1.7 Vapor phase coatings

Coatings formed at reduced pressure (<1 atm) are generally termed 'vapor deposited'. These coatings may be formed by physical vapor deposition, chemical vapor deposition or combinations thereof. Physical vapor deposition such as evaporation is probably the oldest technique for depositing thin films and involves generating a vapor from a source material at reduced pressure. The vapor subsequently condenses on the object to be coated. This technique suffers from a number of limitations such as only line-of-sight coating is possible. In the case of a carbon source, which does not evaporate but rather only sublimes at extreme temperatures, the object to be coated is exposed to direct thermal radiation from the subliming source. Few materials can withstand the intense thermal radiation for any great length of time. Hence coating thickness is limited as is the choice of substrate material to be coated. Much has been written on physical vapor deposition such as the comprehensive text by Maissel and Glang (1970).

More versatile coating techniques are broadly termed chemical vapor deposition (CVD). Coatings are formed through chemical reactions in the vapor phase or through the thermal decomposition or reduction of gases generally at reduced pressures. It is interesting to note that the process used to form pyrolytic carbon is a CVD process but is generally carried out at ambient pressures. The low temperature CVD processes are usually assisted by means of catalysts, glow discharge plasmas, ion beams and the like to activate gas reactions. In fact, production of diamond films is now almost routine through ion beam assisted disassociation of selected hydrocarbons in the presence of excess hydrogen. On the other hand, amorphous carbon films with little or no detectable crystallinity can also be produced by CVD. Thus chemical vapor deposition techniques are extremely versatile and consequently films and coatings produced by CVD must be carefully characterized and identified. An extensive and comprehensive review of thin film deposition technologies can be found in Bunshah (1982).

10.1.8 Composites

Even more complex than the materials described above are a family broadly termed 'composites'. Three-dimensional structures can be formed by combining a filler material with an appropriate matrix. Herein lies the difficulty with composites; all too often, the starting materials are not adequately described and the resultant structure characterized.

Carbon–carbon composites can be produced with a multitude of structures. The simplest have two-dimensional order and consist of stacked plies of carbon fabric held together by a carbon matrix. The fabric fibers may be any of those described previously, prepared from the pyrolysis of polyacrylonitrile and the like. The matrix could be derived from petroleum pitch or be infiltrated pyrolytic carbon or even silicon carbide. The latter are generally referred to as SiC/C composites. From two-dimensional, the next progression in structure is three-dimensional on to n-dimensional. This terminology refers to fiber orientation within the matrix.

Filament wound carbon composites have also been developed. In this case the desired shape is, as the name implies, wound using carbon fibers onto a suitable mandrel. The fibers are bonded using an epoxy type or thermoset resin. The bonding of the matrix to the fibers and direction of fiber orientation in large part determine the mechanical properties of the composite. The biological properties are generally governed by the selection of matrix.

10.2 HISTORICAL OVERVIEW – *IN VIVO* APPLICATIONS

Encouraged by the success of the LTI form of pyrolytic carbon in the demanding mechanical heart valve application, other carbon materials and usages were explored. Different carbon materials have been evaluated because pyrolytic carbon was patented on the one hand and processing constraints limited its versatility on the other hand. Shown in Table 10.2 are examples that demonstrate medical and engineering ingenuity in attempts to expand the use of carbons in the biological environment. Although the attempts are numerous and varied, only the use of carbon as components for artificial heart valves has achieved widespread usage.

10.2.1 Dental

One of the earliest applications of carbon as an implant material was in restorative dentistry. The first devices were bulky posts fabricated from glassy carbon that were implanted in the maxilla or mandible to serve as artificial tooth roots. Because of the inherent lack of strength of glassy carbon, they were bulky and poorly accepted. As a further complication, the stainless steel post on which a crown was cemented formed a galvanic couple *in vivo* leading to complications caused by accelerated corrosion of the stainless steel.

In another attempt, artificial tooth roots in the form of blades were fabricated from pyrolytic carbon. Although they were less bulky than the glassy carbon implants, they were difficult to place. Improper seating of the blade caused micromotion after implantation that ultimately caused the prosthesis to fail. The success rate of 60% after 5 years was judged inadequate. Metal blades coated with carbon fared a similar fate.

Metallic mandibular reconstruction trays coated with a vapor deposited film of carbon generally performed well. The application was complicated by the fact that the trays were custom and many times fashioned directly in the operating room, making the logistics of coating with carbon unacceptable.

10.2.2 Vascular

Graft prostheses >6mm diameter are generally considered to work well and improvements in performance as a result of modifying the biochemical nature of the graft lumen with carbon coatings are difficult to quantify and

Table 10.2 Applications of Carbon in Medical Devices

Active Component in Hemodetoxifier
Alveolar Ridge Maintenance Particles
Carbon Fiber Patch Fabrics
Cathether Tips
Coated Components for Membrane Oxygenators
Coated Emboli Filters
Coated Mandibular Trays
Coated Tracheal Prosthesis
Coated TMJ Condyle Prosthesis
Coated Prosthetic Fabrics and Polymers
Coated Aneurysm Clips
Coating on Angioplasty Stents
Coatings on Heart Valve Suture Rings
Coatings on Indwelling Catheters and Delivery Systems
Coatings on Vortex Blood Pumps
Coatings in Vascular Grafts
Components for Centrifugal Blood Pumps
Composites Soft Tissue Replacement

Dental Implants
- Posts
- Blades
- Coating on metallic implants

Electrodes
- Solid
- Coated

Ex vivo Blood Filters
Femoral Stems
- Coated
- Composite

Femoral Condyle Replacements
Femoral Heads
- Coated

Fracture Fixation Devices
Left Ventricular Apex Inlet Tubes
Ligaments and Tendons
Mechanical Heart Valve Components
Ossicular Replacement Prosthesis
Particles for Filling Periodontal Defects
Percutaneous Access Devices
Small Joint Replacements
- Hand
- Wrist
- Elbow
- Foot

Tibial Plateau Replacements
Vascular Attachment Prosthesis

Carbon forms

	Young's Modulus (GPa)	*Flexural Strength (MPa)*	*Hardness (DPH 500 g)*	*Density (g/cm³)*	*Fracture Toughness (Mpa√m)*	*Wear Resistance*
Diamond	760–1040	600–2000	5700–10400 Knoop	2.9–3.5	5–7	Potentially excellent
Pure pyrolytic carbon	28	486	>230	1.5–2.1	1.67	Excellent
Si-alloyed pyrolytic Carbon	31	389	>230	2.0–2.2	1.17	Excellent
Glassy or Polymeric Carbons	21	175	150	<1.54	0.5–0.7	Poor
Artificial Graphites	4–12	65–300	50–120	1.5–1.8	1.5	Poor
Carbon fibers	172–517	896–2585	*	1.6–1.8	*	*
Charcoal	NA	NA	NA	NA	NA	NA
Vapor phase coatings	17			1.8		
Composites	*	*	*	*	*	*

* Dependent upon matrix.

not significant enough to justify the cost of carbon coating. Improvements in the patency of small diameter grafts (<4 mm) as a result of carbon coating have been reported but even with the improvement, these grafts ultimately failed as a result of intimal hyperplasia proliferation at the anastomoses. While the carbon coating may retard clotting of certain grafts, the coating does little to ameliorate intimal hyperplasia formation. Carbon vascular attachment prostheses have also been reported to perform poorly, not as a result of poor biocompatibility, but rather the result of mechanical complications.

10.2.3 Orthopedics

Femoral stems fabricated from carbon composites fitted with a femoral head fabricated from pyrolytic carbon have been reportedly used successfully by some for over 10 years (Chen, 1986). Others have experienced disastrous failures through a lack of attention to engineering and material property details. Such failures naturally lead to questions on the suitability of 'carbon' for use in such medical devices. Attempts are underway to design and fabricate other joint replacements.

Ligaments and tendons have been fabricated from carbon fibers (Béjui and Drouin, 1988). These fibers in the initial stage perform well as a scaffolding material that aids in the regeneration of tendons and ligaments *in vivo*; but in the long term the fibers fracture and migrate to, for example, the lymph nodes.

Fracture fixation devices that are fabricated from stainless steel are unsuitable for coating or coupling with carbon because of galvanic effects (Haubold *et al.*, 1986). Carbon composite devices have been used reportedly with good results but such usage has not become widespread presumably because of an unaccepted cost/benefit ratio.

10.2.4 Other

Many applications of devices listed in Table 10.2, while successful, are not in widespread use because, even in their non-carbon form, usage is limited. For example, left ventricular apex tubes (Haubold *et al.*, 1979) are used successfully in the construction of a prosthesis to correct idiopathic hypertrophic subaortic stenosis but fortunately in man, such a medical condition is rare.

10.3 NEW DIRECTIONS/FUTURE TRENDS

LTI pyrolytic carbons, since their introduction in the late 1960s, have become the material of choice for use in the fabrication of mechanical prosthetic heart valves. Over 90% of the mechanical valves implanted worldwide utilize such carbon components. To date, more than 2 million valves have been implanted which amounts to an accumulated experience in excess of 12 million patient years. While this material has proven to be the most successful carbon biomaterial, it can be improved. Recently, advances in process control methodologies have allowed refinements in the pyrolytic carbon coating preparation. These improvements allow the elimination of the potentially thrombogenic silicon carbide from the biomedical coatings. Furthermore, this pure pyrolytic carbon can be produced with substantially improved mechanical properties relative to the silicon alloyed material (Emken *et al.*, 1993; Ely *et al.*, 1994,). Such improvements in the material open possibilities for improvements in heart valve prosthesis design and performance.

Results from investigations on the suitability of other forms of carbon for *in vivo* use yielded mixed and often seemingly contradictory results. Some of the confusion developed because of misunderstanding of carbon structure and misunderstanding of the relationship of carbon properties to such structures. The use of the generic label 'carbon' compounded the problem. A similar situation exists with 'polyurethanes'. There are polyether urethanes, polyester urethanes, polyether urethane ureas and even polyester urethane ureas – all misappropriately called simply 'urethanes'. Thus it is not surprising that the biological responses of 'carbon' (Table 10.1) are so varied.

Biocompatibility claims for a particular form of 'carbon' based on published results for a totally different form or structure should be carefully scrutinized. For example, to claim that carbon fibers have the same biological properties as bulk pyrolytic carbons or even that all pyrolytic carbons behave similarly is unjustified. In the case of fibers, geometry plays a significant role. It is well known that bulk materials may be well tolerated when the same material in particulate form may not. The lack of characterization and standardization can be devastating.

More and more entrants are anticipated into the field of carbon biomaterials. In the past, because of technology, patent or cost constraints, there were only several sources for, for example, pyrolytic carbon. A number of the earlier constraints have now been removed. Consequently, these materials are being produced in limited but increasing quantities in many countries, using a multiplicity of fabrication techniques. The challenge for the future is to be precise in material identification, characterization and to avoid generalization.

REFERENCES

Béjui, J. and Drouin, G. (1988). Carbon Fiber Ligaments. In *CRC Critical Reviews in Biocompatibility*, **4**(2), 79–108.

Benson, J. (1969). *Pre-Survey on the Biomedical Applications of Carbon*, North American Rockwell Corporation Report R-7855.

Bokros, J.C. (1969). Deposition, Structure, and Properties of Pyrolytic Carbon. In *Chemistry and Physics of Carbon*, Vol. 5 (Walker, P.L., ed.). Dekker, New York, pp. 1–118.

Bokros, J.C. LaGrange, L.D. and Schoen, F.J. (1972). Control of Structure of Carbon For Use in Bioengineering. In *Chemistry and Physics of Carbon*, Vol. 9 (Walker, P.L., ed.). Dekker, New York, 103–171.

Bokros, J.C., Akins, R.J., Shim, H.S., Haubold, A.D. and Agarwal, N.K. (1975). Carbon in Prosthetic Devices. In *Petroleum Derived Carbons* (Deviney, M.L., and O'Grady, T.M., eds). American Chemical Society, Washington, DC, pp. 237–265.

Bunshah, R.F. (ed.) (1982). *Deposition Technologies for Films and Coatings.*, Noyes Publications, Park Ridge.

Chen, Lan-Tian (1986). Carbon–Titanium Combined Joints. In *Chinese Journal of Biomedical Engineering* **3,** 55–61.

Ely, J., Haubold, A., Bokros, J. and Emken, M. (1994), New Unalloyed Pyrolytic Carbon with Improved Properties for Implant Applications, *XXI Congress European Society for Artificial Organs*, Oct. 20–22, Barcelona Spain. Also US Patent 5 514 410.

Emken, M., Bokros, J., Accuntis, J. and Wilde, D., (1993) Precise Control of Pyrolytic Carbon coating, *Extended Abstracts & Program Proceedings of the 21st Biennial Conference on Carbon*, Buffalo New York, June 13–18, pp. 531–532. Also US Patent 5 284 676.

Haubold, A.D., Shim, H.S., and Bokros, J.C. (1979). Carbon Cardiovascular Devices. In *Assisted Circulation* (Unger, F., ed.) Springer Verlag, Berlin, Heidelberg, New York, pp. 520–532.

Haubold, A.D. (1977). Carbon in Prosthetics. In *Annals of the New York Academy of Sciences*, Vol. 283, *The Behavior of Blood and its Components at Interfaces*, (Vroman, L. and Leonard E.F., eds). New York Academy of Sciences, New York.

Haubold, A.D., Shim, H.S., and Bokros, J.C. (1981). Carbon in Medical Devices. In *Biocompatibility of Clinical Implant Materials*, Vol II (Williams, D.F., ed.). CRC Press, Boca Raton, pp. 3–42.

Haubold, A.D., Yapp, R.A., and Bokros, J.C. (1986). Carbons for Biomedical Applications. in *Encyclopedia of Materials Science and Engineering* (Bever, M.B., ed.) Pergamon Press, Oxford, New York, Toronto, Sydney, Frankfurt, pp. 514–520.

Jenkins, G.M. and Kawamura, K. (1976). *Polymeric Carbons – Carbon Fibre, Glass and Char.* Cambridge University Press, Cambridge. London, New York, Melbourne.

Lewis, J.C. and Redfern, B., and Cowland, F.B. (1963). Vitreous Carbons as Crucible Materials for Semiconductors. In *Solid State Electronics*, **6,** 251.

Maissel, L.I. and Glang, R. (1970). *Handbook of Thin Film Technology*, McGraw-Hill, New York.

May, P.W. (1995), CVD Diamond – a new Technology for the Future?, *Endeavor Magazine* **19**(3), 101–106.

Pauling, L. (1964), *College Chemistry*, W.H. Freeman and Co., San Francisco.

Pierson, H.O. (1993) *Handbook of Carbon, Graphite, Diamond and Fullerenes*, Noyes Publications, Park Ridge, New Jersey.

Sittig, M. (1980). Carbon and Graphite Fibers. Noyes Data Corporation, Park Ridge. Mechanical Behavior of Diamond and Other Forms of Carbon, *Materials Research Society Symposium Proceedings*, Vol. 383, ed. Dory M.D. *et al.*, Materials Research Society, Pittsburgh, Pennsylvania, 1995.

PART III

General Concepts of Biocompatibility

1

D.F. Williams

1.1 INTRODUCTION

The host responses to biomaterials are extremely varied, involve a range of different mechanisms and are controlled by factors that involve characteristics of host, material and surgical procedure. These responses themselves constitute a significant component of the phenomenon of biocompatibility. In this section, the broad concepts of biocompatibility are critically reviewed with particular reference to the role that the human host response plays in determining the performance of the biomaterial and of the device in which it is used. Particular emphasis is given to the influence of biocompatibility in the clinical applications of devices. It should be remembered, however, that biocompatibility phenomena are extremely difficult to interrogate remotely or to study in an active way, so that accurate information of the details of biomaterial–human tissue interactions is not readily available. As Black (1) has pointed out with reference to observations on the host response in general, we are usually limited to detecting events long after they have occurred by examining end-points, usually histopathologically, after the host is dead. This is largely the case with experiments on biocompatibility in animals, but is an even more relevant observation with the human clinical experience. All comments in this section must therefore be interpreted with this in mind.

Handbook of Biomaterial Properties. Edited by J. Black and G. Hastings.
Published in 1998 by Chapman & Hall, London. ISBN 0 412 60330 6.

1.2 THE DEFINITION OF BIOCOMPATIBILITY

Etymologically, the term 'biocompatibility' sounds simple to interpret since it implies compatibility, or harmony, with living systems. This concept, however, is a little too simple to be useful and the meaning of compatibility has to be explored further.

It is intuitively obvious that a biomaterial or implanted medical device should cause no harm to the recipient by intent or by accident. This is the underlying principle of biological safety but is not the totality of biocompatibility. A material may well be entirely safe in the human body but unless it actually does something useful, it is not necessarily appropriate for a medical device. For many years during the evolution of biomaterials, this was not really taken into account and the 'requirements' of biomaterials were dominated by the perceived necessity to be safe, which was interpreted as a requirement that a biomaterial should be totally inert in the physiological environment and should itself exert no effect on that environment. In other words, there should be no interaction between biomaterials and the host, in the latter case implying that the material should be non-toxic, non-irritant, non-allergenic, non-carcinogenic, non-thrombogenic and so on.

This concept of biocompatibility, which equates the quality to inertness and biological indifference, has resulted in the selection of a portfolio of acceptable or standard biomaterials which have widespread usage. These range from the passivatable alloys such as stainless steel and titanium alloys, the noble metals gold and platinum, to some oxide ceramics such as alumina and zirconia, various forms of carbon and a range of putatively stable polymeric materials including silicone elastomers (polysiloxanes), polyolefins, fluorocarbon polymers and some polyacrylates. Of course, if this was all there was to biocompatibility, there would be few problems other than optimizing inertness and there would be little to write about.

In practice, biocompatibility is far more complex. There are at least four reasons for this. The first is that inertness in the physiological sense requires a great deal more than resisting degradation at the atomic or molecular level and the second is that even if it were so, this goal is extremely difficult to achieve. Indeed it is now recognized that no material is totally inert in the body. Even those very stable materials mentioned above will interact to some extent with tissues; titanium, although one of the most corrosion resistant engineering alloys, corrodes in the body, as judged by the presence of the metal in the surrounding tissues as well as serum and urine. With many materials, while the main component itself may be exceptionally inert, there are often minor components, perhaps impurities or additives which can be released under some circumstances. The leaching of plasticizers and other additives from plastics provide good examples of interactions which are not related to the molecular breakdown of the material but which confer a degree of instability to the product. Moreover, in the context of interactions which affect the overall performance of the material in the physiological environment, it is important to note that an interfacial reaction involving a physicochemical process such as protein adsorption will take place with the vast majority of materials, further emphasizing the fact that inertness is a very relative term and there is indeed no such thing as an inert biomaterial.

The third reason why biocompatibility cannot be equated with inertness is that there are several, and indeed an increasing number, of applications which involve intentionally degradable materials. The two most widely quoted situations here are absorbable sutures and implantable drug delivery systems but many more circumstances where degradable scaffolds and matrices could form an essential component of a device are envisaged. If biocompatibility is predicated on inertness, then degradable materials cannot, by definition, be biocompatible. This clearly does not make sense and suggests that the concept of biocompatibility needs to be altered.

The fourth reason is even more compelling, especially when considering biomaterials used in devices for tissue reconstruction. If a device is made from materials which are inert and which do not interact with the body in any way, then it is unlikely that it can be truly incorporated into the body. For effective long term performance in the dynamic tissue environment, it is far more preferable for there to be functional incorporation, which implies that the device should be stimulating the tissues to be reactive to it positively rather than negatively. Thus biocompatibility should not be concerned with avoiding reactions but selecting those which are the most beneficial to device performance.

On the basis of these ideas, biocompatibility was redefined a few years ago (2), as ‘the ability to perform with an appropriate host response in a specific situation.’ Clearly this definition encompasses the situation where inertness is still required for the most appropriate response in some situations is indeed no response. A traditional bone fracture plate is most effective when it is attached mechanically to the bone and does not corrode; no response of the tissue to the material is normally required. Even here, however, we have to concede that a material that could actively encourage more rapid bone healing might be beneficial so that a specific osteoinductive response would be considered appropriate.

More importantly, the definition allows a material to stimulate or otherwise favour a specific response, including cell activation, where that response optimizes the performance of the device. It will be obvious that the required response will vary with the particular application, which clearly implies that the response, both desired and actual, will vary with the different types of tissue encountered by biomaterials.

The above definition also stipulates that the biocompatibility of a material has to be qualified by reference to the specific application. The response to some very common and popular biomaterials may vary quite considerably and some of the major problems of implantable medical devices have been caused by a misunderstanding about transferability of biocompatibility data. To recognize the very effective performance of a material under one set of conditions but then to assume that the same material can perform equally well under entirely different circumstances is inherently dangerous since it takes into account neither the variations one might expect to see in the host response from site to site nor the fact that what is appropriate for one situation may not be appropriate for another.

1.3 COMPONENTS OF BIOCOMPATIBILITY

The above definition of biocompatibility helps to explain the subject area but cannot describe exactly what it is. For this purpose we have to consider the various components that are involved in biocompatibility processes. Biocompatibility refers to the totality of the interfacial reactions between biomaterials and tissues and to their consequences. These reactions and consequences can be divided into four categories. These involve different mechanisms and indeed quite separate sectors of science but are, nevertheless, inter-related.

The first component is that of the protein adsorption mentioned above. This process is initiated as soon as a material comes into contact with tissue fluids such that relatively quickly the surface of the biomaterial is covered with a layer of protein. The kinetics and extent of this process will vary from material to material which will in any case be a dynamic phenomenon with adsorption and desorption processes continuously taking place. Under some circumstances, this layer is extremely important in controlling the development of the host response since cell behavior near the material may depend on interactions with these proteins. For example, thrombogenicity is controlled by a number of events including the interaction between plasma proteins and surfaces, these proteins being able to influence the attachment of platelets to the surface. In other circumstances, the effects of this protein layer are far from clear.

The second component of biocompatibility is that of material degradation. It is emphasized here that degradation is a component of biocompatibility rather than a separate phenomena. There is still confusion over this since it is often perceived that degradation, which occurs on the material side of the interface, is the counterpart to biocompatibility which is equated with the other (tissue) side. This is not correct since degradation is the counterpart to the local host response, both being contributory to the biocompatibility of the system.

Degradation phenomena are covered elsewhere in this *Handbook* and will not be discussed in detail here. It is necessary to point out, however, that descriptions of material degradation mechanisms have to take the special, and indeed unique, features of the tissue environment into account. Whatever its location, a biomaterial will continuously encounter an aqueous environment during its use. This is not simply a saline solution, however, but a complex solution containing a variety of anions and cations, a variety of large molecules some of which are very reactive chemically, and a variety of cells which again may be in passive or active states. There are occasions when a degradation process can be explained, mechanistically and qualitatively, by the presence of an electrolyte. This is the situation with most metals when they suffer from corrosion in physiological environments(3). Even here, however, it is known that the kinetics of corrosion may be influenced by the organic species present, especially the proteins, and it is even possible for the corrosion mechanism to be somewhat different to that found in non-biological situations.

With other groups of materials, however, and especially with polymers, kinetics, mechanisms and consequences of the degradation are fundamentally related to the details of the environment. Although hydrolysis remains the substantive mechanism for degradation of most heterochain polymers, including polyurethanes, polyamides and polyesters, this hydrolysis may be profoundly influenced by the active species present in the tissue, especially in the tissue of the inflammatory response to materials. Included here are the influences of lysosomal enzymes (4). Moreover the hydrolysis may be supplemented by oxidative degradation, again occurring not only by virtue of passively dissolved oxygen in body fluids, but (and probably far more importantly) by active oxidative species such as superoxides, peroxides and free radicals, generated by activated inflammatory cells such as macrophages. It is thus possible for homochain polymers not particularly susceptible to hydrolysis and not normally oxidized at room temperature, to undergo oxidative degradation upon implantation (5). Polyolefins such as polyethylene and polypropylene come into this category.

The term 'biodegradation' is often used to describe degradation which occurs in such situations although the circumstances of and requirements for degradation to be so described have not been entirely clear. A recently agreed definition of biodegradation (6) states quite simply that it is the breakdown of a material mediated by a biological environment. The interpretation of 'biological' is left to the reader.

The purpose of explaining the role of the biological, or physiological environment in degradation phenomena, was to emphasize the crucial significance of the interaction between degradation and the host response, for not only can degradation be influenced by the host response but also it can control that response.

To explain this in a little more detail, let us consider the evolution of the local host response, which is the third component of biocompatibility, using a model that involves inflammatory and repair processes (7). Whenever a material is implanted into the tissues of the body, there has to be a degree of trauma associated with the insertion process. This will inevitably establish an acute inflammatory response, which is the body's natural defence mechanism to any injury. The inflammation is totally desirable and helpful since it is the precursor to the second phase of the response, which is that of tissue repair. The response to a surgical incision is acute inflammation followed by repair, the consequences of which are a zone of fibrous (collagenous) scar tissue. If a biomaterial is placed within the tissue, this response will be modified by its presence, but the extent to which that modification occurs depends on many factors.

Considering first the role of the material, if that material were totally inert chemically and unable to react at all with the tissues, and if the device were not able to irritate the tissues in any way, the perturbation to the inflammation/repair sequence is minimal, and the result will be the formation of a zone of fibrous tissue analogous to the scar, but oriented in such a way as to envelope the implant. The classical response to an implant is its encapsulation by soft fibrous tissue. On the other hand, if the material is able to react with the tissues, chemically, mechanically or any other way, it will act as a persistent stimulus to inflammation. While there is nothing inherently harmful about inflammation as a response to injury, persistent inflammation occurring as a response to a persistent injury is less acceptable. At the very least, this results in a continued stimulus to fibrosis such that the capsule is far more extensive and may intervene between the material and tissue it is meant to be in contact with (for example bone in the case of joint prostheses) but perhaps more importantly it can change the immediate tissue environment from one of quiescent fibrosis to that of active chronic inflammation. This is rarely the appropriate response and, as noted above, is likely to generate an even more aggressive environment.

In the context of the definition of biocompatibility, therefore, it is important that the interaction between the material and the tissues is one which leads to an acceptable balance between inflammation and repair. A few points may serve to explain this further and qualify appropriateness. First, the nature of the host response and those features which constitute acceptability will vary very considerably from one host to another and from one location (or set of circumstances) to another within a particular host. It is often forgotten that host variables are as important as material variables in the determination of biocompatibility. This is particularly important when the wide variety of tissue characteristics is considered. Obviously bone is very different from nerve tissue or a vascular endothelium and there will be very considerable difference in the details of their responses. Not all tissues of the same variety will be able to respond in the same way and it should always be remembered that host variables such as age and overall health status will have a major effect.

Secondly, the importance of time and the sequence of events should never be underestimated. While the above model describes the sequence from surgical intervention to inflammation to repair, such that the process may undergo rapid resolution, with a resulting long lasting equilibrium, the inflammation may be restimulated at any time and rarely can we guarantee long term survival. In this context the third point becomes important, for any feature of the interaction between material and tissue and material can be responsible. In many situations it is the chemical reactivity, represented by degradation processes, which drives the inflammatory response, but it can equally well be a process by which fragments of the material are extracted by physical or mechanical means. The release of wear debris from orthopaedic prostheses is a good example here, since the presence of such particles in sufficient numbers can have a profound effect on the tissue response, which is mediated by the mechanisms of inflammation but where the clinical results, manifest by loosening of the prostheses, may not be seen for quite some time(8). As far as the response to debris is concerned, in general the effects of released fragments will be quite different to those of bulk materials, both by virtue of physical factors as well as changed chemical factors.

Thirdly, the identification of these events and their importance leads to various possibilities for the control of biocompatibility. In the balance of inflammation and repair we have the possibilities of controlling that balance by aiming to eliminate or at least minimize those events which are undesirable for one set of conditions or alternatively enhancing or optimizing those events which are most desirable. This has led to the emergence of the concept and indeed introduction of bioactive materials which have been defined as biomaterials that are designed to elicit or modulate biological activity.

As a final point about the local host response, it has to be recognized that there are significant regional and tissue-specific variations to the phenomena. These cannot be described here, but it is important to mention the particular case with blood. When a biomaterial comes into contact with blood, there are many different mechanisms by which the blood can interact with the material, most of which are preferably avoided. The most important of these are those processes, alluded to in an earlier paragraph, that are responsible for the clotting of blood. This is a vital defense mechanism which prevents death by uncontrolled bleeding under everyday circumstances, but unfortunately in the context of biomaterials, the two processes which can, either separately or together, initiate the formation of a blood clot, that is contact phase activation of clotting proteins and platelet activation, are themselves initiated by contact with foreign surfaces. Thrombogenicity, defined as the property of a material which promotes and/or induces the formation of a thrombus, is clearly an important feature of biocompatibility.

Turning now to the last component of biocompatibility, we have to recognize that if there is an interfacial reaction, there is no reason why the products of that reaction and their effects have to be confined to the locality of that interface and the presence of a benign local response is not necessarily indicative of the absence of any systemic or remote site effects. The possibility of systemic effects arising from the presence of biomaterials has long been recognized, although extreme difficulties exist with their identification and interpretation. Indeed, at the present time, there are few systemic effects that can be readily identified with biomaterials. The transformation of a thrombus into an embolus derived from an intravascular device has obvious implications and we can imagine and often demonstrate the systemic consequences of using overtly cytotoxic materials. However, the more intriguing speculations refer to the putative implant-related carcinogenicity and even more speculative implant-related immune responses. At this stage we have to be concerned about such possibilities but have to put the subject into context. While we cannot deny that there are possible mechanisms for biomaterials to induce tumors, the evidence that they do so in human clinical experience is very sparse. While it is possible for some hypersensitivity responses to be seen to implants, the evidence for any clinically ignificant response from the immune system to biomaterials is even less available.

1.4 CONCLUSIONS

This review attempts to outline the main concept that currently prevail in the subject area of biocompatibility. Clearly it is a complex subject, about which we are still relatively ignorant, not least because it involves a juxtaposition between two quite different sectors of science, the materials sciences and the molecular/cellular biological sciences. Based on these concepts, however, a better understanding is now emerging so that our biomaterials can be chosen, and where necessary treated, in order to determine that the tissues of the host do indeed respond appropriately to them.

ADDITIONAL READING

Black, J. (1992) *Biological Performance of Materials – Fundamentals of Biocompatibility*, 2nd edn, Marcel Dekker, Inc., New York.

A recently updated introductory text describing the basic principles of the performance of biomaterials in biological environments and the relevance of the biomaterial-tissue interactions.

Hench, L.L. and Etheridge, E.C. (1982) *Biomaterials: An Interface Approach*, Academic Press, New York.

An early text describing concepts of biomaterials and their interactions with tissues, concentrating on the interface and based on the authors' experiences with bioceramics.

Williams, D.F. (ed.) (1981) *Fundamental Aspects of Biomaterials*, Volumes I & II, CRC Press, Boca Raton.

An edited collection of contributions dealing with the major components of biocompatibility mechanisms, including corrosion and degradation phenomena, toxicology and the local tissue response.

REFERENCES

1. Black, J. (1984) Systemic effects of biomaterials. *Biomaterials*, **5,** 11–18.
2. Williams, D.F. (1987) *Definitions in Biomaterials*, Elsevier, Amsterdam, pp. 49–59.
3. Williams, D.F. (1985) Physiological and microbiological corrosion. *CRC Critical Reviews in Biocompatibility*, **1**(1), 1–24.
4. Williams, D.F., Smith, R. and Oliver, C. (1987) The enzymatic degradation of polymers *in vitro*. *Journal of Biomedical Materials Research*, **21,** 991–1003.
5. Williams, D.F. and Zhong, S.P. (1991) Are free radicals involved in the biodegradation of implanted polymers? *Advanced Materials*, **3,** 623–626.
6. Williams, D.F., Black, J. and Doherty, P.J. (1992), in Doherty, P.J., Williams, R.L., Williams, D.F. *et al.* (eds.) *Biomaterial-Tissue Interfaces, Advances in Biomaterials*, Volume 10. Elsevier, Amsterdam, pp. 525–533.
7. Williams, D.F. (1989) A model for biocompatibility and its evaluation. *Journal of Biomedical Engineering*, **11,** 185–192.
8. Williams, D.F. (1976) Biomaterials and biocompatibility. *Med. Prog. Tech.*, **4**(1/2), 31–42.

2 Soft tissue response

J.M. Anderson

2.1 INTRODUCTION

Soft tissue responses to biomaterials for medical devices are generally viewed from the inflammation and wound healing perspectives and are usually considered as parts of the tissue or cellular host responses to injury. Placement of a biomaterial or medical device in the soft tissue environment involves injection, insertion, or surgical implantation, all of which injure the tissues or organs involved. Early host responses are dynamic and change with time (Table 2.1). It is important to consider this time variable in determining the host response or biocompatibility of a material.

2.2 TYPES OF RESPONSE

Four general types of response may occur following the implantation of a biomaterial. These are a minimal response, a chemically induced response, a physically induced response, and cellular/tissue necrosis [1].

A minimal response is generally called fibrous encapsulation and the implant is encapsulated within fibrous tissue containing mainly collagen with a few fibroblasts. At the tissue/implant interface, a one to two cell layer of macrophages and foreign body giant cells is present which constitutes the foreign body reaction.

Chemically induced responses may range from an acute, mild inflammatory response to a chronic, severe inflammatory response. These responses may be the result of leaching of biomaterial additives or degradation products.

Handbook of Biomaterial Properties. Edited by J. Black and G. Hastings.
Published in 1998 by Chapman & Hall, London. ISBN 0 412 60330 6.

Table 2.1 Sequence of Local Events Following Implantation

Injury
Acute Inflammation
Chronic Inflammation
Granulation Tissue
Foreign Body Reaction
Fibrosis

Physically induced responses are usually the result of the size, shape, porosity, and other geometric factors of the biomaterial or device. The form and topography of the surface of the biomaterial may determine the composition of the foreign body reaction. With biocompatible materials, the composition of the foreign body reaction and the implant site may be controlled by the surface properties of the biomaterial, the form of the implant, and the relationship between the surface area of the biomaterial and the volume of the implant. High surface to volume implants such as fabrics, porous materials, or particulate, will have higher ratios of macrophages and foreign body giant cells at the implant site than will smooth-surface implants, which will have fibrosis as a significant component of the implant site [2–5]. These three general types of responses are generally found with biocompatible materials.

The fourth type of response, i.e., cellular necrosis, is a toxic reaction which leads to cell death. It is generally taken as a sign of the incompatibility of a material and is generally the response to highly toxic additives, residual monomer, or degradation products released from the biomaterial [6]. The similarity between chemically induced responses leading to chronic, severe inflammatory responses and cellular/tissue necrosis should be considered in determining the biocompatibility of a biomaterial.

Mechanical factors and edge effects may modify the response to a biomaterial. Implant motion or micromotion can lead to variations in the fibrous capsule thickness and the composition of the fibrous capsule and the interfacial foreign body reaction. Edges and sharp changes in surface features may lead to a variation in fibrous capsule thickness and the presence of variable concentrations of chronic inflammatory cells, i.e., monocytes and lymphocytes.

Immune and neoplastic responses are specialized responses which are rarely seen with biomaterials and medical devices. Immune responses are generally created by the phagocytosis of particulate by macrophages which biochemically process the material and communicate with lymphocytes to produce the immune response. The metal sensitivity response is a well-known immune response to metallic corrosion products. Neoplastic, i.e., tumor formation, responses are generally considered to be an example of solid state tumorigenesis. Solid state tumorigenesis is generally linked to the extent or degree of fibrous capsule formation and the potential for solid state tumorigenesis is reduced with increasing foreign body reaction.

2.3 INFLAMMATION

Inflammation is defined as the reaction of vascularized living tissue to local injury (Table 2.1) [7,8]. The size, shape, and intended application of a biomaterial or medical device determine the implantation procedure which in turn determines the extent or degree of initial injury. The size, shape, and chemical and physical properties of the biomaterial may be responsible for variations in the intensity and time duration of the inflammatory and wound healing processes. Figure 2.1 illustrates the temporal sequence of inflammation and wound healing. The inflammatory response is a series of complex reactions involving various types of cells whose implant site concentrations (densities), activities and functions are controlled by various endogenous and autogenous mediators [9]. The predominant cell type present in the inflammatory response varies with the age of the injury, i.e., the time since the implant was inserted. Neutrophils, which are the characteristic cell type of acute inflammation, predominate during the first several days following implantation and are replaced by monocytes as the predominant cell type. Acute inflammation is of relatively short duration, lasting from minutes to days, depending on the extent of injury. The main characteristics of acute inflammation are the exudation of fluid and plasma proteins (edema) and the immigration of leukocytes (predominantly neutrophils). Following localization of leukocytes at the implant site, phagocytosis and the release of enzymes, reactive oxygen intermediates (ROI), and other agents occur following activation of neutrophils and macrophages. Agents released from activated leukocytes, hydrogen ions (acid), enzymes, ROIs and others, may effect the biodegradation of biomaterials [10,11]. The major role of the neutrophils in acute inflammation is to phagocytose and destroy microorganisms and foreign material.

Acute inflammation is of relatively short duration, lasting from minutes to days, and is dependent on the extent of injury. As the acute inflammatory response subsides, monocytes and lymphocytes predominate in the implant site and are the characteristic cells of chronic inflammation [7,8]. Monocytes, migrating from the blood, in the acute and chronic inflammatory responses differentiate into macrophages within the tissue in the implant site. These macrophages will fuse or coalesce into foreign body giant cells (Figure 2.1). Macrophages and foreign body giant cells are prominent at the tissue/implant interface, even with biocompatible materials. In Figure 2.1, the intensity and time variables are dependent upon

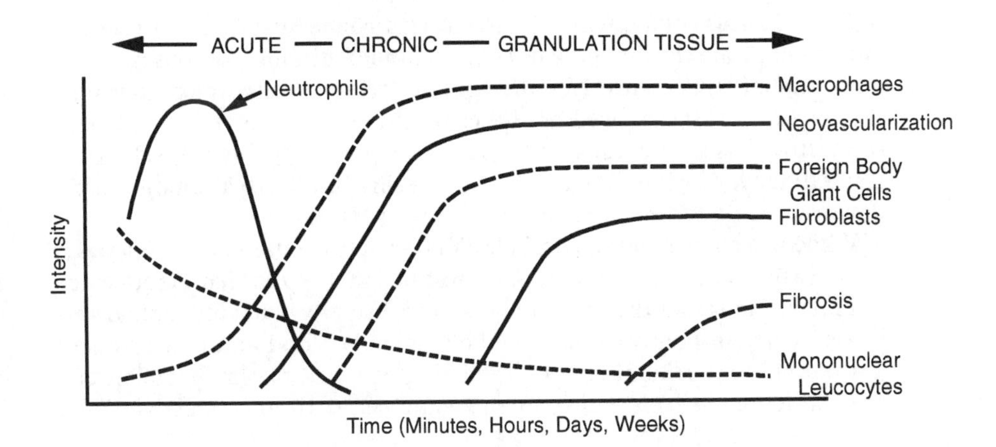

Figure 2.1 The temporal variation in the acute inflammatory response, chronic inflammatory response, granulation tissue development, and foreign body reaction to implanted biomaterials. The intensity and time variables are dependent upon the extent of injury created in the implantation and the size, shape, topography, and chemical and physical properties of the biomaterial.

the extent of injury created in the implantation and the size, shape, topography, and chemical and physical properties of the biomaterial.

In the phagocytosis process, recognition and attachment of neutrophils and monocytes/macrophages are expedited when the biomaterial is coated by naturally occurring blood serum factors called opsonins. The two major opsonins are IgG and the complement-activated fragment C3b. Both of these plasma-derived proteins are known to adsorb to biomaterials and neutrophils and macrophages have corresponding cell membrane receptors for these opsonization proteins. These receptors may also play a role in the activation of the attached neutrophils, monocytes, macrophages, or foreign body giant cells. Small particles, of the order of 5 μm in largest dimension, may undergo the phagocytosis or engulfment process by neutrophils, monocytes/macrophages, or specialized cells in the reticuloendothelial system (liver, spleen, etc.). Medical devices with surface areas of biomaterial many times greater than the size of the cell may stimulate frustrated phagocytosis. Frustrated phagocytosis does not involve engulfment of the biomaterial but rather the extracellular release of leukocyte products in an attempt to degrade or destroy the biomaterial [12]. Macrophages and foreign body giant cells adherent to the surface of the biomaterial may undergo frustrated phagocytosis with the release of hydrogen ion (acid) enzymes, ROIs, and others. Little is known regarding the extent or time period of frustrated phagocytosis and its dependence on the chemical and physical properties of the biomaterial.

The cells and components of vascularized connective tissue (Table 2.2) are involved in the inflammatory and wound healing responses. Thus, injury to soft tissues involves the specific types of cells which constitute the organ or tissue as well as the cells and components of vascularized connective tissue. Vascularized connective tissue can be viewed as the general network which holds together specific cell types in unique three-dimensional patterns to constitute organs or tissues.

While it is convenient to consider blood–material interactions separately from tissue–material interactions, it must be emphasized that blood–material interactions and the inflammatory response are intimately linked and, in fact, early responses to injury involve mainly blood and blood vessels. Therefore, both cellular and humoral elements, i.e., plasma proteins, etc., are considered as cells and components of vascularized connective tissue.

2.4 WOUND HEALING AND FIBROSIS

The wound healing response is initiated by the action of monocytes and macrophages, followed by proliferation of fibroblasts and vascular endothelial cells, i.e., capillaries, at the implant site. The proliferation of fibroblasts and the formation of capillaries constitute granulation tissue. Modified fibroblasts, i.e., myofibroblasts, which have contractile properties which assist in wound site closure are transiently present in granulation tissue. As fibroblasts predominate over macrophages in the healing response, collagens and other extracellular matrix molecules are deposited in the implant site. The extent of the wound healing response is generally dependent on the extent or degree of injury or defect created by the implantation procedure. Wound healing progresses by primary union (or first intention) if the healing is clean such as a surgical incision in

Table 2.2 Cells and Components of Vascularized Connective Tissue

Intravascular (blood) cells	Blood plasma proteins
Erythrocytes (RBC)	Coagulative Proteins
Neutrophils	Complement Proteins
Monocytes	Albumin
Eosinophils	Fibrinogen
Lymphocytes	Gamma-Globulins
Basophils	Others
Platelets	Extracellular matrix components
Connective tissue cells	Collagens
Mast Cells	Elastin
Fibroblasts	Proteoglycans
Macrophages	Fibronectin
Lymphocytes	Laminin

which the wound edges have been approximated by surgical sutures, clips, or staples. Healing under these conditions occurs with a minimal loss of tissue. Wound healing by secondary union (or secondary intention) occurs when there is a large tissue defect that must be filled or there has been an extensive loss of cells and tissue. In wound healing by second intention, regeneration of specific organ or tissue cells cannot completely reconstitute the original architecture and more granulation tissue is formed resulting in larger areas of fibrosis or scar formation. Thus, the surgical procedure to create the implant site may influence the extent or degree of the wound healing response.

The end-stage healing response to biomaterials and medical devices is generally fibrous encapsulation by collagenous fibrous tissue. This has been previously described as the minimal response. In the minimal response, the tissue/implant interface has a layer of macrophages and foreign body giant cells, i.e., foreign body reaction, on the surface of the biomaterial and this is surrounded or encapsulated by a fibrous capsule which is composed of collagen, proteoglycans, and other extracellular matrix molecules. Fibroblasts may be present in the fibrous capsule.

2.5 REPAIR OF IMPLANT SITES

Repair of implant sites involves two distinct processes: regeneration, which is the replacement of injured tissue by parenchymal cells of the same type, or replacement by fibrous connective tissue that forms a capsule [7]. These processes are generally controlled by either (i) the proliferative capacity of the cells in the tissue or organ receiving the implant and the extent of injury as it relates to tissue destruction or (ii) persistence of the tissue framework of the implant site. The regenerative capacity of cells permits their classification into three groups: labile, stable (or expanding), and permanent (or static) cells. Labile cells continue to proliferate throughout life, stable cells retain this capacity but do not normally replicate, and permanent cells cannot reproduce themselves after birth of the host.

Perfect repair, with restitution of normal structure, theoretically occurs only in tissues consisting of stable and labile cells, whereas all injuries to soft tissues composed of permanent cells may give rise to fibrosis and fibrous capsule formation with very little restitution of the normal tissue or organ structure. Tissues composed of permanent cells (e.g., nerve cells, skeletal muscle cells, and cardiac muscle cells) most commonly undergo an organization of the inflammatory exudate, leading to fibrosis. Tissues composed of stable cells (e.g., parenchymal cells of the liver, kidney, and pancreas), mesenchymal cells (e.g., fibroblasts, smooth muscle cells, osteoblasts, and chondroblasts), and vascular endothelial and labile cells (e.g., epithelial cells and lymphoid and hematopoietic cells) may also follow this pathway to fibrosis or may undergo resolution of the inflammatory exudate, leading to restitution of the normal tissue structure. The condition of the underlying framework or supporting stroma of the parenchymal cells following an injury plays an important role in the restoration of normal tissue structure. Retention of the framework may lead to restitution of the normal tissue structure, whereas destruction of the framework most commonly leads to fibrosis. It is important to consider the species-dependent nature of the regenerative capacity of cells. For example, cells from the same organ or tissue but from different species may exhibit different regenerative capacities and/or connective tissue repair. An example of species differences in cell proliferation and regeneration is the endothelialization process, proliferation of endothelial cells, on the luminal surface of vascular grafts which does not occur in humans but does occur in other mammals including other primates.

Following injury, cells may undergo adaptations of growth and differentiation. Important cellular adaptations are atrophy (decrease in cell size or function), hypertrophy (increase in cell size), hyperplasia (increase in cell number), and metaplasia (change in cell type). Hyperplasia of smooth muscle cells at blood vessel/vascular graft anastomoses may lead to failure of the graft by stenosis or occlusion, i.e., narrowing of the lumen, and thrombosis. Other adaptations include a change in which cells stop producing one family of proteins and start producing another (phenotypic change) or begin a marked overproduction of protein. This may be the case in cells producing various types of collagens and extracellular matrix proteins in chronic inflammation and fibrosis. Causes of atrophy may include decreased workload (e.g., stress-shielding by implants), as well as diminished blood supply and inadequate nutrition (e.g., fibrous capsules surrounding implants).

Local and system factors may play a role in the wound healing response to biomaterials or implants. Local factors include the site (tissue or organ) of implantation, the adequacy of blood supply, and the potential for infection. Systemic factors may include nutrition, hematologic and immunologic derangements, glucocortical steroids, and pre-existing diseases such as atherosclerosis, diabetes, and infection.

2.6 SUMMARY

Inflammation, wound healing, foreign body response, and repair of implant sites are usually considered components of the general soft tissue response to biomaterials or medical devices. The extent or degree and temporal variations in these responses are dictated by the inherent biocompatibility characteristics of the biomaterial or medical device. Factors which may play a role in the soft tissue response include the size, shape, topography, and chemical and physical properties of the biomaterial. As the implantation procedure involves injury to vascularized connective tissue, blood responses and interactions may play a role in the general soft tissue response. The extent, degree or type of soft tissue response is generally considered to be tissue-specific, organ-specific, and species-specific. Thus, a given biomaterial may be considered to be biocompatible in one shape or form but not in another and in one tissue but not in another depending on the given application.

ADDITIONAL READING

Black, J. (1992) *Biological Performance of Materials – Fundamentals of Biocompatibility*, 2nd edn, Marcel Dekker, New York.

This volume is an excellent tutorial text for the engineer/biomaterial scientist/biologist/and others who have little or no knowledge in the area of biomaterials and medical devices. The text is divided into four parts: General considerations, material response: function and degradation of materials *in vivo*, host response: biological effects of implants, and methods of test for biological performance. The fourth part, Methods of test for biological performance, is unique to biomaterials texts and provides the reader with *in vitro* and *in vivo* test models and methods as well as perspectives on the design, selection, standardization, and regulation of implant materials.

Cohen, I.K., Diegelmann, R.F. and Lindblad, W.J. (eds) (1992) *Wound Healing: Biochemical and Clinical Aspects*, W.B. Saunders Co., Philadelphia.

This is an edited volume containing 35 chapters. The volume addresses the following areas: Biological processes involved in wound healing (6 chapters), structural and regulatory components of wound healing (7 chapters), factors affecting tissue repair (7 chapters), repair of specific tissues (7 chapters), and clinical management of healing tissues (7 chapters). This is an excellent volume which provides an up-to-date and in-depth perspective of various aspects of wound healing. The references lists provided at the end of each chapter are extensive. The strength of the volume is its biological perspective and little is provided on biomaterials. The chapter by Frederick Grinnell on cell adhesion does offer a biomaterial perspective.

Gallin, J.A., Goldstein, I.M. and Snyderman, R. (eds) (1992) *Inflammation: Basic Principles and Clinical Correlates*, 2nd ed, Raven Press, New York.

This is an edited volume containing 58 chapters by individual authors. The volume is divided in the following areas: Soluble components of inflammation (10 chapters), cytokines (5 chapters), cellular components of inflammation (21 chapters), responses to inflammation (3 chapters), clinical correlates (13 chapters), and pharmacologic modulation of inflammation (4 chapters). Each chapter is a critical, in-depth review of the indicated subject and the references are extensive. This is an excellent volume for those wanting an in-depth overview of the inflammatory process and its components. No information is provided on biomaterial/inflammation interactions.

Greco, R.S. (ed.) (1994) *Implantation Biology: The Host Response and Biomedical Devices*, CRC Press, Boca Raton.

This is an edited volume containing 23 chapters. Three chapters deal with biomaterials in general, 6 chapters address specific blood and tissue interactions with biomaterials, 10 chapters address the use of biomaterials in specific surgical disciplines, and 3 chapters address tissue engineering and genetic manipulation of cells. The reference list for each chapter is extensive. This is an excellent overview of how biomaterials interact with the host and the specific use of biomaterials in indicated applications.

Harker, L.A., Ratner, B.D. and Didisheim, P. (eds) (1993) *Cardiovascular Biomaterials and Biocompatibility: A Guide to the Study of Blood–Tissue–Material Interactions, Cardiovascular Pathology*, **2** (3 Suppl), 1S–224S.

This is the third edition of a standard National Institutes of Health reference previously entitled *Guidelines for Blood–Material Interactions – Report of the National Heart, Lung, and Blood Institute Working Group*. The volume contains 20 chapters and 3 appendices. The chapters address the following areas: Pathophysiologic mechanisms, materials and their physicochemical characterization, safety testing of materials and devices, and blood-vessel–material interactions. The appendices are entitled: NIH Primary Reference Materials, International Standards for Biological Evaluation of Medical Devices, and Blood Analog Fluid for Medical Device Evaluation. This volume provides an in-depth perspective on cardiovascular materials and state-of-the-art information is provided regarding biomaterials. This is an excellent review, however, the editors limited the length and number of references for each chapter due to space considerations.

REFERENCES

1. Williams, D.F. and Roaf, R. (1973) *Implants in Surgery*, W.B. Saunders Company Ltd., London, pp. 233–35.
2. Anderson, J.M. (1993) Mechanisms of inflammation and infection with implanted devices. *Cardiovascular Pathology*, **2** (3 Suppl.), M319–M321.
3. Anderson, J.M. (1994) *In vivo* biocompatibility of implantable delivery systems and biomaterials. *European Journal of Biopharmaceutics*, **40,** 1–8.
4. Anderson, J.M. (1994) Inflammation and the foreign body response. *Problems in General Surgery*, **11**(2), 147–160.
5. Black, J. (1992) The inflammatory process, in *Biological Performance of Materials -Fundamentals of Biocompatibility*, 2nd edn, Marcel Dekker, Inc., New York, pp. 125–147.
6. Marchant, R.E., Anderson, J.M. and Dillingham, E.O. (1986) *In vivo* biocompatibility studies. VII. Inflammatory response to polyethylene and to a cytotoxic polyvinylchloride. *Journal of Biomedical Materials Research*, **20,** 37–50.
7. Cotran, R.Z. *et al.* (1994) Inflammation and repair, in *Pathologic Basis of Disease*, 5th edn, Cotran, R.Z., Kumar, V. and Robbins, S.L. (eds), W.B. Saunders Co., Philadelphia, pp. 51–92.

8. Gallin, J.I., Goldstein, I.M. and Snyderman, R. (eds) (1992) *Inflammation. Basic Principles and Clinical Correlates*, 2nd edn, Raven Press, New York.
9. Spector, M., Cease, C. and Tong-Li, X. (1989) The local tissue response to biomaterials. *CRC Critical Reviews in Biocompatibility*, **5** (4), 269–295.
10. Weissman, G., Smolen, J.E. and Korchak, H.M. (1980) Release of inflammatory mediators from stimulated neutrophils. *New England Journal of Medicine*, **303,** 27–34.
11. Henson, P.M. (1980) Mechanisms of exocytosis in phagocytic inflammatory cells. *American Journal of Pathology*, **101,** 494–511.
12. Henson, P.M. (1971) The immunologic release of constituents from neutrophil leukocytes: II. Mechanisms of release during phagocytosis, and adherence to nonphagocytosable surfaces. *Journal of Immunology*, **107,** 1547–57.

3 Hard tissue response

T. Albrektsson

3.1 INTRODUCTION

The initial tissue response when a biomaterial is implanted in the body is dependent on release of specific growth factors. It has been indicated by Frost [1] that the inevitable bone injury resulting from surgery and the presence of an implant will release various types of growth factors that will sensitize cells and promote cellular mitosis. This is a general healing response that will result in growth of all sorts of local connective tissues, bone as well as various types of soft tissue.

The balance between these tissue varieties is controlled by the action of chemical mediators which issue 'instructions' for the amount of bone and soft tissue to be formed as an appropriate healing response. This delicate balance can easily be disturbed inadvertently and may cause the undesirable end-result of an interfacial soft tissue embedment of the implant or, in the case of fracture healing, formation of a pseudoarthrosis. The discussion in this section will focus on various modes of implant fixation, such as cementation, ingrowth and osseointegration (Figure 3.1).

3.2 FIXATION BY CEMENTATION

Bone cement, a two component acrylic, is frequently used for implant fixation in the cases of hip and knee arthroplasties. Bone cement is toxic with localized as well as general adverse tissue reactions [2]. Therefore, the good long-term results reported with cemented arthroplasties seem to be quite puzzling. However, it must be understood that the strength of

Handbook of Biomaterial Properties. Edited by J. Black and G. Hastings.
Published in 1998 by Chapman & Hall, London. ISBN 0 412 60330 6.

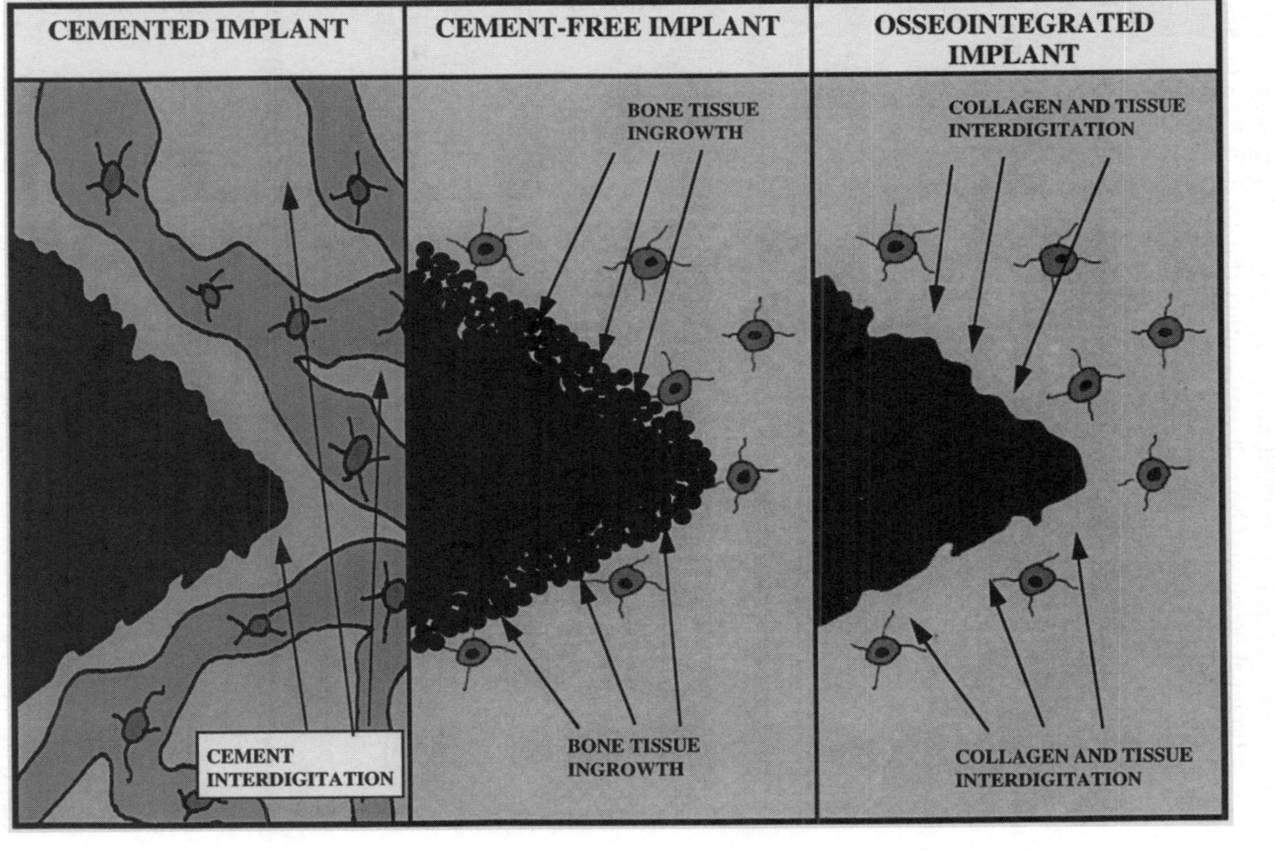

Figure 3.1 Different classification criteria are used for implants in bone. Here we distinguish between cemented implants, which are dependent upon cure in place luting or filling agents; cement-free (ingrowth implants) which are dependent on bone tissue growth into surface features for fixation; and osseointegrated implants, which are dependent upon collagen and cellular processes and their physiochemical interactions with the implant surface for fixation. In each case, a 'ridge' feature on the implant surface is shown in cross-section; the width of each band of the diagram is several millimeters (cells (osteocytes) are shown larger than actual size).

the cemented bone interface is not related to the live state of bone tissue: in reality, the curing bone cement invading the trabecular network results in a substantial cancellous bone interdigitation (Figure 3.1). The interfacial bone usually dies from the combined trauma of heat and monomer leakage. The width of this necrotic zone varies depending on the extent of the surgical trauma and the type of bone cement used, but is at least a few millimeters [2]. Ironically, a revitalization of the interfacial bone may prove disastrous, as the bone will then run an increased risk of resorption. In examining interfacial tissues reactions to retrieved cemented orthopaedic implants, most studies have examined the tissue after removal of the implant. This leads to an uncertainty in examining the proportion of true bone to implant contact.

We have been able to investigate bone implants *in situ*, at the resolution level of light microscopy, utilizing the techniques developed by Donath *et al.* [3]. Computer assisted calculations, using custom developed software, permit determination of the proportion of bone to implant contact, the amount of bone in the region adjacent to the implant and comparisons of the bone density adjacent to and in the immediate region of the implant ('outfolded mirror image') (Figure 3.2).

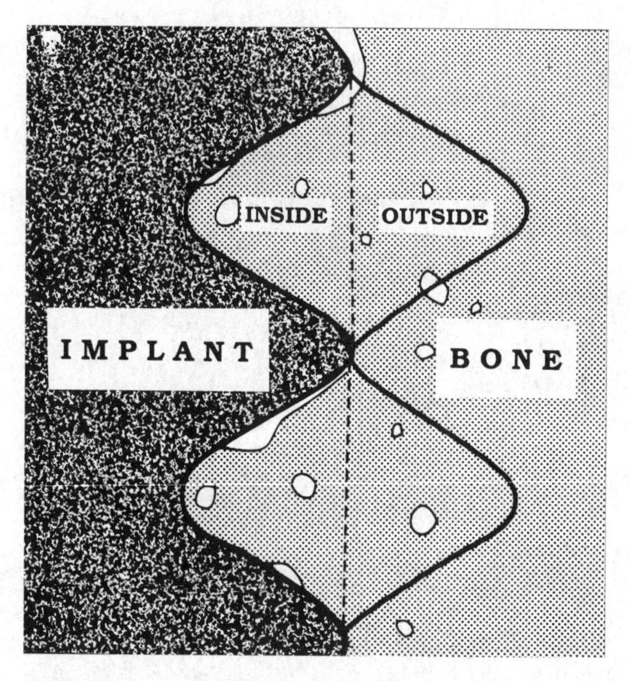

Figure 3.2 Computerized histomorphometric approach to evaluation of the bone–implant interface. The bone-to-implant contact percentage is the linear contact area between bone and implant in the inside zone; percent bone ingrowth is the ratio of bone 'inside' to that 'outside' in the 'mirror' zone.

These data correlate positively to biomechanical tests: the more bone in the interfacial region of the implant, the greater the torque necessary to remove the implant when we apply controlled rotational forces to the implant body. Specimens of 10 μm thickness have been investigated at the light microscopic level of resolution [4]. Other studies using cutting and grinding techniques have investigated the implant *in situ*, but ended up with sections of a final thickness of 40 μm or more leading to clear overestimates of the true bone to implant contact. In a retrieval study of cemented resurface arthroplasties, Morberg [2] was able to overcome these methodological problems and verify a very poor bone to cement contact, even though he found bone fragments with disturbed mineralization bordering the cement.

3.3 FIXATION BY INGROWTH (CEMENT-FREE IMPLANTS IN BONE)

In the absence of cement, fixation may be obtained by active bone tissue ingrowth into the implant surface irregularities of medullary stems (Figure 3.2). As pointed out by Black [5], one disadvantage of cement-free implants is the 3–4 week waiting time before the bone–implant interface can support significant shear loading; this is in contrast to a cemented interface which, if successful, has adequate shear strength within one hour of implantation. Osseointegrated implants have even lower interfacial shear strength at the the same 3–4 week post operative time point [6].

In the clinical experience, however, the results of cement-free joint arthroplasties utilizing ingrowth fixation have not matched those of cemented devices. The appropriate bone ingrowth is often disturbed and incomplete, leading to early failure of fixation. Cement-free knee arthroplasty components have been observed to migrate by up to 2 mm in the first post-operative year, while cemented devices of the same design migrate only half as much or less [7]. The failure rates of cement-free hip arthroplasties have been so substantial in comparison to cemented devices that the former mode of implant insertion has been restricted to young patients for whom cemented devices give poorer results at most clinics [8].

The outcome of cement-free orthopaedic implants depends, as does the outcome of craniofacial osseointegrated implants, on the more or less simultaneous control of a number of different factors including biocompatibility, design and surface conditions of the implant, the state of the host bed, the surgical technique and the loading conditions after implant insertion.

Herein is the explanation for the dubious results of many current designs of cement-free hips and knees: the implant material used, the design and surface finish have been well adapted to engineering demands, but not so well matched to the biological needs.

Ideal implant characteristics with respect to bone anchorage are quite different from those of gliding surfaces. The surgical technique utilized when inserting a cement-free hip or knee of current designs is, of necessity, traumatizing: resulting in an impaired bone healing response. Current stem-type cement-free hips migrate when loaded, as do tibial components of artificial knees, leading to a change in the chemical mediators and subsequent increase of soft tissue formation. It is, therefore, not surprising to learn from studies of retrieved cement-free hips that there is, as a rule, only sparse bony ingrowth into retrieved acetabular cups [9], femoral cups [2, 10] or femoral stems [9, 11, 12]. More modern types of cement free hip prostheses with titanium meshwork or HA-coated surfaces have had slightly better clinical results than those implanted and retrieved during the 1980s and it may well be possible that there is more abundant bone ingrowth in some of the more recent designs. Nevertheless, from multicenter studies it seems quite clear that summed five-year failure rates for cement-free arthroplasties are greater than those for cemented devices [8]. This observation illustrates that the anchorage problems associated with cement free arthroplasties are far from solved.

3.4 OSSEOINTEGRATION

Osseointegration is a term introduced by Brånemark *et al.* [13] to describe a loaded, stable implant in direct contact with bone (no apparent intervening soft tissue under light microscopic examination). Osseointegrated implants differ from ingrown ones that are dependent upon bone growth into surface macroscopic features or irregularities. By contrast, osseointegration is dependent on tissue ingrowth into minute surface features, such as the fundamental asperities of a 'smooth' surface or, as postulated for surfaces of various crystalline calcium phosphates (such as calcium hydroxyapatite) or amorphous, bioactive glasses, on direct chemical bonding between tissue and implant. Irrespective of the type of interfacial contact – chemical bonding or mechanical interdigitation – an important difference is that while the former requires only limited tissue elements, the latter requires complete, mature bone elements for appropriate function. Theoretically, an ingrown interface may also be osseointegrated as well but experimental evidence for this, from examination of thin sections, is virtually nonexistent. Macroscopic features on implant surfaces designed for ingrowth fixation include sintered beads, rough plasma sprayed coatings and sintered meshes, since bone requires features of minimum dimensions of about 100 μm for successful ingrowth [14, 15].

However, surface irregularities only in the nanometer to micrometer range are necessary for osseointegration when implant stability is dependent on cellular and/or collagen ingrowth, rather than bone ingrowth. Since this ingrowth (perhaps better termed 'ongrowth') of tissue elements occurs in a three dimensional manner, the osseointegrated implant will, from a biomechanical viewpoint, be a directly bone-anchored device. In fact, Wennerberg [16] has demonstrated that implant surfaces with a CLA (center line average) roughness of ~1 μm will experience more rapid bony incorporation, through osseointegration, than ones with CLAs of 0.1 or 2 μm. This observation leads to the hypothesis that too smooth surfaces (CLA ~0.1) may not permit proper collagen attachment while rougher ones (CLA ≥ 2 μm) may release too many metal ions that disturb cellular functions necessary for anchorage.

There is no doubt that osseointegration has resulted in a clinical breakthrough in oral implants. Soft tissue embedded load-carrying devices do not function adequately in the jaw. In sharp contrast, properly osseointegrated implants do. However, this does not necessarily imply that every functioning bone implant in other parts of the body need to be osseointegrated. On the contrary, cemented hip arthroplasties with a bone-cement interface consisting of soft tissue or mostly dead bone have demonstrated significant clinical longevity, in many cases exceeding ten to fifteen years.

Furthermore, the so called osseointegrated interface is still in need of a proper definition. First described by Brånemark [17] as a bone response that occurred everywhere around the implant circumference of c.p. titanium screws in placed in bone, osseointegration is regarded today as a more nonspecific tissue response resulting in a mix of interfacial soft and hard tissues. In reality, bone anchorage of foreign bodies is a more general type of tissue response that occurs to c.p. titanium alone [3]. The only definition of osseointegration that has stood up to a critical analysis is based on a clinical finding of implant stability: 'A process whereby clinically asymptomatic rigid fixation of alloplastic materials is achieved and maintained, in bone, during functional loading' [18]. The continued usage of a term such as osseointegration is motivated by the proven clinical results in the case of craniofacial implants and the hope to replicate these findings in the case of orthopaedic implants in the future. However, from a strict histological point of view osseointegration remains poorly defined.

Osseointegrated implants have resulted in a clinical breakthrough in two different clinical applications in the craniofacial skeleton: one of these being oral implants, irrespective of whether treating total or partial edentulousness [19, 20]; the other being skin penetrating extra-oral implants. The clinical results of screw-type, c.p. titanium oral implants in mandibles or maxillas for 5 years or more of follow up have been in the 90–99% range[21]. The results of skin penetrating implants in the temporal bone region have been similar, but not in the orbit region, where the host bed has been irradiated. Now, 20 years since their clinical introduction in 1977, permanent skin-penetrating, osseointegrated, screw-shaped titanium implants are regarded as routine clinical treatments for facial disorders or certain types of hearing impairments [22, 23].

Press-fit fixation represents one approach to the osseointegration of orthopedic implants. The design of press-fit joint replacements is based on three dimensional geometric data with the intention of fitting the implant as closely as possible to the host bone. The objective of this design approach is to transfer load across the implant–bone interface to as wide an area of the bone as possible [24]. In theory, press-fit fixation may lead to osseointegration of the implanted device. However, as it is difficult to mimic precisely the resulting intravital loading patterns, osseointegration of initially stable press-fit components is threatened by subsequent bone remodeling processes. Too stiff a device may cause 'stress shielding,' leading to bone resorption. Conversely, too high local stresses may lead to pressure necrosis and resorption prior to remodeling. Finally, bone resorption may lead to local interfacial movements: these predispose to soft-tissue formation and may cause a subsequent failure of fixation.

Polymers are not one hundred percent stable under biological conditions, leading to highly variable clinical durability. Ultrahigh molecular weight polyethylene (UHMWPE), although relatively stable, has shown poor outcomes when press-fitted in knee replacement arthroplasties [25]. The poor fixation of such devices may relate both to intrinsic properties of the polymers involved as well as to differences in their elastic moduli from that of bone. For instance, the Young's modulus of UHMWPE is approximately 2% of that of cortical bone (0.3 GPa vs. 17 GPa). This leads to a quite different loading pattern for both the polymer and the surrounding tissue than that encountered in the case of c.p. titanium, which is approximately 7 times as stiff as cortical bone (127 GPa vs. 17 GPa).

Ceramics are still stiffer, with moduli up to 30 times that of cortical bone. Bulk ceramics, such as aluminum oxide (alumina) are well tolerated by bone but are generally insufficiently strong and tough to serve as load bearing implants, especially in the presence of tensile or bending loads. Calcium phosphates, such as calcium hydroxyapatite (CaHAP), although much weaker still, are an interesting class of biomaterials due to their assumed capability for 'bone bonding'. Søballe *et al.* [26] has observed that the addition of a CaHAP coating induces proliferating bone to bridge gaps in the bone–implant interface, in the presence of dynamic loading, which would be filled with soft tissue around uncoated metallic implants. He also suggests that such coatings enhance bone growth from osteopenic tissue, utilizing an experimental animal arthritis model with substantial pre-implantation loss of bone density.

In experimental studies, c.p. titanium has been demonstrated to induce a stronger bone response than most other pure metals or alloys, including

Ti6Al4V [4, 27]. However, there is substantial evidence that CaHAP leads to a still more rapid healing response [28]. This may be due to a direct positive influence on interfacial bone from the calcium phosphate material and/or a relatively rough surface topography resulting from the manufacturing process in combination with the reduction of metal ion release by the presence of the CaHAP coating. Long term experimental and dental clinical data from CaHAP coated implants has been disappointing [29]. However, CaHAP remains a very interesting biomaterial with efforts underway to explore functional improvement through changes in crystallinity, coating thickness, method of application, etc.

Retrieval data [30–32] have contributed to our current knowledge of oral implants. Steflik and co-workers [32] reviewed 51 retrieved oral implants of different designs. They claimed that implants inserted 10 years ago or more fail generally due to loss of bone support and other biological features while more recently placed oral implants also fail secondary to intrinsic biomaterial failure such as implant fracture. One hundred stable (uncoated) Brånemark System® 'Nobelpharma' implants were retrieved and studied at our laboratories: 33% were removed because of therapy-resistant pain or progressive bone resorption, 26% were removed after death from unrelated causes, 24% were fractured implants and 17% were removed for psychological reasons. The implants had been in situ and functioning for 1–18 years. There was on average 82% bone-to-implant contact and a similar percentage of bone within the threads of these retrieved implants (evaluated over the three best consecutive threads on both sides of the implant). Whenever possible, the entire bone to implant contact percentages were also calculated and found to be ~ 70%. In almost every case, there was >60% bone to implant contact. In fact, such extensive bone to implant contact percentages may represent a histological correlate to osseointegration.

3.5 HOW BONE–BIOMATERIAL INTERFACES FAIL

The implant–bone interface can fail for various reasons but the most common is so-called 'aseptic loosening': i.e. loosening not associated with infection. The causative factors for aseptic loosening may be classified as mechanical or biological. For example, early post-operative failures of cemented, cement-free (ingrown) as well as osseointegrated implants may be attributed to lack of initial fixation due to mechanical failure of the bone-cement (when present) or bone–implant interface. Such failures may relate to incidents of overload. However, early failures may also occur subsequent to overheating of the tissues during surgery, leading to bony necrosis, collapse and subsequent mechanical loosening. Overheating due to a combination of surgical trauma and polymerization heat release may occur at bone–cement interfaces; surgical trauma, with associated heating, alone may prevent bone and other tissue elements from invading cement-free implant–bone interfaces, whether designed for ingrowth or osseointegration. Biological failure is also possible in the longer term, associated with generation or release of cytotoxic products, such as cement monomer or metallic corrosion products or through induction of specific immune responses [33] (Figure 3.3).

In clinical use, cylindrical shaped oral implants which lack any additional retention features, such as threads, grooves, etc., are prone to gradual failure due to ongoing bone 'saucerization' (gradual loss of bone at the implant–bone–mucosal boundary) [21]. In the case of orthopaedic implants with medullary structural elements (such as a femoral stem), Willert and Semlitsch were first to propose that bone loss occurred secondary to biological response to small particles, such as wear debris. [34] Macrophages (MP) and foreign body giant cells (GC) ingest these undigestible particles of metal, polymer or ceramic and release factors which stimulate osteolytic activity by cells in membranes associated with the implant–bone interface (Figure 3.3) [35]. With modern histological staining techniques, especially the use of oil red O [33], it has now become possible to appreciate the large amounts of small and submicron UHMWPE particles found in the vicinity of loose orthopaedic joint replacement implants. Many investigators believe that biological response to these particles is the leading biological cause of osteolysis leading to gradual, late implant failure.

3.6 CONCLUSIONS

The major advantage of the osseointegrated interface is its remodelling capacity. Gradual adaptation to load has been verified in retrieval studies; the implants are known to have almost no bone to implant contact during the first few weeks after placement but then demonstrate an increasing amount of interfacial bone tissue. The main proportion of osseointegrated implant failures occur during the first one or two years and result from failure to achieve a proper osseointegration. This trend is quite different from most orthopaedic studies reported in the literature, which show clinical failure rates increasing with time. Cemented arthroplasties of today have resulted in a significantly better clinical outcome than cement-free ones. It must be pointed out that the results of orthopaedic implants published in the literature are generally based on the number of revisions alone. This means that the actual number of successful arthroplasties is lower than the figures quoted in the literature. Furthermore, there is a patient drop-out of more than 20% in most clinical reports. From a biological viewpoint it is important to strive for improved cement-free implants

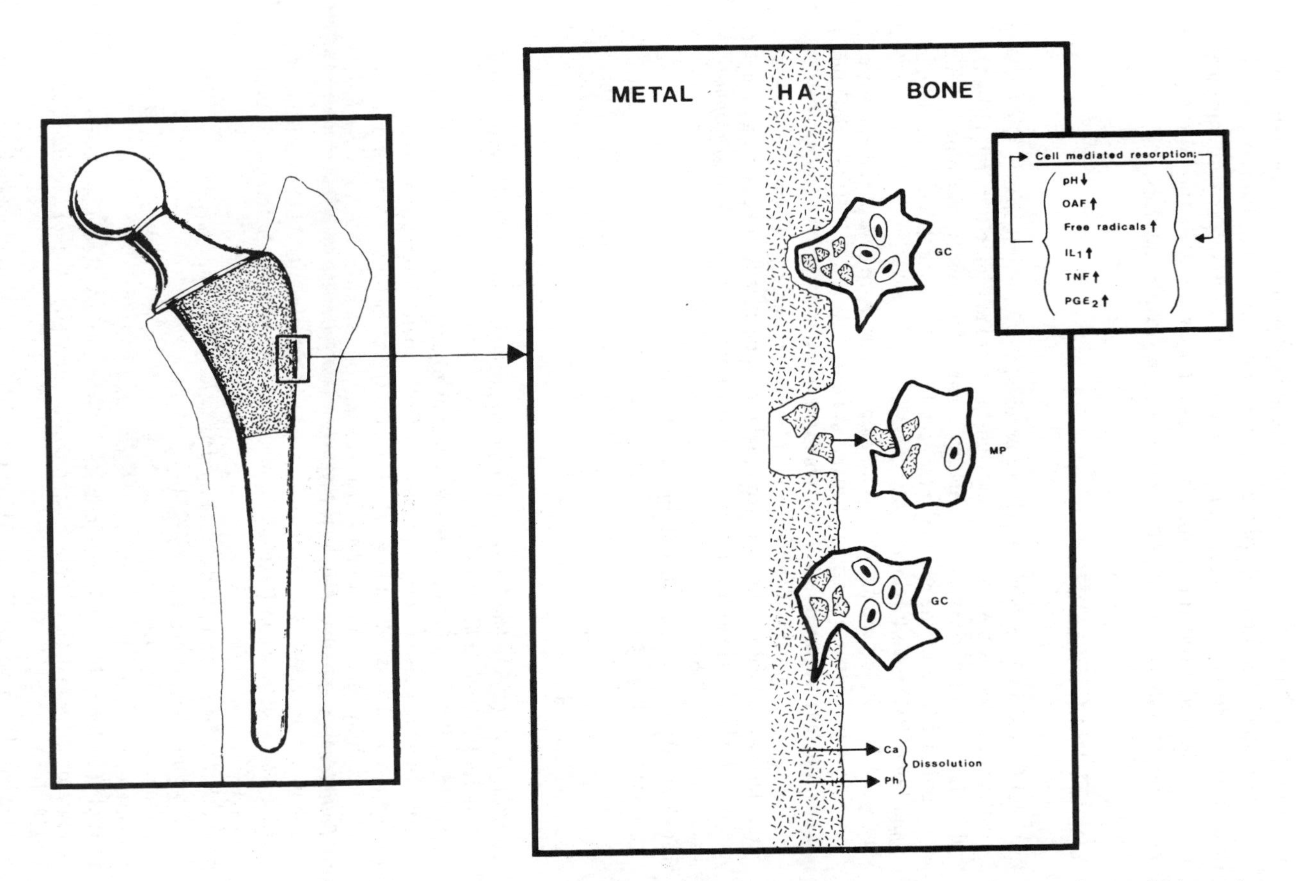

Figure 3.3 Theoretical failure modes for an osseointegrated calcium hydroxyapatite-coated femoral stem of a total hip replacement prosthesis [29; by permission]. Key: GC: multinucleated giant cell; MP: macrophage; Ca: calcium; Ph: phosphorous; OAF: osteoclastic activating factor; IL_1: interleukin 1, TNF: tumor necrosis factor; PGE_2: prostaglandin E_2.

so that their clinical results will at least match those of the cemented arthroplasties. New types of osseointegrated hip and knee constructions have been designed and are presently in clinical trials. Altering prosthetic design (in comparison with current practice), and improving surgical instruments and procedures may well overcome some of the hurdles in the development of new osseointegrated arthroplasty devices.

ADDITIONAL READING

Lee, A.J.C. and Ling, R.S.M. (1984): Loosening, in *Complications of Total Hip replacement*, (ed. R.S.M. Ling), Churchill-Livingstone, Edinburgh, pp. 110–145.

Still useful account of the biological and mechanical features of loosening leading to clinical failure of the various interfaces formed between rigid biomaterials and bone. Extensive bibliography.

Manley, M.T. (1993): Calcium phosphate biomaterials: A review of the literature, in *Hydroxylapatite Coatings in Orthopaedic Surgery*, (eds G.T.R. Geesink and M.T. Manley), Raven Press, New York, pp. 1–24.

The title speaks for itself. Additional chapters in the same book provide experimental and clinical results of osseointegration, specifically adhesion fixation.

Spector, M. (1987): Historical review of porous-coated implants. *J. Arthroplasty*, **2**(2), 163–177, 1987.

Historical review of experimental and clinical results of ingrowth fixation, with extensive bibliography.

REFERENCES

1. Frost, H.M. (1989) The biology of fracture healing. *Clinical Orthopaedics and Related Research*, **248**, 283–293.
2. Morberg, P. (1991) On bone tissue reactions to acrylic cement. PhD Dissertation, Biomaterials Group, University of Göthenberg, Sweden, pp. 1–142.
3. Donath, K., Laass, M. and Günzl, H.-J. (1992) The histopathology of different foreign body reactions in oral soft tissue and bone tissue. *Virchows Archiv A Pathologia Anatomica*, **420**, 131–137.
4. Johansson, C. (1991) On tissue reactions to metal implants. PhD Dissertation, Biomaterials/Handicap Research, University of Göteborg, Göteborg, Sweden, pp. 1–232.
5. Black, J. (1988) *Orthopaedic Biomaterials in Research and Practice*. New York, Churchill Livingstone, pp. 267–284.
6. Steinemann, S.G., Eulenberger, J., Maeusli, P.-A. *et al.* (1986) Adhesion of bone to titanium. *Adv. in Biomaterials* **6**, 40–44.
7. Ryd, L. (1986) Micromotion in knee arthroplasty. A Roentgen stereophotogrammetric analysis of tibial component fixation. *Acta Orthop. Scand.*, Suppl. **220**, 1–80.
8. Malchau, H., Herberts, P. and Anhfelt, L. (1993) Prognosis of total hip replacement in Sweden. Follow-up of 92,675 operations performed in 1978–1990, *Acta Orthop Scand.*, **64**, 497–506.

9. Collier, J.P., Mayor, M.B., Chae, J.C. *et al.* (1988) Macroscopic and microscopic evidence of prosthetic fixation with porous coated materials. *Clin. Orthop. Rel. Res.*, **235**, 173–180.
10. Willems, W.J., Eulderbrink, F., Rozing, P.M. *et al.* (1988) Histopathologic evaluation in failed Gerard double cup arthroplasty. *Clin. Orthop. Rel. Res.*, **228**, 123–133.
11. Engh, C.A., Bobyn, J.D. and Glassman, A.H. (1987) Porous coated hip replacement. The factors governing bone ingrowth, stress shielding and clinical results. *J. Bone Joint Surg.*, **69B**, 45–55.
12. Cook, S.D., Thomas, A.K. and Haddad, R.J. (1988) Histologic analysis of retrieved human porous coated joint components. *Clin. Orthop. Rel. Res.*, **234**, 90–101.
13. Brånemark, P.-I., Hansson, B.-O., Adell, R. *et al.* (1977) Osseointegrated implants in the treatment of the edentulous jaw. *Scand. J. Plastic Reconst. Surg.*, Suppl **16**, 1–116.
14. Albrektsson, T. (1979) Healing of bone grafts. *In vivo* studies of tissue reactions at autografting of bone in the rabbit tibia. PhD Dissertation, Laboratory for Experimental Biology, Göteborg University, Göteborg, Sweden, pp. 1–90.
15. Pilliar, R.M. (1986) Implant stabilization by tissue ingrowth. In *Tissue Integration in Oral and Maxillofacial Reconstruction*, D. van Steenberghe (ed.), Amsterdam, Excerpta Medica, pp. 60–76.
16. Wennerberg, A. (1995) On surface topography of implants. PhD Dissertation, Biomaterials/Handicap Research, University of Göteborg, Göteborg, Sweden, pp. 1–202.
17. Brånemark, P.-I. (1985) Introduction to osseointegration, in *Tissue Integrated Prostheses* (eds P.-I. Brånemark, G. Zarb and T. Albrektsson), Quintessence Co, Chicago, pp. 11–76.
18. Zarb, G. and Albrektsson, T. (1991) Osseointegration – A requiem for the periodontal ligament? – An editorial. *Int. J. Periodontal and Restorative Dent.*, **11**, 88–91.
19. Albrektsson, T., Dahl, E., Enbom, L. *et al.* (1988) Osseointegrated oral implants. A Swedish multicenter study of 8139 consecutively inserted Nobelpharma implants. *J. Periodont.*, **59**, 287–296.
20. Lekholm, U., vanSteenberghe, D., Herrmann, I. *et al.* (1994) Osseointegrated implants in partially edentulous jaws: A prospective 5-year multicenter study. *Inter. J. Oral & Maxillofacial Implants*, **9**, 627–635.
21. Albrektsson, T. (1993) On the long-term maintenance of the osseointegrated response. *Australian Prosthodontic J.*, **7**, 15–24.
22. Tjellström, A. and Granström, G. (1994) Long-term follow-up with the bone anchored hearing aid: A review of the first 100 patients between 1977 and 1985. *Ear Nose and Throat J.*, **2**: 138–140.
23. Jacobsson, M., Tjellström, A., Fine, L., *et al.* (1992) A retrospective study of osseointegrated skin-penetrating titanium fixtures used for retaining facial prostheses. *Int. J. Oral & Maxillofacial Implants*, **7**, 523–528.
24. Poss, R., Robertson, D.D., Walker, P.S. *et al.* (1988) Anatomic stem design for press-fit and cemented application. In *Non-cemented Total Hip Arthroplasty*, R. Fitzgerald, Jr (ed.), New York, Raven Press, pp. 343–363.

25. Freeman, M.A.R., McLoed, H.C. and Levai, J.P. (1983) Cementless fixation of prosthetic components in total arthroplasty of the knee and hip. *Clin. Orthop. Rel. Res.*, **176**, 88–94.
26. Søballe, K. (1993) Hydroxyapatite ceramic coating for bone implant fixation. *Acta Orthop. Scand.* (Suppl 225), **64**, 1–58.
27. Han, C.H., Johansson, C., Wennerberg, A. *et al.* (1995) A quantitative comparison of commercially pure titanium and titanium-6 aluminum-4 vanadium implants in rabbit bone. *Proc. Fifth Biomaterials Club Meeting*, Ischgl, Austria, Albrektsson T. and Tjellström, A. (eds), p. 25.
28. Søballe, K., Hansen, E.S., Rasmussen, H.B. *et al.* (1993) The effect of osteoporosis, bone deficiency, bone grafting, and micromotion on fixation of porous coated vs. hydroxyapatite-coated implants. In *Hydroxyapatite Coatings in Orthopedic Surgery*, Geesink, R.G.T. and Manley, M.T. (eds), New York, Raven Press, pp. 107–136.
29. Gottlander, M. (1994) On hard tissue reactions to hydroxyapatite-coated titanium implants. PhD Dissertation, Biomaterials/Handicap Research, University of Göteborg, Göteborg, Sweden, pp. 1–202.
30. Lemons, J.E. (1991) Bone–biomaterial interfaces in retrieved implants, in *The Bone Biomaterial Interface* (ed. J.E. Davies), University of Toronto Press, Toronto, pp. 419–424.
31. Albrektsson, T., Eriksson, A.R., Friberg, B., *et al.* (1993) Histologic investigations on 33 retrieved Nobelpharma implants. *Clinical Materials* **12** (1), 1–9.
32. Steflik, D.E., Parr, G.R., Singh, B.B. *et al.* (1994) Light microscopic and scanning electron microscopic analyses of dental implants retrieved from humans. *J. Oral Implantol.*, **20**(1), 8–24.
33. Campbell, P. (1995) On aseptic loosening of total hip replacements: The role of UHMWPE wear particles. PhD Dissertation, Biomaterials/Handicap Research, Göteborg University, Göteborg, Sweden, pp. 1–225.
34. Willert, H., Semlitsch, M. (1976) Reactions of the articular capsule to joint prostheses. In *Biocompatibility of Implant Materials*, D.F. Williams (ed.), London, Sector Publishing, pp. 157–169.
35. Goldring, S.R., Schiller, A.L., Roelke, M., *et al.* (1983) The synovial-like membrane at the bone–cement interface in loose total hip replacements and its proposed role in bone lysis. *J. Bone Joint Surg.*, **65A**, 575–584.

Immune response

4

K. Merritt

4.1 INTRODUCTION

There is increasing concern about the role of specific immune response to implanted materials. This section discusses the general principles governing immune responses and outlines techniques for their measurement and evaluation. This is a necessarily brief presentation of the issues, and the reader is encouraged to pursue the topic through relevant references provided for further study.

4.2 OVERVIEW OF THE SPECIFIC IMMUNE RESPONSE

The specific immune response is the normal response of vertebrates when a foreign substance is introduced into the body. This is a desirable protective response which detoxifies, neutralizes, and helps to eliminate such substances.

However, in some cases, responses to seemingly innocuous substances may cause harm to the host. Such effects are usually termed allergic or hypersensitivity responses. The responses have been classified into four types: Type I, Type II, Type III, Type IV.

These four responses share elements of a common mechanism, triggered by the presence of a foreign material termed an *antigen*. The antigen is initially processed by a cell, usually either a monocyte or macrophage, but occasionally a skin dendritic cell also referred to as an *antigen processing cell* (APC). The APC engulfs the antigen, processes it (usually by enzymatic digestion or attempted digestion), and transfers or presents

Handbook of Biomaterial Properties. Edited by J. Black and G. Hastings.
Published in 1998 by Chapman & Hall, London. ISBN 0 412 60330 6.

it to another cell, usually a *lymphocyte* termed a *T helper cell.* The T helper cell then presents the processed antigen to another T lymphocyte, called the *T cytotoxic cell,* or to a B lymphocyte. The receiving cell, whether T- or B-type, initiates a response for interaction with the processed antigen, forming a less biologically active complex. In the former case, the immune response is a Type IV or cell mediated immunity while in the latter case, the final result is release of free antibody, which may lead to a humoral Type I, II, or III response. T-cell responses result in accumulation of T-cells at the site where the foreign material is present. B-cells remain at remote depots of lymphoid tissue while the antibody circulates and appears at the site of the foreign material.

The main features of the four types of responses are described in the following table:

Type:	*Antibody:*	*Cells involved:*	*Mediator:*	*Consequences:*
I	IgE	B-lymphocytes	Histamine, vasoactive amines	Itching, rhinitis, vascular collapse
II	IgG, IgM	B-lymphocytes	Histamine, vasoactive amines	Vascular collapse
III	IgG, IgM	B-lymphocytes	Vasoactive amines	Pain, swelling, some vascular plugging and collapse
IV	none	T-lymphocytes	Cytokines	Pain, swelling

Both the T- and B-cells are small lymphocytes, which circulate in the blood, and are found in lymphoid tissue. They arise from a common stem cell and then undergo processing in the thymus to become T-cells or an unknown site, probably the bone marrow, to become B-cells. They are difficult to distinguish and a great deal of work has been done to facilitate identification of these cells in order to elucidate specific immune responses. Identification of T-cells has been greatly aided by the recognition that there are unique substances on the cell surface that can be recognized by the use of monoclonal antibodies generated using murine cells. These antigens are referred to as *cluster differentiation markers* (CDs) and are given numbers. There are a large number of them, more are being identified, and the importance of each is being evaluated. However, all T-cells express CD3 which is consequently referred to as a Pan (= all) T-cell marker. CD2 may also be a Pan T-cell marker. Additionally, the T helper cell expresses CD4 while the T cytotoxic cell expresses CD8. New CDs continue to be identified and their importance evaluated.

The B-cell retains small amounts of antibody on its surface which can be used for identification. The B-cell response results in further differentiation to plasma cells which produce antibody in large quantities. Antibody is a four chain immunoglobulin which has combining sites specific for a single antigen. Antibody is soluble, circulates in the plasma, and the plasma or serum drawn from a vertebrate, or the antibody produced in cell culture for monoclonal antibodies, can be stored frozen and will last virtually forever.

There are five general classes of immunoglobulins produced as antibodies. In order of concentration in normal human blood from highest to lowest are IgG, IgM, IgA, IgE, and IgD. IgD is a surface marker on B-cells and will not be discussed further. IgE is the antibody associated with Type I responses. IgA is a secretory immunoglobulin, found in high concentrations in saliva, GI contents, and milk and in the associated organs. IgG and IgM are present in high concentrations in blood and are excellent antibodies for immunological testing since they can participate in Type II and III responses.

Type I responses and Type II responses have the same consequences, but the mechanisms are different. Type I responses are best known as hay fever and dust allergies and are immune responses to these antigens mediated by a skin fixing antibody (IgE).

Type II responses involve the reaction of IgG, rarely IgM, antibody with a cell surface antigen. The result is lysis of the cell with release of products. If the cell contains vasoactive amines, then the consequences are signs and symptoms described here. This is commonly seen in allergies to drugs which bind to blood platelets.

Type III responses are referred to as *immune complex* reactions and occur when both antigen and antibody are present in large quantities at the same time. In the normal immune response, the antigen is processed, the immune response is initiated, and the antigen disappears shortly. However, if the antigen is persistent, then significant amounts of immune complexes can form, plug small vessels, and result in tissue or organ damage.

Type IV responses are those most usually associated with chronic presence of a foreign body, such as an implanted biomaterial. They are typified by the common contact dermatitis caused by poison ivy.

In each case, an antigen stimulates the immune response and the immune response in turn reacts specifically with the antigen. T-cells, B-cells and circulating antibody each recognize only one antigen. For a substance to be antigenic, it must be foreign to the host, of high molecular weight (> 3000), and processable by an APC. However, some small substances become antigenic by binding to larger carrier molecules, usually proteins, found in the host. Such a small substance is called a *hapten* and the immune response is mounted to the hapten–carrier complex.

4.3 DETECTION OF ANTIBODY

To evaluate whether or not a patient has produced antibody against a substance, such as an implant, a blood sample needs to be drawn, tested and the results compared to those from controls. A pre-implantation sample is an ideal control but usually this is not available. The choice of appropriate controls is a major problem. The test procedure itself requires a known positive control (often difficult to obtain for evaluating responses to biomaterials), and a known negative control (usually saline, tissue culture media, or bovine or equine serum used for tissue culture). The controls for the patient population under study are generally obtained from normal individuals without implants and without underlying disease, individuals with the disease (e.g. arthritis) but without the implant (e.g. total joint replacement), individuals with the implant and without problems, and individuals with diagnosed implant failure. The results for all of these need to be analyzed in order to ascertain whether or not antibody is increased in the patient population and whether or not its presence can be correlated with failure of the device.

Most current tests are based on immobilization of the antigen to a solid surface such as polystyrene. The general procedure is outlined in Figure 4.1. Detection of bound antibody involves the use of enzyme (EIA or ELISA assays) or a radioisotope labeled antibody (RIA). (The tests are simple to perform, but great care is needed to wash away excess materials and use the appropriate concentrations. Individuals wishing to initiate such testing procedures are encouraged to attend workshops (often offered by American Society for Microbiology, American Type Culture Collection, etc.) or obtain training in a clinical immunology lab, and also explore detailed manuals on procedures.) Antiserum to human antibodies, (all classes or individual types) with enzyme labels, can be purchased from several biological supply houses. Isotope labeled antibody is available to licensed laboratories.

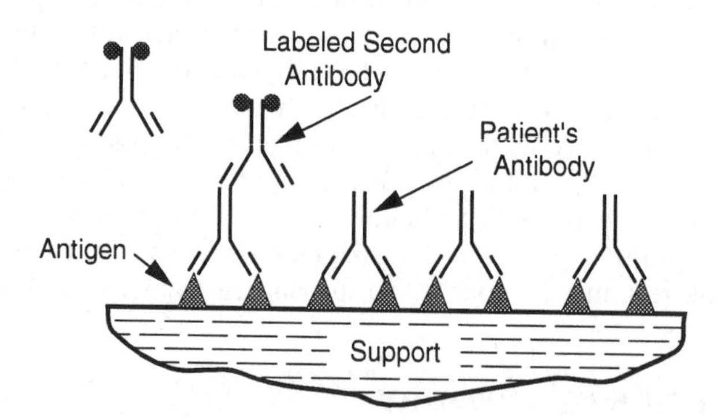

Figure 4.1 Standard immunoassay for antibody. An antigen is fixed (attached) to a solid support and binds a specific antibody from solution. The bound antibody is detected by binding a second, labeled (enzyme, isotope, etc.) antibody.

Problems with interpretation of results:

Positive results

If negative controls are negative and patient samples are positive, then the interpretation is that the patient made antibody to that antigen. However, the question remains as to whether or not the antigen is the correct one and if contaminating antigens are contributing to the reaction. This is difficult to determine but inhibition studies with well characterized antigens are helpful.

In vivo testing

Type I sensitivity is associated with histamine and vasoactive amine release with vascular responses. Often such sensitivity is determined by 'patch' (skin) testing. The positive reaction will occur in a few minutes as a wheal and erythematous (reddening) flare response in the skin. This test is hampered by availability of antigen for testing but the biomaterial applied directly to skin or a mucosal surface may stimulate a response. Caution needs to be taken in interpreting these tests, however, since this is a short term application.

Negative results

Negative results are the desired response in evaluating biomaterials for clinical use, but they are also difficult to evaluate. If there are no responses recorded except in the positive control sample, this is indicative that patient does not produce antibody to that antigen. Again the question of appropriateness of the antigen and its concentration on the solid support remains.

In vivo testing

A negative skin test presents the same problem: Was the antigen correct and/or was it applied to a correct site?

4.4 DETECTION OF CELL MEDIATED RESPONSES (TYPE IV)

The procedures for detecting cell mediated responses are much more complicated and difficult than for antibody determination. Most of the assays require the use of living cells and thus tests must be done shortly after obtaining the cells. Controls may have to be done at a different time which complicates the comparisons.

The two most common *in vitro* test procedures used are lymphocyte proliferation and cell migration inhibition tests. The basic theory behind both of these is that T-cells have receptors on their surface which will each respond to a specific antigen. In the course of the response, soluble substances (cytokines or lymphokines), principally blastogenic factor and migration inhibition factor, which act on other cells, including other T-cells, are produced and released.

Blastogenic factor (lymphocyte transformation factor)

This causes other lymphocytes to transform and divide. If cell counts are done, an increased number is seen. If a radioactive cell proliferation precursor (such as tritiated thymidine) is added to the culture, the isotope is taken up by dividing cells and the 'counts' increase. This test, usually called LTT for lymphocyte transformation test, requires living cells to produce and respond to the factor. This takes several days, with 7 days being the general time for response to antigen. Some control stimulants (mitrogens) such as PHA (phytohemagglutinin) act in 4–5 days. Interpretation of the tests presents the same problems as with tests for antibody: Are the appropriate controls included, what was the antigen used, were the cells viable; if the results are negative, were the culture conditions correct?

Migration inhibition factor

Migration inhibition factor (MIF) is produced by the stimulated T-cell and acts on cells that are normally motile. The two cell types are the monocyte/macrophage line and polymorphonuclear leukocytes (polys). Thus the test, usually called LIF test (leukocyte inhibition test) requires living lymphocytes and living migrating cells which may be obtained from fresh, whole blood. The results of the LIF test are available in 18–24 hours. Blood does not contain enough monocytes to evaluate inhibition of their migration and this indicator cell is usually obtained from the peritoneal cavity of other animals, typically the mouse or the guinea pig. It is possible to stimulate human lymphocytes in culture for 24–48 hours and then harvest the culture fluid and add it to the macrophages obtained from the animals. Migration (or inhibition of migration) of cells is observed by placing them into tissue culture medium solidified with purified agarose and observing them with a microscope in 18–24 hours or by packing them into capillary tubes and observing migration from the tubes in a few hours giving the appearance of 'ice cream cones'. The factor for LIF and the one for MIF may be slightly different and thus the two separate terms remain.

Choice of test

There is no evidence that one test is better than the other. The choice is usually based on laboratory preference. This author uses blood cells and migration in agarose since it requires little equipment, is rapid, and small breaks in aseptic procedure are tolerated. The evidence is that the stimulated T-cells produce a group of cytokines. Thus detecting migration inhibition factor or lymphocyte proliferation implies the presence of the others and one is not more specific or sensitive.

Direct testing for lymphokines or cytokines

It would seem from the above studies that the ideal test would be for the lymphokines without the use of a viable indicator cell. These substances are produced in low levels, and thus the cell based assays such as LTT and LIF or MIF are required. Although ELISA based or RIA based assays can be used to detect and quantitate cytokines, reagents are not yet available for these human lymphokines (LIF, MIF, LTT) specifically.

Testing for production of cytokines

There is a current explosion of studies on production of cytokines in response to biomaterials, especially to particles produced by wear and degradation. Thus it seems pertinent to discuss these assays briefly. The assays are generally done by inhibition of ELISA or RIA based assays. This concept is shown in Figure 4.2. Many of these assays are available as complete 'kits' from emerging biotechnology companies. (There are

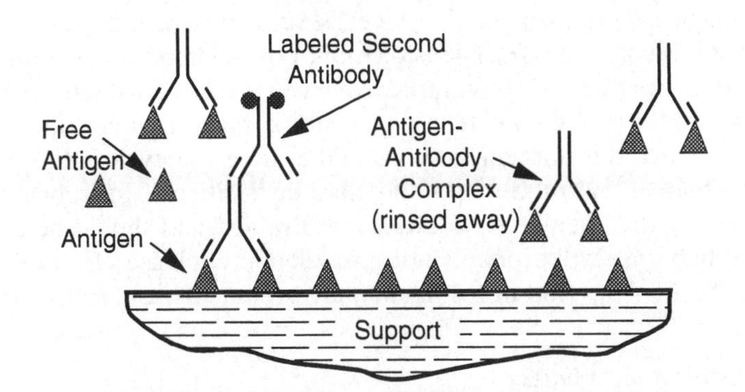

Figure 4.2 Quantitation of antigen by competitive (inhibition) assay. An antigen is fixed (attached) and binds a specific antibody from solution. However, additional antigen is provided in solution and antibody binding to the bound antigen is reduced in direct proportion to the concentration of free antigen. The bound antibody is then detected by binding a second, labeled (enzyme, isotope, etc.) antibody.

many companies, each doing only a few of the cytokines; thus no specific reference will be given. A glance at the methods section in an article reporting on assays will give their source. In addition, a glance at a biotechnology based journal and *Science* will give ads, or an immunologist's mail box will give you a plethora of choices). These tests are easy to perform, but have technical difficulties and must be done carefully. Interpretation of the results involves being sure that the control studies were done successfully. Again, as with most studies, a positive test can be evaluated but a negative test is difficult to interpret until you are confident of the laboratory doing the testing.

In vivo studies

The classical test for *cell-mediated immunity* (CMI) (Type IV) in the early days of immunology was the skin test. Antigens were applied to the skin or injected under the skin and swelling was observed in 24–72 hours if there was CMI. This was differentiated from Type I, IgE mediated responses, which occur rapidly (in minutes) and usually disappears in 24 hours. CMI begins in 24 hours, has a swelling with some resemblance to the wheal but does not show a flare. This author does not advocate skin testing for responses to biomaterials since the testing is difficult to do correctly, has the potential for producing sensitivity to the test agents and the results are easily misinterpreted. In general, the use of the actual biomaterial (rather than extracts, corrosion products or constituents) is contraindicated since mechanical irritation may be read as a false positive or or the biomaterial may fail to release the antigen and thus produce a false negative.

Skin testing is an excellent diagnostic procedure in patients with clinical suspicion of hypersensitivity. However, skin testing with haptens, such as metal ions, involves a risk of sensitization. For the immune response to be detected, the hapten must bind to dermal cells or proteins. However, such binding produces a complete antigen which may stimulate an immune response. Since this immune response takes time to develop, the skin test will be negative, but future tests may then be positive. Thus repeated testing increases the likelihood of inducing sensitivity and should be avoided. Bulk biomaterials will probably not give adequate release of soluble materials in the 24–48 period of testing so may produce false negative results.

Histochemical techniques

There are a number of studies now examining tissues removed from sites adjacent to implants. It is possible, using immunological techniques resembling those outlined in Figure 4.1, to identify cell types and perhaps cell products produced at the site. The major interest is in the detection and typing of lymphocytes by use of antisera prepared against the CD markers described earlier. The same type of assay is being initiated for detection of the cytokines in the tissue. The techniques are simple but not all antisera work and thus a variety of antisera are used. The required antisera are available commercially.

Interpretation of the results is again a problem. Tests using 'home made' monoclonal antibodies are suspect until the antisera is made available to other investigators for conformation. The use of well characterized antisera from companies which supply to others is better at this stage. Since the tissue section is examined and scored by an observer, the 'data' from these studies are not really available for analysis by the reader. Computerized image analysis techniques are still not widely used. Thus, in evaluating the results, possible bias of the investigator must be taken into account.

4.5 DETECTION OF IMMUNE RESPONSES TO HAPTENS

Detection of immune responses to haptens is the same as that described above, but there are some special techniques now being used. A hapten–carrier complex can be prepared *in vitro* by combination in solution with a large protein such as albumin or a smaller molecule such as glutathione. These can then be used to coat a solid substrate. Alternatively, the protein carrier can be coated onto a substrate, the hapten added, and then the assay performed. This probably increases the amount of hapten that is available for antibody binding and minimizes that which is lost in the tertiary folding of the protein.

4.6 HUMAN IMMUNE RESPONSE TO MATERIALS

4.6.1 Latex

The term 'latex' actually is confusing since the name is given to some materials because of the way they are processed and not because of their source. The biomaterial latex used to fabricate gloves, condoms, etc. is a rubber (elastomer) extracted from a plant (Hevea brasiliensis). As such, there is a great deal of antigenic protein contamination. Allergies to latex are usually of the Type I, IgE mediated response, with an immediate reaction (in minutes) that can be life threatening. Since latex is encountered in many household objects such as household gloves, balloons, etc., sensitivity to it is a frequent pre-existing condition. Latex material cleaned of protein seems to be nonallergenic. Other types of immune response to latex have not been as frequent or of much concern. Latex is not used as a long term implanted material and thus the long term responses are not noted. The population at greatest risk are the health care workers with the increased use of examining and surgical gloves.

4.6.2 Collagen

This is another material that is an extract of material of natural origin with bovine and orvine skin or tissue the favored source. This is a foreign protein and thus capable of stimulating a variety of immune responses. Antibodies of IgE, IgM, and IgG classes have been observed. Cell mediated immune responses have also been observed. As with latex, the important precaution is to remove as much foreign material as possible. Since collagen across mammalian species has a similar structure, it is possible to remove contaminating proteins and leave a relatively nonallergenic material. Chemical treatment and cross linking of the collagen can further reduce antigenicity. Collagen products need to be carefully evaluated for their ability to initiate immune responses, but it is possible to produce safe products.

4.6.3 Synthetic polymers

The use of chemically defined synthetic polymers is associated with minimal human immune responses. These materials are based on carbon, hydrogen, nitrogen and oxygen which are basic building blocks of the biological system. Thus the generation of antigenic material would be unlikely. Nevertheless, there are some polymeric materials with additional chemical moieties that are of concern.

A. Polysiloxane (silicone elastomer)

There is abundant lay press comment and little scientific material on this topic. It is apparent that there can be binding of silicone to foreign protein with stimulation of the immune response. The use of a simple hapten test, as described in section 4.5, has added greatly to our knowledge of this. It is also apparent that silicone gel is a potent adjuvant enhancing immune responses to unrelated materials. Whether this is of relevance to the use of gel filled implants remains unknown. The possible stimulation of related and unrelated immune responses remain a major concern in the use of these materials.

B. Polyurethanes

This is a complex group of polymers. Their propensity to stimulate an immune response is very small since there are few molecular groups which would be perceived as foreign by the host, perhaps explaining why clinical immune responses to polyurethanes have not been reported.

C. Poly(methyl)methacrylate

Acrylics are in widespread use in activities of daily living. As with metals, there are documented cases of contact dermatitis from the use of these materials, especially self curing glues containing methacrylate monomer that is very skin sensitizing, usually stimulating a Type IV response. The use of these materials for implants generally exposes the patient to the monomer for only a brief period of time as the bone cement or dental acrylic cures *in situ*. Acrylics which are fully polymerized before use will not be associated with an allergic response. Reports of sensitization responses of patients to acrylics are rare and the health care workers at most risk are the personnel, such as the surgeon and dental laboratory technician, handling the monomer frequently.

D. Metals

A number of metallic elements and alloys are used extensively in implants, external medical devices and are encountered in activities of daily living. Allergy to metals as a contact dermatitis (Type IV response) is well known in individuals in contact with metal salts, corroding metals, and jewelry or snaps and fasteners. Reactions have been seen to metals used in dental, orthopaedic, and general surgery. The contact dermatitis from topical use resolves when the device is removed. The role of the immune response in reactions to metals implanted into the deep tissue remains controversial. Cell mediated immune responses have been associated, in some studies but not in others, with pain and swelling at the implant site and loosening of the device. Antibodies to metals in patients with metallic implants have recently been reported, but again the consequences of this response remain unknown. Concern remains about the chronic use of metals that are known human sensitizers, such as chromium, nickel and cobalt.

4.7 CONSEQUENCES OF AN IMMUNE RESPONSE

The immune response is apparently intended to neutralize, detoxify, and help eliminate a foreign material. However, sometimes the immune response can inadvertently cause harm. This will be discussed in various categories in the next section.

1. Damage to the implant. The inflammation which is part of the initiation of the immune response is an oxidative response. Materials subject to oxidative attack, such as polyethylenes and polyurethanes, may be degraded.

2. Damage to adjacent tissues. Products, particularly from Type II and IV responses, may initiate swelling and other vascular responses at the site. This may resolve with no further harm, or it may cause tissue necrosis and/or loss of tissue mass with loosening or movement of the device.
3. Systemic responses. Immune responses of Type I and II generate vasoactive substances which may circulate and cause vascular collapse. This is seen in response to latex materials and drugs which bind to platelets, mast cells, or eosinophils, resulting in an immune response and release of these vasoactive substances.
4. Autoimmune diseases: This is the most controversial area of consequences of immune response to implants. Autoimmune diseases are technically the result of an immune response to host tissue. Autoimmune diseases such as arthritis, glomerulonephritis, etc., occur in individuals with an unknown cause of onset although some have an association with a preceding infection (especially *streptococci*). Proving cause and effect is an epidemiological problem with surveys of large populations. It is important to refine our immunological testing techniques to prove cause and effect associated with implants and do thorough epidemiological studies.

These responses, if present in clinical populations, may arise from several mechanisms. The two most likely ones associated with the use of implants are (i) binding of the material to host tissue making it a foreign substance such as with hapten–carrier complexes or (ii) altering the host tissue through folding of proteins, degradation of cells or proteins thus making then antigenic for the host. This is the main issue now with the silicone breast implants. This is difficult to prove and massive studies as controlled as possible are needed.

4.8 CONCLUSIONS

There has been a rapid growth in our knowledge of the immune response and how to evaluate and quantitate it. As these techniques are applied to the population in contact with biomaterials, we will learn more about its importance in performance of the material. We will also learn more about how to process the materials to minimize the immune response. However, it is important to remember that the immune response is a protective response and detection of immune responses to products of biomaterials does not necessarily indicate clinical problems. On the other hand, implants are foreign material and will stimulate host responses, some of which may cause harm to the host or implant.

Thus the important issue is to distinguish between those immune responses which are normal and help to render antigens less biologically active from those which are harmful to the host. It is clear that IgE (Type I) responses are harmful. Detection of a Type I response to products of biomaterials indicates potential problems in the clinical setting. Responses of the IgG type are generally protective and may not be predictive of further problems unless there is continual release of antigenic material leading to a Type III-response. Biomaterial wear and degradation products that bind to platelets or mast cells pose a potential for adverse Type II responses.

The most commonly observed is the Type IV (cell-mediated) response. This is a protective response in walling off the stimulating agent and in killing cells which have the antigen on the surface, thus eliminating the antigen. However, the tissue reaction accompanying this response may cause harm to the host through soft and hard tissue necrosis. The difference between protection and allergy from Type IV responses is still unclear and careful evaluation of patients is required.

ADDITIONAL READING

General Immunology

Golub, E.S. and Green, D.R. (1990) *Immunology, A Synthesis*, 2nd Edition, Sinauer Associates, Inc., Sunderland: Good general text.

Roitt, I. (1971) *Essential Immunology*, Blackwell Scientific Publications, London: Good description of types I–IV reactions.

Annual Review of Immunology, Annual Reviews Inc., Palo Alto, CA: Yearly publication with timely reviews.

Immunology Today: Elsevier Science Inc. Tarrytown, NY: Monthly: Good review articles.

Antigen Presentation

Celada, A. and Nathan, C. (1994) Macrophage activation revisited. *Immunology Today*, **15**, 100–102: good review of macrophages.

Chicz, R.M. and Urban, R.G. (1994). Analysis of MHC presented peptides: applications in autoimmunity and vaccine development. *Immunology Today*, **15**, 155–160: good review on a complicated subject.

CD markers

Kemeny, D.M., Noble, A. Holmes, B.J. *et al.* (1994) Immune regulation: a new role for the CD8+ T cell. *Immunology Today*, **15**, 107–110: Good description of the function of the CD8+ T-cell which is a key cell in Type IV responses.

Sclossman, S.F., Boumsell, L., Gilkes, L.W. *et al.* (1994) CD antigens 1993. *Immunology Today*, **15**, 98–99: good description of recently reported CDs.

Cytokines/interleukins

Miyajima, A., Kitamura, T., Harada, N. *et al.* (1992) Cytokine receptors and Signal Transduction. *Annual Reviews of Immunology*, **10**, 295–331: Review of function and methods of stimulation.

Mizel, S.B. (1989) The interleukins. *FASEB J.* **3**, 2379–2388: good detailed review.

Effects of cytokines/interleukins

Goldring, M.B., and Goldring, S.R. (1990) Skeletal tissue response to cytokines. *Clin. Orthop. Rel. Res.*, **258**, 245–278: review of cytokines and orthopaedics.

Stashenko, P., Obernesser, M.S., and Dewhirst, F.E. (1989) Effect of immune cytokines on bone. *Immuno Invest.*, **18**, 239–249: one of the few reviews focussing on bone.

Immune response to metals/metallic implants

Agrup, G. (1968) Sensitization induced by patch testing, *Brit. J. Derm.*, **80**, 631–634: points out problem of routine skin testing in nonallergic individual.

Benson, M.K.D., Goodwin, P.G. and Brostoff, J. (1975) Metal sensitivity in patients with joint replacement arthroplasties, *Brit. Med. J.*, **4**, 374–375: third of the original 1975 articles pointing to a possible problem. Skin test used.

Black J. (1988) Does corrosion matter? *J. Bone Jt. Surg.*, **70B** (4), 517–520: discusses issues of importance of understanding corrosion, minimizing it, and recognizing it can be important for the patient.

Brown, G.C., Lockshin, M.D., Salvati, E.A. *et al.*, (1977) Sensitivity to metal as a possible cause of sterile loosening after cobalt–chromium total hip-replacement arthroplasty, *J. Bone Joint Surg.*, **59A**(2), 164–168: Denies existence of metal allergy in orthopaedics. Complete misinterpretation of data. Uses negative results of an invalid test to draw conclusions. Limited patient population deliberately selected to prove lack of allergy.

Burholm, A.; Al-Tawil, N.A.; Marcusson, J.A. *et al.* (1990): The lymphocyte response to nickel salt in patients with orthopedic implants. *Acta Orthop. Scand.*, **61**(2): 248–250: Example of use of LTT test.

Elves, M.W., Wilson, J.N. and Kemp, H.B.S. (1975) Incidence of metal sensitivity in patients with total joint replacements. *Brit. Med. J.*, **4**, 376–378: Second one of the original 1975 articles pointing to a possible problem. Skin test used.

Evans, E.M., Freeman, M.A.R., Miller, A.J. *et al.* (1974) Metal Sensitivity as a Cause of Bone Necrosis and Loosening of the Prosthesis in Total Joint Replacement, *J. Bone and Joint Surg.*, **56B** (4), 626–642: One of the original articles pointing to a possible problem. Skin test used.

Goh, C.L. (1986) Prevalence of contact allergy by sex, race, and age. *Contact Dermat.*, **14**, 237–240: discusses normal population

Grimsdottir, M.R., Gjerdet, N.R. and Hensten-Pettersen, A. (1992) Composition and *in vitro* corrosion of orthodontic appliances. *Am. J. Orthod. Dentofac. Orthop.*, **101**, 525–532: Discusses sensitivity and stainless steels. Release of nickel related to many metallurgical aspects and not necessarily to nickel content of the metal.

Lalor, P.A., Revell, P.A., Gray, A.B. *et al.* (1991) Sensitivity to titanium. *J. Bone and Joint Surg.*, **73B**(1), 25–28: Description of possible titanium sensitivity. Patch test vehicle of unknown composition, larger cobalt–chromium component than titanium component in device. Of interest and important, but not conclusive.

Menne, T.; and Maibach, H.I. (1989) Systemic contact allergy reactions. *Immunol Allergy Clin. N.A.*, **9**, 507–522: Discusses extension from contact dermatitis to systemic reactions.

Merritt, K. (1984) Role of medical materials, both in implant and surface applications, in immune response and in resistance to infection. *Biomaterials*, **5** (1), 47–53.: Review article. Out of date now but covers literature through 1983.

Merritt, K. (1986) Biochemistry/hypersensitivity/clinical reactions. in: Lang B, Morris, J. and Rassoog, J. (eds). *Proc. International Workshop on Biocompatibility, Toxicity, and Hypersensitivity to Alloy Systems used in Dentistry*. Ann Arbor, U. MI; pp 195–223.: Review article. Covers the literature through 1984. Good discussion of the problem in the discussion section of the symposium.

Merritt, K. (1986) Chapter 6. Immunological testing of biomaterials, *Techniques of Biocompatibility Testing*, D.F. Williams (ed.), Vol. II, CRC Press, Boca Raton: Description of possible test methods.

Merritt, K.; and Brown, S.A. (1980): Tissue reaction and metal sensitivity: An animal study. *Acta Orthop. Scand.* **51** (3), 403–411: Example of use of LIF test.

Rostoker, G., Robin, J., Binet, O. *et al.* (1987) Dermatitis due to orthopaedic implants. *J. Bone Joint Surg.*, **69A**, 1408–1412: Example of a reaction to implant.

Rudner, E.J., Clendenning, W.E., Epstein, E. *et al.* (1975) The frequency of contact dermatitis in North America 1972–1974. *Contact Derm.* **1**, 277–280: Incidence of contact dermatitis.

Shirakawa, T., Kusaka, Y. and Morimoto, K. (1992) Specific IgE antibodies to nickel in workers with known reactivity to cobalt. *Clin. Exp. Allergy*, **22** (2), 213–218: Measuring IgE and nickel cobalt interactions.

Trobelli, L., Virgili, A., Corassa, M. *et al.* (1992) Systemic contact dermatitis from an orthodontic appliance. *Contact Dermatitis*, **27**, 259–260: Example of reaction to dental application of metals.

Yang, J., and Merritt, K. (1994) Detection of antibodies against corrosion products in patients after Co–Cr total joint replacements. *J. Biomed. Mater. Res.*, **28**, 1249–1258: Method for measuring antibodies to metals

Immune response to latex, collagen, silicones

Belsito, D.V. (1990) Contact urticaria caused by rubber. Analysis of seven cases. *Dermatol. Clin.* **8**, 61–66: Questions whether increased demand for latex may have decreased quality with more allergens leachable.

Hanke, C.W., Higley, H.R., Jolivette, D.M. *et al.* (1991) Abscess formation and local necrosis after treatment with Zyderm or Zyplast collagen implant. *J. Amer. Acad. Dermatol.* **25**, 319–326: Deals with some adverse responses to collagen materials which may be related to the immune response. Points to possible problems.

Meade, K.R., Silver, F.H. (1990) Immunogenicity of collagenous implants. *Biomaterials*, **11**, 176–180: Discusses immunogenicity problem and cross linking. Good place to begin reading.

Naim, J.O., Lanzafame, R.J. and van Oss, C.J. (1993). The adjuvant effect of silicone gel on antibody formation in rats. *Immunol Inv.*, **22**, 151–161: Shows that the gel is better than Freund's adjuvant in stimulating the response to BSA in rats. Caution on use of gel.

Slater, J.E. (1989) Rubber anaphylaxis. *New Eng. J. Med.* **320**, 1126–1130: Good methods. Good literature review, real cases reacting to anaesthesia mask.

Sussman, G.L., Tarlo, S. and Dolovich, J. (1991). The spectrum of IgE responses to latex. *J. Am. Med. Assoc.* **265**, 2844–2847: Latex gloves on health workers causing allergic responses in patients. Can do skin test with latex to check patients or use non-latex gloves.

Warpinski, J.R., Folgert, J., Cohen, M. *et al.* (1991) R.K. Bush. Allergic reaction to latex: a risk factor for unsuspected anaphylaxis. *Allergy Proc.* **12**, 95–102: Clinical symptoms of Type I allergy. Identifies IgE antibodies against latex (gloves, balloons, condoms). IgE against proteins from latex.

Wolk, L.E., Lappe, M., Peterson, R.D. *et al.* (1993) Immune response to polydimethylsiloxane (silicone): screening studies in a breast implant population. *FASEB J.*, **7**, 1265–1268: Very important study with a good technique. Hopefully more studies will be done with this technique. Valid test of antibody to silicone.

Oxidative damage of implants

Carter, W.O., Narayanan, P.K. and Robinson, J.P. (1994). Intracellular hydrogen peroxide and superoxide anion detection in endothelial cells. *J. Leukocyte Biol.* **55**, 253–258: Good method for detecting H_2O_2 release and superoxide production. Example of biologically produced oxidizing species.

Kao, W.J., Zhao, Q.H., Hiltner, A. *et al.* (1994) Theoretical analysis of *in vivo* macrophage adhesion and foreign body giant cell formation on polymethylsiloxane, low density polyethylene, and polyetherurethanes. *J. Biomed. Mater. Res.*, **28** (1), 73–80: Recent article on macrophages on polymers and references some articles on oxidative events.

Kaplan, S.S., Basford, R.E., Jeong, M.H. *et al.* (1994) Mechanisms of biomaterial-induced superoxide release by neutrophils. *J. Biomed. Mater. Res.*, **28**, 377–86: Discusses the release of reactive oxygen species stimulated by biomaterials. Not all materials are activating.

Consequences of immune responses to materials

Angell, M. (1994) Do Breast implants cause systemic disease? Science in the courtroom *New Eng. J. Med.*, **330** (24), 1748–1749: Editorial in response to article by Gabriel *et al.* (1994) Reiterates the necessity of doing detailed studies. Indictment of patients, manufacturers and government jumping to conclusions using inadequate data. Doesn't say how we get the adequate data though.

Gabriel, S.E., O'Fallon, W.M., Kurland, L.T. *et al.* (1994) Risk of connective tissue diseases and other disorders after breast implantation. *New Eng. J. Med.*, **330** (24), 1697–1702: Excellent study. Shows problems of doing studies on long term consequences. Example of how it ought to be done.

Cancer

5

M. Rock

5.1 INTRODUCTION

The widespread use of temporary and permanent implants in the post World War II era has had a dramatic impact on the practice of medicine and on the life of disabled and ill individuals. Nowhere has this been more obvious than in the frequent use of implants to stabilize fractures and replace diseased joints which has revolutionized orthopedic practice and afforded millions of patients levels of function that previously could not be achieved. Although the metal alloys used in these implants exhibit excellent resistance to corrosion, oxidation of these large components ultimately produce free ions, chlorides, oxides, and hydroxides which, in combination with particulate metal matter released by wear and fretting, are released into the surrounding environment. Efforts to improve these alloys have included compositional as well as processing changes. Additionally, modifications have been made to the plastic articulating components in efforts to produce a much more consistent ultrahigh molecular weight polyethylene. The perceived need to improve implant wear and corrosion resistance and alter design has been largely motivated by the excessive soft tissue staining noted by orthopedic surgeons at the time of removal or revision of clinically failed joint arthroplasty. The presence of particulate metal matter, polyethylene, and even fragments of polymethyl methacrylate in local tissue has been confirmed histologically and by direct analysis [1–4]. In spite of all of the modifications made in implant composition, implant fixation, and articulation, biomaterial degradation and release of these products persist [4–7].

Handbook of Biomaterial Properties. Edited by J. Black and G. Hastings.
Published in 1998 by Chapman & Hall, London. ISBN 0 412 60330 6.

5.2 RELEASE AND DISTRIBUTION OF DEGRADATION PRODUCTS

The body's response to the local presence of debris is dependent on the size, amount, and composition as well as rate of accumulation. The body attempts to neutralize these foreign particles by precipitating granulomatous foreign body reactions and/or removal through local lymphatic channels. If the local accumulation of debris exceeds the body's ability to neutralize and/or transport, the debris migrates from the site to remote areas including the bone–implant interface, possibly contributing to if not initiating the phenomena of loosening and osteolysis (Figure 5.1).

Of equal or possibly even greater concern is the detection of metal ions, metallic debris, polyethylene, and even methylmethacrylate in areas remote from the implant including circulating serum, excreted urine, and regional draining lymph nodes. Elevated serum levels of metal ions consistent with the composition of the implanted alloy have been confirmed in animal models [8] and in human patients after total hip arthroplasty [9]; identifying serum levels of cobalt, chromium, nickel, and titanium that are two and three fold higher than preoperative determinations. These figures represent significant elevations both over means for contemporary control groups and for the individual patients before operation [9]. However, since they are within the widely accepted normal range for these metallic ions in the unimplanted human controls, it is assumed that toxic levels of these foreign materials do not materialize. However, when analyzing the serum to urine concentration in patients subjected to conventional total hip arthroplasty, it has become apparent that the urinary concentration of chromium in particular does not rise with the same magnitude and time course as the serum level [9]. This observation parallels that made in the accounts of industrial overexposure to Cr^{6+} and suggests that metal ions accumulate in organs and tissues remote from implantation. Such accumulation is unlike that resulting from normal

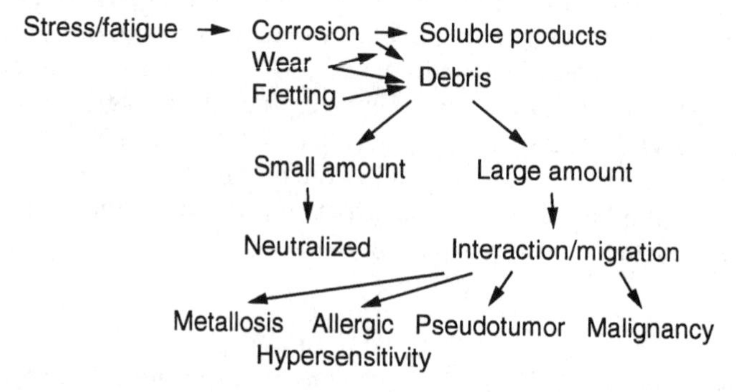

Figure 5.1 Tissue Reaction to Implant Degradation Products.

systemic circulation. This was previously suggested by Steineman [10] who calculated the potential release of metallic ions of 0.15 to 0.3 micrograms per cm^2 per day which would translate to between 11 and 22 milligrams per year in patients with total hip replacement. This incidentally coincides with or exceeds the total body burden of such metallic ions in a 70 kilogram man [11].

Evidence for metallic debris accumulating in distant organs has also been confirmed by Langkamer *et al.* [12] who identified wide spread dissemination of particulate wear debris from hip prosthesis to lymph nodes, liver, and spleen. He reported increases above normal levels in these organs of 30 fold for aluminum, chromium, and iron in the lymph node, and 10 fold in the spleen and liver.

These findings suggest that concentrations of metal ions and debris at remote sites may reach such proportions as to precipitate altered cellular dynamics in organs principally of the lymphoreticular system. It would only be logical to assume that local concentrations of such debris at the site of implantation would be even higher, although attempts at quantifying the effects of local concentrations have been fraught with inaccuracies mostly due to sampling error and the need to distinguish between bioavailable and non bioavailable metal species.

What is potentially more disturbing is that these figures for serum concentrations and the identification of this debris in remote organs have come primarily from patients who have received conventional polymethyl methacrylate cemented components. With the advent of using uncemented porous coated implants, particularly in younger patients, these figures would be expected to increase, creating the distinct possibility of toxic levels in the serum, tissues and organs that will respond with altered cellular dynamics and function.

5.3 NEOPLASIA

Perhaps one of the greatest concerns with debris dissemination locally and within the systemic circulation is the possibility of inducing malignant neoplasia. This is thought to be possible by one of two mechanisms:

(i) A 'solid-state' mechanism has been proposed, whereby a large foreign object implanted *in vivo* possibly stimulates mutagenesis of local cells, thereby creating tumor by its mere presence. Most large foreign objects upon implantation will initiate a very marked fibrous reaction. The cells within this fibrous reaction ultimately mutate and become cancer growths.

(ii) The other possibility is that particulate metal matter or other debris have an innate capacity, upon corrosion or dissolution, to induce cancer through a more traditional chemical route.

Cancer, the end product of carcinogenesis, is the result of transformation of a normal cells to ones which grow in an uncontrolled or malignant manner. Cancer is a genetic disease, which may result from expression of genetic pre-dispositions present from birth or from later insults to cells of many different types. In particular, the phagocytosis or pinocytosis of foreign matter (in an attempt to neutralize or eliminate it) may cause or precipitate malignant conversion. Such conversion, if not lethal to the cell, may then persist through cell duplication, creating first a cluster of cells with altered DNA and eventually a clinical malignant tumor. Malignancy is characterized by rapid, uncontrolled growth, invasion in surrounding tissues and seeding to form tumors (metastases) in other anatomical locations such as the lung.

Some of the more common malignant tumors of musculoskeletal origin are osteosarcoma (OS) of bone and malignant fibrous histiocytoma (MFA) of soft tissue.

Osteosarcoma is the most common tumor of bone: it occurs in children, adolescents and, less frequently, in adults. OS may also occur as a consequence of radiation therapy or in Paget's disease, an ostensibly benign bone embrittling disease of the elderly. It frequently appears about the knee (distal femur; proximal tibia), and in the proximal femur and proximal humerus.

MFA is the most common primary malignant tumor of soft tissues and can occur in bone in adults over the ages of 50–55. The more common soft tissue type usually involves the large muscular areas of the body, including the thigh, buttock and upper arm and shoulder.

5.4 EVIDENCE FOR CARCINOGENICITY OF IMPLANTED MATERIALS

Well-documented cases of carcinoma and sarcoma have developed in refinery workers who inhaled nickel and chromium and in miners who were exposed to iron or even at local injection sites of iron dextran [13]. Aluminum has been linked to a high rate of lung and bladder cancer in exposed individuals and titanium has been associated with experimental induction of lymphoreticular tumors and leukemia. Although the results have not been universally accepted, many animal experiments have shown a direct correlation between the initiation of sarcomas and the injection of particulate metal debris. This appears to be related to the concentration, as well as the physical nature, of the metal implanted [14]. Metal ions, particularly cobalt, chromium, and nickel, are known to induce infidelity of DNA synthesis by causing the pairing of non-complimentary nucleotides and thereby creating a misinterpretation of the genetic code which may lead to neoplasia.

Furthermore, it must be remembered that particulate metal matter may not be the only solid-form material that can be, and has been proven to be, carcinogenic in appropriate environments. In 1954 long before the first total hip arthroplasty was performed, Laskin [15] observed the carcinogenic capabilities of polymethylmethacrylate after subcutaneous introduction of this material in mice. His conclusions suggested that similar occurrences of tumor may appears in humans that were being treated at that time with methylmethacrylate for dental deficiencies and that this evolution of cancer may take up to 20 years of exposure given the proportional time exposure before tumors were seen in the mice. A similar conclusion was reached [16] on the use of polyethylene plastic before it was conventionally used in the management of arthritic joints. Regardless of form, whether powder or large solid segments, polyethylene plastic produced sarcomas in 25 percent and 35 percent of rats, respectively. Their conclusions also suggested a latent period, after exposure, of 20 years in humans before such an event could be expected to occur.

It is, therefore, with interest that investigators were forewarning the medical community of the carcinogenic effect of metals and polymers years before the development and introduction of joint replacement using these very same materials. In 1961, Sir John Charnley introduced total hip arthroplasty as an alternative in the management of arthritic hips. No other orthopedic procedure has been adopted with such enthusiasm. Thirty-five years later we are still witnessing an incremental increase in the yearly utilization of this operation, attesting to the obvious success associated with it. According to some investigators, we may be coming into an era of increased tumor activity in the vicinity of or possibly remote from implantation sites of these orthopedic appliances.

5.5 CASE REPORTS OF IMPLANT RELATED TUMORS

In 1976, Harris *et al.* [17] were the first to describe an aggressive granulomatous lesion around a cemented femoral stem in a total hip replacement. This was a condition of localized tumor-like bone resorption that appeared radiographically as large lytic defects within the femur, approximating the cement mantle of the implant. Initially thought to be neoplastic, these lesions were surgically biopsied and found to be consistent with well-organized connective tissue containing numerous histiocytes, monocytes, and fibroblastic reactive zones. Immunohistologic evaluation revealed multinucleated giant cells and nonspecific esterase-positive monocyte macrophages. These findings suggest a foreign-body type reaction, and with the subsequent isolation of polyethylene, polymethyl methacrylate, and metal debris, it was theorized that these constituents of the construct likely migrated down around the implant cement mantle in cemented prostheses and implant–bone interface in non-circumferentially coated ingrowth implants. Such a reaction suggests an excessive accumulation of debris at the site of articulation that surpasses the body's ability to neutralize and/or transport the material resulting in migration of debris to sites remote from the source. This rapid appearance of bone loss radiographically which is often associated with a deteriorating clinical course has been termed type-II aseptic loosening [17].

In 1978, two years after the recognition of pseudo tumors of bone induced by the degradation products of total hip arthroplasty, Arden and Bywaters [20] (Table 5.1) reported a case of a 56-year-old patient who developed a high-grade fibrosarcoma of soft tissue 2.5 years after receiving a metal-on-metal McKee–Farrar hip prosthesis. The tumor apparently did not have a direct association with the underlying bone or any components of the total hip arthroplasty. No formal analysis of the tumor for debris

Table 5.1 Malignancies Associated with Joint Replacements (published)

Author	*Year*	*Implant*	*Time interval (yrs)*	*Tumor type*
Castleman and McNeely [18]	1965	Austin–Moore	1	M.F.H.*
Rushforth [19]	1974	McKee–Farrar	0.5	Osteosarcoma
Arden and Bywaters [20]	1978	McKee–Farrar	2.5	Fibrosarcoma
Bagó-Granell *et al.* [21]	1984	Charnley–Muller	2	M.F.H.
Penman and Ring [22]	1984	Ring	5	Osteosarcoma
Swann [23]	1984	McKee–Farrar	4	M.F.H.
Weber [26]	1986	Cemented TKA	4.5	Epithelioid sarcoma
Ryu *et al.* [27]	1987	Uncemented Vitallium**	1.4	M.F.H.
Vives *et al.* [28]	1987	Charnley–Muller	2	M.F.H.
Van der List [29]	1988	Charnley–Muller	11	Angiosarcoma
Lamovec *et al.* [30]	1988	Charnley–Muller	11	Synovial sarcoma
Lamovec *et al.* [31]	1988	Charnley–Muller	10	Osteosarcoma
Tait *et al.* [32]	1988	Charnley–Muller	11	M.F.H.
Martin *et al.* [33]	1988	Charnley–Muller	10	Osteosarcoma
Haag and Adler [34]	1989	Weber–Huggler	10	M.F.H.
Mazabraud *et al.* [35]	1989	unknown	9	Epidermoid sarcoma
Brien *et al.* [36]	1990	Charnley	8	Osteosarcoma
Troop *et al.* [37]	1990	Charnley–Muller	15	M.F.H.
Kolstad and Högstorp [38]	1990	Freeman TKA	0.25	Metastatic adenocarcinoma
Jacobs *et al.* [39]	1992	AML cementless	0.5	M.F.H.
Solomon and Sekel [40]	1992	Charnley–Muller	7	M.F.H.

* *M.F.H. = malignant fibrous histiocytoma.*
** Trademark, Howmedica, Inc. (Cobalt–Chromium alloy).

products was performed. This case drew attention to the possibility of tumors being initiated in the presence of large orthopedic appliances. It was not until 1984 when this concept became fashionable in large part due to three articles that appeared simultaneously in the *Journal of Bone and Joint Surgery* recounting two malignant fibrous histiocytomas and one osteosarcoma at the site of a total hip arthroplasty [21–23].

This sudden and rather unexpected evolution prompted editorials [24, 25] in the same journal addressing the issue of sarcoma and total hip arthroplasty and encouraged the orthopedic community worldwide to report such cases to a central registry to obtain more accurate figures on the incidence of such a problem. These tumors occurred 2, 4, and 5 years after hip replacement that was performed with various femoral and acetabular components, some with metal-on-metal articulations and others with metal on polyethylene. In two of these cases, the proximal femur was extensively involved with tumor that was in direct contact with the component. The remaining case was a soft-tissue sarcoma not in direct approximation to the prosthesis. Two of these tumors were malignant fibrous histiocytomas, one of bone and one of soft tissue. The remaining tumor was osteosarcoma. In this particular case, there was evidence of gray-brown pigmentation both intra- and extracellularly between the tumor and femoral component. No formal metal analysis was performed. Three additional cases emerged prior to 1988 at 15 months, 4.5 years, and 2.0 years after implantation [26–28].

In 1988, five cases were reported occurring at 10 [29, 30] and 11[29, 31, 32] years after implantation. The sarcomas included two osteosarcomas, two malignant fibrous histiocytomas, and one synovial sarcoma. Two of these were soft tissue in a location with no direct association with the implant, yet in the case reported by Tait *et al.* [32] there was evidence of nickel within tumor cells. The remaining three patients all had direct contact with either the cement or implant with the tumor originating in bone.

In 1990 there were three additional reports in the literature which included an osteosarcoma developing at the site of a Charnley total hip arthroplasty 8 years [36] after implantation, malignant fibrous histiocytoma developing 15 years after a Charnley–Muller total hip arthroplasty [37], and metastatic adenocarcinoma developing at the site of a Freeman total knee arthroplasty three months after implantation [38]. In 1992, Jacobs *et al.* [39] presented a malignant fibrous histiocytoma developing one half year after implantation of a cementless AML total hip arthroplasty.

In that same journal volume, unpublished but submitted reports of five tumors occurring around implants were brought to the attention of the orthopedic community [41] (Table 5.2). These included malignant fibrous histiocytomas around a Thompson and a Muller total hip arthroplasties, an osteosarcoma around a Charnley total hip arthroplasty, a rhabdomyosarcoma of soft tissue in the vicinity of a Christiansen total hip arthroplasty, and a chondrosarcoma developing in a patient with Maffucci syndrome having a Charnley total hip arthroplasty. The intervals from implantation to tumor detection were 9, 3, 10, 9 and 1 years respectively. To this, we add two previously unreported additional patients, neither of whom had their joint replacement done at the Mayo Clinic (Table 5.2). The first is that of a 79-year-old man who nine months previously came to total hip replacement with an uncemented Harris–Galante component who was found to have a large malignant fibrous histiocytoma engulfing the proximal femur and extending to the implant. There was, however, no evidence of any particulate debris within the tumor cells removed. The second case was that of a 56-year-old man who developed a soft tissue osteosarcoma 14 months after a left total knee arthroplasty with conventional cemented components. The tumor extended down to both the femoral and patellar components.

5.6 CRITICAL ANALYSIS OF TUMORS

As such, 28 tumors have been reported in direct contact or in close proximity to joint arthroplasty. The vast majority of these appeared with total hip arthroplasty [27] with a smaller contribution from total knee arthroplasty [3]. There have been no reported cases of malignant degeneration occurring in the vicinity of total shoulder and/or total elbow arthroplasty. Of the reported 26 cases, 8 tumors were of soft tissue origin, 19 were of primary bone pathology, and 1 metastatic gastric carcinoma. The histogenesis of the soft tissue tumor included 3 malignant fibrous histiocytomas, 1 synovial sarcoma, 1 soft tissue osteogenic sarcoma, 1 fibrosarcoma, 1 epidermoid sarcoma and 1 rhabdomyosarcoma. The histogenesis of the primary bone tumors included 10 malignant fibrous histiocytomas,

Table 5.2 Malignancies Associated with Joint Replacements (unpublished)[41]

Author	*Year*	*Implant*	*Time interval (yrs)*	*Tumor type*
Harris	1992	Charnley	1	Chondrosarcoma
Surin	1992	Christiansen	9	Rhabdomyosarcoma
Lightowler	1992	Charnley	10	Osteosarcoma
Rees, Thompson, Burns	1992	Thompson	3	M.F.H.*
Nelson	1992	Muller	9	M.F.H.
Rock	1992	HG ingrowth	0.8	M.F.H.
Rock	1992	PCA TKA	1.2	Osteosarcoma

* *M.F.H. = Malignant Fibrous Histiocytoma.*

6 osteosarcomas, 1 chondrosarcoma, 1 angiosarcoma, 1 fibrosarcoma. Direct contact with the underlying tumor was noted in 15 of the 19 cases in which sufficient information is known from which to make such determinations. In three of the cases, particulate metal matter was determined to be present in the tumor including one case of a soft tissue sarcoma that appeared on image and exploration to be remote from the implant but had obvious evidence of nickel present within the tumor cells.

Many of these tumors have not had an appropriate latent interval between implantation and development to be seriously considered implant induced. Given that the interval to tumor induction from bone stimulation should be at least as long as the accepted five year interval from radiation therapy to sarcoma degeneration, 15 of the 28 patients would qualify, all of whom have had tumours around total hip arthroplasties.

Apart from tumors developing at the site of prosthetic replacement, there have been ten known malignant tumors that have developed at the site of previous internal fixation (Table 5.3). To date there have been no malignancies noted around a titanium implant. The vast majority (> 80%) of malignancies both in the prosthetic and internal fixation groups have occurred in the vicinity of Vitallium™ (cobalt–chromium alloy) implants. This is not, however, to exonerate stainless steel because tumors in the proximity of the implants made of this alloy have been reported in the animal literature [52] as well as the human experience utilizing stainless steel as fixation devices for traumatology [42, 44, 50, 51]. It is interesting to note that in 1976 veterinarians were encouraged within their own literature to report similar experiences of tumors around implants nearly eight years before such concern was voiced with the application of these same metallic alloys in humans [52].

Table 5.3 Malignancies Associated with Internal Fixation of Fractures

Author	*Year*	*Implant*	*Time interval (yrs)*	*Tumor type*
McDougall [42]	1956	Stainless steel	30	Ewings
Delgado [43]	1958	Unknown	3	Undifferentiated
Dube and Fisher [44]	1972	Stainless steel	36	Angiosarcoma
Tayton [45]	1980	Vitallium*	7.5	Ewings
McDonald [46]	1981	Vitallium	17	Lymphoma
Dodion *et al.* [47]	1982	Vitallium	1.2	Lymphoma
Lee *et al.* [48]	1984	Vitallium	14	M.F.H.*
Hughes *et al.* [49]	1987	Vitallium	29	M.F.H.
Ward *et al.* [50]	1990	Stainless steel	9	Osteosarcoma
Khurana *et al.* [51]	1991	Stainless steel	13	M.F.H.

* *Trademark, Howmedica, Inc. (cobalt–chromium alloy).*
** *M.F.H. = malignant fibrous histiocytoma.*

5.7 SIGNIFICANCE OF CLINICAL REPORTS

As impressive as these cases may be, they must be put into perspective given the global use of internal fixation and prosthetic devices. Approximately 300 000 to 350 000 total hip joint replacements are performed worldwide on a yearly basis [53]. It can be assumed that approximately four million people will have had total hip arthroplasties performed by the end of 1995. To date, there have been 28 reports of malignant tumor arising in close proximity to these implants (25 total hip and three total knee arthroplasties). No direct contact was noted in four. If we assume a minimal latency of five years to suggest association between presence of implant and tumor, 15 of the 28 could have association. As such, the incidence of sarcomas in total joint replacement would be approximately 1 in 250 000. There are approximately 3000 new primary bone tumors and 5000 soft-tissue sarcomas in the United States per year. This would give an incidence of approximately 1 in 100 000 for the general population to develop a primary bone sarcoma and 1 in 40 000 to develop a soft tissue sarcoma a year. This is obviously not stratified for age given that many primary bone tumors develop in the second and third generation of life, yet it does afford the opportunity of putting this rather unusual event in perspective.

The prevalence of osteosarcoma among the osseous malignancies in this series is not entirely unexpected. Of the total osteosarcoma population 15 percent to 20 percent occur after the age of 50 years. Most of these cases are superimposed on Paget's disease or in previously irradiated tissue, yet *de novo* cases of osteosarcoma do occur in this age group. Malignant fibrous histiocytoma of bone is somewhat less common. A review of the Mayo Clinic files reveals 71 cases with more than half of these occurring after age 55. Malignant fibrous histiocytoma of soft tissue is the most common soft-tissue sarcoma. It is not surprising, therefore, that two of six soft-tissue tumors in the combined series are of this histogenesis. As such, the distribution of sarcomas in the combined series could have been predicted from general population data given the age of the patients and anatomical distribution.

There have been two separate reports that have critically analyzed the cancer risk after total hip arthroplast [54, 55]. The combined person years of exposure after operation between the two series was 20 015. The overall cancer incidence among total hip replacement procedure in both series did not appear to be any different than what was expected or anticipated. The cancer-observed/expected ratio was especially low for the first two years following surgery in both series, implying that patients undergoing this procedure are otherwise generally healthy. In both series, the observed/expected ratio of developing lymphoma or leukemia was two to three times higher in patients who had total hip arthroplasty. Additionally, there was a two fold decrease in breast carcinoma among patients who had total hip arthroplasty.

Of interest, Gillespie *et al.* [54] suggested a similar decrease in the incidence of rectal, colon, and lung cancer among total hip arthroplasty patients. The results suggest or are possibly compatible with the hypothesis of chronic stimulation of the immune system, thereby potentially allowing for malignancies to occur within the lymphoreticular system. We have already determined a predilection for particulate metal matter to accumulate in the reticuloendothelial system [12]. This has been further supported by studies in animals subjected to metal implants, especially those containing nickel, in which there was an increase in malignancies of the lymphoretinacular systemic [52]. Additionally, due to the added immune surveillance, tumors of the breast, possibly colon, rectal, and lung may be decreased. A hyper immune state is not unexpected given the dissemination of debris locally at implantation sites as well as the well-recognized and documented capacity of this material to gain access to the systemic and possibly storage sites including the reticuloendothelial system. This trend obviously needs continued surveillance.

A recent extensive analysis of the cancer risk in a cohort of 39 154 patients with at least one hip replacement operation has been performed by the Swedish Nationwide In-Patient Registry [56]. Patients were identified by means of a linkage to the Swedish Cancer Registry. The overall results, although showing a significant 3% increase in cancer, were judged by the authors not to be of clinical significance. Increases of cancer of kidney, skin and brain in women and of prostate in men were found, accompanied by a decrease in gastric cancer for women. The study showed no increase in lymphoreticular cancers as previously reported [54,55] nor a decrease in colon, breast or rectal cancers. The authors' judgement is that the overall cancer risk associated with total hip replacement arthoplasty is negligible and should not distract from the obvious benefits of the procedure.

A similar extensive review of the relationship between metallic implants and cancer in dogs was performed by Li *et al.* [57]. This case controlled study of 1857 dogs from 22 veterinary medical centers failed to reveal significant association between stainless steel fracture fixation devices and the development of bone and soft tissue sarcomas.

5.8 SUMMARY

In summary, careful examination of the scientific and clinical literature suggests that implant materials commonly used for fixation and joint reconstruction are not entirely inert. Accumulation of particulate debris is to some extent going to occur in all patients who have large prosthetic devices. This necessarily includes the distinct possibility of systemic and remote site exposure to these foreign objects that the body attempts to neutralize and excrete. Due to the heightened immunologic surveillance and/or possible storage of particulate metal matter in sites remote from the implantation site, patients with total hip arthroplasty may be at added risk for remote malignancies, particularly of the lymphoreticular system. The incidence of primary mesenchymal tumors in close proximity to implants appears to be consistent with the incidence in the general public. The frequency of occurrence and the associated individual and group risks of systemic and remote site malignancy remains unresolved.

ADDITIONAL READING

Nyren, O., McLaughlin, J.K. *et al.* (1995) Cancer risk after hip replacement with metal implants: A population based study. *J. National Can. Inst.* **87,** 28–33.

An extensive review of risk of cancer in 39 154 total hip replacement patients who appeared in the Swedish National Cancer Registry between 1965 and 1983. A review of 60 cancer-specific sites showed an overall, not clinically significant increase of 3% in incidence, slight increases noted for kidney cancer, prostate cancer (in men) and melanoma accompanied by a continuous decline in gastric cancer for both sexes. This would appear to be the definitive review of the risk for developing cancers after total hip replacement arthroplasty.

Brand, K.G. and Brand, I. (1980) Risk assessment of carcinogenesis at implantation sites. *Plastic Reconst. Surg.* **66**, 591–595.

Review of possible foreign body cancer initiation in humans based upon published case reports. The authors conclude that, since the clinical use of prosthetic implants has been popular for more than twenty years and since, extrapolating from animal experience, at least 25% if not 50% of foreign body tumors should have appeared by the time of their publication, there is little risk of such non-chemically mediated tumors occuring in patients.

Gillespie, W.J., Frampton, C.M.A., Henderson, R.J. *et al.* (1988) The incidence of cancer following total hip replacement. *J. Bone Joint Surg.*, **70B**, 539–542.

A New Zealand study of 1358 patients with total hip arthroplasty, for a total of 14 286 patient years. A significant increase in tumors of the hemopoetic and lymphatic systems, accompanied by a significant decrease of cancers of breast (in women), colon and bowel was observed. The authors suggest that these data are evidence for increased immune surveillance, allowing or precipitating hemopoetic and lymphatic tumors but at the same time providing better resistance to the development of soft tissue tumors. The first large scale study of this question.

Visuri, T. and Koskenvuo, M. (1991) Cancer risk after McKee-Farrar total hip replacement. *Orthopedics*, **14**, 137–142.

A study similar to that of Gillespie *et al.* but on a Finnish patient group (433 patients; 5729 patient years) leading to the same general conclusions. Includes a historical discussion of the carcinogenic properties of various trace elements.

Jacobs, J.J., Rosenbaum, D.H., Hay, R.M. *et al.* (1992): Early sarcomatous degeneration near a cementless hip replacement. A case report and review. *J. Bone Joint Surg.*, **74B**, 740–744.

A review of a patient who developed a malignant fibrous histiocytoma at the site of a cementless total hip replacement five months after implantation and succumbed of diffuse metastases, as is typical for such patients, within one year of presentation. Includes an extensive review of world literature on sarcomas in the vicinity of total hip replacement and suggest the need for an international registry of such case reports.

REFERENCES

1. Coleman, R.R., Herrington, S. and Scales, J.T. (1973) Concentration of wear products in hair, blood, and urine after total hip arthroplasty. *Brit. Med. J.* **1** 1527–1529.
2. Lux, F. and Zeisler, R. (1974) Investigations of the corrosive deposition of components of metal implants and of the behavior of biologic trace elements in metallosis tissue by means of instrumental, multi-element activation analysis. *J. Radiol. Anal. Chem.*, **19,** 289–297.
3. Rock, M.G. and Hardie, R. (1988): Analysis of local tissue response in 50 revision total hip arthroplasty patients. *Trans. Soc. Biomater.*, **XI,** 43.
4. Agins, H.J., Alcock, N.W., Bansal, M. et al. (1988) Metallic wear in failed titanium alloy total hip replacements. A histological and quantitative analysis. *J. Bone Joint Surg.* **70A,** 347–356.
5. Buchert, B.K., Vaughn, B.K., Mallory, T.H. *et al* (1986): Excessive metal release due to loosening and spreading of sintered particles on porous coated hip prosthesis. Report of two cases. *J. Bone Joint Surg.*, **68A,** 606–609.
6. Jacobs, J.J., Skipor, A.K., Black, J. *et al.* (1991), Release in excretion of metal in patients who have a total hip replacement component made of titanium-base alloy. *J. Bone Joint Surg.* **73A,** 1475–1486.
7. Witt, J.D. and Swann, M. (1991) Metal wear and tissue response in failed titanium alloy total hip replacements. *J. Bone Joint Surg.* **73B,** 559–563.
8. Woodman, J.L., Jacobs, J.J., Galante, J.O., et al. (1984), Metal ion release from titanium-based prosthetic segmental replacements of long bones in baboons. A long term study. *J. Orthop. Res.*, **1,** 421–430.
9. Bartolozzi, A. and Black, J. (1985) Chromium concentrations in serum, blood clot and urine from patients following total hip arthroplasty. *Biomaterials*, **6,** 2–8.
10. Steineman, S.G. (1985) Corrosion of Titanium and Titanium Alloys For Surgical Implant. in: Lutergering, G., Swicker, U., Bunk, W. (eds), *Titanium, Science, and Technology*, Volume 2, DG für Metal. e.V. Oberuresel, Berlin, 1373–1379.
11. Harvey, A.M., Johns, R.S., Owens, A.H. *et al.* (1972) *The Principles and Practice of Medicine*. New York: McGraw-Hill, pp. 68–102.
12. Langkamer, V.G., Case, C.P., Heap, P. *et al.* (1992) Systemic distribution of wear debris after hip replacement. A cause for concern? *J. Bone Joint Surg.*, **74B,** 831–839.

13. Doll, R. (1958) Cancer of lung and the nose. Nickel workers. *Brit. J. Indust. Med.*, **15,** 217–223.
14. Swanson, S.A.V., Freeman, M.A.R. and Heath, J.C. (1973) Laboratory tests on total joint replacement prosthesis. *J. Bone Joint Surg.*, **55B,** 759–773.
15. Laskin, D.M. (1954): Experimental production of sarcomas by methylacrylate implant. *Proc. Soc. Exper. Biol. Med.*, **87,** 329–333.
16. Carter, R.L. and Rowe, F.J.C. (1969): Induction of sarcomas in rats by solid and fragmented polyethylene; Experimental observations and clinical implications. *Brit. J. Cancer*, **23,** 401–407.
17. Harris, W.H., Schiller, A.L., Scholler, J.M. *et al.* (1976) Extensive localized bone resorption in the femur following total hip replacement. *J. Bone Joint Surg.* **58A,** 612–618.
18. Castleman, B., McNeely, B.U. (eds) (1965) Case 38-1965, Case records of the Massachusetts General Hospital. *New Engl. J. Med.*, 273, 494–504.
19. Rushforth, G.F. (1947) Osteosarcoma of the pelvis following radiotherapy for carcinoma of the cervix. *Brit. J. Radiol.* **47,** 149–152.
20. Arden, G.P. and Bywaters, E.G.L. (1978), in *Surgical Management of Juvenile Chronic Poly Arthritis*. Arden, G.P., Ansel, B.M. (eds), Academic Press, London, pp. 269–270.
21. Bágo-Granell, J., Aguirre-Canyadell, M., Nardi, J. *et al.* (1984) Malignant fibrous histiocytoma of bone at the site of a total hip arthroplasty. A case report. *J. Bone Joint Surg.* **66B,** 38–40.
22. Penman, H.G. and Ring, P.A. (1984) Osteosarcoma in association with total hip replacement. *J. Bone Joint Surg.* **66B,** 632–634.
23. Swann, M. (1984) Malignant soft tissue tumor at the site of a total hip replacement. *J. Bone Joint Surg.* **66B,** 269–231.
24. Hamblen, D.L. and Carter, R.L. (1984) Sarcoma and Joint Replacement (Editorial). *J. Bone Joint Surg.* **66B,** 625–627.
25. Apley, A.G. (1989) Malignancy and joint replacement. The tip of an iceberg? (Editorial). *J. Bone Joint Surg.* **71B,** 1.
26. Weber, P.C. (1986) Epithelioid sarcoma in association with total knee replacement. *J. Bone Joint Surg.* **68B,** 824–826.
27. Ryu, R.K.N., Bovill, E.G. Jr, Skinner, H.B. *et al.* (1987) Soft tissue sarcomas associated with aluminum oxide ceramic total hip arthroplasty. A case report. *Clin. Orthop.* **216,** 207–212.
28. Vives, P., Sevestre, H., Grodet, H. *et al.* (1987) Histiocytome fibreux malin du fémur après prosthèses totale de hanche (Malignant fibrous histiocytoma of the femur following total hip replacement). *Rev. Chir. Orthop.* **73,** 407–409.
29. Van der list, J.J.J. (1988) Malignant epithelioid hemangioendothelioma at the site of a hip prosthesis. *Acta Orthop. Scand.* **59,** 328–330.
30;31. Lamovec, J., Zidar, A., Cucek-Plenicar, M. *et al.* (1988): Synovial sarcoma associated with total hip replacement. A case report. Addendum: Osteosarcoma associated with a Charnley–Muller hip arthroplasty. *J. Bone Joint Surg.* **70A,** 1558–1560.
32. Tait, N.P., Hacking, P.M. and Malcolm, A.J. (1988) Case report, malignant fibrous histiocytoma occurring at the site of a previous total hip replacement. *Brit. J. Radiol.*, **61,** 73–76.

33. Martin, A., Bauer, T.W., Manley, M.T. *et al.* (1988) Osteosarcoma at the site of a total hip replacement. *J. Bone Joint Surg.* **70A,** 1561–1567.
34. Haag, M. and Adler, C.P. (1989) Malignant fibrous histiocytoma in association with hip replacement. *J. Bone Joint Surg. (Brit)*, **71B,** 701.
35. Mazabraud, A., Florent, J. and Laurent, M. (1989) (A case of epidermoid carcinoma developed in contact with a hip prosthesis)(Fr.)(au. transl.). *Bull. Cancer*, **76,** 573–581.
36. Brien, W.W., Salvati, E.A., Healey, J.H. *et al.* (1990) Osteogenic sarcoma arising in the area of a total hip replacement. A case report. *J. Bone Joint Surg.*, **72A,** 1097–1099.
37. Troop, J.K., Mallory, T.H., Fisher, D.A., *et al.* (1990) Malignant fibrous histiocytoma after total hip arthroplasty: A case report. *Clin. Orthop. Rel. Res.*, **253,** 297–300.
38. Kolstad, K. and Högstorp, H. (1990): Gastric carcinoma metastasis to a knee with a newly inserted prosthesis: A case report. *Acta Orthop. Scand.* **61,** 369–370.
39. Jacobs, J.J., Rosenbaum, D.H., Hay, R.M. *et al.* (1992): Early sarcomatous degeneration near a cementless hip replacement. A case report and review. *J. Bone Joint Surg.*, **74B,** 740–744.
40. Solomon, M.I. and Sekel, R. (1992) Total hip arthroplasty complicated by a malignant fibrous histiocytoma. A case report. *J. Arthroplasty*, **7**, 549–550.
41. Goodfellow, J. (1992) Malignancy and joint replacement (Editorial). *J. Bone Joint Surg.*, **74A,** 645.
42. McDougall, A. (1956) Malignant tumor at site of bone plating. *J. Bone Joint Surg.* **38B,** 709–713.
43. Delgado, E.R. (1958) Sarcoma following a surgically treated fractured tibia: A case report. *Clin. Orthop.* **12,** 315–318.
44. Dube, V.E. and Fisher, D.E. (1972) Hemangioendothelioma of the leg following metallic fixation of the tibia. *Cancer* **30,** 1260–1266.
45. Tayton, K.J.J. (1980) Ewing's sarcoma at the site of a metal plate. *Cancer* **45,** 413–415.
46. McDonald, I. (1981) Malignant lymphoma associated with internal fixation of a fractured tibia. *Cancer* **48,** 1009–1011.
47. Dodion, P., Putz, P., Amiri-Lamraski, M.H. *et al.* (1983) Immunoblastic lymphoma at the site of an infected vitallium bone plate. *Histopathol.*, **6,** 807–813.
48. Lee, Y.S., Pho, R.W.H. and Nather, A. (1984) Malignant fibrous histiocytoma at site of metal implant. *Cancer* **54,** 2286–2289
49. Hughes, A.W., Sherlock, D.A., Hamblen, D.L. *et al.* (1987) Sarcoma at the site of a single hip screw. A case report. *J. Bone Joint Surg.* **69B,** 470–472.
50. Ward, J.J., Thornbury, D.D., Lemons, J.E. *et al.* (1990) Metal-induced sarcoma: A case report and literature review. *Clin. Orthop.* **252,** 299–306.
51. Khurana, J.S., Rosenberg, A.E., Kattapuram, S.V. *et al.* (1991) Malignancy supervening on an intramedullary nail. *Clin. Orthop.* **267,** 251–254.
52. Sinibaldi, K. (1976): Tumors associated with metallic implants in animals. *Clin. Orthop. Rel. Res.*, **118,** 257–266.

53. Moss, A.J. (1991) Use of selected medical devices in the United States. *Advance Data from Vital and Health Statistics of the National Center for Health Statistics*, **191,** 1–24.
54. Gillespie, W.J., Frampton, C.M., Henderson, R.J. *et al.* (1988) The incidence of cancer following total hip replacement. *J. Bone Joint Surg.* **70B,** 539–542.
55. Visuri, T. (1992) Cancer risk after McKee–Farrar total hip replacement. *Orthopedics*, **14,** 137–142, 1992.
56. Nyren, O., McLaughlin, J.K. *et al.* (1995) Cancer risk after hip replacement with metal implants: A population based study. *J. National Can. Inst.* **87**, 28–33.
57. Li, X.Q., Stevenson, S., Hom, D.L. *et al.* (1993): Relationship between metallic implants and cancer: A case-control study in a canine population. *Vet. Comp. Orthop. Traumatol.* **6**, 70–74.

Blood–material interactions | 6

S.R. Hanson

6.1 INTRODUCTION

The importance of understanding mechanisms of blood–material interactions is emphasized by the increasingly widespread use of cardiovascular devices; hence, this field has been the subject of intense inquiry as described in several excellent reviews [1–4]. Unfortunately, it is still not possible to simply rank or classify materials with respect to their suitability for particular blood-contacting applications. Nor is it possible to predict in any general way, based on the properties of devices and of their blood-contacting surfaces, the behavior of blood in contact with materials or the propensity of devices to produce clinically adverse events. Despite many attempts to correlate biologic responses to physicochemical property measurements, our success in understanding blood–material interactions, and the clinical application of many blood-contacting devices, has been largely empirical. It is not appropriate to discuss in detail this large and controversial literature, which has been reviewed elsewhere [1, 2]. Rather, this section will focus on the available experimental data in humans, or results which may likely be extrapolated to humans from relevant animal studies, that may guide in the development of new designs for blood-contacting devices. Cardiovascular device applications in humans have also been the subject of an excellent review [5].

6.2 EXPERIMENTAL DIFFICULTIES

Before summarizing relevant experimental findings, it is appropriate to review briefly the theoretical and practical limitations to our understanding of blood–material interactions.

Handbook of Biomaterial Properties. Edited by J. Black and G. Hastings.
Published in 1998 by Chapman & Hall, London. ISBN 0 412 60330 6.

There are several factors which have precluded the rational engineering design of devices based on first principles. While thousands of materials have been put forward as 'biocompatible' or non-thrombogenic, based on *in vitro* studies and animal testing, the relevance of these tests for outcomes in humans remains uncertain. Device responses *in vivo* depend upon actual device configuration and resulting flow geometry as well as upon intrinsic materials' properties. In many applications, mechanical and physical property requirements may dominate materials' selection. For example, membranes used in dialyzers and oxygenators must be both solute and gas permeable; chronic vascular grafts and heart valves must be mechanically durable and chemically stable for years; heart assist devices require flexible pumping chambers. Thus, the use of *in vitro* assays or simplified *in vivo* flow geometries, as in many animal models, has not proven adequate to predict actual device performance in patients. Furthermore, most animals and humans, as individuals, differ markedly from one another in both blood chemistry and in blood response to foreign materials [6]. It is deemed unethical to perform screening tests in humans, hence relatively few materials have undergone clinical evaluation and only limited human comparative data are available. In the case of chronic implants, devices removed at autopsy provide only a single set of observations which cannot be related to dynamic blood–material interactions prior to explantation.

Another limitation is our recognition that all blood–material interactions of clinical consequence are preceded by complex interactions between the biomaterial surface and circulating blood proteins. Plasma contains more that 100 identified proteins with specific functions and varying biologic properties [7]. These proteins interact with surfaces in a complex, interdependent and time-dependent fashion that remains poorly understood, except in low dilution, simplified model systems [8]. These reactions may vary from individual to individual depending upon coagulation status, the use antithrombotic or other drug therapies, or the administration of contrast media for fluoroscopic imaging. A partial listing of variables which may affect device outcomes following blood exposure is given in Table 6.1.

Despite these limitations, the design engineer may be guided by previous successful applications of materials in a variety of device configurations, and by certain generalizations which have resulted from these studies. Devices which are commonly used include catheters, cannulae, guide wires, stents, shunts, vascular grafts, heart valves, heart and ventricular assist devices, oxygenators, and dialyzers. With respect to these devices it is important to consider those events which can lead to serious clinical complications. These complications include: (1) thrombosis, (2) thromboembolism, (3) consumption (ongoing destruction) or activation of circulating hemostatic blood elements, and (4) activation of inflammatory

Table 6.1. Variables influencing blood interactions with cardiovascular devices

Device Properties
Size and shape
Surface composition
Texture or roughness
Mechanical properties
Blood Flow Phenomena
Shear forces
Convection and diffusion of reactants, products, cofactors and inhibitors
Disturbed flow and turbulence
Blood Chemistry-related Effects
Coagulation status
Antithrombotic and other therapies
Contrast media
Other Variables
Duration of device blood exposure
Tissue injury
Infection

and immunologic pathways. An appreciation for the biologic mechanisms of these events is essential for understanding the blood-compatibility of devices, and may be briefly described as follows. Thrombus forms as the localized accumulation of blood elements on, within, or associated with a device, and thrombus which is actively deposited can accumulate to the extent of producing device dysfunction or blood vessel occlusion. Interruption of normal blood flow may produce ischemia (relative lack of oxygen) and infarction (tissue death due to total oxygen deprivation) in distal circulatory beds leading to heart attacks and strokes. Thrombus structure may be complex, and is distinguished from that of whole blood clots which are often formed under static flow conditions. Thus, clots are relatively homogeneous structures containing red blood cells and platelets trapped in a mesh of polymerized protein (fibrin), while thrombus formed under arterial flow conditions and high fluid shear rates ('white thrombus') may be composed primarily of layers of fibrin and platelets (small procoagulant cells occupying only about 0.3% of the total blood volume). Under conditions of low fluid shear, as found in veins, thrombus may more closely resemble the structure of whole blood clots ('red thrombus'). Thromboembolism is the dislodgement by blood flow of a thrombus which is then transported downstream, ultimately blocking vessels which are too small for the thrombus to traverse. Thromboembolism is a common cause of stroke (cerebrovascular infarction) and peripheral limb ischemia. Often the balance between dynamic processes of thrombus deposition and its removal by embolic and lytic mechanisms will produce platelet consumption (ongoing destruction) and a net reduction in circulating platelet levels. Other clotting factors may be consumed as well [9]. Finally, certain devices, particularly those having large surface areas, may activate enzyme systems (e.g., complement) leading to inflammatory or immunologic responses [10]. With these issues in mind we will now review the performance of various classes of biomaterials in actual device configurations.

6.3 CONVENTIONAL POLYMERS

Conventional polymers, such as polyethylene (Intramedic™), poly (vinyl chloride)(Tygon™), polytetrafluoroethylene (Teflon™), and poly (dimethyl siloxane)(Silastic™), and certain polyurethanes, have been used for many decades in short-term applications including catheters, cannulas, arteriovenous shunts for hemodialysis, and tubing components of extracorporeal circuits. When used for periods of only a few hours, and most often in patients receiving systemic anticoagulation agents, the performance of such materials has usually been clinically acceptable. For example, although thrombus on angiographic catheters can be demonstrated in about half of all cases, most thromboembolic or occlusive events are clinically silent and significant complications occur in less than 1% of procedures [5]. Even total occlusion of small peripheral veins, by short term catheters used for venous sampling or drug administration, is usually inconsequential. However, longer-term indwelling catheters in a variety of configurations and polymer compositions, particularly in infants and children, are now recognized to produce a significant risk of thrombosis which can ultimately lead to organ or limb damage, and even death [11]. Comparative, quantitative studies with different polymer formulations remain to be performed in humans.

Polyurethanes, due in part to their flexibility and toughness, are perhaps the polymer of choice for ventricular assist devices and blood pumps. Consequently, they have received considerable interest as blood-contacting materials. In nonhuman primates, those polyurethanes, such as Pellethane™, which exhibit the most hydrophobic surface chemistry produce the least platelet consumption [12]. In dogs, early platelet interactions with polyurethanes vary considerably although relationships to polymer surface chemistry remain unclear [13]. Thus while polyurethanes are chemically versatile and possess many desirable mechanical properties, it is generally not possible to predict their biologic responses in humans.

6.4 HYDROPHILIC POLYMERS

These materials, which preferentially adsorb or absorb water (hydrogels), were initially postulated to be blood compatible based on the view that many naturally occuring phospholipids, comprising the cell membranes of blood contacting tissues, are also hydrophilic. Thus, water, as a biomaterial, was expected to show minimal interaction with blood proteins and cells [14, 15]. Interestingly, in animal studies highly hydrophilic polymers based on acrylic and methacrylic polymers and copolymers, as well as poly(vinyl alcohol) are all found to consume platelets excessively although they accumulate little deposited thrombus [12, 16]. The materials have variable thrombogenicity, but little capacity to retain adherent thrombus, i.e., they shed deposited platelets as microemboli. Thus, while surface-grafted hydrogels (which are mechanically weak) are currently used to improve catheter lubricity and as reservoirs for drug delivery, they have not received widespread application for improving blood-compatibility.

Another hydrophilic polymer that has received considerable attention is poly(ethylene oxide) [17, 18]. While poly(ethylene oxide) surfaces have been shown (like hydrogels) to have relatively low interactions with blood proteins and cells in *in vitro* studies and in some animal models, the suitability of such polymers for actual device applications and long-term implants has not been established.

6.5 METALS

Metals, as a class, tend to be thrombogenic, and are most commonly applied in situations requiring considerable mechanical strength, such as in the struts of mechanical heart valves and as endovascular stents [3, 19] or electrical conductivity, as in pacing electrodes. Stents are metallic mesh devices placed within blood vessels to preserve vessel patency after procedures to expand the vessel lumen diameter (e.g., after balloon angioplasty). Metals most commonly employed are stainless steel (316L type) and tantalum; however, both are thrombogenic [19, 20]. Catheter guide wire thrombogenicity, although readily documented, has been less of a clinical problem because of the usually short period of blood exposure involved in most procedures.

In early canine implant studies, the thrombogenicity of a wide series of metallic implants was seen to be related to the resting electrical potential of the metal which was generated upon blood contact [21]. Metals with negative potentials tend to be antithrombogenic, while stainless steel tends to be neutral. Copper, silver, and platinum are positive and extremely thrombogenic. Indeed, the use of copper coils inserted into canine arteries continues to be a widely used model for inducing a thrombotic response [22].

Theoretically, reduced thrombogenicity of metallic stents and heart valve components might be achieved by thin film polymer coatings, although the clinical effectiveness of this strategy has not been demonstrated. Thus, chronic systemic anticoagulation is generally employed in patients with prosthetic heart valves (with metallic components) and stents.

6.6 CARBONS

Cardiac valves with components fabricated from low temperature isotropic carbons (pyrolytic carbon) are successfully used clinically [23]. These materials are appropriate for such applications as mechanical valves which require long-term chemical inertness, smoothness, and wear-resistance. The reasons for the marked improvement in the performance (reduced thrombosis and thromboembolic stroke rates) of these newer vs. older style heart valves are not entirely understood, but are undoubtedly multifactorial and related to improved patient management and valve design, as well as to the nature of the carbon surface. The specific benefits conferred by pyrolytic carbons with respect to blood cell and protein interactions, resulting in a very low frequency of clinical complications, remain to be defined. The use of carbon coatings has been proposed for other devices, i.e., vascular grafts, although such devices have not yet been used clinically.

6.7 ULTRA-THIN FILM COATINGS

Polymeric thin films of widely varying chemical composition may be deposited onto polymers, metals, and other surfaces using the method of plasma polymerization (also called 'glow-discharge' polymerization) [24]. This method is advantageous since very thin films (e.g., 100 nm) may selectively modify the surface chemistry of devices, but not their overall mechanical properties or surface texture. Plasma polymers form highly cross-linked, covalent, inert barrier layers which may resist the adsorption of proteins, lipids, and other blood elements. Plasma reacted coatings, based on hydrocarbon monomers such as methane, may produce durable diamond like coatings. Plasma polymer coatings have been proposed for vascular grafts and stents, based on promising animal studies [25], but are not used clinically at the present time.

6.8 MEMBRANES

Blood contacting membranes are used for gas exchange (e.g., blood oxygenators) or solute exchange (e.g., dialyzers). The large membrane surface area, which may exceed $2\,m^2$, and the complexity of cardiopulmonary bypass circuits can produce consumption and dysfunction of circulating blood elements such as platelets, leading to an increased risk of bleeding as well as thromboembolism [26]. The activation of inflammatory and immune response pathways (complement system) by dialysis and oxygenator membranes may also produce significant complications

[27]. Complement activation by dialysis membranes may be related in part to the availability of surface hydroxyl groups, particularly on cellulosic membranes. Complement activation may be greatly attenuated by the use of other membrane materials such as polysulfone and polycarbonate. Complement activation by biomaterial membranes has been reviewed [27].

6.9 BIOLOGICAL SURFACES

The use of biological and bioactive molecules as device surface coatings may confer thromboresistance. Such coating materials include phospholipids and heparin. Phospholipids such as phosphorylcholine, a normal constituent of cell membranes, may orient polar head groups towards the aqueous phase and locally organize water molecules, much like hydrogel surfaces. These surfaces may minimize protein and complement interactions [28]. In preliminary animal studies, phosphorylcholine coated stents, guide wires, and vascular grafts have shown improved thromboresistance. This approach is being actively developed for clinical applications.

Heparin, a naturally occuring anticoagulant glycosaminoglycan, has been considered an attractive surface coating based on its ability to directly catalyze the inactivation of procoagulant enzymes, and thus suppress thrombus development. Recently, the reduced thrombogenicity and improved biocompatibility of heparinized metallic stents has been demonstrated in animals [29]. In these studies, heparin was covalently attached to a polymer surface coating. This method has also been used clinically for the heparin coating of catheters and other devices, although it remains unclear whether the improved biocompatibility is a function of heparin's anticoagulant activity, nonspecific physicochemical properties, or both.

With biomolecule modified surfaces, there may also be important questions regarding the possible deleterious effects of sterilization procedures required before implantation.

6.10 SURFACE TEXTURE

Surface 'smoothness' is a generally desirable feature of blood contacting surfaces. In this context, a smooth surface is one with irregularities with typical dimensions less than those of cells (< 1 μm). However, in certain applications, device incorporation by tissue is desirable, or the texturing of polymers may increase mechanical flexibility and durability. Thus, the sewing ring of mechanical heart valves is typically composed of poly(ethylene terephthalate) (Dacron™) fabric to permit tissue in growth and healing, which is associated with a reduction in thromboembolic events. Vascular grafts used to replace diseased blood vessels are most commonly fabricated from woven or knitted Dacron™ or textured (expanded) polytetrafluoroethylene (ePTFE) (Goretex™). In tubular form, these textured polymers remain flexible and stable for many years following implantation. Smooth-walled vascular grafts have generally not been considered attractive for long-term applications since smooth surfaces may not permit tissue ingrowth or flow surface healing. Textured flow surfaces are initially thrombogenic upon blood contact, although ePTFE appears less thrombogenic and thromboembolic than fabric Dacron™ prostheses [30]. These grafts perform acceptably in man when the graft diameter exceeds about 6 mm since the layer of thrombus that forms does not significantly restrict blood flow. Interestingly, both smooth-walled and textured ventricular assist devices have also performed successfully in clinical trials [31, 32].

6.11 CONCLUSION

Because the variables affecting cardiovascular device responses are sufficiently numerous and complex, those properties of blood-contacting surfaces which would be desirable to minimize adverse reactions cannot, in most instances, be predicted with confidence. The choice of material is usually constrained by mechanical property considerations and by variable requirements for material durability and chemical stability. Cardiovascular device engineering must therefore be guided by previous experience in successful clinical applications.

ADDITIONAL READING

Colman, R.W., Hirsch, J., Marder, V.J. and Salzman, E.W. (eds)(1994) *Hemostasis and Thrombosis: Basic Principles and Clinical Practice*, 3rd edn, J.B. Lippincott, Philadelphia.

This book is highly recommended. This state-of-the-art text covers in detail essentially all important hematological aspects of cardiovascular device blood compatibility. In particular, Chapter 76, Interaction of blood with artificial surfaces, which considers many theoretical, experimental, and animal studies, and Chapter 77, Artificial devices in clinical practice, which describes clinical device thromboembolic complications, are of great practical value.

Harker, L.A., Ratner, B.D. and Didisheim, P. (eds)(1993) Cardiovascular Biomaterials and Biocompatibility, *Cardiovascular Pathology*, **2**(3) (suppl.), 1S–224S.

In this volume, 20 chapters by expert authors treat all aspects of biomaterials and blood compatibility including pathologic mechanisms, material characterization, blood-material interactions and device performance. This volume updates an excellent earlier book *Guidelines for Blood-Material Interactions*, National Institutes of Health, Washington, DC, Publication No. 85–2185 (1985).

Szycher, M. (ed.) (1983) *Biocompatible Polymers, Metals, and Composites*, Technomic Publishing Co., Lancaster, Pennsylvania.

Many of the same issues of blood–material interactions are broadly covered while selected polymer and device applications are described in additional detail. Of particular interest are Section I (Fundamental Concepts in Blood/Material Interactions) and Section II (Strategies for Hemocompatibility).

ACKNOWLEDGEMENT

This work was supported by Research Grant HL 31469 from the Heart, Lung and Blood Institute, the National Institutes of Health.

REFERENCES

1. Salzman, E.W., Merrill, E.W. and Kent K.C. (1994) Interaction of blood with artificial surfaces, in *Hemostasis and Thrombosis: Basic Principles and Clinical Practice*, 3rd edn, R.W. Colman, J. Hirsch, V.J. Marder, and Salzman, E.W. (eds), J.B. Lippincott, Philadelphia, pp. 1469–85.
2. Harker, L.A., Ratner, B.D. and Didisheim, P. (eds) (1993) Cardiovascular Biomaterials and Biocompatibility, *Cardiovascular Pathology* **2**(3)(supplement), 1S–224S.
3. Szycher, M. (ed.) (1983) *Biocompatible Polymers, Metals, and Composites*, Technomic Publishing Co., Lancaster, Pennsylvania.
4. Williams, D.F. (ed) (1981) *Biocompatibility of Clinical Implant Materials*, CRC Press, Boca Raton, Florida.
5. Clagett, G.P. and Eberhart, R.C. (1994) Artificial Devices in Clinical Practice, in *Hemostasis and Thrombosis: Basic Principles and Clinical Practice*, 3rd edn R.W. Colman, J. Hirsch, V.J. Marder, and Salzman, E.W. (eds), J.B. Lippincott, Philadelphia, pp. 1486–1505.
6. Grabowski, E.F., Didisheim, P., Lewis, J.C. *et al.* (1977) Platelet adhesion to foreign surfaces under controlled conditions of whole blood flow: human vs. rabbit, dog, calf, sheep, pig, macaque, and baboon. *Transactions – American Society for Artificial Internal Organs*, **23**, 141–51.
7. Lentner, C. (ed.) (1984) *Geigy Scientific Tables* (vol. 3): *Physical Chemistry, Composition of Blood*, Hematology, Somatometric Data, Ciby-Geigy, Basle.
8. Brash, J.L. and Horbett, T.A. (eds) (1987) *Proteins at Interfaces. Physicochemical and Biochemical Studies*, American Chemical Society, Washington, DC.
9. Harker, L.A. and Slichter, S.J. (1972) Platelet and fibrinogen consumption in man. *New England J Med.* **287**(20), 999–1005.
10. Bennett, B., Booth, N.A., Ogston D. (1987) Potential interactions between complement, coagulation, fibrinolysis, kinin-forming, and other enzyme systems, in: *Haemostasis and Thrombosis* (2nd edn), A.L. Bloom and D.P. Thomas (eds), Churchill Livingstone, New York, pp. 267–82.

11. Andrew, M. (1995) Developmental hemostasis: relevance to thromboembolic complications in pediatric patients. *Thrombosis and Hemostasis*, **74**(1), 415–25.
12. Hanson, S.R., Harker, L.S., Ratner, B.D. *et al.* (1980) *In vivo* evaluation of artificial surfaces using a nonhuman primate model of arterial thrombosis. *J Laboratory Clinical Med.* **95**, 289–304.
13. Silver, J.H., Myers, C.W., Lim, F. *et al.* (1994) Effect of polyol molecular weight on the physical properties and haemocompatibility of polyurethanes containing polyethylene oxide macroglycols. *Biomaterials* **15**(9), 695–704.
14. Hoffman, A.S. (1974) Principles governing biomolecular interactions at foreign surfaces. *J. Biomedical Materials Res.* (Symp.) **5**(1), 77–83.
15. Andrade, J.D., Lee, H.B., Jhon, M.S. *et al.* (1973) Water as a biomaterial. *Transactions – American Society for Artificial Internal Organs* **19**, 1–7.
16. Strzinar, I. and Sefton, M.V. (1992) Preparation and thrombogenicity of alkylated polyvinyl alcohol coated tubing. *J. Biomedical Materials Research* **26**, 577–92.
17. Merrill, E.W. (1993) Poly(ethylene oxide) star molecules: synthesis, characterization, and applications in medicine and biology. *J. Biomaterials Science, Polymer Edition* **5**(1–2), 1–11.
18. Llanos, G.R. and Sefton, M.V. (1993) Does polyethylene oxide possess a low thrombogenicity? *J. Biomaterials Science, Polymer Edition*, **4**(4), 381–400.
19. Sigwart, U., Puel, J., Mirkovitch, V. *et al.* (1987) Intravascular stents to prevent occlusion and restenosis after transluminal angioplasty. *New England J. Med*, **316**(12), 701–6.
20. Scott, N.A., Nunes, G.L., King, S.B. *et al.* (1995) A comparison of the thrombogenicity of stainless steel and tantalum coronary stents. *American Heart J.*, **129**, 866–72.
21. Saywer, P.N., Stanczewski, B., Lucas, T.R., *et al.* (1978) Physical chemistry of the vascular interface, in *Vascular Grafts*, P.N. Sawyer and M.J. Kaplitt (eds), Appleton-Century-Crofts, New York, pp. 53–75.
22. Rapold, H.J., Stassen, T., Van de Werf, F., *et al.* (1992) Comparative copper coil-induced thrombogenicity of the internal mammary, left anterior descending coronary, and popliteal arteries in dogs. *Arteriosclerosis and Thrombosis*, **12**(5), 634–44.
23. Schoen, F.J. (1983) Carbons in heart valve prostheses: Foundations and clinical performance, in M. Szycher (ed.), *Biocompatible Polymers, Metals, and Composites*, Technomic Publishing Co., Lancaster, Pennsylvania, pp. 239–61.
24. Yasuda, H.K. (1985) *Plasma Polymerization*, Academic Press, Orlando.
25. Yeh, Y.S., Iriyama, T., Matsuzawa, Y., *et al.* (1988) Blood compatibility of surfaces modified by plasma polymerization. *J. Biomedical Materials Research*, **22**, 795–818.
26. Harker, L.A., Malpass, T.W., Branson H.E., *et al.* (1980) Mechanism of abnormal bleeding in patients undergoing cardiopulmonary bypass: acquired transient platelet dysfunction associated with selective alpha-granule release. *Blood*, **56**(5), 824–34.
27. Hakim, R. (1993) Complement activation by biomaterials. *Cardiovascular Pathology*, **2**(3)(suppl), 187S–198S.

28. Yu, J., Lamba, N.M., Courtney J.M., *et al.* (1994) Polymeric biomaterials: Influence of phosphorylcholine polar groups on protein adsorption and complement activation. *International Journal of Artificial Organs*, **17**(9), 499–504.
29. Hardhammer, P.A., van Beusekom H.M., Emanuelsson, H.U., *et al.* (1996) Reduction in thrombotic events with heparin-coated Palmaz–Schatz stents in normal porcine coronary arteries. *Circulation*, **93**(3), 423–30.
30. Schneider, P.A., Kotze, H.F., Heyns, A. duP., *et al.* (1989) Thromboembolic potential of synthetic vascular grafts in baboons. *J. Vascular Surgery*, **10**, 75–82.
31. Dasse, K.A., Poirier, V.L., Menconi, M.J., *et al.* (1990) Characterization of TCPS textured blood-contacting materials following long-term clinical LVAD support. In: *Cardiovascular Science and Technology: Basic and Applied: II*, JC Norman (ed.), Oxymoron Press, Boston, MA, pp. 218–220.
32. Kormos, R.L., Armitage, J.M., Borovetz, H.S., *et al.* (1990) Univentricular support with the Novocor left ventricular assist system as a bridge to cardiac transplantation: An update in *Cardiovascular Science and Technology: Basic and Applied: II*, JC Norman (Ed), Oxymoron Press, Boston, MA, pp. 322–324.

7 Soft tissue response to silicones

S.E. Gabriel

7.1 SILICONES USED IN MEDICINE

Although the term 'silicone' refers to a group of organic silicone compounds, the one most commonly used in medicine is composed of a polymer known as dimethypolysiloxane (DMPS). In silicone gel the polymer is cross-linked; the more cross-linking, the more solid is the gel. Liquid silicone consists of glucose-linked DMPS polymer chains. Silicones first became commercially available in 1943, with the first subdermal implantation of silicone occurring in the late 1940s [1–3]. Silicones have since been developed for a wide variety of medical applications, most notably in joint and breast prostheses.

There is a large body of literature attesting to the chemical and physical inertness of silicone [4–12]. Recently, there has been increasing interest in the possible adverse effects of silicones used in implantation. Much of the literature describing the adverse effects of silicone has been in reference to direct silicone injection. The following discussion will review the immunologic effects of prostheses used in breast reconstruction and augmentation.

7.2 LOCAL IMMUNOLOGIC REACTIONS TO SILICONE

Immunologic reactions to silicone can be local, regional due to silicone migration, or systemic. Local cutaneous and subcutaneous reactions to

Handbook of Biomaterial Properties. Edited by J. Black and G. Hastings.
Published in 1998 by Chapman & Hall, London. ISBN 0 412 60330 6.

injected silicone or gel have been reported [13–18]; and it has become apparent that these reactions are not due to impurities in the silicone, as was originally suspected. Subcutaneous injection of silicone liquid in experimental animals provokes an acute inflammatory response characterized by a primarily polymorphonuclear reaction, followed by a chronic inflammatory response with lymphocytes, fibroblasts, and plasma cells [19]. The late response is characterized by a small amount of cellular infiltrate and an increase in extracellular material. Macrophages with clear vacuoles have been observed and are suspected to contain silicone. Occasionally, multinucleated foreign body giant cells have also been observed [16, 20–23].

In humans, liquid silicone has been injected subcutaneously for cosmetic reasons. Granulomatous reactions have been reported to occur in some instances [14–17]. Similar reactions have been noted in two case reports following the rupture of silicone gel-filled breast prostheses [24,25]. Clinically, these reactions have the characteristics of an inflammatory response, i.e., redness, swelling, and pain. Histologic examination shows chronic inflammatory reactions, occasionally with the presence of refractile material resembling silicone [24].

Migration of silicone has been documented on numerous occasions in the literature. Following experimental intra-peritoneal injection in mice, silicone was demonstrated to be present in the liver, spleen, ovaries, and kidneys [26]. Other investigators have documented the migration of subcutaneously injected silicone to the lung, associated with an increased incidence of respiratory problems in experimental animals [27]. Pneumonitis was reported in 3 patients several days following liquid silicone injection, and silicone was demonstrated in macrophages obtained by pulmonary lavage from these patients [27]. The presence of silicone was confirmed by atomic absorption and infra-red spectrophotometry. Another case report described a patient with silicone-induced granulomatous hepatitis; analysis of liver biopsy specimens revealed quantifiable amounts of silicone [28]. Subcutaneous masses or nodules, hepatic granulomas have also been reported following injections into humans [23,24,28]. Regional lymphadenopathy is a frequently reported finding [29–35]. In rare cases, this has progressed to malignant lymphoma [29,32,33]. The relevance of these reports to silicone breast implants is uncertain.

7.3 SYSTEMIC IMMUNOLOGIC REACTIONS TO SILICONE

Systemic reactions have been reported following the introduction of silicone into the body. In one instance, a severe systemic reaction consisting of a febrile illness, acute renal insufficiency, respiratory compromise, pulmonary infiltration, delirium, anemia, and thrombocytopenia has been reported following implantation of a silicone gel envelope prosthesis. Improvement followed implant removal. Silicone was identified by mass spectrophotometry in this case [36]. Another case involved the injection of a large quantity of free silicone under the breasts by an unauthorized individual. The patient expired within 10 hours of injection. Silicone was identified by absorption spectrophotometry in large quantities in the lung, kidney, liver, brain and serum [28].

The mechanism underlying the systemic immunologic reactions to silicone has not been thoroughly investigated. A marked local granulomatous reaction to silicone has been noted in guinea pigs; however, an antibody response to silicone by Ouchterlony gel diffusion or passive cutaneous anaphylaxis was not demonstrated [37]. Other investigators have studied macrophage migration inhibition [38]. In these studies, pigs were sensitized by subcutaneous injection of silicone. Harvested macrophages demonstrated inhibition of migration in the presence of silicone, suggesting specific antigen recognition. In addition, silicone was demonstrated in the cytoplasmic bridges joining macrophages and lymphocytes. Alternatively, it has been suggested that the immune system does not respond with a specific recognition of silicone but that silicone promotes the immune response to other antigens, i.e., acts as an adjuvant. Hypergammaglobulinemia has been noted by some investigators, and silicon dioxide has been reported to have adjuvant effects [39]. A disorder which has been termed, 'human adjuvant disease', was described following injection of paraffin for breast augmentation mammoplasty [40]. In Japan, in 1973, Yoshida reviewed seven cases of human adjuvant disease in Japan following injections of paraffin or silicone for augmentation mammoplasty [41]. The symptoms included arthritis, arthralgia, lymphadenopathy, hypergammaglobulinemia, elevated erythrocyte sedimentation rates and positive rheumatoid factor. Removal of the injected materials resulted in improvement of the condition in some patients [41].

In 1979, Kumagai reported four cases of classical systemic sclerosis following cosmetic surgery [42]. Five years later, the same investigator described a series of 46 patients with signs and symptoms of connective tissue disease following injection of either silicone or paraffin [43]. Definite connective tissue diseases, based on American Rheumatism Association Criteria, were diagnosed in 24 patients. These conditions included systemic lupus erythematosus, mixed connective tissue disease, rheumatoid arthritis, Sjögren's syndrome, and systemic sclerosis. Another group of 22 patients were described as having human adjuvant disease, with signs, symptoms, and laboratory abnormalities suggestive but not diagnostic of a connective tissue disease. In 1984, three patients from Singapore were reported who developed autoimmune disease following injection augmentation mammoplasty [44]. In the same year, a 52-year-old woman who developed systemic sclerosis, primary biliary cirrhosis and Sjögren's syndrome following silicone/paraffin injection mammoplasty was reported [45].

In 1982, the first case series describing autoimmune disorders following augmentation mammoplasty with gel-filled prostheses was reported. This was followed by other reports involving both gel-filled implants and saline-filled silicone implants [46–49]. The most frequently reported connective tissue disease associated with silicone breast implants is systemic sclerosis. Table 7.1 summarizes the clinical and laboratory characteristics of 19 cases of systemic sclerosis associated with silicone breast augmentation published in the English language literature. Eleven of these cases received implantation in the United States [35]. Eleven of the 19 patients were ANA positive, 15 had Raynaud's, and 10 had diffuse systemic sclerosis. The interval between augmentation to diagnosis of systemic sclerosis varied from 1 to 25 years, with a mean of 13 years. Fourteen of the 19 patients were exposed to silicone (11 silicone gel and 3 silicone injection), the remainder being exposed to paraffin injection. In two cases, histopathologic demonstration of multinucleated giant cells, vacuoles with refractile droplets, and intracytoplasmic asteroid bodies in lymph nodes draining the prostheses suggested leakage of silicone from the implants and its dissemination in lymphoid tissues. The authors used energy-dispersive X-ray analysis to confirm that the macrophage inclusions in the lymphatic tissue contain silicone.

Although systemic sclerosis is the most commonly reported disorder occurring following silicone breast implantation, there have also been reports of systemic lupus erythematosus [43,44,46,50], Sjögren's syndrome [45], keratoconjunctivitis sicca [45], rheumatoid arthritis [4,34,43], polymyositis [43], overlap syndromes (including human adjuvant disease) [34,43,46,50,51], morphea [35,43], Hashimoto's thyroiditis [43,52], anticardiolipin antibody syndrome [53], primary biliary cirrhosis [45] and toxic shock syndrome [54]. Unfortunately, it is impossible to tell, on the basis of case reports, whether the frequency of these events is greater than might be expected on the basis of chance alone (Table 7.1).

7.4 EVIDENCE FOR CAUSATION

It has been estimated that two million American women have undergone breast augmentation or reconstruction since the introduction of the silicone gel-filled elastomer envelope-type prosthesis in the early 1960s [60,61]. The reported cases of systemic sclerosis among this population raise the important question of whether the association between systemic sclerosis and silicone breast implants is a real one. Unfortunately, almost all of the evidence to date is derived from case reports, which are the

Table 7.1 Cases of Systemic Sclerosis after Augmentation Mammoplasty Reported in the English-Language Literature

Patient	*Age at Diagnosis, y*	*Age at Mammoplasty, y*	*Type of Implant*	*Interval to Onset, y*	*Extent of Systemic Sclerosis*	*Raynaud Phenomenon*	*Systemic Involvement*	*Antinuclear Antibodies**	*Reference*
1	52	50	Silicone bag gel	2	Diffuse	No	No	-	(55)
2	41	20	Silicone bag gel	21	Diffuse	Yes	Pulmonary, gastrointestinal	+	(55)
3	63	53	Silicone bag gel	10	Limited	Yes	Pulmonary	+	(55)
4	37	32	Silicone bag gel	5	Diffuse	No	Pulmonary	+	(55)
5	45	25	Paraffin injection	19	Diffuse	Yes	No	-	(42)
6	49	20	Paraffin injection	16	Diffuse	Yes	Pulmonary, gastrointestinal	-	(42)
7	51	25	Paraffin injection	17	Limited	Yes	No	-	(43)
8	36	24	Paraffin injection	9	Limited	Yes	Pulmonary	-	(43)
9	55	30	Paraffin injection	25	Limited	Yes	Pulmonary	-	(44)
10	50	31	Silicone injection	19	Limited	Yes	Pulmonary, gastrointestinal, primary biliary cirrhosis	+	(45)
11	59	34	Silicone injection	25	Diffuse	Yes	No	+	(56)
12	38	26	Silicone bag gel	7	Limited	Yes	Gastrointestinal	+	(56)
13	47	32	Silicone bag gel	15	Diffuse	Yes	Pulmonary	+	(35)
14	59	50	Silicone gel	9	Diffuse	No	Pulmonary, gastrointestinal	+	(35)
15	44	34	Silicone gel	10	Limited	Yes	Pulmonary, gastrointestinal	+	(35)
16	43	37	Silicone gel	6	Diffuse	Yes	Gastrointestinal	+	(35)
17	44	43	Silicone gel	1	Limited	Yes	Malignant hypertension	+	(57)
18	44	19	Silicone injection	25	Diffuse	Yes	Malignant hypertension/ renal failure	+	(58)
19	46	34	Silicone gel	12	Limited	No	No	-	(59)

- negative.
+ positive.
* Determined using immunofluorescence.

very weakest form of data bearing on the question of causality (Table 7.2). Indeed, the most important evidence for establishing a cause–effect relationship is the strength of the research design used to study that relationship [62]. Randomized control trials provide the strongest evidence but are seldom ethical in studies of causation because they involve randomly assigning individuals to receive or not to receive a potentially harmful intervention. In addition, the long latent periods and large numbers of subjects needed to answer most cause and effect questions in clinical medicine make it impractical to utilize this research design.

Well conducted prospective cohort studies are the next strongest design because they minimize the effects of selection bias, measurement bias, and known confounders. Such a study would involve following a large population of women, preferably for one or more decades, looking for the outcomes of interest (e.g., connective tissue disorders). A relative risk for connective tissue disorders among those women who elect to have breast implantation compared to those who do not can then be calculated. Although this is a powerful research design, it is usually impractical because of the necessary long follow-up period. This problem can be circumvented by a retrospective cohort study, which is similar with the exception that the population and the exposure (breast implantation) is identified in the past, allowing the patients to be followed to the present for the outcomes of interest. Although this is a very attractive research design, it requires that the complete exposed and unexposed populations be identifiable and that follow-up information be available on all individuals.

Case-control studies retrospectively compare the frequency of breast implantation in women with and without the outcomes of interest. If, for example, connective tissue disorders were more likely to occur among women with breast implants, this would constitute some evidence for causation. Case-control studies typically require less time and resources than cohort studies. However, they are susceptible to many more biases than cohort studies [62]. The primary reason not to perform a case-control study here, however, is that a separate case-control study would be required for each of the outcomes of interest, i.e., a case-control study of systemic sclerosis, a case-control study of rheumatoid arthritis, etc. The

Table 7.2 Strength of Research Designs Used to Determine Causation

Strongest	Randomized controlled trials
↓	Prospective cohort studies
↓	Case control studies
↓	Ecological survey
Weakest	Case series

retrospective cohort design is much more efficient since it can evaluate multiple outcomes in a single study, as is the need here.

A set of eight criteria has been proposed as a guide to formulate decisions regarding cause and effect relationships (Table 7.3). The relationship between breast implants and connective tissue disorders does fulfill the criterion of *temporality* since, at least in the published case reports, the connective tissue disorders all followed breast implantation. There is no evidence describing the magnitude of the *relative risk* in this relationship. There is also no evidence for a *dose response* relationship, i.e., that women with bilateral implants perhaps have an increased likelihood of connective tissue disorders compared to women with unilateral implants. The evidence regarding the *reversibility* of these disorders with removal of implants is variable. Although there have been some reports of improvement of connective tissue disorders following removal of the implants, this is not consistent and the number of patients involved is small. The relationship does appear to be consistent, i.e., it has been observed repeatedly by different persons in different places, circumstances, and times, however it has not yet been assessed using adequate study designs. Perhaps the most compelling evidence is the *biologic plausibility* of this relationship due to the hypothesis of silicone acting as an immune adjuvant. The relationship does not appear specific, as silicone implants have lead to not just one effect, but several, albeit somewhat related, effects. Finally, a cause and effect relationship is strengthened if there are examples of well established causes that are analogous to the one in question. Adjuvant induced arthritis can be considered analogous [63].

In summary, in spite of the anecdotal evidence, until very recently there was a lack of evidence to either support or refute a cause-and-effect relationship between silicone breast implants and connective tissue/ autoimmune disorders.

Table 7.3 Evidence that an Association is Causal[62]

Characteristic	*Definition*
Temporality	Cause precedes effect
Strength	Large relative risk
Dose-response	Larger exposures to cause associated with higher rates of disease
Reversibility	Reduction in exposure associated with lower rates of disease
Consistency	Repeatedly observed by different persons, in different places, circumstances, and times
Biologic plausibility	Makes sense, according to biologic knowledge of the time
Specificity	One cause leads to one effect
Analogy	Cause-and-effect relationship already established for a similar experience

7.5 CONTROLLED STUDIES EXAMINING THE RELATIONSHIP BETWEEN BREAST IMPLANTS AND CONNECTIVE TISSUE DISEASE.

At least seven controlled studies have now been published (Table 7.4), each of which provided a quantitative assessment of the risk of connective tissue diseases among women with breast implants [64–70]. The first of these was a case-control study of augmentation mammoplasty and scleroderma [68]. The aims of this study were to compare the frequency and temporal relationship of augmentation mammoplasty among scleroderma cases and matched controls. Scleroderma patients and age stratified general practice controls were interviewed using a pretested telephone questionnaire. Self-reported dates of augmentation mammoplasty were ascertained as were dates of scleroderma symptoms and diagnoses as relevant. Frequencies of nonaugmentation mammoplasty silicone exposure between interviewed cases and controls were expressed in terms of rate ratios and 95% confidence intervals. Rate ratios were also adjusted for socioeconomic status.

A total of 315 cases and 371 controls were interviewed, of whom 251 and 289, respectively, were female. The unadjusted rates for augmentation mammoplasty among interviewed cases and controls were 4/251 (1.59%) and 5/289 (1.73%), respectively. The socioeconomic status adjusted rate of augmentation mammoplasty in scleroderma patients was 1.54% (95% CI: 0.03–3.04) which is very similar to the 1.73% rate in interviewed controls. These results indicate that augmentation mammoplasty rates were comparable in cases and controls. In addition, the rates of exposure to nonmammoplasty silicone mastectomy and breast lumpectomy were comparable in interviewed cases and controls. This study failed to demonstrate an association between silicone breast implantation and the subsequent development of scleroderma to a relative risk as low as 4.5 with 95% statistical power.

In June of 1994, a population-based retrospective cohort study was published which examined the risk of a variety of connective tissue diseases and other disorders after breast implantation [65]. In this study, all women in Olmsted County, Minnesota who received a breast implant between 1 January 1964 and 31 December 1991 (the case subjects) were studied. For each case subject, two women of the same age (within three years) from the same population who had not received a breast implant and who underwent a medical evaluation within two years of the date of the implantation in the case subject were selected as control subjects. Each woman's complete inpatient and outpatient medical records were interviewed for the occurrence of various connective tissue diseases (i.e., rheumatoid arthritis, systemic lupus erythematosus, Sjögren's syndrome, dermatomyositis, polymyositis, systemic sclerosis, ankylosing spondylitis,

Table 7.4 Summary of controlled studies examining the relationship between breast implants (BI) and connective tissue diseases (CTD)

Reference	*Study Design*	*Study Population*		*Outcome(s) Examined*	*Main Result*	*Conclusions*
		Cases (exposed)	*Controls (unexposed)*			
68	Case control	315	371	Systemic sclerosis (SS, scleroderma)	Rates of BI among cases and controls were 1.59% and 1.73%	Rates of BI were similar in cases and controls.
65	Retrospective cohort	749	1498	Connective tissue and other autoimmune diseases	Relative risk (cases:controls) of developing any of these diseases was 1.06 (95% CI: 0.34–2.97).	There was no association between BI and the connective tissue and other disorders studied.
67	Case control	195	143	Systemic lupus erythematosus (SLE)	One (0.8%) of the SLE cases and 0 (0%) of the controls reported having a BI (p=0.57).	No association was shown between BI and SLE.
64	Case control	349	1456	Rheumatoid arthritis (RA)	Relative risk for a history of BI (cases:controls) was 0.41 (95% CI: 0.05–3.13).	No increased risk for RA among women with BI was demonstrated.
60	Multi-center case control	869	2061	SS (scleroderma)	Odds ratio for BI surgery (cases:controls) was 1.25 (95% CI: 0.62–2.53).	No significant causal relationship was demonstrated between BI and the development of SS.
70	Nested case control	121 700		Connective tissue disease	Five cases with BI were identified among 300 patients with RA; 0 cases with BI among 123 with SLE, 20 patients with SS, 3 with Sjögren's syndrome, 13 with dermato/polymyositis, and 2 with mixed connective tissue disease.	No association was found between BI and CTD.
69	Case control (preliminary results)	592	1184	SS (scleroderma)	Odds ratio for BI (cases:controls) was 0.61 (95% CI: 0.14–2.68)	No significant association between BI and SS was found.

CI = confidence interval

psoriatic arthritis, polymyalgia rheumatica, vasculitis, arthritis associated with inflammatory bowel disease, and polychondritis), certain other disorders thought to have an autoimmune pathogenesis (i.e., Hashimoto's thyroiditis), and cancer other than breast cancer. In addition, this study itemized the results of ten related symptoms and the abnormal results of four related laboratory tests. A total of 749 women who had received a breast implant were followed for a mean of 7.8 years and the corresponding 1498 community controls were followed for a mean of 8.3 years. The relative risk of developing any one of these specified connective tissue and other diseases among case subjects compared to controls was 1.06 (95% CI: 0.34–2.97). This study, therefore, found no association between breast implants and the connective tissue diseases and other disorders that were studied [65].

In the summer of 1994, Strom and colleagues published a case-control study which addressed the risk of systemic lupus erythematosus among women with breast implants [67]. A total of 219 eligible cases who met the American Rheumatism Association criteria for systemic lupus erythematosus [71] were identified from the medical practices of cooperating rheumatologists in the Philadelphia metropolitan area. One hundred ninety-five (89%) of these were enrolled in the study. Friends of the cases, matched to the cases on sex and age (±5 years), served as controls. Using a short telephone interview, cases and controls were contacted and asked to provide information on any surgery that they had prior to the index date, i.e., the date of diagnosis of systemic lupus erythematosus, in the cases and the same year for the age-matched friend controls. Specific questions were asked about plastic surgery in general and breast implants in particular. One hundred forty-eight (75.9%) of the 195 systemic lupus erythematosus being sought and 111 (77.6%) of the 143 controls agreed to be reinterviewed for this study. Only 1 (0.8%) of the 133 female systemic lupus erythematosus cases reported having a breast implant eight years prior to the diagnosis of systemic lupus erythematosus. This compared to 0 out of the 100 female friend controls (Fisher exact one-tailed p-value = 0.57). These authors concluded, based on this very large case-control study of systemic lupus erythematosus, that no association existed between silicone breast implants and the subsequent development of systemic lupus erythematosus. However, the modest statistical power of the study was only able to provide sufficient evidence against a very large association.

Three additional controlled studies have been presented and are published in abstract form [64,66,70]. As part of a prospective case-control study of the risk of rheumatoid arthritis, Dugowson *et al.* recruited 349 women with new-onset rheumatoid arthritis and 1456 similarly aged control women. Information about breast implants was obtained on both cases and controls and age-adjusted risk for a history of breast implants among cases was compared to that of controls. The relative risk, i.e., comparing the rate of a history of breast implants among rheumatoid arthritis cases compared to a similar history among controls, was 0.41 (95% CI: 0.05–3.13) [64]. These data did not support an increased risk for rheumatoid arthritis among women with silicone breast implants.

A multi-center, case-controlled study was performed to examine the association between scleroderma and augmentation mammoplasty [66]. A total of 869 women with systemic sclerosis recruited from three university-affiliated rheumatology clinics and 2061 local community controls matched on age in three strata (ages 25–44, 45–64, and ≥65); race and sex were identified by random-digit dialing. Data on exposure and potential confounding variables were collected from cases and controls by self-administered questionnaires and telephone interviews, respectively. The frequency of breast implant surgery was compared in both groups and the odds ratio and 95% confidence intervals for the association of augmentation mammoplasty with systemic sclerosis, adjusted for age, race, marital status, and site, was 1.25 (95% CI: 0.62–2.53). These data failed to demonstrate a significant causal relationship between augmentation mammoplasty and the development of systemic sclerosis.

Using a nested case-control study, Sanchez–Guerrero *et al.* examined the association between silicone breast implants and connective tissue diseases among a cohort of 121 700 registered American nurses followed since 1976 [70]. In 1992, a questionnaire was sent to nurses who had reported any rheumatic disease from 1976 to 1990 asking about rheumatic symptoms and silicone exposure. The complete medical records were obtained on all participants who confirmed any rheumatic or musculoskeletal symptoms. Connective tissue disease cases were classified according to the American College of Rheumatology or other published criteria. Ten age-matched controls per case were randomly selected among nurses with no rheumatic or musculoskeletal complaints. Odds ratios and 95% confidence intervals were used as a measure of association. This study identified 448 cases with definite connective tissue diseases and 1209 nurses with silicone breast implants. Five patients had silicone breast implants and any connective tissue disease. The mean time since implantation was 139 ± 95.81 months among these five patients and 119.17 ± 76.64 months among all nurses with silicone breast implants. These five patients were identified among 300 patients with rheumatoid arthritis. No case with a silicone breast implant was identified among 123 patients with systemic lupus erythematosus, 20 patients with scleroderma, three with Sjögren's syndrome, 13 with dermato/polymyositis, and two with mixed connective tissue diseases. In conclusion, this study found no association between silicone breast implants and connective tissue diseases.

Finally, Burns and Schottenfeld are conducting a population-based case-control study examining the relationship between this condition and prior history of breast implant surgery [69,72]. The cases and normal population controls are being assembled from the states of Michigan and Ohio. The cases are being identified using several sources: a computerized data base of hospital discharge diagnostic listings during the period 1980–1991; a collaborative network of major medical centers; a postal survey of certified rheumatologists; and from patient members of the United Scleroderma Foundation. Although this study is still underway, preliminary results demonstrate a crude odds ratio of 0.61 (95% CI: 0.14–2.68) for breast implants among cases compared to controls. These results do not support a causal relationship between breast implants and systemic sclerosis.

In summary, although numerous anecdotal case reports have suggested an association between silicone breast implants and connective tissue diseases, all seven controlled epidemiologic studies conducted to date have failed to confirm such an association. Whether silicone breast implants cause a new and previously undescribed condition is yet to be determined.

REFERENCES

1. Williams, D.F. (1981) *Biocompatibility of clinical implant materials*. Vol 2. Boca Raton: CRC Press, pp. 1–272.
2. Blocksma. R. and Braley, S. (1965) The silicone in plastic surgery. *Plast. Reconstr. Surg.*, **35**(4), 366–370.
3. Braley, S.A., Jr (1964) The medical silicones. *Trans. Am. Soc. Artif. Int. Organs,* **10**, 240–243.
4. Weiner, S.R. and Paulus, H.E. (1986) Chronic arthropathy occurring after augmentation mammaplasty. *Plast. Reconstr. Surg.,* **77**(2), 185–192.
5. Ward, T.C. and Perry, J.T. (1981) Dynamic mechanical properties of medical grade silicone elastomer stored in simulated body fluids. *J. Biomed. Mater. Res.*, **15** 511–525.
6. Homsy, C.A. (1970). Bio-compatibility in selection of materials for implantation. *J. Biomed. Mater. Res.*, **4,** 341–356.
7. Rigdon, R.H. and Dricks, A. (1975) Reaction associated with a silicone rubber gel: An experimental study. *J. Biomed. Mater. Res.*, **9,** 645–659.
8. Robertson, G. and Braley, S. (1973) Toxicologic studies, quality control, and efficacy of the silastic mammary prosthesis. *Med. Instrum.*, **7**(2), 100–103.
9. Boone, J.L. and Braley, S.A. (1966) Resistance of silicone rubbers to body fluids. *Rubber Chem. Technol.*, **39**(4), 1293–1297.
10. Boone, J.L. (1966) Silicone rubber insulation for subdermally implanted devices. *Med. Res. Eng.*, **5,** 34–37.
11. Roggendorf, E. (1976) The biostability of silicone rubbers, a polyamide, and a polyester. *J. Biomed Mater. Res.*, **10,** 123–143.
12. Speirs, A.C. and Blocksma, R. (1963) New implantable silicone rubbers. An experimental evaluation of tissue response. *Plast. Reconstr. Surg.*, **31**(2), 166–175.

13. Symmers, W.StC. (1968) Silicone mastitis in 'topless' waitresses and some other varieties of foreign-body mastitis. *Br. Med J.*, **3,** 19–22.
14. Ortiz-Monasterio, F. and Trigos, I. (1972) Management of patients with complications from injections of foreign materials into the breasts. *Plast. Reconstr. Surg.*, **50**(1) 42–47.
15. Parsons, R.W. and Thering, H.R. (1977) Management of the silcone-injected breast. *Plast. Reconstr. Surg.*, **60**(4), 534–538.
16. Wilkie, T.F. (1977) Late development of granuloma after liquid silicone injections. *Plast. Reconstr. Surg.*, **60**(2), 179–188.
17. Pearl, R.M., Laub, D.R., and Kaplan, E.N. (1978) Complications following silicone injections for augmentation of the contours of the face. *Plast Reconstr Surg*, **61**(6): 888–891.
18. Kozeny, G.A., Barbato, A.L., Bansal, V.K. *et al.* (1984) Hypercalcemia associated with silicone-induced granulomas. *N. Engl. J. Med.*, **311**(17), 1103–1105.
19. Andrews, J.M. (1966) Cellular behavior to injected silicone fluid: A preliminary report. *Plast. Reconstr. Surg*, **38**(6), 581–583.
20. Ballantyne, D.L., Rees, T.D. and Seidman, I. (1965) Silicone fluid: Response to massive subcutaneous injections of dimethylpolysiloxane fluid in animals. *Plast. Reconstr. Surg.*, **36**(3), 330–338.
21. Ben-Hur, N. and Neuman, Z. (1965) Siliconoma – another cutaneous response to dimethylpolysiloxane. Experimental study in mice. *Plast. Reconstr. Surg.*, **36**(6), 629–631.
22. Rees, T.D., Platt, J., and Ballantyne, D.L. (1965) An investigation of cutaneous response to dimethylpolysiloxane (silicone liquid) in animals and humans – A preliminary report. *Plast. Reconstr. Surg.*, **35**(2), 131–139.
23. Travis, W.D., Balogh, K. and Abraham, J.L. (1985) Silicone granulomas: Report of three cases and review of the literature. *Hum. Pathol.*, **16**(1), 19–27.
24. Mason, J. and Apisarnthanarax, P. (1981) Migratory silicone granuloma. *Arch. Dermatol.*, **117,** 366–367.
25. Apesos, J. and Pope, T.L., Jr (1985) Silicone granuloma following closed capsulotomy of mammary prosthesis. *Ann. Plast. Surg.*, **14**(5), 403–406.
26. Rees, T.D., Ballantyne, D.L., Seidman, I. *et al.* (1967) Visceral response to subcutaneous and intraperitoneal injections of silicone in mice. *Plast. Reconstr. Surg.*, **39**(4), 402–410.
27. Chastre, J., Basset, F., Viau, F. *et al.* (1983) Acute pneumonitis after subcutaneous injections of silicone in transsexual men. *N. Engl. J. Med.*, **308**(13), 764–767.
28. Ellenbogen, R. and Rubin, L. (1975) Injectable fluid silicone therapy: Human morbidity and mortality. *J. Am. Med. Assoc.*, **234**(3), 308–309.
29. Murakata, L.A. and Rangwala, A.F. (1989) Silicone lymphadenopathy with concomitant malignant lymphoma. *J. Rheumatol.*, **16**(11), 1480–1483.
30. Christie, A.J., Weinberger, K.A. and Dietrich, M. (1977) Silicone lymphadenopathy and synovitis. Complications of silicone elastomer finger joint prostheses. *J. Am. Med. Assoc.,* **237**(14), 1463–1464.
31. Kircher, T. (1980) Silicone lymphadenopathy. A complication of silicone elastomer finger joint prostheses. *Hum. Pathol.*, **11**(3), 240–244.

32. Benjamin, E. and Ahmed, A. (1982) Silicone lymphadenopathy: A report of two cases, one with concomitant malignant lymphoma. *Diagn. Histopathol.*, **5,** 133–141.
33. Digby, J.M. (1982) Malignant lymphoma with intranodal silicone rubber particles following metacarpophalangeal joint replacements. *Hand*, **14**(3), 326–328.
34. Endo, L.P., Edwards, N.L., Longley, S. *et al.* (1987) Silicone and rheumatic diseases. *Semin. Arthritis Rheum.*, **17**(2), 112–118.
35. Varga, J., Schumacher, H.R. and Jimenez, S.A. (1989) Systemic sclerosis after augmentation mammoplasty with silicone implants. *Ann. Intern. Med.*, **111**(5), 377–383.
36. Uretsky, B.F., O'Brien, J.J., Courtiss E.H. *et al.* (1979) Augmentation mammaplasty associated with a severe systemic illness. *Ann. Plast. Surg.*, **3**(5), 445–447.
37. Nosanchuk, J.S. (1968) Injected dimethylpolysiloxane fluid: A study of antibody and histologic response. *Plast. Reconstr. Surg.*, **42**(6), 562–566.
38. Heggers, J.P., Kossovsky, N. and Parsons, R.W. *et al.* (1983) Biocompatibility of silicone implants. *Ann. Plast. Surg.*, **11,** 38–45.
39. Pernis, B. and Paronetto, F. (1962) Adjuvant effect of silica (tridymite) on antibody production. *Proc. Soc. Exp. Biol. Med.*, **110,** 390–392.
40. Miyoshi, K., Miyamura, T. and Kobayashi, Y. (1964) Hypergammaglobulinemia by prolonged adjuvanticity in man. Disorders developed after augmentation mammaplasty. *Jpn Med. J.*, **2122,** 9.
41. Yoshida, K. (1973) Post mammaplasty disorder as an adjuvant disease of man. *Shikoku Acta Med.*, **29,** 318.
42. Kumagai, Y., Abe, C. and Shiokawa, Y. (1979) Scleroderma after cosmetic surgery. Four cases of human adjuvant disease. *Arthritis Rheum.*, **22**(5), 532–537.
43. Kumagai, Y., Shiokawa, Y. and Medsger, T.A., Jr (1984) Clinical spectrum of connective tissue disease after cosmetic surgery. *Arthritis Rheum.*, **27**(1), 1–12.
44. Fock, K.M., Feng, P.H., Tey, B.H. (1984). Autoimmune disease developing after augmentation mammoplasty: Report of 3 cases. *J. Rheumatol*, **11**(1), 98–100.
45. Okano, Y., Nishikai, M. and Sato, A. (1984) Scleroderma, primary biliary cirrhosis, and Sjogren's syndrome after cosmetic breast augmentation with silicone injection: A case report of possible human adjuvant disease. *Ann. Rheum. Dis.*, **43,** 520–522.
46. van Nunen, S.A., Gatenby, P.A. and Basten, A. (1982) Post-mammoplasty connective tissue disease. *Arthritis Rheum.*, **25**(6), 694–697.
47. Baldwin, C.M., Jr, and Kaplan, E.N. (1983) Silicone-induced human adjuvant disease? *Ann. Plast. Surg.*, **10,** 270–273.
48. Byron, M.A., Venning, V.A. and Mowat, A.G. (1984) Post-mammoplasty human adjuvant disease. *Br. J. Rheumatol.*, **23**(3), 227–229.
49. Vargas, A. (1979) Shedding of silicone particles from inflated breast implants. *Plast. Reconstr. Surg.*, **64**(2), 252–253.
50. Walsh, F.W., Solomon, D.A., Espinoza, L.R. *et al.* (1989) Human adjuvant disease. A new cause of chylous effusions. *Arch. Intern. Med.*, **149,** 1194–1196.
51. Ziegler, V.V., Haustein, U.F., Mehlhorn, J. *et al.* (1986) Quarzinduzierte sklerodermie sklerodermie-ahnliches syndrom oder echte progressive sklerodermie? *Dermatol. Mon. Schr.*, **172**(2), 86–90.

52. Taura, N., Usa, T. and Eguchi, K. (1976) A case of human adjuvant disease. *J. Jap. Soc. Intern. Med.*, **65,** 840–841.
53. Alusik, S., Jandova, R. and Gebauerova, M. (1989) Anticardiolipin syndrome in plastic surgery of the breast. *Cor. Vasa*, **31**(2), 139–144.
54. Olesen, L.L., Ejlertsen, T. and Nielsen, J. (1991) Toxic shock syndrome following insertion of breast prostheses. *Br. J. Surg.*, **78**(5), 585–586.
55. Spiera, H. (1988) Scleroderma after silicone augmentation mammoplasty. *J. Am. Med. Assoc.*, **260**(2), 236–238.
56. Brozena, S.J., Fenske, N.A., Cruse, C.W. *et al.* (1988) Human adjuvant disease following augmentation mammoplasty. *Arch. Dermatol.*, **124,** 1383–1386.
57. Gutierrez, F.J. and Espinoza, L.R. (1990) Progressive systemic sclerosis complicated by severe hypertension: Reversal after silicone implant removal. *Am. J. Med.*, **89**(3), 390–392.
58. Hitoshi, S., Ito, Y., Takehara, K. *et al.* (1991) A case of malignant hypertension and scleroderma after cosmetic surgery. *Jpn J. Med.*, **30**(1), 97–100.
59. Sahn, E.E., Garen, P.D., Silver, R.M. *et al.* (1990) Scleroderma following augmentation mammoplasty. Report of a case and review of the literature. *Arch. Dermatol.*, **126,** 1198–1202.
60. Deapen, D.M., Pike, M.C., Casagrande, J.T. *et al.* (1986) The relationship between breast cancer and augmentation mammaplasty: An epidemiologic study. *Plast. Reconstr. Surg.*, **77(3),** 361–367.
61. May, D.S. and Stroup, N.E. (1991) The incidence of sarcomas of the breast among women in the United States, 1973–1986. *Plast. Reconstr. Surg.*, **87**(1), 193–194.
62. Fletcher, R.H., Fletcher, S.W. and Wagner, E.H. (1988) Cause. In: Collins, N., Eckhart, C., Chalew, G.N., eds. *Clinical Epidemiology: The Essentials.* Baltimore: Williams & Wilkens, pp. 208–225.
63. Pearson, C.M. (1963) Experimental joint disease. Observations on adjuvant-induced arthritis. *J. Chron. Dis.*, **16,** 863–874.
64. Dugowson, C.E., Daling, J., Koepsell, T.D. *et al.* (1992) Silicone breast implants and risk for rheumatoid-arthritis. *Arthritis Rheum.*, **35,** S66. (Abstract)
65. Gabriel, S.E., O'Fallon, W.M., Kurland, L.T. *et al.* (1994) Risk of connective-tissue diseases and other disorders after breast implantation. *N. Engl. J. Med.*, **330,** 1697–1702.
66. Hochberg, M.C., Perlmutter, D.L., White, B. *et al.* (1994) The association of augmentation mammoplasty with systemic sclerosis: Results from a multi-center case-control study. *Arthritis Rheum.*, **37** (Supplement): S369 (Abstract).
67. Strom, B.L., Reidenberg, M.M., Freundlich, B. *et al.* (1994) Breast silicone implants and risk of systemic lupus erythematosus. *J. Clin. Epidemiol.* (in press).
68. Englert, H.J., Brooks, P. (1994) Scleroderma and augmentation mammoplasty – a causal relationship? *Aust. NZ J. Med.*, **24,** 74–80.
69. Burns, C.J., Laing, T.J., Gillespie, B.W. et al. (1996) The epidemiology of scleroderma among women: Assessment of risk from exposure to silicone and silica. *J. Rheumatol.*, **23**(11), 1904–1911.
70. Sanchez-Guerrero, J., Karlson, E.W., Colditz, G.A. *et al.* (1994) Silicone breast implants (SBI) and connective tissue disease (CTD). *Arthritis Rheum*, **37** (Supplement): S282 (Abstract).

71. Tan, E.M., Cohen, A.S., Fries, J.F. *et al.* (1982) The 1982 revised criteria for the classification of systemic lupus erythematosus. *Arthritis Rheum*, **25** (11), 1271–1277.
72. Schottenfeld, D., Burns, C.J., Gillespie, B.W. *et al.* (1995) The design of a population-based case-control study of systemic sclerosis (scleroderma): Commentary on the University of Michigan Study. *J. Clin. Epidemiol.* **48**(4), 583–586.

Index

Page numbers in **bold** refer to figures; those in *italics* refer to tables